MOUNT SINAI
EXPERT GUIDES

Hepatology

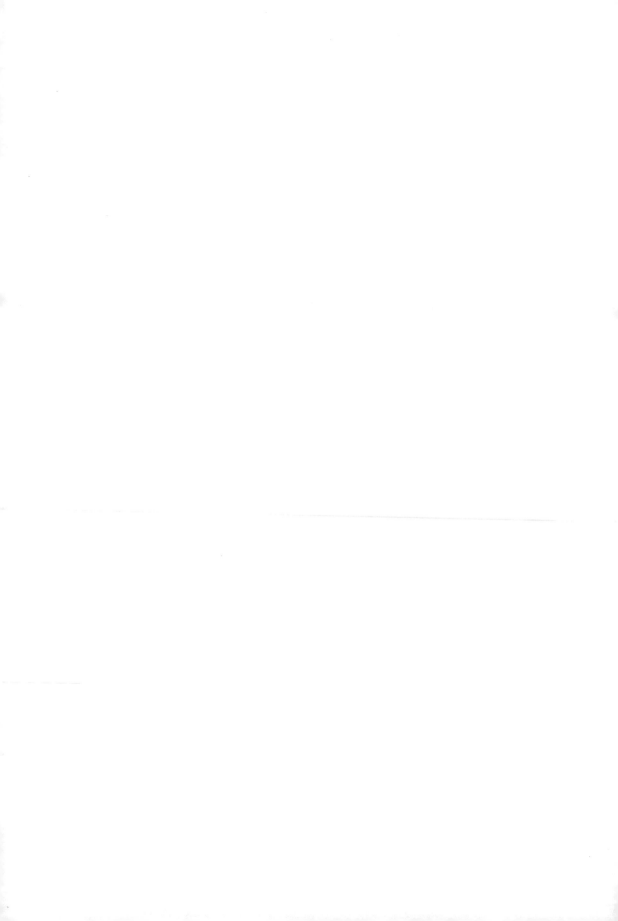

MOUNT SINAI EXPERT GUIDES

Hepatology

EDITED BY

Jawad Ahmad MD
Associate Professor of Medicine
Division of Liver Diseases
Icahn School of Medicine at Mount Sinai
New York, NY, USA

Scott L. Friedman MD
Fishberg Professor of Medicine
Dean for Therapeutic Discovery
Chief, Division of Liver Diseases
Icahn School of Medicine at Mount Sinai
New York, NY, USA

Henryk Dancygier MD, PhD
Professor of Medicine
Chair, Departments of Medicine II and IV
Sana Klinikum Offenbach, Goethe University
Frankfurt am Main, Germany;
Adjunct Professor of Medicine
Department of Medicine, Division of Liver Diseases
Icahn School of Medicine at Mount Sinai
New York, NY, USA

Icahn
School of
Medicine at
**Mount
Sinai**

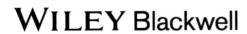

This edition first published 2014 © 2014 by John Wiley & Sons, Ltd

Registered office: John Wiley & Sons, Ltd, The Atrium, Southern Gate, Chichester, West Sussex, PO19 8SQ, UK

Editorial offices: 9600 Garsington Road, Oxford, OX4 2DQ, UK
The Atrium, Southern Gate, Chichester, West Sussex, PO19 8SQ, UK
111 River Street, Hoboken, NJ 07030-5774, USA

For details of our global editorial offices, for customer services and for information about how to apply for permission to reuse the copyright material in this book please see our website at www.wiley.com/wiley-blackwell

The right of the author to be identified as the author of this work has been asserted in accordance with the UK Copyright, Designs and Patents Act 1988.

Designations used by companies to distinguish their products are often claimed as trademarks. All brand names and product names used in this book are trade names, service marks, trademarks or registered trademarks of their respective owners. The publisher is not associated with any product or vendor mentioned in this book. It is sold on the understanding that the publisher is not engaged in rendering professional services. If professional advice or other expert assistance is required, the services of a competent professional should be sought.

The contents of this work are intended to further general scientific research, understanding, and discussion only and are not intended and should not be relied upon as recommending or promoting a specific method, diagnosis, or treatment by health science practitioners for any particular patient. The publisher and the author make no representations or warranties with respect to the accuracy or completeness of the contents of this work and specifically disclaim all warranties, including without limitation any implied warranties of fitness for a particular purpose. In view of ongoing research, equipment modifications, changes in governmental regulations, and the constant flow of information relating to the use of medicines, equipment, and devices, the reader is urged to review and evaluate the information provided in the package insert or instructions for each medicine, equipment, or device for, among other things, any changes in the instructions or indication of usage and for added warnings and precautions. Readers should consult with a specialist where appropriate. The fact that an organization or Website is referred to in this work as a citation and/or a potential source of further information does not mean that the author or the publisher endorses the information the organization or Website may provide or recommendations it may make. Further, readers should be aware that Internet Websites listed in this work may have changed or disappeared between when this work was written and when it is read. No warranty may be created or extended by any promotional statements for this work. Neither the publisher nor the author shall be liable for any damages arising herefrom.

Library of Congress Cataloging-in-Publication Data
Mount Sinai expert guides. Hepatology / edited by Jawad Ahmad, Scott L. Friedman, Henryk Dancygier.
       p. ; cm.
   Hepatology
   Includes bibliographical references and index.
   ISBN 978-1-118-51734-5 (alk. paper) – ISBN 978-1-118-74251-8 (emobi) – ISBN 978-1-118-74252-5 (epub) – ISBN 978-1-118-74253-2 (epdf) – ISBN 978-1-118-74862-6
   I. Ahmad, Jawad (Hepatologist), editor of compilation. II. Friedman, Scott L., editor of compilation. III. Dancygier, Henryk, editor of compilation. IV. Title: Hepatology.
   [DNLM: 1. Liver Diseases.   2. Liver Transplantation. WI 700]
   RC845
   616.3'62–dc23
                                        2013024785

A catalogue record for this book is available from the British Library.

Wiley also publishes its books in a variety of electronic formats. Some content that appears in print may not be available in electronic books.

Cover image: iStock file File #6124416 © David Marchal
Cover design by Ruth Bateson

Set in 8.5/12 pt Frutiger Light by Toppan Best-set Premedia Limited

1   2014

Contents

List of Contributors

Jawad Ahmad MD
Associate Professor of Medicine
Division of Liver Diseases
Icahn School of Medicine at Mount Sinai
New York, NY, USA

Abdulelah Alhawsawi MD
Surgical Fellow
Recanati/Miller Transplantation Institute
Mount Sinai Hospital
New York, NY, USA

Costica Aloman MD
Associate Professor of Medicine
University of Illinois
Chicago, IL, USA

Ronen Arnon MD, MHA
Associate Professor of Pediatrics and Surgery
Department of Pediatrics
Icahn School of Medicine at Mount Sinai
New York, NY, USA

Nancy Bach MD
Assistant Professor of Medicine
Division of Liver Diseases
Icahn School of Medicine at Mount Sinai
New York, NY, USA

Meena B. Bansal MD
Associate Professor of Medicine
Division of Liver Diseases
Icahn School of Medicine at Mount Sinai
New York, NY, USA

Charissa Y. Chang MD
Assistant Professor of Medicine
Division of Liver Diseases
Icahn School of Medicine at Mount Sinai
New York, NY, USA

Jaime Chu MD
Assistant Professor of Pediatrics
Division of Hepatology
Icahn School of Medicine at Mount Sinai
New York, NY, USA

Alan G. Contreras Saldivar MD
Attending Transplant Surgeon
Instructor of Surgery
Mount Sinai Hospital
Icahn School of Medicine at Mount Sinai;
Recanati/Miller Transplantation Institute
Mount Sinai Hospital
New York, NY, USA

Henryk Dancygier MD, PhD
Professor of Medicine
Chair, Departments of Medicine II and IV
Sana Klinikum Offenbach, Goethe University
Frankfurt am Main, Germany;
Adjunct Professor of Medicine
Department of Medicine
Division of Liver Diseases
Icahn School of Medicine at Mount Sinai
New York, NY, USA

Eric G. Davis MD
Assistant Professor of Surgery
University of Louisville School of Medicine
Louisville, KY, USA

Douglas T. Dieterich MD
Professor of Medicine
Division of Liver Diseases
Icahn School of Medicine at Mount Sinai
New York, NY, USA

Deepti Dronamraju MD
Fellow
Division of Liver Diseases
Icahn School of Medicine at Mount Sinai
New York, NY, USA

Marcelo E. Facciuto MD, MPH
Associate Professor of Surgery
Recanati/Miller Transplantation Institute
Mount Sinai Hospital
New York, NY, USA

Donna J.C. Fanelli CRNP
Division of Liver Diseases
Icahn School of Medicine at Mount Sinai
New York, NY, USA

M. Isabel Fiel MD
Professor of Pathology
Department of Pathology
Icahn School of Medicine at Mount Sinai
New York, NY, USA

Sander S. Florman MD
The Charles Miller, MD Professor of Surgery
Director, Recanati/Miller Transplantation
Institute
Mount Sinai Hospital
New York, NY, USA

Scott L. Friedman MD
Fishberg Professor of Medicine
Dean for Therapeutic Discovery
Chief, Division of Liver Diseases
Icahn School of Medicine at Mount Sinai
New York, NY, USA

Priya Grewal MD
Associate Professor of Medicine
Division of Liver Diseases
Icahn School of Medicine at Mount Sinai
New York, NY, USA

Shirish Huprikar MD
Director, Transplant Infectious Diseases
Program
Associate Professor
Division of Infectious Diseases
Department of Medicine
Icahn School of Medicine at Mount Sinai
New York, NY, USA

Nanda Kerkar MD
Professor of Clinical Pediatrics
Medical Director Liver and Intestinal Program
Director Hepatology Program
Children's Hospital of Los Angeles
University of Southern California
Los Angeles, CA, USA

Vivek Kesar MD
Internal Medicine Resident
Lenox Hill Medical Center
New York, NY, USA

Leona Kim-Schluger MD
Professor of Medicine
Division of Liver Diseases
Icahn School of Medicine at Mount Sinai
New York, NY, USA

Elizabeth A. Kula CRNP
Division of Liver Diseases
Icahn School of Medicine at Mount Sinai
New York, NY, USA

Marie E. Le MD
Surgical Fellow
Recanati/Miller Transplantation Institute
Mount Sinai Hospital
New York, NY, USA

Lawrence U. Liu MD
Assistant Professor of Medicine
Division of Liver Diseases
Icahn School of Medicine at Mount Sinai
New York, NY, USA

Tamir Miloh MD
Director of Pediatric Liver and Liver
Transplant Program
Department of Gastroenterology and
Hepatology
Phoenix Children's Hospital;
Associate Professor of Pediatrics
University of Arizona, College of Medicine
Phoenix, AZ;
Associate Professor in Pediatrics
Mayo Clinic
USA

Joseph A. Odin MD, PhD
Director, Autoimmune Liver Diseases
Program
Associate Professor of Medicine
Division of Liver Diseases
Icahn School of Medicine at Mount Sinai
New York, NY, USA

James S. Park MD, CNSC
Assistant Professor of Medicine
Division of Gastroenterology
NYU School of Medicine
New York, NY, USA

Gopi Patel MD, MS
Assistant Professor
Division of Infectious Diseases
Icahn School of Medicine at Mount Sinai
New York, NY, USA

Ponni V. Perumalswami MD, MS
Assistant Professor of Medicine
Division of Liver Diseases
Icahn School of Medicine at Mount Sinai
New York, NY, USA

Juan P. Rocca MD
Assistant Professor of Surgery
Icahn School of Medicine at Mount Sinai;
Surgical Director, Live Donor Kidney Program
Associate Director, Transplant Surgery
Fellowship
Recanati/Miller Transplantation Institute
Mount Sinai Hospital
New York, NY, USA

Thomas D. Schiano MD
Professor of Medicine
Medical Director, Liver Transplantation
Clinical Director, Hepatology
Division of Liver Diseases
Icahn School of Medicine at Mount Sinai
New York, NY, USA

Hiroshi Sogawa MD, FACS
Assistant Professor of Surgery
Director, Transplant Surgery Fellowship
Program
Thomas E. Starzl Transplantation Institute
University of Pittsburgh Medical Center
Pittsburgh, PA, USA

Alicia C. Stivala NP
Nurse Practitioner
Division of Infectious Diseases
Icahn School of Medicine at Mount Sinai
New York, NY, USA

Matthew Y. Suh MD
Surgical Fellow
Recanati/Miller Transplantation Institute
Mount Sinai Hospital
New York, NY, USA

Marie-Louise C. Vachon MD, MSc
Fellow
Division of Liver Diseases
Icahn School of Medicine at Mount Sinai
New York, NY, USA

Series Foreword

Now more than ever, immediacy in obtaining accurate and practical information is the coin of the realm in providing high quality patient care. The Mount Sinai Expert Guides series addresses this vital need by providing accurate, up-to-date guidance, written by experts in formats that are accessible in the patient care setting: websites, smartphone apps and portable books. The Icahn School of Medicine, which was chartered in 1963, embodies a deep tradition of pre-eminence in clinical care and scholarship that was first shaped by the founding of the Mount Sinai Hospital in 1855. Today, the Mount Sinai Health System, comprised of seven hospitals anchored by the Icahn School of Medicine, is one of the largest health care systems in the United States, and is revolutionizing medicine through its embracing of transformative technologies for clinical diagnosis and treatment. The Mount Sinai Expert Guides series builds upon both this historical renown and contemporary excellence. Leading experts across a range of disciplines provide practical yet sage advice in a digestible format that is ideal for trainees, mid-level providers and practicing physicians. Few medical centers in the US could offer this type of breadth while relying exclusively on its own physicians, yet here no compromises were required in offering a truly unique series that is sure to become embedded within the key resources of busy providers. In producing this series, the editors and authors are fortunate to have an equally dynamic and forward-viewing partner in Wiley Blackwell, which together ensures that health care professionals will benefit from a unique, first-class effort that will advance the care of their patients.

Scott Friedman MD
Series Editor
Dean for Therapeutic Discovery
Fishberg Professor and Chief, Division of Liver Diseases
Icahn School of Medicine at Mount Sinai
New York, NY, USA

Preface

The last 20 years has seen hepatology emerge as a distinct discipline, separate from gastroenterology, reflecting the profound advances in our understanding of the pathophysiology, diagnosis and management of liver diseases. Concurrently, academic centers throughout the world now have faculty who function exclusively as hepatologists, and even in these institutions there is often further distinction between non-transplant and transplant hepatologists, with a similar trend emerging in pediatrics.

In recognition of these trends, international liver societies in the US (American Society for the Study of Liver Diseases), Europe (European Association for the Study of the Liver) and Asia (Asian Pacific Association for the Study of the Liver), seek evidence-based guidelines to standardize management of the most common liver diseases. This expert guide is intended to address this need for a concise and practical guide to patient management. While many textbooks provide detailed descriptions of pathophysiology, they may not be well suited to provide practical, accessible treatment options in the clinical setting where information is urgently needed and time is short. For students and trainees, a basic understanding of epidemiology and pathogenesis of disease entities is important, but guidance for the management of a specific clinical condition is the real world need.

This book is separated into three sections: hepatology, pediatrics and transplantation, with each chapter organized in a standardized format. The first section of each chapter provides the reader a bottom-line of 'take home' points that emphasizes the most important aspects of the chapter. This is followed by sections on background, prevention and diagnosis. Key features across the chapters are: easily accessible evidence-based management algorithms, with appropriate laboratory and imaging tests and commonly used medications with dosages. Short reading lists with society guidelines complete the text. Also accompanying the book is a companion website which provides the reader with case histories and multiple choice questions for those preparing for specialty exams. An additional multimedia resource available for purchase is an app with highlights of each chapter for smartphone users.

We have sought to provide a comprehensive list of diseases and situations that clinicians will confront in general hepatology and transplant hepatology practices. The pediatric and surgical chapters have been included to ensure that adult hepatologists understand problems they are likely to encounter in these related specialities in practice, but not as a guide specifically for pediatricians and surgeons.

We thank the staff at Wiley Blackwell, particularly Oliver Walter and Jennifer Seward, for ensuring such a smooth publication process. We also gratefully acknowledge the many Mount Sinai residents and hepatology fellows for their enthusiasm, dedication to their patients and candid feedback throughout the preparation of this text.

Finally, we are indebted to our Mount Sinai colleagues in the Divisions of Liver Diseases and Infectious Diseases, the Departments of Pediatrics and Pathology, and in the Recanati/Miller Transplantation Institute. The editors are fortunate to work with such superb physicians, but what truly distinguishes our colleagues is their selfless dedication to mentoring the next generation of trainees in caring for patients with liver disease. This book reflects their exceptional generosity as clinicians, teachers and role models.

Jawad Ahmad
Scott L. Friedman
Henryk Dancygier

Abbreviation List

AAP	American Academy of Pediatrics
AASLD	American Association for the Study of Liver Diseases
AAT	alpha-1 antitrypsin
ABG	Arterial blood gas
ABW	Adjusted body weight
ACE	Angiotensin-converting enzyme
ACR	Acute cellular rejection
ADH	Alcohol dehydrogenase
AD-PCLD	Adult polycystic liver disease
ADV	Adefovir
AFLP	Acute fatty liver of pregnancy
AFP	Alpha-fetoprotein
AH	Alcoholic hepatitis
AIDs	Acquired immunodeficiency syndrome
AIH	Autoimmune hepatitis
ALA	Amebic liver abscess
ALF	Acute liver failure
ALT	Alanine aminotransferase
AMA	Antimitochondrial antibodies
ANA	Antinuclear antibody
ANA	Antinuclear autoantibodies?
anti-HAV	Antibodies to the hepatitis A virus
anti-HBc	Antibodies to the hepatitis B core antigen
anti-HBs	Antibodies to the hepatitis B surface antigen
anti-LKM	Anti-liver kidney microsomal (antibody)
AP	Alkaline phosphatase
AR	Acute rejection
ARDS	Acute respiratory distress syndrome
ARF	Acute renal failure
ART	Antiretroviral therapy
ARV	Antiretroviral
ASMA	Anti-smooth muscle antibody
AST	Aspartate aminotransferase
AUDIT	Alcohol Users Disorders Indentification Test
BCLC	Barcelona Clinic Liver Cancer Staging System
BCS	Budd–Chiari syndrome
BMI	Body mass index
BOC	Boceprevir
BRTO	Balloon retrograde transvenous obliteration

CBC	Complete blood count
CDC	Centres for Disease Control and Prevention
cEVR	Complete early virological response
CHB	Chronic hepatitis B
CHF	Congestive heart failure
CK	Creatine kinase
CKD	Chronic kidney disease
CMV	Cytomegalovirus
CNI	Calcineurin inhibitors
CNS	Central nervous system
CO	Cardiac output
COPD	Chronic obstructive pulmonary disease
CR	Chronic rejection
CRP	C-reactive protein
CSF	Cerebrospinal fluid
CT	Computed tomography
CTP	Child-Pugh-Turcotti Score
CVP	Central venous pressure
CVVH	Continuous veno-venous hemofiltration
CVVHD	Continuous veno-venous hemodialysis

DAA	Direct acting antiviral agent
DDLT	Deceased donor liver transplant
DGF	Delayed graft function
DHHS	Department of Health and Human Services
DIC	Disseminated intravascular coagulation
DILI	Drug-induced liver injury
DVR	Delayed virological response

EBV	Epstein-Barr virus
ECG	Electrocardiogram
EEG	Electroencephalogram
eEVR	Extended early virological response
EGD	Esophagogastroduodenoscopy
EHBA	Extrahepatic biliary atresia
ELISA	Enzyme-linked immunosorbent assay
ERC	Endoscopic retrograde cholangiography
EOT	End of treatment
ERCP	Endoscopic retrograde cholangiopancreatography
eRVR	Extended rapid virological response
ESLD	End-stage liver disease
ESR	Erythrocyte sedimentation rate
ESRD	End-stage renal disease
ETV	Entecavir
EUS	Endoscopic ultrasound
EV	Esophageal varices
EVR	Early virological response

FDA	Food and Drug Administration
FEV1	Forced expiratory volume in one second
FHF	Fulminant hepatic failure
FNA	Fine needle aspiration
FNH	Focal nodular hyperplasia
FVC	Forced vital capacity
GABA	Gamma-aminobutyric acid
GFR	Glomerular filtration rate
GGT	Gamma glutamyl transpeptidase
GI	Gastrointestinal
GIB	Gastrointestinal bleeding
HAART	Highly active antiretroviral therapy
HAT	Hepatic artery thrombosis
HBcAb IgG	Hepatitis B core antibody immunoglobulin G
HBcAb IgM	Hepatitis B core antibody immunoglobulin M
HBIg	Hepatitis B immune globulin
HBsAb	Hepatitis B surface antibody
HBsAg	Hepatitis B surface antigen
HBV	Hepatitis B virus
HCC	Hepatocellular carcinoma
HCT	Hematocrit
HCV	Hepatitis C virus
HDL	High density lipoprotein
HE	Hepatic encephalopathy
HELLP	Hemolytic anemia, Elevated Liver enzymes and Low Platelet count
HEV	Hepatitis E virus
HFE	Hemochromatosis
HG	Hyperemesis gravidarum
HH	Hereditary hemochromatosis
HHT	Hereditary hemorrhagic telangiectasia
HIC	Hepatic iron concentration
HIDA	Hepatobiliary immunodiacetic acid (scan)
HII	Hepatic iron index
HIV	Human immunodeficiency virus
HLA	Human leukocyte antigen
HLH	Hemophagocytic lymphohistiocystosis
HOMA	Homeostasis model assessment
HPS	Hepatopulmonary syndrome
HRS	Hepatorenal syndrome
HSV	Herpes simplex virus
HVPG	Hepatic venous pressure gradient
IAIHG	International Autoimmune Hepatitis Group
IBD	Inflammatory bowel disease
IBW	Ideal body weight
ICH	Intracranial hypertension

ICP   Intrahepatic cholestasis of pregnancy
ICU   Intensive care unit
IDUs   Intravenous drug users
IEF   Isoelectric focusing
IFN   Interferon
IgG   Immunoglobulin G
IgM   Immunoglobulin M
IHA   Indirect hemagglutination
INR   International normalized ratio
IPVDs   Intrapulmonary vascular abnormalities or dilatations
IRI   Ischemia reperfusion injury
ISC   Incomplete septal cirrhosis
IV   Intravenous
IVC   Inferior vena cava
IVIG   Intravenous immunoglobulin

KF   Kayser–Fleischer (rings)

LCHAD   Long-chain 3-hydroxyacylcoenzyme A dehydrogenase
LCT   Long-chain triglycerides
LDH   Lactate dehydrogenase
LDLT   Live donor liver transplantation
LFT   Liver function tests
LKM-1   Liver kidney microsomal type 1
LKM-3   Liver kidney microsomal types 3
LLOD   Lower limit of detection
LLOQ   Lower limit of quantification
LPS   Lipopolysaccharide
LR   Likelihood ratio
LT   Liver transplantation
LV   Left ventricle
LVP   Large volume paracentesis
LVRS   Lung volume reduction surgery

MAP   Mean arterial pressure
MARS   Molecular Adsorbent Recirculating System
MCT   Medium-chain triglycerides
MCV   Mean cell volume
MDR   Multi-drug resistant
MELD   Model for end stage liver disease (score)
MHE   Minimal hepatic encephalopathy
MI   Myocardial infarction
MICU   Medical intensive care unit
MMR   Measles mumps rubella
MPAP   Mean pulmonary artery pressure
MRA   Magnetic resonance angiogram
MRCP   Magnetic resonance cholangiopancreatography
MRI   Magnetic resonance imaging

MSM	Men who have sex with men
MTCT	Mother-to-child transmission
NAC	N-acetylcysteine
NAFLD	Non-alcoholic fatty liver disease
NASH	Non-alcoholic steatohepatitis
NASPGHAN	The North American Society for Pediatric Gastroenterology, Hepatology and Nutrition
NCA	N-acetylcysteine
NCPH	Non-cirrhotic portal hypertension
99TcMAA	Technetium labeled macro-aggregated albumin
NG	Nasogastric
NR	Null response
NRH	Nodular regenerative hyperplasia
NRTIs	Nucleoside reverse transcriptase inhibitors
NSAIDs	Non-steroidal anti-inflammatory drugs
OCP	Oral contraceptive pill
OLT	Orthotopic liver transplant
OPV	Obliterative portal venopathy
PALF	Pediatric Acute Liver Failure (study group)
P-ANCA	Perinuclear-staining antineutrophil cytoplasmic antibody
PAP	Pulmonary artery pressure
PAS	Period acid Schiff
PASP	Pulmonary artery systolic pressure
PBC	Primary biliary cirrhosis
PBS	Primary biliary sclerosis
PCLD	Polycystic liver disease
PCP	Primary care provider
PCR	Polymerase chain reaction
PCWP	Pulmonary capillary wedge pressure
PDH	Pyruvate dehydrogenase
PEG-IFN	Pegylated interferon
PELD	Pediatric end-stage liver disease
PEM	Protein energy malnutrition
PFIC	Progressive familial intrahepatic cholestasis
PFT	Pulmonary function tests
PHT	Portal hypertension
PHTN	Pulmonary hypertension
PI	Protease inhibitor
PKD	Polycystic kidney disease
PMN	Polymorphonuclear leukocytes
PNF	Primary non-function
PO	Per oram
POD	Post-operative day
PPHTN	Portopulmonary hypertension

PPI	Proton-pump inhibitor
PR	Partial non-response
PREP-C	Psychosocial Readiness Evaluation and Preparation for Hepatitis C
PSC	Primary sclerosing cholangitis
PSE	Portal systemic encephalopathy
PT	Prothrombin time
PTC	Percutaneous transhepatic cholangiography
PTLD	Post-transplant lymphoproliferative disorder
PTT	Partial thromboplastin time
PVR	Pulmonary vascular resistance
PVS	Peritoneovenous shunt
PVT	Portal vein thrombosis

RAI	Rejection activity index
RBV	Ribavarin
RCT	Randomized controlled trial
RDA	Recommended daily allowance
RES	Reticuloendothelial system
RFA	Radiofrequency ablation
RGT	Response-guided therapy
ROS	Reactive oxygen species
RUQ	Right upper quadrant
RVR	Rapid virological response

SAAG	Serum-ascites albumin gradient
SBP	Spontaneous bacterial peritonitis
SC	Subcutaneous
SFSS	Small for size syndrome
SGA	Subjective global assessment
SICU	Surgical intensive care unit
SIRS	Systemic inflammatory response syndrome
SLA/LP	Soluble liver antigen/liver pancreas
SLE	Systemic lupus erythematosus
SMA	Smooth muscle antibody
SNP	Single nucleotide polymorphism
STD	Sexually transmitted disease
SVR	Sustained virological response

TACE	Transarterial chemoembolization
TDF	Tenofovir disoproxil fumarate
TIBC	Total iron binding capacity
TIPS	Transjugular intrahepatic portosystemic shunting
TNF	Tumour necrosis factor
TPGS	D-alpha-tocopheryl-polyethylene-glycol-succinate
TPN	Total parenteral nutrition
TSB	Total serum bilirubin

TSH	Thyroid-stimulating hormone
TTG	Transglutaminase antibody
TVR	Telaprevir
UCSF	University of California San Francisco
UD	Undetected
UDCA	Ursodeoxycholic acid
UGT	Uridine-diphosphoglucuronate glucuronosyltransferase
ULN	Upper limit of normal
UNOS	United Network for Organ Sharing
UTI	Urinary tract infection
VLDL	Very low density lipoprotein
VZV	Varicella-zoster virus
WBC	White blood cells
WCC	White cell count
WD	Wilson disease
WHO	World Health Organization

About the Companion Website

This series is accompanied by a companion website:

www.mountsinaiexpertguides.com

The website includes:
- Video clips
- Case studies
- ICD codes
- Interactive MCQs
- Patient advice

PART 1

HEPATOLOGY

CHAPTER 1

Approach to the Patient with Abnormal Liver Tests

Charissa Y. Chang
Division of Liver Diseases, Icahn School of Medicine at Mount Sinai, New York, NY, USA

OVERALL BOTTOM LINE

- A detailed medical history is the single most important step in the evaluation of a patient with abnormal liver tests.
- Evaluation of liver enzyme elevation can be categorized into hepatocellular injury, cholestatic injury, or mixed injury based on patterns of relative elevation of different liver enzymes.
- Serum chemistries which are used to diagnose liver disease can be divided into laboratories which evaluate liver function (INR, albumin), those which primarily evaluate integrity of hepatocytes (AST, ALT) and those which predominantly assess abnormalities of bile ducts and bile flow (bilirubin, AP, GGT).
- The differential diagnosis of abnormal liver tests is broad and includes infectious (viral hepatitis), metabolic (NAFLD, Wilson disease, hemochromatosis, alpha-1 antitrypsin deficiency), toxin- and drug-induced (alcohol, herbal products), immunologic (autoimmune hepatitis, primary biliary cirrhosis, primary sclerosing cholangitis, overlap syndromes), infiltrative, vascular and neoplastic diseases.
- Non-hepatic causes of elevated liver enzymes, such as congestive hepatopathy, shock liver, muscle diseases, thyroid disorders, celiac disease, or adrenal insufficiency must be excluded.

Section 1: Background
Definition of disease

Tests which are used to assess for liver injury and liver function

	Normal function	Significance of abnormal value
Tests of liver injury:		
ALT, formerly SGOT	Catalyzes transfer of amino groups of alanine	Elevated in: • Hepatocellular injury
AST, formerly SGPT	Catalyzes transfer of amino groups of L-aspartic acid	Elevated in: • Hepatocellular injury • Myocyte injury (rhabdomyolysis, exercise, myocardial infarction)
		(Continued)

Mount Sinai Expert Guides: Hepatology, First Edition. Edited by Jawad Ahmad, Scott L. Friedman, and Henryk Dancygier.
© 2014 John Wiley & Sons, Ltd. Published 2014 by John Wiley & Sons, Ltd.
Companion website: www.mountsinaiexpertguides.com

	Normal function	Significance of abnormal value
AP	Enzyme found on canalicular membrane of hepatocytes, function unknown. Also found in bone, small intestine, placenta	Elevated in: • Cholestatic liver disease of various etiology (biliary obstruction, biliary injury, drug induced) • Infiltrative diseases of the liver (sarcoidosis, amyloidosis) • Neoplastic diseases of the liver • Congestive hepatopathy • Bone disorders, normal bone growth, pregnancy
GGT	Found in cell membranes of many tissues (liver, kidney, pancreas, spleen)	Sensitive but non-specific indicator of hepatobiliary injury. An elevated GGT is not specific for alcohol use. Clinical utility is in differentiating origin of AP elevation (GGT elevated in liver disease, normal in bone disease)
Tests of liver function:		
Total bilirubin	Normal breakdown product of heme	Elevated in biliary obstruction, disorders of bilirubin metabolism, hepatitis, cirrhosis and acute liver failure
Indirect bilirubin	Unconjugated form of bilirubin which is insoluble in plasma and converted to excretable conjugated form by hepatocytes	Elevated in: • Increased heme breakdown (i.e. hemolysis) • Inherited disorders of bilirubin metabolism (Gilbert's disease)
Direct bilirubin	Conjugated form of bilirubin which is excreted by hepatocytes across canalicular membrane into bile	Elevated in: • Obstruction of bile ducts • Impaired hepatocyte function (chronic liver disease, cirrhosis, liver failure) • Genetic syndromes (Rotor syndrome, Dubin–Johnson syndrome)
PT	Measurement of clotting time	Elevated in disease states causing impaired liver function and decreased hepatic production of clotting proteins (cirrhosis, acute liver failure)
Albumin	Protein synthesized by hepatocytes	Decreased in hepatocellular dysfunction/chronic liver disease

- ALT and AST are enzymes found in hepatocytes. High serum levels reflect hepatocellular injury. AST is found in other cells including in the heart, skeletal muscle, brain and other organs. In contrast, ALT is found mostly in liver which makes it a more specific marker of liver injury compared with AST. Revised upper limits of ALT have been proposed (30 IU/L for men and 19 IU/L for women) after excluding individuals with probable NASH and hepatitis C from the "normal" population used to determine range limits.

- Normal ALT serum levels have a high negative predictive value (>90%) in excluding a clinically significant liver disease.
- GGT is present in decreasing quantities in the kidneys, liver, pancreas and intestine. It is a sensitive indicator of hepatobiliary disease, but lacks specificity. GGT levels are increased in cholestatic liver diseases, NAFLD, space-occupying liver lesions and venous hepatic congestion. GGT may be induced by many drugs and alcohol.
  - GGT is not a marker of alcoholic liver disease.
    - Decreasing enzyme activities during abstinence from alcohol are diagnostically more helpful than the presence of an elevated GGT per se.
  - Normal GGT levels have a high negative predictive value (>90%) in excluding hepatobiliary disease.
  - An isolated elevation of GGT should not lead to an exhaustive work-up for liver disease.
- Liver AP is a sensitive indicator of cholestasis of various etiologies, but AP does not discriminate between intra- and extrahepatic cholestasis. Elevation in 5'nucleotidase, GGT and liver isoenzyme fractionation of AP can be used to confirm hepatic origin of AP.
- Mild elevations of serum AP levels may be found in viral hepatitis, drug induced, granulomatous and neoplastic liver disease.
- Bilirubin is formed from breakdown of heme. It is carried bound to albumin to hepatocytes where UGT1A1 (bilirubin-UDP-glucuronosyltransferase) conjugates bilirubin. The conjugated bilirubin is then exported through a transporter into bile canaliculi and excreted through bile ducts. Transport of bilirubin through the canalicular membrane into the canaliculus is the rate limiting step ("bottle neck") of bilirubin excretion. Causes of hyperbilirubinemia include excess heme breakdown, disorders of conjugation and bilirubin transport, hepatocellular damage and obstruction of bile ducts.
  - Increases in conjugated bilirubin are highly specific for hepatobiliary disease.

Disease classification

Enzyme patterns of liver injury	
Enzyme pattern	**ALT:AP ratio[a]**
Hepatocellular	≥5
Cholestatic	≤2
Mixed	>2 to <5

[a] All enzymes expressed as multiples of ULN

Etiology
See "Definition of disease."

Pathology/pathogenesis
See "Definition of disease."

Section 2: Prevention

Not applicable for this topic.

Section 3: Diagnosis

BOTTOM LINE/CLINICAL PEARLS
- A detailed history is the key to the correct interpretation of abnormal liver tests. History taking should include information including alcohol use, recent use of acetaminophen, herbal products or other medications, and risk factors for viral hepatitis transmission.
- Physical examination should include assessment for jaundice and encephalopathy which can indicate acute liver failure in a patient with no prior history of underlying liver disease. Stigmata of cirrhosis (spider angiomata, ascites, muscle wasting, Dupuytren's contracture, splenomegaly) should be noted on physical examination.
- Elevated INR and bilirubin in a patient with encephalopathy and no underlying liver disease indicates acute liver failure and should prompt consideration of referral to a transplant center.
- Further laboratory investigations and imaging to diagnose the cause of elevated liver tests should be driven by clinical history and the pattern of liver test elevation (see Table: Enzyme patterns of liver injury and algorithms shown in Algorithm 1.1 and Algorithm 1.2).

- Viral and metabolic causes (i.e. hemochromatosis and Wilson disease) can be diagnosed with confirmatory laboratory tests. However, alcoholic liver disease, NASH and DILI rely on careful history taking and clinical diagnosis. Herbal preparations can be overlooked as a cause of hepatotoxicity unless an accurate history is obtained. Causes of elevated tests that are unique to pregnancy are discussed at the end of the chapter and in a separate chapter.

Hepatocellular/mixed elevation of liver tests
- The diagnostic approach to aminotransferase or mixed aminotransferase/cholestatic liver test elevation is shown in Algorithm 1.1 and selection of testing is largely driven by the clinical presentation and the degree of AST and ALT elevation. Aminotransferase elevation above 10 times the ULN reflects severe acute injury and is observed in shock liver, toxic- or drug-induced injury, acetaminophen toxicity, and acute viral hepatitis A, B (± D) and E. A detailed history eliciting recent toxin or drug exposure, or a recent period of hypotension is important in making the diagnosis. An acetaminophen level may be helpful for confirmation of suspected acetaminophen injury.
- Acute liver injury in the setting of suspected recent viral hepatitis exposure (hepatitis B, C and A) should prompt specific testing (HBV core IgM, HBV DNA, HCV RNA, hepatitis A IgM) due to absence of antibodies in the window phase of acute infection. Failure to send the proper tests can result in a missed or delayed diagnosis.
- Lesser degrees (up to 5 × ULN) of aminotransferase elevation can be caused by chronic viral hepatitis, alcoholic hepatitis, autoimmune hepatitis, Wilson disease, hemochromatosis, Budd–Chiari syndrome, and infiltrative diseases. Serologic testing is available for autoimmune hepatitis, Wilson disease, hemochromatosis and alpha-1 antitrypsin deficiency whereas diagnosis of alcoholic hepatitis, NASH and drug-induced liver injury relies on careful history taking.
- Alcoholic hepatitis often causes elevations of AST and ALT in a 2:1 ratio. This is because patients with alcoholic liver disease are deficient in pyridoxal 5′-phosphate, which is required for synthesis of ALT more so than AST. Additional features of alcoholic hepatitis include leukocytosis, fever and jaundice.
- NASH, the most common cause of abnormal liver tests in the developed world, is diagnosed after excluding other causes of elevated liver tests and after taking a history to exclude excess

alcohol use (20 g/day in women, 40 g/day in men). Diagnosis is supported by a history of metabolic syndrome and can be confirmed with liver biopsy and/or imaging demonstrating steatosis. Cirrhosis in the absence of steatosis can develop as a late complication of NASH.

- DILI is diagnosed based on a history of exposure and after excluding other causes of liver enzyme elevation. Often the diagnosis is made by observing normalization of liver tests after discontinuation of a drug. A liver biopsy may be helpful in certain instances of specific pathologic findings seen with certain drugs (i.e. pseudoalcoholic hepatitis with amiodarone, sinusoidal obstructive syndrome with chemotherapeutic agents, nodular regenerative hyperplasia with azathioprine).
- Budd–Chiari syndrome, primary and secondary malignancies, and infiltrative diseases such as amyloidosis can cause elevated liver tests and are diagnosed through imaging and/or liver biopsy. Sarcoidosis may cause liver enlargement and is associated with AP elevation; diagnosis is confirmed with a liver biopsy demonstrating non-caseating granulomas.

Laboratory features of selected conditions leading to elevated liver enzymes

Differential diagnosis	Features
Shock liver	AST and ALT in the thousands range, peak rise 2–3 days following hypotensive injury, prompt decline after restoration of blood flow
Alcoholic hepatitis	AST:ALT ratio > 2:1, jaundice, elevated GGT, leukocytosis
NASH	ALT > AST, elevated GGT, history of obesity or metabolic syndrome, alcohol intake < 20–40 g/day
Wilson disease	AP disproportionately low compared with other liver tests, AST:ALT ratio > 4:1 (fulminant Wilson disease), unconjugated hyperbilirubinemia/hemolysis
Acute liver failure from HSV	Bilirubin disproportionately normal compared with other liver tests

Cholestatic elevation of liver tests

- AP, a canalicular enzyme, and GGT, found in hepatocytes and biliary epithelial cells, are elevated in instances of biliary obstruction and hepatocellular injury and can help distinguish liver-related causes of hyperbilirubinemia from non-liver related causes.
- The diagnostic approach to hyperbilirubinemia starts with assessing whether the conjugated (direct) or unconjugated (indirect) form of bilirubin predominates. Causes of predominantly unconjugated hyperbilirubinemia are hemolysis, disorders of bilirubin metabolism and drug-induced impairment of conjugation and transport. Isolated indirect hyperbilirubinemia in the absence of aminotransferase or AP elevation should prompt an investigation for hemolysis. If hemolysis is ruled out, the differential diagnosis includes drug-induced causes and Gilbert's syndrome. Gilbert's syndrome is a benign condition due to a congenital mutation in UGT1A1 and is characterized by asymptomatic isolated indirect hyperbilirubinemia. Drugs that can cause an isolated indirect hyperbilirubinemia include indinavir and atazanivir (competitively inhibit UGT1A1) and drugs such as rifampin, chloramphenicol and gentamicin which affect uptake of bilirubin by hepatocytes.
- Conjugated hyperbilirubinemia can result from obstruction of bile ducts. Abdominal imaging starting with ultrasound to assess for biliary dilation is essential. Causes of biliary obstruction include choledocholithiasis, cholangiocarcinoma and tumors involving the head of the pancreas. Imaging which shows dilated bile ducts may prompt further diagnostic studies including

ERCP or EUS (EUS is the most sensitive method in the diagnosis of common bile duct stones). Absence of biliary dilation does not rule out the presence of bile duct stone(s).
- If no biliary obstruction is seen on imaging and choledocholithiasis is excluded, PSC and PBC should be considered. PSC is diagnosed by MRCP or ERCP showing beading of intrahepatic ducts caused by periductal fibrosis. Small duct PSC may not show abnormalities on gross imaging and may require a liver biopsy for diagnosis. PBC usually affects women and is associated with positive antimitochondrial antibodies (M2) and elevated IgM levels. A liver biopsy is helpful for diagnosis and staging. Inherited causes of conjugated hyperbilirubinemia are Dubin–Johnson syndrome (caused by a mutation in the canalicular transporter of bilirubin) and Rotor syndrome. Both have a benign course and can be differentiated by liver biopsy findings.

Typical presentation
- Patients with elevated liver tests due to acute liver failure may present with jaundice, encephalopathy or non-specific symptoms such as fatigue, nausea, or abdominal pain from hepatomegaly. Prompt recognition and diagnosis of acute liver failure with timely referral to a transplant center can be lifesaving.
- In contrast to acute liver failure, most patients with chronic liver disease are asymptomatic. Abnormal laboratory results in patients with chronic liver disease are often detected after blood tests during routine visits or during investigation of unrelated symptoms. Patients with later stages of cirrhosis may present with symptoms of hepatic decompensation such as ascites, encephalopathy, variceal bleeding or jaundice.

Clinical diagnosis
History
- History should include:
  - Alcohol use.
  - Recent use of medications, including herbal products.
  - Family history of liver disease (hemochromatosis, Wilson disease, alpha-1 antitrypsin deficiency).
  - Duration of jaundice (new onset jaundice in a patient with no underlying liver disease suggests acute liver failure).
  - Risk factors for viral hepatitis transmission (needle drug use, unprotected intercourse, tattoos, blood transfusions, hemodialysis).

Physical examination
Pertinent components of physical examination assessment include:
- Neurologic examination to assess for asterixis and/or encephalopathy (acute liver failure), stigmata of cirrhosis (spider angiomata, splenomegaly, ascites, muscle wasting).
- Presence of ascites (Budd–Chiari syndrome, cirrhosis).

Laboratory diagnosis
List of diagnostic tests
- Specific further tests which can aid in diagnosis:
  - Acetaminophen toxicity – acetaminophen level.
  - Hepatitis B – hepatitis B surface antigen, HBV DNA, HBV core IgM (acute infection and some cases of reactivation).

- Hepatitis C – HCV antibody, HCV RNA.
- Hepatitis A – hepatitis A IgM (positive in acute infection).
- Hepatitis Delta – hepatitis Delta antibody (in a patient with underlying hepatitis B).
- Hepatitis E – hepatitis E antibody (travel to endemic areas, pregnancy, immunosuppression).
- Autoimmune hepatitis – ANA, ASMA, anti-LKM, SLA/LP, IgG.
- PBC – AMA (M2), IgM.
- Wilson disease – ceruloplasmin, 24 hour urine copper, slit lamp examination to assess for Kayser–Fleischer rings.
- Hemochromatosis – iron studies, HFE gene mutation analysis (C282Y, H63D).
- Alpha-1 antitrypsin deficiency – alpha-1 antitrypsin phenotype
- A liver biopsy may be useful in making or confirming a diagnosis of autoimmune hepatitis, PBC, small duct PSC, Wilson disease, drug-induced liver injury, and alcoholic/non-alcoholic steatohepatitis. Infiltrative diseases such as sarcoidosis, amyloidosis and lymphoma may require liver biopsy for diagnosis.

List of imaging techniques
- Diagnoses which can be made by imaging:
  - Budd–Chiari syndrome – hepatic vein thrombosis on ultrasound, CT, MRI or venogram.
- PSC – MRCP (ERCP) showing beaded ducts.
- Biliary obstruction due to stones, stricture, cholangiocarcinoma, or pancreatic head neoplasm – MRI/MRCP, EUS, ERCP.
- Infiltrative diseases of the liver (sarcoidosis, malignancies) – ultrasound, CT, MRI.
- Non-alcoholic fatty liver disease – ultrasound, CT or MRI may show evidence of hepatic steatosis.

Diagnostic algorithm
See Algorithms 1.1 and 1.2 which outline the diagnostic approach to hepatocellular/mixed versus cholestatic liver test elevations.

Potential pitfalls/common errors made regarding diagnosis of disease
Errors made in evaluating patients with elevated liver enzymes
- Inadequate history.
- Haphazard use of a wide net of assorted tests instead of a directed approach guided by the history and the clinical context.
- Failure to consider extrahepatic causes for elevated liver enzymes.
  - AP can be elevated in bone diseases, celiac disease or pregnancy.
  - Isolated elevations in bilirubin (predominantly indirect) can be due to hemolysis.
  - AST can be elevated in muscle injury (as seen following strenuous exercise or in the setting of rhabdomyolysis or myocardial infarction). CK and aldolase are elevated in muscle injury.
- To initiate an exhaustive investigation for liver disease based on an isolated elevation of GGT

Section 4: Treatment
When to hospitalize
- Acute liver failure, defined as coagulopathy (INR > 1.5, encephalopathy, and new onset jaundice within 8 weeks of presentation in a patient with no underlying liver disease should prompt hospitalization and transfer to a liver transplant center.

Algorithm 1.1 Diagnostic algorithm for evaluation of hepatocellular/mixed liver enzyme elevation

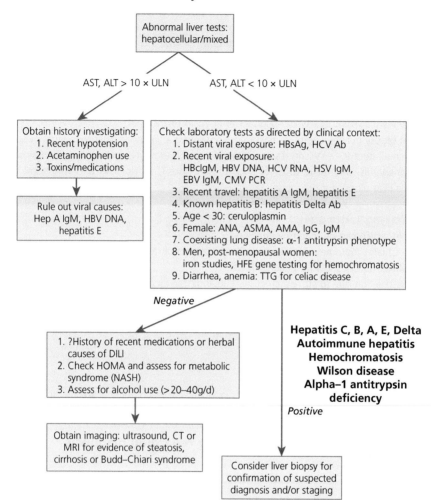

Section 5: Special Populations
Pregnancy
Abnormal liver tests during pregnancy (see also Chapter 25)
- Hyperemesis gravidarum occurs during the first trimester and is characterized by intractable vomiting along with elevated liver tests in 50% of cases. Management is supportive care including intravenous fluids to correct volume depletion.
- Intrahepatic cholestasis of pregnancy is characterized by pruritis during the second half of pregnancy. Jaundice occurs in 10–20% of cases and aminotransferase elevation can be mild to 10–20 times normal.
- Pre-eclampsia occurs during the third trimester and is diagnosed by the triad of hypertension, edema and proteinuria. Liver tests can be elevated up to 10–20-fold.

Algorithm 1.2 Diagnostic algorithm for investigation of cholestatic liver test elevation

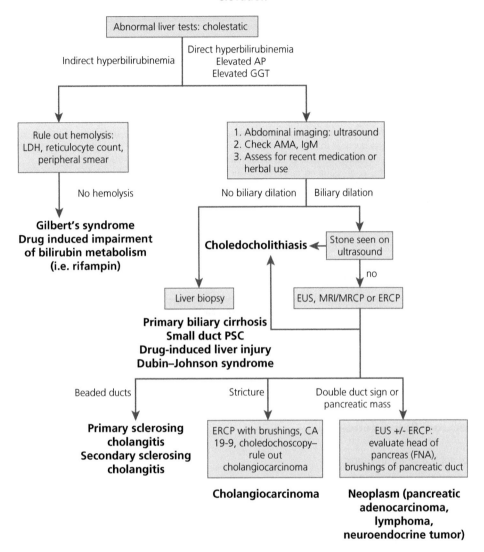

- HELLP syndrome is defined by hemolysis, elevated liver tests and low platelets. It usually occurs in the third trimester but can also occur post-partum.
- Acute fatty liver of pregnancy occurs in the third trimester and can present as abnormal liver tests with elevated aminotransferases (up to 500 IU/L) and bilirubin (up to 5 mg/dL). Liver biopsy shows microvesicular fatty infiltration. However, coagulopathy in the setting of acute liver failure may preclude biopsy. Cases can progress to acute liver failure, therefore INR assessment is critical in timely management.

Section 6: Prognosis

Not applicable for this topic.

Section 7: Reading List

Ahmed A, Keefe E. Liver chemistry and function tests. In Feldman M, Friedman L, Brandt L (eds) Sleisenger and Fordtran's Gastrointestinal and Liver Disease, 8th edition. Philadelphia: Saunders Elsevier, 2006:1575–86

American Gastroenterological Association Medical Position Statement: Evaluation of liver chemistry tests. Gastroenterology 2002;123:1364–66

Fabris L, Cadamuro M, Okolicsanyi L. The patient presenting with isolated hyperbilirubinemia. Dig Liver Dis 2009;41:375–81

Hay E. Liver disease in pregnancy. Hepatology 2008;47:1067–76

O'Brien C. The hospitalized patient with abnormal liver function tests. Clin Liver Dis 2009;13:179–92

Piton A, Poynard T, Imbert-Bismut F, et al. Factors associated with serum alanine transaminase activity in healthy subjects: consequences for the definition of normal values for selection of blood donors and for patients with chronic hepatitis C. MULTIBIRC Group. Hepatology 1998;27:1213–19

Prati D, Taioli E, Zanella, et al. Updated definitions of healthy ranges for serum alanine aminotransferase levels. Ann Intern Med 2002;137:1–10

Pratt D, Kaplan M. Evaluation of abnormal liver enzyme results in asymptomatic patients. N Engl J Med 2000;342:1266–71

Section 8: Guidelines
National society guidelines

Guideline title	Guideline source	Date
American Gastroenterological Association Medical Position Statement: Evaluation of liver chemistry tests	American Gastroenterological Association (AGA) http://download.journals.elsevierhealth.com/pdfs/journals/0016-5085/PIIS0016508502002408.pdf	2002

Section 9: Evidence

Not applicable for this topic.

Section 10: Images

Not applicable for this topic.

Additional material for this chapter can be found online at:
www.mountsinaiexpertguides.com.
This includes case studies and multiple choice questions

CHAPTER 2

Approach to the Patient with Jaundice

Jawad Ahmad
Division of Liver Diseases, Icahn School of Medicine at Mount Sinai, New York, NY, USA

OVERALL BOTTOM LINE
- Jaundice occurs when there is an elevation in the plasma total bilirubin level that is visible clinically.
- There are several methods of classifying jaundice in the adult patient that provide some indication of the etiology, the simplest being to separate jaundice into unconjugated versus conjugated hyperbilirubinemia.
- In the adult patient, the main causes of jaundice are related to intrinsic liver disease or interruption of bile flow due to obstruction of the biliary tree.
- The approach to jaundice should include a thorough history and physical examination, appropriate laboratory studies and further directed investigation including imaging and liver biopsy.

Section 1: Background
Definition of disease
- Jaundice occurs when there is an elevation in the serum total bilirubin level that can be detected clinically. In adults the normal upper limit for total bilirubin level is 1.2 mg/dL. Jaundice only becomes clinically apparent when the total bilirubin rises to greater than 2 mg/dL, and is first visible in the sclera and sublingual area.
- The vast majority of total bilirubin exists in serum in the unconjugated form but acute or chronic liver disease can affect multiple steps in bilirubin processing and can lead to mainly unconjugated, conjugated or mixed hyperbilirubinemia.
- Since bilirubin is the end-product of the metabolism of heme and is conjugated in the liver and then excreted into the biliary tree, jaundice can occur from dysfunction at any of these three steps.

Disease classification
- There are several methods of classifying jaundice, the simplest being to differentiate into unconjugated (indirect) and conjugated (direct) hyperbilirubinemia. This is an oversimplification as hyperbilirubinemia can be mixed.

Mount Sinai Expert Guides: Hepatology, First Edition. Edited by Jawad Ahmad, Scott L. Friedman, and Henryk Dancygier.
© 2014 John Wiley & Sons, Ltd. Published 2014 by John Wiley & Sons, Ltd.
Companion website: www.mountsinaiexpertguides.com

- Another classification system splits jaundice into pre-hepatic, hepatic and post-hepatic depending on where the pathological process is occurring.

Incidence/prevalence
- There is no reliable data on the incidence of jaundice in the general adult population.
- In adult patients presenting with jaundice, the incidence of different etiologies depends on several demographic factors, mainly age and geography, and risk factors for underlying liver disease.

Etiology
- There are multiple causes of jaundice in adults and the classification into unconjugated and conjugated bilirubin can be useful in determining the etiology.
- Causes of predominantly unconjugated hyperbilirubinemia:
  - Inherited (e.g. Gilbert's syndrome) or acquired (e.g. drug-induced) bilirubin conjugation disorders.
  - Intravascular and extravascular hemolysis (e.g. autoimmune, toxic, infectious, mechanical).
  - Impaired red cell production (dyserythropoiesis) or increased red cell destruction (e.g. sickle cell anemia and other hemoglobinopathies).
- Causes of mixed hyperbilirubinemia:
  - Acute or chronic liver disease.
- Causes of predominantly conjugated hyperbilirubinemia:
  - Intrahepatic cholestasis:
    - inherited (e.g. Dubin–Johnson syndrome, Rotor syndrome, PFIC disorders).
    - primary biliary cirrhosis.
    - any cause of chronic liver disease.
    - toxic/drug-related.
    - sepsis.
    - infiltrative (sarcoid, amyloidosis) or sequestrative (sickle cell hepatic crisis) diseases.
    - pregnancy.
    - malignancy (lymphoma).
    - post-operative.
  - Extrahepatic cholestasis:
    - intrinsic biliary obstruction:
      - cholelithiasis (choledocholithiasis).
      - malignant (cholangiocarcinoma).
      - primary sclerosing cholangitis.
      - sclerosing cholangitis from other causes (chemotherapy, autoimmune).
    - infectious – parasitic infections.
    - HIV- and AIDS-related cholangiopathy.
    - extrinsic biliary obstruction:
      - malignant:
        - pancreatic cancer.
        - lymphoma.
        - metastatic lymphadenopathy.
      - benign:
        - acute and chronic pancreatitis and its sequelae.
        - post-surgical complications.

- ◆ Mirizzi's syndrome.
- ◆ developmental anomalies.

Pathology/pathogenesis

- Unconjugated hyperbilirubinemia is typically due to increased bilirubin production or impaired uptake or conjugation of bilirubin in the liver.
  - Bilirubin is produced by catabolism of heme which is found in several proteins, notably hemoglobin, myoglobin and cytochromes.
  - The initial step is the oxidation of heme, catalyzed by heme oxygenase, found in the reticuloendothelial system and in Kupffer cells in the liver.
  - This leads to the formation of biliverdin which in turn is converted to bilirubin by biliverdin reductase.
  - Bilirubin is poorly soluble in water and is reversibly bound to albumin in plasma which prevents it crossing the blood–brain barrier. It is the unbound unconjugated bilirubin that leads to toxic effects.
  - Clinically, any condition leading to increased red cell destruction as in hemolysis or dyserythropoiesis results in increased unconjugated bilirubin production.
  - Bilirubin bound to albumin is transported to the liver sinusoids where the bilirubin is actively taken up by the hepatocytes. Inherited disorders can affect several steps in the process, and the formation of portosystemic collaterals in portal hypertension can lead to bypass of the liver, leading to unconjugated hyperbilirubinemia.
  - Bilirubin undergoes conjugation inside the endoplasmic reticulum in the hepatocyte. It is catalyzed by the enzyme family termed UGT and leads to the formation of bilirubin glucuronides, mainly the diglucuronide. Inherited deficiency of UGT is seen in Gilbert's syndrome and in the Crigler–Najjar syndromes. Conjugation can be affected by liver disease and several drugs, notably antibiotics such as gentamicin, chloramphenicol and rifampin, and HIV protease inhibitors such as indinavir.
- Conjugated hyperbilirubinemia is caused by impaired excretion of conjugated bilirubin in the liver from inherited causes or acquired liver disease and from obstruction of the biliary tree.
  - Conjugated bilirubin is actively transported across the bile canalicular membrane and excreted into bile.
  - This process can be affected by several inherited disorders (Dubin–Johnson and Rotor syndromes) and by several drugs (e.g. ethinyl estradiol, chlorpromazine).
  - Liver injury secondary to toxins typically leads to conjugated hyperbilirubinemia through a variety of postulated mechanisms. Pyrrolizidine alkaloids such as comfrey and bush teas cause damage to the endothelium of the central vein leading to sinusoidal obstruction syndrome. The resultant hepatic congestion interferes with bilirubin excretion.
  - Acute and chronic liver disease can cause conjugated hyperbilirubinemia. Viral hepatitis can acutely lead to jaundice as well as cholestatic variants seen after liver transplantation. The mechanism is multifactorial but involves impaired excretion.
  - Parasites are a cause of conjugated hyperbilirubinemia due to intrahepatic cholestasis. In ascariasis, the adult worm migrates into the biliary tree leading to obstruction. Similarly the eggs of *Clonorchis sinenis* and *Fasciola hepatica* (liver flukes) can obstruct the biliary tree.
  - Obstruction of the extrahepatic biliary tree can be caused by injury to the bile duct at surgery but typically is seen with obstruction of the extrahepatic bile duct by stone disease or malignancy involving the head of the pancreas or cholangiocarcinoma as well as benign disease of the pancreas.

Section 2: Prevention

- No interventions have been demonstrated to prevent the development of the disease.

Section 3: Diagnosis

> **BOTTOM LINE/CLINICAL PEARLS**
> - In the jaundiced patient, a detailed history is critical and can often point to the diagnosis.
> - On physical examination it is important to look for stigmata of chronic liver disease.
> - Initial investigations should include a total and fractionated bilirubin, liver enzymes (ALT, AST, AP, GGT), and tests of liver synthetic function.
> - Imaging should be obtained in the jaundiced patient and a right upper quadrant ultrasound is a reasonable first test.

Typical presentation
- The clinical presentation of the jaundiced patient will depend on the etiology. Typically patients have minimal symptoms and it is usually diagnosed when the patient (or family and friends) recognizes scleral icterus but can be preceded by pruritis and dark urine, particularly in patients with conjugated hyperbilirubinemia. If the jaundice is related to intrinsic liver disease, this can be associated with constitutional symptoms such as fatigue, malaise and myalgia. The presence of fever and abdominal pain can point to cholangitis, suggesting biliary obstruction from choledocholithiasis. Malignant causes of jaundice are classically painless but can present with concomitant weight loss.

Clinical diagnosis
History
- The history in the jaundiced patient is critical and should include the onset of jaundice, any associated symptoms such as pruritis, dark urine, pale stool, fever, abdominal pain, malaise, arthralgias/myalgias and weight loss. Prior episodes of jaundice and history of abdominal surgery (particularly liver or biliary surgery) are important. A detailed medication history is essential and should include over the counter and herbal medications and supplements. Risk factors for viral hepatitis and alcohol history should be documented as well as family history of liver disease or hemoglobinopathies. Any travel history and the patient's ethnic background are important. The patient's HIV status and occupation can also point to the etiology.

Physical examination
- The physical examination in the jaundiced patient should focus on identifying the possibility of underlying liver disease or malignancy. Stigmata of chronic liver disease include palmar erythema, leuconychia, parotid enlargement, multiple spider nevi (in the distribution of the superior vena cava, i.e. above the nipple line), gynecomastia, loss of axillary hair, ascites, dilated abdominal veins, hepatomegaly, splenomegaly, a venous hum in the epigastric area, and testicular atrophy. Tenderness in the right upper quadrant might indicate cholangitis, and an enlarged, palpable gallbladder (Courvoisier's sign) can be seen in malignant biliary obstruction. Excoriations and shiny finger nails can suggest pruritis.

Laboratory diagnosis

Diagnostic tests

- The initial laboratory tests in the jaundiced patient should include:
  - Total and fractionated bilirubin.
  - ALT and AST (transaminases).
  - AP and GGT (cholestatic enzymes).
  - Total protein, prothrombin time and albumin.
  - Complete blood count.
- Depending on the ratio of conjugated and unconjugated bilirubin, follow-up studies should include:
  - Hemolysis investigation if the liver enzymes are normal and the bilirubin is unconjugated.
  - Tests for underlying liver disease if the liver enzymes are elevated:
    - viral hepatitis serology:
      - hepatitis C: anti-HCV and consider HCV RNA.
      - hepatitis B: HBsAg, anti-HBs, anti-HBc (IgM), HBV DNA.
      - hepatitis A: anti-HAV (IgM).
    - autoimmune disease:
      - ANA, SMA, anti-LKM antibody, serum immunoglobulins.
      - if mainly cholestatic enzymes: AMA (or M2 fraction) for primary biliary cirrhosis. For primary sclerosing cholangitis P-ANCA can be checked and IgG4 for autoimmune pancreatitis/cholangitis.
    - metabolic disease:
      - iron studies: iron saturation and ferritin for hemochromatosis. If elevated ferritin and iron saturation (>50%) genetic testing for hemochromatosis (HFE genetic testing) can be ordered.
      - serum ceruloplasmin for Wilson disease.
      - alpha-1 antitrypsin level (and phenotype if decreased) for alpha-1 antitrypsin deficiency.
    - Miscellaneous:
      - HIV testing is suspected by history.
      - serum ACE level if cholestatic enzymes elevated (for sarcoidosis).
  - If bilirubin is conjugated and cholestatic enzymes are increased serum tumor markers can be checked:
    - CA19-9 (for cholangiocarcinoma or pancreatic cancer).
  - Percutaneous liver biopsy is indicated if the diagnosis is still in doubt after laboratory studies and imaging, particularly if there is the possibility of therapeutic intervention. We perform this at the bedside with ultrasound guidance but this can be performed by the radiologist. If there is concern for bleeding risk due to a prolonged prothrombin time or low platelet count, the biopsy can be performed by the transjugular route although the samples obtained are smaller but it has the advantage of allowing portal pressure measurement.

List of imaging techniques

- The initial imaging study in the jaundiced patient will depend on local availability and expertise. In all patients with jaundice an imaging study would not be unreasonable but is mandatory when biliary obstruction is suggested by conjugated hyperbilirubinemia.
- Non-invasive imaging studies include:
  - Abdominal ultrasound is relatively inexpensive and more readily available and can even be performed at the bedside. It is relatively sensitive in detecting biliary ductal dilation (implying

obstruction) and cholelithasis but is operator dependent. Overlying bowel gas can obscure the distal biliary tree.
- Abdominal CT scan is more expensive and newer technology scanners have better resolution but radiation exposure is not insignificant. It is equally as sensitive as ultrasound in detecting biliary ductal dilation and provides better assessment of the distal bile duct, hilar region and pancreas.
- MRI and MRCP is expensive but is the most sensitive non-invasive technique for detecting ductal dilation.
- Invasive imaging studies include:
  - ERCP provides assessment of the biliary tree and pancreatic duct and permits therapy such as stone extraction or stenting. It is expensive and associated with several complications, notably pancreatitis and should not be used for diagnostic purposes alone.
  - EUS is equally as effective as ERCP as a diagnostic tool but does not afford therapy.
  - PTC provides an alternative to ERCP when access to the ampulla of Vater is precluded due to prior surgery.
- My preference is for an initial ultrasound in all patients unless there is a high probability of biliary obstruction based on history and laboratory studies. In that situation MRI/MRCP is the test of choice since it can reliably detect primary sclerosing cholangitis. CT scan can be substituted based on local expertise and availability.

Diagnostic algorithm
See Algorithm 2.1.

Potential pitfalls/common errors made regarding diagnosis of disease
- It is important to make sure the total bilirubin is fractionated to determine the degree of conjugated hyperbilirubinemia.
- Lack of biliary ductal dilation on imaging does not exclude obstruction as a cause particularly if the clinical suspicion is high.

Section 4: Treatment
Treatment rationale
- The approach to treatment of the jaundiced patient will depend on the etiology and is documented elsewhere in this book.
- Unconjugated hyperbilirubinemia due to hemolysis will require consultation with hematology.
- Jaundice caused by underlying liver disease can be treated but in most situations the jaundice will resolve spontaneously as in viral hepatitis.
- Autoimmune hepatitis is an exception and is treated with immunosuppressive therapy.
- Obstructive jaundice is typically treated with endoscopic drainage and surgery where appropriate.

When to hospitalize
- Hospitalization is rarely required for the jaundiced patient unless there is concern for urgent intervention as in acute liver failure or biliary obstruction leading to cholangitis.

Algorithm 2.1 Management of the jaundiced patient

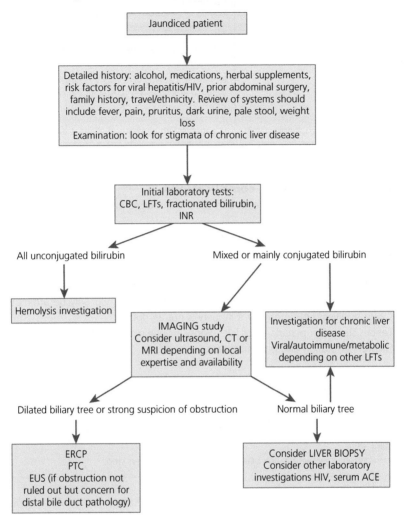

Table of treatment

Treatment	Comment
Conservative treatment	If a drug or toxic insult is suspected and liver tests are improving
	If acute viral hepatitis A or C or atypical viral hepatitis suspected
Medical (this will depend on the etiology). For example:	
Steroids for autoimmune hepatitis	Typically given orally at a dose of 40 mg and tapered over several months
Prednisolone/ pentoxifylline for alcoholic hepatitis	Given over several weeks or months in patients with a high discriminant function (see Chapter 10 on alcoholic hepatitis).
	(Continued)

Treatment	Comment
Surgical:	
Endoscopic retrograde cholangiography	In patients with benign or malignant biliary obstruction from stones, cancer, etc.
Surgical resection	In selected patients with biliary obstruction (e.g. Whipple procedure for pancreatic cancer)
Radiological:	
Percutaneous transhepatic cholangiography	In patients with benign or malignant biliary obstruction

Prevention/management of complications

- The complications of the various treatments for the jaundiced patient can be found in other relevant chapters.
- If intervention with ERCP is required complications can include acute pancreatitis, post-sphincterotomy bleeding, infection and rarely perforation.
- A recent study has suggested that routine ERCP for biliary drainage prior to surgery for cancer of the head of the pancreas is associated with more complications than surgery alone (although does not affect mortality). Hence, biliary drainage should only be attempted for patients with significant symptoms or if surgery is not an option.
- Complications seen after percutaneous liver biopsy include pain, bleeding, bile leak and occasionally bowel perforation and pneumothorax.

CLINICAL PEARLS
- The treatment of the jaundiced patient will depend on the etiology.
- Determining whether there is conjugated or unconjugated hyperbilirubinemia is the first important step.
- Determining whether there is any biliary obstruction is the next step.

Section 5: Special Populations

Pregnancy

- The approach to jaundice in pregnancy depends largely on the trimester. Diseases that are unique to pregnancy such as acute fatty liver of pregnancy, HELLP syndrome and intrahepatic cholestasis of pregnancy typically occur in the third trimester. Intrinsic liver disease can occur in pregnancy as can biliary obstruction from gallstones.
- These disorders are covered in the Chapter 25.

Children

- The approach to jaundice in children is covered in Chapter 36.

Elderly

- Does not differ from the approach in all adults.

Section 6: Prognosis

BOTTOM LINE/CLINICAL PEARLS
- The prognosis in the jaundiced patient depends on the etiology.
- Infectious causes can be self-limiting and can be treated.
- Removing the offending drug or toxic insult typically leads to improvement.
- Obstructive causes can be relieved endoscopically or surgically.

Natural history of untreated disease
- Depends on etiology.

Prognosis for treated patients
- Depends on etiology.

Follow-up tests and monitoring
- Depends on etiology.

Section 7: Reading List

American Gastroenterological Association. American Gastroenterological Association medical position statement: evaluation of liver chemistry tests. Gastroenterology 2002;123:1364–6

Pratt DS, Kaplan MM. Evaluation of abnormal liver-enzyme results in asymptomatic patients. N Engl J Med 2000;342:1266–71

Ramachandran R, Kakar S. Histological patterns in drug-induced liver disease. J Clin Pathol 2009;62: 481–92

Trauner M, Meier PJ, Boyer JL. Molecular pathogenesis of cholestasis. N Engl J Med 1998;339:1217–27

van der Gaag NA, Rauws EA, van Eijck CH, et al. Preoperative biliary drainage for cancer of the head of the pancreas. N Engl J Med 2010;362:129–37

Section 8: Guidelines
National society guidelines

Guideline title	Guideline source	Date
American Gastroenterological Association medical position statement: evaluation of liver chemistry tests	American Gastroenterological Association (AGA) http://download.journals.elsevierhealth.com/pdfs/journals/0016-5085/PIIS0016508502002408.pdf	2002

Section 9: Evidence

See individual chapters dealing with various different diseases.

Type of evidence	Title, date	Comment
Randomized trial	Preoperative biliary drainage for cancer of the head of the pancreas. N Engl J Med 2010;362:129–37	Demonstrated that routine ERCP for pancreatic head cancer not necessary

Section 10: Images

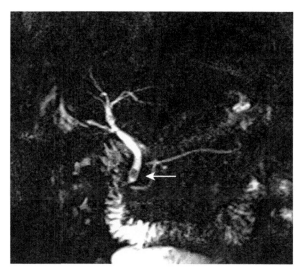

Figure 2.1 MRCP of a 62-year-old male presenting with conjugated hyperbilirubinemia 8 months after cholecystectomy. The study shows a non-dilated bile duct with an ovoid distal filling defect (white arrow) in the distal duct. The patient underwent ERCP with sphincterotomy and removal of the stone

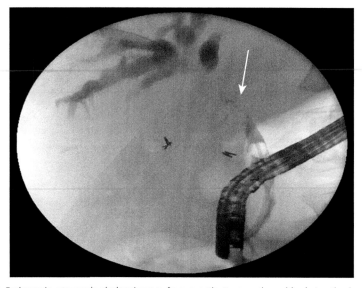

Figure 2.2 Endoscopic retrograde cholangiogram from a patient presenting with obstructive jaundice demonstrating very dilated intrahepatic ducts and a long stricture at the hilum of the biliary tree extending into the bile duct (white arrow). This patient had cholangiocarcinoma

Additional material for this chapter can be found online at:
www.mountsinaiexpertguides.com
This includes a case study and multiple choice questions

CHAPTER 3

Drug-Induced Liver Injury

Ponni V. Perumalswami
Division of Liver Diseases, Icahn School of Medicine at Mount Sinai, New York, NY, USA

OVERALL BOTTOM LINE
- DILI is the most common cause of acute liver failure in the USA.
- DILI can be caused by prescription medications, over-the-counter medications, vitamins, hormones, herbs, illicit ("recreational") drugs and environmental toxins.
- Typically, there are three signature patterns of DILI: hepatocellular, cholestatic, and mixed.
- The diagnosis of DILI often is clinically challenging and therefore providers should maintain a high index of suspicion. It is important to exclude other potential causes of liver injury.
- The treatment of DILI involves discontinuation of the offending agent and supportive care. Patients who develop hepatic failure as a result of DILI should be considered for liver transplant.

Section 1: Background
Definition of disease
- Drug induced liver injury is liver injury due to medications or other toxic agents.

Disease classification
- Jaundice associated with aminotransferase elevation portends a worse prognosis compared with aminotransferase elevation alone.
- Typically, three signature patterns of liver test abnormalities are recognized with DILI: hepatocellular, cholestatic, and mixed. These patterns are generally defined as follows:
  - Hepatocellular ALT/ULN ÷ AP/ULN $\geq$5
  - Cholestatic ALT/ULN ÷ AP/ULN $\leq$2
  - Mixed ALT/ULN ÷ AP/ULN >2 to <5

Incidence/prevalence
- DILI is the leading cause of acute liver failure in the USA.
- DILI is infrequent (one in 10 000 to 100 000 persons exposed).
- The majority of patients with symptomatic acute DILI are expected to completely recover with supportive care after discontinuation of the suspect drug.
- Patients with DILI that progress to acute liver failure have only a 25% chance of spontaneous recovery.

Mount Sinai Expert Guides: Hepatology, First Edition. Edited by Jawad Ahmad, Scott L. Friedman, and Henryk Dancygier.
© 2014 John Wiley & Sons, Ltd. Published 2014 by John Wiley & Sons, Ltd.
Companion website: www.mountsinaiexpertguides.com

Economic impact

- DILI has broad implications for not only patients and healthcare providers but the pharmaceutical industry and policy makers.
- DILI is the major determinant of drug-related regulatory action and can therefore have a tremendous economic impact on the pharmaceutical industry. DILI is the leading cause for termination of clinical drug trials, failure to obtain US Food and Drug Administration (FDA) approval and post-marketing decisions for drug withdrawal.

Etiology

- Many drugs and toxins are capable of evoking some degree of liver injury.
- Drugs that are implicated in DILI include not only prescription medications but also herbal and over-the-counter supplements.
- The liver represents a primary target for adverse drug reactions due to its pivotal role in biotransformation and excretion of drugs and their by-products.

Pathology/pathogenesis

- There are many different proposed mechanisms of action in DILI including: cell membrane disruption, canalicular alterations, formation of drug adducts, apoptosis and formation of free fatty acids.
- Others factors that likely play a role in the development of DILI include genetic and environmental associations.
- The risk factors, pathogenesis and outcomes of idiosyncratic DILI are inadequately understood.
- DILI has been difficult to understand due to the heterogeneity of its clinical presentation and course of injury, ranging from asymptomatic transient elevations in liver enzymes to liver failure and in rare cases chronic liver disease.
- Susceptibility to DILI is thought to be influenced by certain patient characteristics, predominantly age (adults > children) and sex (female > male), although there have been insufficient data to define increased risk in any given patient subpopulation. Other factors including nutrition, concomitant diabetes mellitus or alcohol use may be associated with increased risk of DILI as well as severity.
- Genetic factors may further influence an individual's susceptibility to adverse drug reactions. There are reports of a relationship between adverse reactions and HLA polymorphisms.

Predictive/risk factors

- Age (adults > children; e.g. isoniazid, halothane, valproic acid).
- Sex (female > male; e.g. halothane, minocycline, nitrofurantoin).
- Malnutrition and fasting (e.g. acetaminophen).
- Concomitant diabetes mellitus (e.g. methotrexate).
- Concomitant alcohol use (e.g. acetaminophen).
- Genetic factors including HLA polymorphisms (e.g. (HLA)-B5701 genotype as a major determinant of flucloxacillin DILI).
- Dose (e.g. acetaminophen).

Section 2: Prevention
Screening

- Having a high index of suspicion for the culprit drug, based on circumstantial evidence and exclusion of other confounding causes of liver injury, usually supports the diagnosis.

Primary prevention

- Avoiding any drugs that are not indicated would be a method of primary prevention.
- Restricted availability and blister packaging of over-the-counter medications.
- Physician and public education about possible drug side effects and dose limitations as well as monitoring for adverse drug reactions.
- Patient adherence to dosing guidelines.
- Baseline and periodic liver tests monitoring for select agents with known increased risk of hepatotoxicity.
- One difficulty associated with prevention of DILI is the relatively underpowered nature of clinical trials.

Secondary prevention

- Avoiding re-exposure to drugs that have precipitated DILI previously.

Section 3: Diagnosis

> **CLINICAL PEARLS**
> - Diagnosing DILI can be quite challenging as there is presently no specific diagnostic test or marker for DILI. The diagnosis of DILI is established based on the clinical history, chronology of exposure and injury, exclusion of competing etiologies and subjective assessment based on clinical experience and published data wherever available.
> - Idiosyncratic drug reactions are particularly problematic given that these are generally not dose or even time dependent and are instead characterized as reactions unique to the patient.
> - Clinically significant DILI is often defined as ALT > 3 times the ULN.
> - Clinical features by patient's history include symptoms of fever, pharyngitis, malaise, headache, rash, dark urine.
> - Physical examination findings in severe DILI can include icteric sclerae. In cases of fulminant hepatic failure, signs of hepatic encephalopathy will be present.
> - A temporal association between the onset of drug therapy and biochemical evidence of liver injury is helpful as is a temporal association between cessation of drug therapy and improvement in liver biochemistry; and the exclusion of alternative diagnoses.
> - Idiosyncratic drug reactions are particularly problematic given that these are generally not dose or even time dependent and are instead characterized as reactions unique to the patient.
> - The exclusion of competing etiologies of liver disease is integral to the evaluation of suspected DILI.

Differential diagnosis

Differential diagnosis	Features
Viral/infectious	Evidence of serologic markers or viremia, consistent with viral liver disease
	Liver biopsy evidence of periportal, not pericentral, mononuclear leukocyte infiltration
Autoimmune hepatitis	Presence of serum autoimmune markers and elevated gamma globulin
	Liver biopsy with plasma cell infiltration and immune cells, interface hepatitis

(Continued)

Differential diagnosis	Features
Biliary obstruction ̇	Acute obstruction can lead to liver tests abnormalities
	Imaging to evaluate for biliary obstruction including ultrasound, EUS, MRI/MRCP, ERCP
Metabolic liver diseases	Wilson disease: evidence of serum/urine copper abnormalities, low alkaline phosphatase
	Alpha-1 antitrypsin deficiency: genetic testing
Vascular disorders of liver	Imaging to assess vasculature
Alcoholic hepatitis	Evidence of leukocytosis, elevated liver tests
	Liver biopsy with features of alcoholic steatohepatitis

Typical presentation

- In DILI, the latency period may provide valuable clues for the correct diagnosis of the potential hepatotoxin. The latency period is variable and may be short (hours to days); intermediate or delayed (1–8 weeks); or long (1–12 months). The diagnosis of DILI is often clinically challenging. Providers should maintain a high index of suspicion for the culprit drug based on circumstantial evidence and exclusion of other confounding causes of liver injury. Often multiple drugs are involved, making it very difficult to determine the culprit. The physician must empirically decide which, if any, treatments to discontinue or substitute when DILI is suspected.

Clinical diagnosis (Algorithm 3.1)

History

- A careful and thorough history is key in diagnosing DILI. Providers should ascertain a complete list of all medications from patients suspected with DILI including prescription, over-the-counter and herbal medications. It is important to note that most patients do not consider over-the-counter and herbal medications as drugs and therefore directed questions regarding these preparations should be asked. Careful consideration should also be taken regarding when drugs were initiated and or dose modifications made. Prior history of DILI can also be helpful in identifying culprit agents.
- Clinical features by patient's history include symptoms of fever, pharyngitis, malaise, headache, rash, dark urine.

Physical examination

- A careful physical examination is imperative in patients with DILI. Fever and rash can be seen in drug hypersensitivity reactions. Icteric sclerae can be an indication of more severe DILI. In cases of fulminant hepatic failure, signs of hepatic encephalopathy will be present.

Useful clinical decision rules and calculators

- Identify "clinical drug signature" which is the term used to describe characteristic patterns of liver test abnormality, latency to onset of symptoms, presence or absence of immune hypersensitivity, and course of reaction after drug withdrawal. Individual variations do exist for each drug, and clinical signatures are not always consistent, but identifying these signatures can be helpful, especially when multiple potentially hepatotoxic drugs are being considered.
- Typically, three patterns of liver test abnormalities are recognized: hepatocellular, cholestatic, and mixed (see "Disease classification" in Section 1)

Disease severity classification

- The clinical spectrum of DILI is quite variable ranging from asymptomatic elevation in liver tests to fulminant hepatic failure. The predominant form of DILI is hepatocellular injury (90%) and is characterized by an initial early increase in ALT.
- Observation made by Hyman Zimmerman which was validated by larger studies. Hy's Law is utilized by the FDA in assessing hepatotoxicity in drugs that are being developed.

> Hy's Law: Persons who have drug-induced hepatocellular jaundice have the worst prognosis, with a 10% or greater chance of progressing to acute liver failure that ultimately may result in liver transplantation or death

- King's College Criteria identify two groups of patients that have a poor prognosis with acetaminophen-induced liver failure:
  - Arterial pH <7.3 (taken by sampling of blood from an artery).
  - All three with an INR of >6.5, serum creatinine >300 μmol/L and the presence of encephalopathy (of grade III or IV).

Laboratory diagnosis

List of diagnostic tests

- Liver tests should be obtained along with viral hepatitis serologies and autoimmune markers.
- Coagulation parameters to determine if there are signs of hepatic failure.
- Serum acetaminophen level along with serum and urine toxicology.
- Arterial blood gas and lactate to help determine predictors for spontaneous recovery.
- A liver biopsy is not required but can be helpful when the diagnosis is in doubt. There is limited data on the impact of histology on the clinical outcome in DILI. Liver histology can be helpful to identify the presence of confluent lobular necrosis, submassive necrosis, and massive necrosis which when combined are associated with a poor prognosis.

List of imaging techniques

- Ultrasound with Doppler to exclude vascular obstruction around the liver as a cause of abnormal liver tests.
- Imaging with a CT scan can be helpful to rule out stigmata of portal hypertension in patients who are suspected of having concomitant underlying chronic/advanced liver disease.

Algorithm 3.1 Clinical diagnosis

Step 1. Exclude other causes of liver injury (serologies for viral/infectious and autoimmune hepatitis, abdominal ultrasonography, and identification of potential confounders such as hypotension, sepsis, heart failure and use of total parenteral nutrition)

Step 2. Identify "clinical drug signature" (characteristic patterns of liver test abnormality, latency to onset of symptoms, presence or absence of immune hypersensitivity, and the course of the reaction after drug withdrawal)

Potential pitfalls/common errors made regarding diagnosis of disease

- Need to exclude other causes of liver injury including infectious hepatitis, autoimmune hepatitis, acute biliary obstruction and other causes of liver test abnormalities.
- DILI is a diagnosis of exclusion of other causes of liver disease.

Section 4: Treatment

Treatment rationale (Algorithm 3.2)

- The most important management in patients with DILI is early recognition and discontinuation of suspected culprit drug(s). The prognosis of DILI is generally good if the drug treatment is stopped. After culprit drugs are discontinued, most DILI reactions will resolve spontaneously, rapidly and most often completely. Patients who develop hepatic failure as a result of DILI should be considered for liver transplant, since such patients have a poor outcome. Patients with DILI who progress to acute liver failure have only a 25% chance of spontaneous recovery. Chronic liver disease, as a result of DILI, including the development of liver cirrhosis and portal hypertension, has been reported rarely.

When to hospitalize

- Patients with mild elevations in liver tests and normal bilirubin and who can adhere to close follow up, can often be managed as an outpatient.
- Patients who are jaundiced and/or who have any signs of fulminant hepatic failure should be managed in hospital.

Managing the hospitalized patient

- Conservative management with supportive care.
  - NAC can be administered to patients with suspected acetaminophen toxicity.
  - Only the 72-hour oral and 21-hour i.v. regimens are FDA-approved. Ideally, in patients with acute acetaminophen ingestion, treatment should begin within 8 hours of ingestion.
  - Oral 72-hour regimen: consists of 18 doses. Total dose delivered: 1330 mg/kg. Loading dose: 140 mg/kg. Maintenance dose: 70 mg/kg every 4 hours.
  - Intravenous 21-hour regimen: consists of three doses. Total dose delivered: 300 mg/kg. Loading dose: 150 mg/kg (maximum: 15 g) infused over 60 minutes. Second dose: 50 mg/kg (maximum: 5 g) infused over 4 hours. Third dose: 100 mg/kg (maximum: 10 g) infused over 16 hours.
- Patients who develop hepatic failure as a result of DILI should be considered for liver transplant, since such patients have a poor outcome.

Table of treatment

Treatment	Comment
Conservative treatment	Close monitoring of liver tests
Medical	NAC for acetaminophen overdose (see dosing in "Managing the hospitalized patient")
Surgical	Liver transplant for cases of fulminant hepatic failure
Radiological	US with Doppler and/or CT or MRI of abdomen
Psychological (includes cognitive, behavioural, etc. therapies)	Careful social work and psychiatric evaluations in patients with suspected suicide attempt or drug overdose

Prevention/management of complications

None.

Algorithm 3.2 Treatment rationale

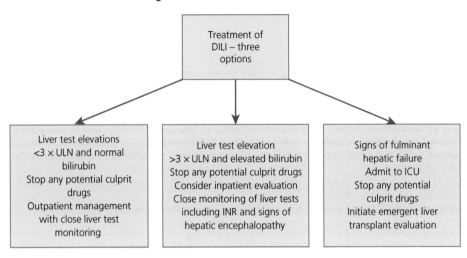

CLINICAL PEARLS
- Discontinuation of drug is most important treatment in DILI.
- The prognosis of DILI is generally good if the drug treatment is stopped.
- After culprit drugs are discontinued, most DILI reactions will resolve spontaneously, rapidly and most often completely.
- Patients who develop hepatic failure as a result of DILI should be considered for liver transplant, since these patients have a poor outcome.

Section 5: Special populations

Not applicable for this topic.

Section 6: Prognosis

CLINICAL PEARLS
- The prognosis of DILI is generally good if the drug treatment is stopped.
- Hy's Law: Persons who have drug-induced hepatocellular jaundice have the worst prognosis, with a 10% or greater chance of progressing to acute liver failure that ultimately may result in liver transplantation or death.
- Patients who develop hepatic failure as a result of DILI should be considered for liver transplant, since such patients have a poor outcome.

Natural history of untreated disease

- The prognosis of DILI is generally good if the drug treatment is stopped.
- Hy's Law: Persons who have drug-induced hepatocellular jaundice have the worst prognosis, with a 10% or greater chance of progressing to acute liver failure that ultimately may result in liver transplantation or death.

Section 7: Reading List

Andrade RJ, Lucerna MI, Fernandez MC, et al. Drug-induced liver injury: an analysis of 461 incidences submitted to the Spanish registry over a 10-year period. Gastroenterology 2005;129:512–21

Bernal W, Donaldson N, Wyncoll D, et al. Blood lactate as an early predictor of outcome in paracetamol-induced acute liver failure: a cohort study. Lancet 2002; 359: 558–63

Bjornsson E, Olsson R. Suspected drug-induced liver fatalities reported to the WHO database. Dig Liver Dis 2005;38:33–8

Black M, Mitchell JR, Zimmerman HJ, Ishak KG, Epler GR. Isoniazid associated hepatitis in 114 patients. Gastroenterology 1975;69:289–302

Chang CY, Schiano TD. Review article: drug hepatotoxicity. Aliment Pharmacol Ther 2007;25:1135–51

Chitturi S, Farrell GC. Drug-induced liver disease. In Schiff's Diseases of The Liver, 11th edition, 2011: 703–84

Ghabrila M, Chalasani N, Björnsson E. Drug-induced liver injury: a clinical update. Curr Opin Gastroenterol 2010;26:222–6

Holt M, Ju C. Drug-induced liver injury. In J. Uetrecht (ed.), Adverse Drug Reactions, Handbook of Experimental Pharmacology. Berlin: Springer-Verlag. 196, DOI 10.1007/978-3-642-00663-0_1

O'Grady JG, Alexander GJ, Hayllar KM, et al. Early indicators of prognosis in fulminant hepatic failure. Gastroenterology 1989;97:439–45

Watkins PB, Seeff, LB. Drug induced liver injury: summary of single topic clinical research conference. Hepatology 2006;43:618–31

Suggested website

DILIN: https://dilin.dcri.duke.edu/

Section 8: Guidelines
National society guidelines

Guideline title	Guideline source	Date
Drug Induced Liver Injury: Summary of Single Topic Clinical Research Conference	American Association for the Study of Liver Diseases (AASLD)	2006

Section 9: Evidence

Not applicable for this topic.

Section 10: Images

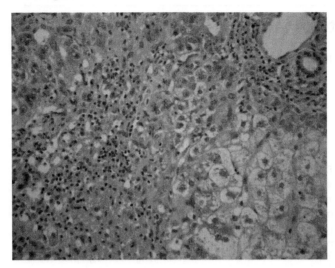

Figure 3.1 A 49-year-old woman with DILI from prophylactic isoniazid therapy for 3 months. There is necrosis and loss of hepatocytes in the centrilobular zone. The hepatocytes that have dropped out are replaced by a mild mononuclear inflammatory infiltrate and red blood cells (left portion). The portal tract on the right upper hand corner is unremarkable. The remaining hepatocytes are swollen and undergoing ballooning degeneration.

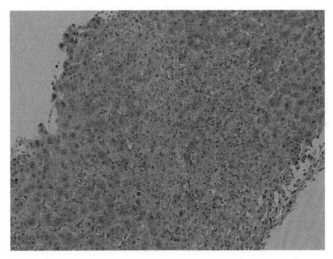

Figure 3.2 DILI from dilantin toxicity. The center of the photomicrograph shows confluent necrosis and many inflammatory cells consisting of lymphocytes and plasma cells. Individual necrotic hepatocytes (apoptotic bodies) may be seen at the periphery of this necrotic focus. The rest of the lobules demonstrate many areas of spotty necrosis.

Additional material for this chapter can be found online at:
www.mountsinaiexpertguides.com
This includes a case study and multiple choice questions

CHAPTER 4

Hepatitis A and E

Ponni V. Perumalswami

Division of Liver Diseases, Icahn School of Medicine at Mount Sinai, New York, NY, USA

OVERALL BOTTOM LINE
- HAV is an RNA picornavirus that infects only primates. HEV is an RNA virus and a member of the Hepeviridae family that infects humans and multiple domestic (e.g. pigs) animals and small mammals (e.g. rats).
- The route of transmission for HAV and HEV is fecal–oral and both are therefore highly endemic in developing nations with poor sanitation.
- The incubation period for HAV and HEV ranges from 15 to 50 days.
- Clinical features of acute HAV and HEV infection range from asymptomatic to fulminant hepatic failure; presence and severity of symptoms is related to the patient's age.
- Diagnosis of HAV or HEV infection is made with HAV or HEV IgM antibody.
- Treatment of hepatitis A or E is supportive.
- HEV can cause chronic hepatitis in immuncompromised patients (particularly after liver transplant) and has a high mortality in pregnant women in the third trimester (20%).

Section 1: Background
Definition of disease
- Hepatitis A is an acute infection caused by HAV.

Incidence/prevalence
- An estimated 1.4 million cases of acute hepatitis A occur worldwide annually.
- HAV infections occur sporadically and via outbreaks or epidemics.
- Hepatitis A is highly endemic in developing nations with poor sanitation, where infection often occurs in children, who are likely to be asymptomatic. Because even asymptomatic infected children may shed virus in their stools for up to 6 months, infection in children often initiates and perpetuates community-wide outbreaks. The prevalence of HEV is about 3 million acute cases annually.

Economic impact
- Acute HAV/HEV infections can occur as large epidemics related to contaminated food or water with significant economic and social impact on communities.

Mount Sinai Expert Guides: Hepatology, First Edition. Edited by Jawad Ahmad, Scott L. Friedman, and Henryk Dancygier.
© 2014 John Wiley & Sons, Ltd. Published 2014 by John Wiley & Sons, Ltd.
Companion website: www.mountsinaiexpertguides.com

Etiology
- HAV is a non-enveloped RNA picornavirus that infects only primates.
- There are five different HAV genotypes.
- HEV is a small (7.2 kb) non-enveloped positive sense, single-stranded RNA with five identified genotypes

Pathology/pathogenesis
- The pathology and pathogenesis of HAV and HEV are very similar.
- The route of transmission is oral inoculation of fecally excreted virus by person-to-person contact. The virus is ingested, traverses the small intestine and reaches the liver via the portal circulation and replicates within the liver in hepatocytes.
- After replication, mature virus reaches the systemic circulation and is released into the biliary tree and subsequently passes into the small intestine and is eventually excreted in the feces.
- Chronic shedding of HAV/HEV in feces does not occur.
- Viremia occurs soon after infection and persists through the period of liver enzyme elevation.
- On rare occasions, HAV/HEV has been transmitted by transfusion of blood products collected during the donor's viremic phase.
- The peak infectivity correlates with the greatest viral excretion in the stool during the 2 weeks before the onset of jaundice or elevation of liver enzyme levels.
- Liver inflammation is due to the host's cell-mediated immune response. HAV-specific CD8[+] lymphocytes and natural killer cells induce liver cell death and apoptosis.

Predictive/risk factors
- Living in areas with poor sanitation.
- Children > adults.
- Not previously vaccinated against HAV.
- Intravenous drug use.
- Household contact with infected person.
- Sexual partner of someone with acute HAV infection.
- Travel to endemic areas.
- Men who have sex with men.
- HIV-positive patients.

Section 2: Prevention

> **CLINICAL PEARLS**
> - Most effective prevention strategies include hepatitis A immunization and improved sanitation. A preventive vaccine for HEV has recently been developed and used in China.
> - A combination vaccine (Twinrix, GlaxoSmithKline) is available for HAV and hepatitis B vaccination in adults. It contains half the adult Havrix dose and 20 μg of recombinant hepatitis B surface antigen protein and is given in three doses at 0, 1, 6 months.

Immunization/vaccine	Age group	Dose	Volume	Doses	Interval/comments
Pre-exposure immunoglobulin	>1 year	0.02–0.06 mL/kg IM		1	Lower dose protects for <3 months, higher for 3–5 months
Post-exposure immunoglobulin (within 2 weeks)	>1 year	0.02 mL/kg IM		1	80–90% effective
Havrix (GlaxoSmithKline)	1–18 years	720 U IM	0.5 mL	2	0, 6–12 months
Havrix (GlaxoSmithKline)	>8 years	1440 U IM	1.0 mL	2	0, 6–12 months
Vaqta (Merck)	1–18 years	25 U IM	0.5 mL	2	0, 6–12 months
Vaqta (Merck)	>18 years	50 U IM	1.0 mL	2	0, 6–12 months

Screening
- No routine screening.

Primary prevention
- Most effective prevention strategies include hepatitis A immunization and improved sanitation.
- Personal hygiene practices, such as regular hand-washing, reduce the spread of HAV/HEV.
- HAV vaccination consists of two doses to ensure long-term protection. Nearly 100% of people will develop protective levels of antibodies to the virus within one month after a single dose of the vaccine.
- Adequate supplies of safe-drinking water and proper disposal of sewage within communities, combined with personal hygiene practices, such as regular hand-washing, reduce the spread of HAV/HEV.

Secondary prevention
- Primary contacts of persons infected with HAV should receive immune globulin administered intramuscularly which provides short-term protection (i.e. 3–5 months) through passive transfer of hepatitis A virus antibody. Immune globulin should be administered within 2 weeks after exposure for maximum protection. There is no evidence that immunoglobulin provides protection against HEV (even if the immunoglobulin is produced in countries where HEV is endemic).
- Even after virus exposure, one dose of the vaccine within two weeks of contact with the virus has protective effects.

Section 3: Diagnosis

> **CLINICAL PEARLS**
> - Hepatitis A and E range from asymptomatic to mild or severe disease. Symptoms and signs can include fever, malaise, loss of appetite, diarrhea, nausea, abdominal discomfort, dark-colored urine and jaundice. Physical signs can include tender hepatomegaly, splenomegaly, bradycardia, and posterior cervical lymphadenopathy.

- The icteric phase, which lasts 4–30 days, begins with hyperbilirubinuria followed within a few days by pale, clay-colored stools and jaundice.
- The anti-HAV or anti-HEV IgM test is the preferred confirmatory test for acute hepatitis A or E. HAV/HEV IgM usually remains positive for approximately 4 months but can occasionally be present for up to 1 year.

Differential diagnosis

Differential diagnosis	Features
Viral (HBV or HCV)/ infectious	Evidence of serologic markers or viremia, consistent with other viral liver disease Liver biopsy evidence of periportal, not pericentral, mononuclear leukocyte infiltration
Autoimmune hepatitis	Presence of serum autoimmune markers and elevated gamma globulin Liver biopsy with plasma cell infiltration and immune cells, interface hepatitis (occasionally plasma cells may predominate in hepatitis A)
Biliary obstruction	Acute obstruction can lead to cholestatic liver tests abnormalities Imaging to evaluate for the presence and cause of biliary obstruction including ultrasound, EUS, MRI/MRCP, ERCP
Metabolic liver diseases	Wilson disease: evidence of serum/urine copper abnormalities, low AP Alpha-1 antitrypsin deficiency: genetic testing
Vascular disorders of liver	Imaging to assess vasculature
Alcoholic hepatitis	Evidence of leukocytosis, elevated liver tests Liver biopsy with features of alcohol steatohepatitis
DILI	Diagnosis of exclusion and culprit drug

Typical presentation

- HAV and HEV have very similar clinical presentations although HEV can be more severe.
- Incubation period for HAV and HEV ranges from 15 to 50 days, with an average of 25–30 days.
- Preicteric phase. Lasts 5–7 days, with abrupt onset of fever, malaise, anorexia, nausea, vomiting, abdominal pain and headache. Less common symptoms include chills, myalgias, arthralgias, cough, diarrhea, constipation, pruritus, and urticaria
- Icteric phase. Lasts 4–30 days. Begins with hyperbilirubinuria followed within a few days by pale, clay-colored stools and jaundice. Upon the development of jaundice the prodromal symptoms usually subside. Fatigue, anorexia and slight nausea may persist. A dull sense of pressure in the right upper quadrant is caused by distention of the liver capsule.
- The presence and severity of symptoms with hepatitis A virus infection is related to the patient's age. Approximately 70% of infected adults develop symptoms, including jaundice. In contrast, only 10–30% of children younger than 6 years of age develop symptoms, which usually are non-specific and flu-like without jaundice.
- Organ transplant recipients. Acute HEV can occur in 5–6% of solid organ recipients. Ingestion of insufficiently cooked game meat or pork is a risk factor. Chronic HEV can occur in up to 50% of solid organ transplant recipients who acquire HEV infection, manifested by elevated AST/ALT levels, detectable serum HEV RNA and chronic viral hepatitis changes on liver biopsy.

Clinical diagnosis

History

- Enquire about:
  - Contact with infected persons (e.g day care centers, men who have sex with men, sexual or household contacts).
  - Travel to endemic regions.
  - Ingestion of contaminated food (e.g. shellfish).

Physical examination

- Look for tender hepatomegaly, splenomegaly, bradycardia, posterior cervical lymphadenopathy, and jaundice.
- Extrahepatic manifestations can occur with HAV infection (see Table: Extrahepatic manifestations of HAV infection).

Disease severity classification

- The presence and severity of symptoms with HAV infection is related to the patient's age. The mortality of hepatitis A, like its clinical attack rate, is age dependent: most infections of infants and young children are unapparent or subclinical, whereas infections of older children and adults are more likely to be clinically significant and this is reflected in the mortality rate of 0.1–2%.
- HEV is more likely to cause jaundice and can cause fulminant hepatic failure with a mortality rate of 0.5–3% but can be as high as 20% in women in the third trimester of pregnancy.
- HEV can also cause acute and chronic infection after solid organ transplant.

Extrahepatic manifestations of HAV infection
GI findings
Acalculous cholecystitis
Pancreatitis
Hematological findings
Aplastic anemia
Autoimmune hemolysis
Autoimmune thrombocytopenic purpura
Hemolysis (glucose-6-phosphate dehydrogenase deficiency)
Red cell aplasia
Neurologic findings
Guillain-Barré syndrome
Mononeuritis
Mononeuritis multiplex
Post-viral encephalitis
Transverse myelitis
Renal findings
Acute tubular necrosis
Interstitial nephritis
Mesangial proliferative glomerulonephritis
Nephrotic syndrome
Other findings
Cutaneous vasculitis
Cryoglobulinemia
Reactive arthritis

Laboratory diagnosis

List of diagnostic tests

- The anti-hepatitis A/E virus IgM test is the preferred confirmatory test for acute hepatitis A/E because it has high sensitivity and specificity when used on specimens from persons with symptoms.
- Serum anti-hepatitis A/E virus IgM usually can be detected 5–10 days before symptom onset, and the level remains elevated for 4–6 months. The anti-hepatitis A/E virus IgG level begins to rise soon after the IgM level and antihepatitis A/E virus IgG is present throughout the person's lifetime, conferring immunity.
- HEV RNA testing by real-time PCR of serum or stool is not commercially available but can be performed in specialized laboratories.
- The initial diagnostic tests include determination of hepatic enzyme and bilirubin levels with follow-up viral serology for hepatitis A, B, and C.
- In patients with hepatitis A/E, serum aminotransferase levels may be as high as 10 000 U/dL or higher, but there is little correlation between enzyme levels and disease severity. The AP level is elevated only minimally (even in cholestatic variants).The bilirubin level usually is elevated to about 5–10 mg/dL, and the prothrombin time is usually is 11 to 26 seconds.
- Despite an ongoing acute inflammatory process ESR and CRP are normal in most patients with acute hepatitis A/E.

List of imaging techniques

- No particular imaging required to diagnose hepatitis A/E.
- Ultrasound should be obtained to rule out any vascular causes of liver test abnormalities and dilation of bile ducts.

Potential pitfalls/common errors made regarding diagnosis of disease

- In order to diagnose acute HAV/HEV infection, it is necessary to check HAV/HEV IgM antibody status rather than HAV/HEV total IgG antibody.
- A positive anti-HAV IgM test in a person without symptoms of acute viral hepatitis and with only mild elevation of aminotransferases (≤100 IU/L) is likely to be false positive.
- It is important to exclude other viral causes for liver disease.

Section 4: Treatment (Algorithm 4.1)

Treatment rationale

- The treatment of hepatitis A/E is supportive.
- Patients with pre-existing chronic liver disease who develop fulminant hepatic failure as a result of hepatitis A/E infection should be considered for liver transplant.

When to hospitalize

- Patients with pre-existing chronic liver disease who develop fulminant hepatic failure as a result of hepatitis A/E infection should be hospitalized and considered for liver transplant.

Table of treatment

Treatment	Comment
Conservative treatment	Majority of patients with acute HAV/HEV infection can be followed closely with conservative management. Patients with signs of fulminant hepatic failure should be managed more aggressively
Medical	Post-exposure prophylaxis for HAV as described in "Secondary prevention"

CLINICAL PEARLS
- The treatment of hepatitis A/E is supportive.
- Patients with pre-existing chronic liver disease who develop fulminant hepatic failure as a result of hepatitis A/E infection should be considered for liver transplant.
- Primary contacts of persons infected with HAV should receive immune globulin administered intramuscularly which provides short-term protection (i.e. 3–5 months) through passive transfer of hepatitis A virus antibody.
- Immune globulin should be administered within 2 weeks after exposure for maximum protection.
- HEV infection should be considered early in the organ transplant recipients with unexplained elevated liver enzymes.

Algorithm 4.1 Treatment algorithm for hepatitis A

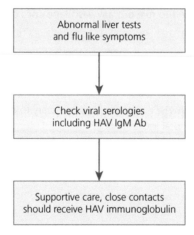

Section 5: Special Populations
Pregnancy
- Acute HAV infection during pregnancy is associated with a high risk of maternal complications and preterm labor.
- Acute HEV has a 20% mortality in the third trimester of pregnancy.

Children
- Of children younger than 6 years of age with acute hepatitis A, 50–90% are asymptomatic.

Section 6: Prognosis

> **CLINICAL PEARLS**
> - HAV/HEV infection is an acute self-limited illness. The vast majority of patients recover completely within 3 months.
> - Immunity is lifelong after recovery from HAV/HEV infection.
> - An asymptomatic HAV carrier state and chronic HAV-induced liver disease do not occur. Chronic HEV can occur in organ transplant recipients.
> - In very rare cases, HAV/HEV infection can cause fulminant hepatic failure. This usually occurs in people with concomitant underlying liver disease.
> - The mortality rate of hepatitis A in adults and in the elderly is 0.1–2%.
> - The mortality rate of HEV-related fulminant hepatic failure is 0.5–3%.

Natural history of untreated disease
- Hepatitis A/E is an acute self-limited disease in most patients. Chronic disease does not occur in HAV but can occur in HEV in immunosuppressed patients.

Clinical variants
- Relapsing hepatitis. A relapse may occur in 10–20% of symptomatic patients (mainly children) after apparent resolution of hepatitis A. Prognosis for complete recovery is excellent, but patients with a relapse should be regarded as potentially infectious.
- Cholestatic hepatitis. Uncommon. Characterized by prolonged jaundice (bilirubin may exceed 20 mg/dL) and pruritus. Prognosis for spontaneous complete resolution is excellent.
- Fulminant hepatitis. A fulminant course occurs in <1% of patients and is characterized by acute liver failure. Fulminant courses with high case-fatality rates primarily occur in patients with underlying liver disease and in elderly patients with comorbid conditions.

Section 7: Reading List

Aggarwal R, Naik S. Epidemiology of hepatitis E: current status. J Gastroenterol Hepatol 2009;24:1484–93

Atkinson W, Wolfe S, Hamborsky J, McIntyre L (eds) Epidemiology and Prevention of Vaccine-Preventable Diseases, 11th edition. Washington DC: Public Health Foundation, 2009

Dalton HR, Bendall R, Ijaz S, Banks M. Hepatitis E: an emerging infection in developed countries. Lancet Infect Dis 2008;8:698–709.

Daniels D, Grytdal S, Wasley A. Surveillance for acute viral hepatitis – United States, 2007. MMWR Surveill Summ 2009;58:1–27

Elinav E, Ben-Dov IZ, Shapira Y, et al. Acute hepatitis A infection in pregnancy is associated with high rates of gestational complications and preterm labor. Gastroenterology 2006;130:1129–34

Kamar N, Selves J, Mansuy JM, et al. Hepatitis E virus and chronic hepatitis in organ-transplant recipients. N Engl J Med 2008; 358:811

Navaneethan U, Al Mohajer M, Shata MT. Hepatitis E and pregnancy: understanding the pathogenesis. Liver Int 2008;28:1190–9

Prevention of hepatitis A through active or passive immunization. MMWR 1996;45(No. RR-15)

Prevention of hepatitis A through active or passive immunization. MMWR 1999;48(No. RR-12)

Prevention of hepatitis A through active or passive immunization: recommendations of the Advisory Committee on Immunization Practices (ACIP). MMWR 2006;55(No. RR-7)

Previsani N, Lavanchy D. World Health Organization. Hepatitis A (WHO/CDS/CSR/EDC/2000.7). 2000

Purcell RH, Emerson SU. Hepatitis E: an emerging awareness of an old disease. J Hepatol 2008;48: 494–503

Sjogren MH. Hepatitis A. In Schiff's Diseases of the Liver, Volume One, 10th edition. Berlin: Springer-Verlag:
    729–35
US Department of Health and Human Services. Estimates of disease burden from viral hepatitis. Atlanta, GA:
    US Department of Health and Human Services, CDC: 2008. Available at http://www.cdc.gov/hepatitis/PDFs/
    disease_burden.pdf
Victor JC, Monto AS, Surdina TY, et al. Hepatitis A vaccine versus immune globulin for postexposure
    prophylaxis. N Engl J Med 2007;357:1685–94

Suggested websites

http://www.who.int/mediacentre/factsheets/fs328/en/

http://www.cdc.gov/hepatitis/HAV/index.htm

Section 8: Guidelines

National society guidelines

Guideline title	Guideline source	Date
Surveillance for Acute Viral Hepatitis – United States, 2007	MMWR, CDC	2007
Hepatitis A Fact Sheet	WHO	2008

Section 9: Evidence

Not applicable for this topic.

Section 10: Images

Not applicable for this topic.

Additional material for this chapter can be found online at:
www.mountsinaiexpertguides.com
This includes a case study and multiple choice questions

CHAPTER 5

Hepatitis B and D

Elizabeth A. Kula, Donna J.C. Fanelli and Douglas T. Dieterich
Division of Liver Diseases, Icahn School of Medicine at Mount Sinai, New York, NY, USA

OVERALL BOTTOM LINE
- HBV infection is a significant global health problem.
- Chronic hepatitis B is a major cause of cirrhosis, fulminant hepatitis and HCC worldwide. Chronic hepatitis B is responsible for over 1 million deaths per year globally.
- HDV is dependent on HBV for its reproduction.
- HDV co-infection is associated with more severe disease with a higher incidence of cirrhosis, hepatic decompensation and HCC compared with those with chronic HBV infection alone.

Section 1: Background
Definition of disease
- Hepatitis B is a 42 nm DNA virus in the Hepadnaviridae family.

Incidence/prevalence
- The burden of chronic HBV infection in the USA is greater among certain populations as a result of earlier age at infection, immune suppression or higher levels of circulating infection. These include persons born in geographic regions with high (>8%) or intermediate (2–7%) prevalence of chronic HBV infection, HIV-positive persons (who might have additional risk factors) and certain adult populations for whom hepatitis B vaccination has been recommended because of behavioral risks (e.g. MSM and people who inject drugs).
- Approximately 5% of the global population is infected with HBV. This translates to over 400 million HBV carriers worldwide.
- It is estimated that 1.4 million people in the USA have chronic hepatitis B with 46 000 documented new HBV infections in 2006.
- Many experts believe that there are two to three times more infected persons in the USA.

Etiology
- HBV is transmitted by vertical transmission (perinatal), or horizontal transmission: percutaneous and mucosal exposure to infectious blood or body fluids, sexual exposure, as well as by close person-to-person contact presumably by open cuts and sores, especially among children in hyperendemic areas. The risk of developing chronic HBV infection after acute exposure ranges from 90% in newborns of HBeAg positive mothers to 25–30% in infants and children under age 5 and to less then 5% in adults.

Mount Sinai Expert Guides: Hepatology, First Edition. Edited by Jawad Ahmad, Scott L. Friedman, and Henryk Dancygier.
© 2014 John Wiley & Sons, Ltd. Published 2014 by John Wiley & Sons, Ltd.
Companion website: www.mountsinaiexpertguides.com

Pathology/pathogenesis

- After exposure to hepatitis B the virus is transported by the bloodstream to the liver, which is the primary site of HBV replication.
- Acute hepatitis B infection can be self-limited, with elimination of virus from blood and subsequent lasting immunity against reinfection, or it can progress to chronic infection with continuing viral replication in the liver and persistent viremia. Rarely, it can present as fulminant hepatitis.

Section 2: Prevention

CLINICAL PEARLS
- The key to prevention is elimination of further spread of infection.
- Offer hepatitis B vaccination to the entire population. Widespread HBV vaccination efforts have lead to a substantial decline in overall incidence of HBV infection in the USA.
- HBIG and vaccination post-delivery has significantly reduced the risk of perinatal transmission, in countries where it is used. Unfortunately it is not 100% effective, and some experts recommend treatment of pregnant women with high viral loads as a preventative measure.
- Increase screening, diagnosis and linkage to care.

Screening

- Screening strategies to diagnose those with hepatitis B include identifying those at risk for HBV infection. Screening begins with a thorough history and physical examination and serum blood sampling for those identified at risk. The CDC 2008 HBV screening guidelines help identify a high risk population that should be tested for HBV (see http://www.cdc.gov/mmwr/preview/mmwrhtml/rr5708a1.htm):
  - Persons born in regions of high and intermediate HBV endemicity (HBsAg prevalence ≥2%).
  - USA born persons not vaccinated as infants and whose parents were born in regions of HBsAg incidence ≥8%.
  - Persons needing immunosuppressive therapy (chemotherapy, post-transplant or treatment of GI/rheumatic disorders).
  - Persons with elevated ALT/AST of unknown etiology.
  - Donors of blood, plasma, organs, tissues, or semen.
  - Persons who are the sources of blood or body fluids resulting in an exposure that might require post-exposure prophylaxis.
  - Household, needle-sharing, or sex contacts of persons know to be HBsAg positive.
  - People who inject drugs, men who have sex with men, inmates of correctional facilities, hemodialysis patients, co-infection with HIV and/or HCV.
  - All pregnant women, infants born to HBsAg-positive mothers.

Primary/secondary prevention

- Primary prevention is directed at identifying those at high risk for transmission and preventing transmission. (All persons should be given HBV vaccination series.)
- Those with serum markers positive for hepatitis B should be counseled on routes and risk of transmission. Their household members and sexual partners should be tested for hepatitis B and offered vaccination if negative for serologic markers.

- Pregnancy is not a contraindication to HBV vaccination. Limited data suggest that developing fetuses are not at risk for adverse events when hepatitis B vaccine is administered to pregnant women. Available vaccines contain non-infectious HBsAg and should cause no risk of infection to the fetus.
- Pregnant women who are identified as being at risk for HBV infection during pregnancy (e.g. having more than one sex partner during the previous 6 months, been evaluated or treated for an STD, recent or current injection drug use, or having had an HBsAg-positive sex partner) should be vaccinated.

Section 3: Diagnosis (Algorithm 5.1)

> **BOTTOM LINE**
> - Serologic markers for HBV infection can help determine acute, chronic or past infection.
> - Serologic markers also help identify subjects who are vaccinated or eligible for vaccination.
> - With accurate diagnosis of infected individuals educational initiatives can be instituted to prevent further transmission of infection.

Typical presentation
- Persons with chronic HBV infection can be asymptomatic and have no evidence of liver disease, or they can have a spectrum of disease, ranging from chronic hepatitis to cirrhosis or liver cancer.

Clinical diagnosis
Acute HBV
- Illness typically begins 2–3 months after HBV exposure (range: 6 weeks–6 months). Infants, children aged <5 years, and immunosuppressed adults with newly acquired HBV infection typically are asymptomatic; 30–50% of other persons aged ≥5 years have clinical signs or symptoms of acute disease after infection.
- Symptoms of acute hepatitis B include fatigue, poor appetite, nausea, vomiting, abdominal pain, low-grade fever, jaundice, dark urine, and light stool color.

Chronic HBV
- Infection can be asymptomatic with no evidence of liver disease, or a spectrum of disease can be present, ranging from chronic hepatitis to cirrhosis or liver cancer. Chronic infection is responsible for the majority of cases of HBV-related morbidity and mortality.
- Physical examination may include the appearance of jaundice, liver tenderness and possibly hepatomegaly or splenomegaly. Fatigue and loss of appetite typically precede jaundice by 1–2 weeks. Acute illness typically lasts 2–4 months.

Laboratory diagnosis
List of serum diagnostic tests
- HBcAb IgG – hepatitis B core antibody immunoglobulin G
- HBcAb IgM – hepatitis B core antibody immunoglobulin M

Algorithm 5.1 Suggested algorithm for patient with serum markers for hepatitis B

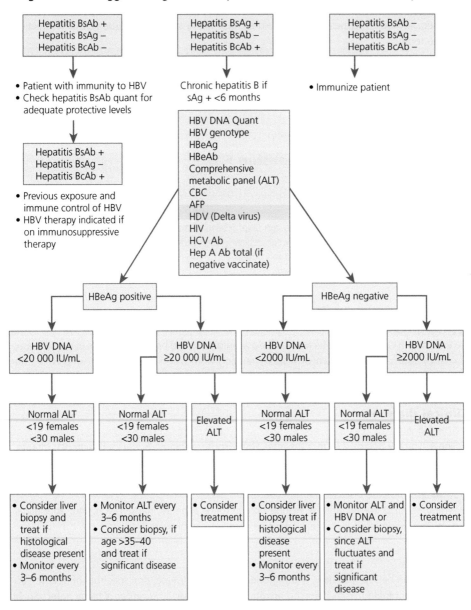

EASL HBV guidelines recommend consideration of treatment when HBV DNA levels are above 2000 IU/mL regardless of eAb or eAg markers and/or the serum ALT levels are above the upper limit of normal.

- HBeAb – hepatitis B e antibody
- HBeAg – hepatitis B e antigen
- HBsAb – hepatitis B surface antibody
- HBsAg – hepatitis B surface antigen
- HBV DNA – hepatitis B virus DNA

Serologic test results	Never infected	Chronic infection – replicating virus	Chronic infection – low level replicating virus	Immune/vaccinated	Acute infection	Acute infection recovery phase	Occult HBV
HBsAg	−	+	+	−	+	−	−
HBsAb	−	−	−	+	−	+	−
HBcAB IgG	−	+	+	−	−	+	+
HBcAB IgM	−	−	−	−	+	−	−/+
HBeAg	−	+	−	−	−	−	−
HBeAb	−	−	+	−	−	+	−
HBV DNA	−	+ ≥20 000 IU/mL	+/− ≥2000 IU/mL	−	+	+/−	+ low level

List of imaging techniques
- The goal of therapy for chronic hepatitis B is to eliminate or significantly suppress the replication of HBV and prevent progression of liver disease to cirrhoisis or HCC eventually leading to death or transplantation.

HCC screening protocol
- AASLD: AFP every 6 months and ultrasound.
- CT and MRI imaging may be preferred by some clinicians (although more expensive they are more sensitive) and in patients who have elevated AFP, cirrhosis or are at high risk for HCC.
- AFP and ultrasound are particularly important for those at high risk:
  - Africans >20 years old.
  - Asian men >40 years old.
  - Asian women >50 years old.
  - Family history of HCC.
  - Persistently elevated ALT/high viral load in person >40 years old.
  - Asians with HBV acquired through vertical transmission.
  - Cirrhosis.

Potential pitfalls/common errors made regarding diagnosis of disease
- Failure to screen all patients undergoing chemotherapy or other immunosuppressive therapy for HBV leading to serious reactivations and flares.
- Failure to consider HBV DNA levels as the major factor for the risk of disease and categorizing a patient as an "asymptomatic carrier" without checking HBV DNA.
- Failure to realize that laboratory normal ALT is not "healthy ALT" nor is it now part of the guidelines shown in Algorithm 5.1.
- Failure to screen for HCC aggressively enough in high risk patients.
- Failure to consider resistance in the long-term treatment of HBV.
- Lack of consensus between Association guidelines leading to delay in start of treatment.
- Need for frequent monitoring as viral levels fluctuate and disease may progress over time.

Section 4: Treatment (Algorithm 5.2)
Treatment rationale
- Treatment of chronic hepatitis B is aimed at viral suppression to reduce damage to the liver and its consequences (cirrhosis and HCC) and improve overall survival rate.
- There are seven drugs currently approved by the FDA for treatment of hepatitis B.

FDA approved therapies for HBV	
Nucleoside analog • Lamivudine (100 mg/daily) • Entecavir (0.5 mg/daily treatment naive, otherwise 1 mg/daily) • Telbivudine (600 mg/daily)	**Immune modulator/antiviral** • Interferon (IFN) alpha (three times a week) • PEG-IFN alpha-2a (180 μg SC injection weekly for 24–48 weeks)
Nucleotide analog • Adefovir (10 mg/daily) • Tenofovir (300 mg/daily)	**Demonstrated efficacy not FDA approved** • Emtricitabine/tenofovir (FDA approved for HIV not HBV) (200/300 mg/daily)

- At present, the preferred first-line treatment choices for treatment of naïve patients are entecavir, PEG-IFN-alpha-2a, and tenofovir because of their superior efficacy, tolerability, superior potency and favorable resistance profiles in patients with HBeAg-positive and HBeAg-negative chronic hepatitis B over comparable drugs in pivotal clinical trials. Treatment with nucleos(t)ide analogs is generally well tolerated and has become the mainstay treatment of chronic HBV infection, resulting in rapid viral suppression, improvement in Child-Pugh scores in patients with cirrhosis, and improved overall survival (Algorithm 5.3). Entecavir should not be used in patients who have previously been treated with lamivudine because of the high rate of resistance associated with its use in that population.

Algorithm 5.2 Treatment goals for chronic HBV

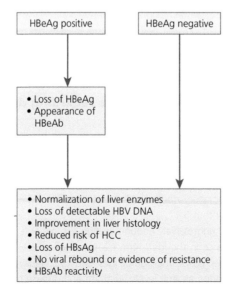

- In HBeAg-positive patients, tenofovir was most effective in inducing undetectable levels of HBV DNA (predicted probability, 88%), normalization of ALT levels (66%), HBeAg seroconversion (20%), and hepatitis B surface antigen loss (5%); it ranked third in histologic improvement of the liver (53%). Entecavir was most effective in improving liver histology (56%), second for inducing undetectable levels of HBV DNA (61%) and normalization of ALT levels (70%), and third in loss of hepatitis B surface antigen (1%). In HBeAg-negative patients, tenofovir was the most effective in inducing undetectable levels of HBV DNA (94%) and improving liver histology (65%); it ranked second for normalization of ALT levels (73%).

Algorithm 5.3 Nucleos(t)ide treatment response

Interferon treatment
- Interferons have antiviral and immunomodulatory effects. IFN-alpha has been shown to be effective in suppressing HBV replication and in inducing remission of liver disease. Its limitations include its efficacy limited to a small amount of patients (those who have low viral loads $<10^7$ IU/mL, elevated ALT > 3× upper limit of normal, high activity on liver biopsy and are either genotype A or B who respond better then genotype C or D) and treatment requires self-administered subcutaneous injection. Benefits of interferon treatment are its finite course of treatment, lack of resistance and PEG-IFN-alpha-2a shows high rates of HBsAg loss of 3–8%. If a patient is unresponsive to IFN-alpha treatment retreatment with interferon has shown very low levels of response and is not recommended. IFN-alpha is contraindicated in patients with decompensated cirrhosis or autoimmune disease, and in those with uncontrolled severe depression or psychosis.

Treatment with IFN-alpha
- Adults (5 MU daily or 10 MU three times weekly subcutaneous injections.
- HBeAg positive 16–24 weeks. Data suggest HBeAg-negative 12 months treatment.
- Should be treated for at least 12 months which may increase rates of response.
- PEG-IFN-alpha: 180 µg subcutaneous injections weekly for 48 weeks.

Definitions of treatment response with IFN-alpha therapy:
- Primary non-response: <1 log IU/mL decreased in HBV DNA from baseline at 3 months.
- Virologic response: HBV DNA less than 2000 IU/mL at 24 weeks of therapy.
- Serologic response: HBe seroconversion in patients with HBeAg- positive chronic hepatitis B

- The combination of PEG-IFN-alpha-2a with lamivudine showed a higher on-treatment response but did not show a higher rate of sustained response.

Prevention/management of complications (viral resistance)
- The major challenge of nucleoside/nucleotide analogue treatment is the considerable risk of developing antiviral resistance.
- The rate of resistance depends on pre-treatment HBV DNA levels, potency of the antiviral agent, prior exposure to oral nucleoside or nucleotide antiviral therapy, duration of treatment and the genetic barrier to resistance of the individual drug.
- Antiviral resistance may lead to loss of clinical benefits, development of multidrug resistance and transmission of resistant virus.
- Loss of clinical benefit is evidenced by loss of initial HBV DNA response with rebound, ALT increase and eventual reversion of histologic improvement with progression of liver disease leading to decompensation and cirrhosis.

Viral resistance nomenclature	
Genotypic resistance	Detection of viral populations bearing amino acid substitutions in the reverse transcriptase region of the HBV genome that have been shown to confer resistance to antiviral drugs in phenotypic assays during antiviral therapy. These mutations are usually detected in patients with virologic breakthrough but can also be present in patients with persistent viremia and no virologic breakthrough

Virologic breakthrough	Increase in serum HBV DNA level by >1 log10 copies/mL above nadir after achieving a virologic response during continued therapy
Viral rebound	Increase in serum HBV DNA level to >20000IU/mL or above pre-treatment level after achieving virologic response during continued therapy
Biochemical breakthrough	Increase in ALT level above the ULN after achieving normalization during continued therapy

Methods to detect resistance

Commercially available standard population-based sequencing	INNO-LiPA
• Less sensitive • Detects variants present at 25% of viral population • Needed to detect "new" substitutions not previously described	• More sensitive • Detects variants present at 5% of viral population • Detects only known mutations

Research

Restriction fragment length polymorphism analysis	Allele-specific PCR
• Detects variants present at 1% of viral population • Like INNO-LiPA, only detects known mutations	

Resistance mutations and preferred management strategies with nucleos(t)ide analogs

Antiviral	Primary resistance rutations	Resistance at 1 year HBeAg positive (%)	Resistance at 1year HBeAg negative (%)	Preferred management
Lamivudine	M204V/I A181V/T	11–32	11–27	Add adefovir or switch to tenofovir
Telbuvidine	M204I	5	2	Add adefovir Add or switch to tenofovir
Entecavir	L180M & M204V +I168T and M250V or T184Gand S202I	0	0	Add or switch to tenofovir Switch to emtricitabine/ tenofovir
Adefovir	A181V/T N236T	0	0	Switch to tenofovir Switch to entecavir
Tenofovir	None yet described	0	0	? (Consider emtricitabine/ tenofovir)

CLINICAL PEARLS
• Don't be confused if you see both eAg and eAb at the same time. Some patients will either flip-flop or they may be in the process of seroconverting. The same is true for sAg and sAb.
• Never drop your guard and get complacent with HBV. It is a very adaptable virus and a formidable foe.

(Continued)

- The only time when you can feel comfortable stopping therapy is when you see the development of sAb. However, you must still monitor for HBV and screen for HCC
- HBV infection after the acute phase presents a lifelong risk.
- When virologic breakthrough occurs in a patient who is adherent to antiviral therapy, the presence of mutations associated with drug resistance should be confirmed.
- If there is no resistance detected in a patient with a high viral load, then suspect non-adherence to treatment.
- Do not use entecavir in lamivudine-treated patient
- Goal of chronic hepatitis B therapy is to suppress the replication of HBV and prevent progression of liver disease to cirrhoisis or HCC eventually leading to death or transplantation.

Section 5: Special Populations
Pregnancy (Algorithm 5.4)

- MTCT of hepatitis B has been the most common mode of transmission worldwide. HBV infection in a pregnant woman poses a serious risk to her infant at birth. Without post-exposure immunoprophylaxis, approximately 40% of infants born to HBV-infected mothers in the USA will develop chronic HBV infection, approximately 25% of whom will eventually die from chronic liver disease. Perinatal HBV transmission can be prevented by identifying HBV-infected (i.e. HBsAg-positive) pregnant women and providing hepatitis B immune globulin and hepatitis B vaccine to their infants within 12 hours of birth. Data indicate a 20.2% immunoprophylaxis failure rate when infants were tested positive for HBsAg at birth.
- New data suggests that MTCT is more likely when HBV DNA levels are greater than 200 000 IU/mL, and elective Caesarean section may lower the rate of transmission.
- Treating hepatitis B in pregnancy has been controversial and several recent studies have demonstrated success in preventing MTCT with treatment as late as the third trimester of pregnancy.
- Decisions regarding initiating or continuing antiviral therapy in pregnant women should depend on the stage of the mother's liver disease and the potential benefit to her versus the risk to the fetus.

Category B	Category C	Category X
Telbivudine	Entecavir	Interferon
Tenofovir	Lamivudine	
	Adefovir	

- Based on the risk of teratogenicity in preclinical evaluation
- Considerable data in HIV positive women who have received tenofovir and/or lamivudine or emtricitabine
- Some data regarding lamivudine during the third trimester of pregnancy in HBsAg positive women with high levels of viremia, i.e >6–8 logs

- Breastfeeding has been a major concern because HBsAg has been detected in 72% of breast milk samples. Breastfeeding is not contraindicated in treatment-naive women with HBV if infants received proper immunoprophylaxis with HBIG and HBV vaccine, ideally within 12 hours of birth. It is safe for a mother infected with HBV to breastfeed her infant immediately after giving birth. There is no need to delay breastfeeding until the infant is fully immunized. All mothers who breastfeed should take good care of their nipples to avoid cracking and bleeding to prevent HBV transmission to the infant. Tenofovir concentrations in breast milk have been reported. The available data suggest that such low tenofovir levels in milk will most likely have no biological effect for the nursing infant.

- Intrauterine transmission is defined as HBsAg in the neonatal blood between 1 and 30 days after birth or detectable HBV DNA in neonatal peripheral venous blood. Immunoprophylaxis with HBIG and HBV vaccine is unlikely to prevent intrauterine transmission.
- Intrapartum infection can occur as a result of maternal–fetal microtransfusion during delivery or due to swallowing of infective fluid. Partial placental leakage during labor and trauma from instrumentation resulting in the mixing of fetal and maternal circulation is also a source of infection. A linear association was observed between the duration of first stage of labor and the presence of HBV antigens in cord blood. HBsAg was detected in 55–98% of vaginal epithelial cells, and HBV DNA in 12.1% of cervico-vaginal cells.
- Vertical transmission occurs despite perinatal immunoprophylaxis, especially in mothers with HBeAg (+) and high viral load (>6 log10 c/mL). Antiviral therapy in the third trimester for highly viremic mothers who have HBeAg (+) may effectively reduce vertical transmission to their infants. Limited data suggested that elective Cesarean-section might have a role on reducing vertical transmission compared to vaginal delivery or emergent Cesarean-section. Missing the opportunity to give HBIG and HBV vaccine remain the major causes for vertical transmission.
- At birth, high levels of HBsAg and the absence of HBsAb predicts failure of passive-active immunization resulting in an established chronic infection of HBV, HBsAg positivity at 12 months of age.

Risk factors and likelihood of HBV (MTCT)							
	Infants receiving HBIg and vaccine within 12 hours of birth				**Infants not receiving HBIg and/or vaccine within 12 hours of birth**		
High risk	HBeAg+	HBsAg+	DNA >200000 IU/ mL	Threaten pre-term labor	HBeAg+ HBsAg+	DNA >200000 IU/mL	High titer of HBsAg
Moderate risk	Genetic factors	Genotype/S mutation	Mother education		HBeAg- HBsAg+	DNA 2000–200000 IU/mL	Breastfeeding
Low risk or inconclusive	Amniocentesis	Forceps/ vacuum delivery	Breastfeeding		Amniocentesis	DNA <2000 IU/mL	Low titer of HBsAg

Serum HBV DNA level has been identified as the single most important predictor and independent risk factor for MTCT

- All infants with immunoprophylaxis failure were born to HBeAg+ mothers with HBV DNA levels >6 log$_{10}$ copies/mL.

**Algorithm 5.4 Proposed algorithm for the risk assessment and prevention
of HBV MTCT**

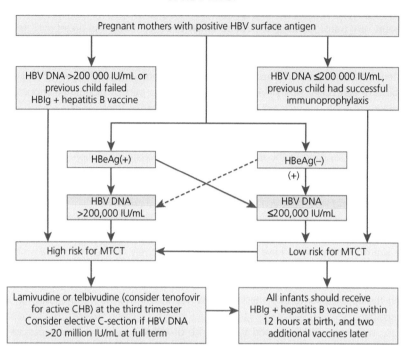

Source: Pan CQ, et al. 2012. Reproduced with permission of Elsevier.

Pre-natal HBsAg testing – CDC recommendations
- Routinely test all pregnant women for HBsAg during an early pre-natal visit in each pregnancy, even if they have been previously vaccinated or tested.
- Incorporate HBsAg testing into standard pre-natal testing panels.
- Women who were not screened pre-natally should be tested at the time of admission to the hospital for delivery.
- The prevention of HBV perinatal transmission, which is considered to occur mainly at delivery, is traditionally based on the combination of passive and active immunization with HBIG and HBV vaccination.

Management of infants born to women who are HBsAg positive
- All infants born to HBsAg-positive women should receive single-antigen hepatitis B vaccine and HBIg (0.5 mL) ≤12 hours of birth, administered at different injection sites. The vaccine series should be completed according to a recommended schedule for infants born to HBsAg-positive mothers. The final dose in the vaccine series should not be administered before age 24 weeks (164 days).
- For pre-term infants weighing <2000 g, the initial vaccine dose (birth dose) should not be counted as part of the vaccine series because of the potentially reduced immunogenicity of hepatitis B vaccine in these infants; three additional doses of vaccine (for a total of four doses) should be administered beginning when the infant reaches age 1 month.
- Post-vaccination testing for anti-HBs and HBsAg should be performed after completion of the vaccine series, at age 9–18 months. Testing should not be performed before age 9 months to avoid detection of anti-HBs from HBIG administered during infancy and to maximize the likeli-

hood of detecting late HBV infection. Anti-HBc testing of infants is not recommended because passively acquired maternal anti-HBc might be detected in infants born to HBV-infected mothers to age 24 months. Infants of HBsAg-positive mothers may be breast fed beginning immediately after birth.

Management of infants born to women with unknown HBsAg status

- Women admitted for delivery without documentation of HBsAg test results should have blood drawn and tested as soon as possible after admission. All infants born to women without documentation of HBsAg test results should receive the first dose of single-antigen hepatitis B vaccine (without HBIg) ≤12 hours of birth.
- If the mother is determined to be HBsAg positive, her infant should receive HBIg as soon as possible but no later than age 7 days, and the vaccine series should be completed according to a recommended schedule for infants born to HBsAg-positive mothers. If the mother is determined to be HBsAg negative, the vaccine series should be completed according to a recommended schedule for infants born to HBsAg.

Hepatitis B vaccine schedules for newborn infants, by maternal HBsAg status (Source: Data from Lee C, et al. 2006.).

Maternal HBsAg status	Single-antigen vaccine		Single antigen + combination vaccine	
	Dose	Age	Dose	Age
Positive	1*	Birth (≤12 hours)	1*	Birth (≤12 hours)
	HBIG†	Birth (≤12 hours)	HBIG	Birth (≤12 hours)
	2	1–2 months	2	2 months
	3§	6 months	3	4 months
			4§	6 month (Pediarix) or 12–15 month (Comvax)
Unknown¶	1*	Birth (<12 hours)	1*	Birth (≤12 hours)
	2	1–2 months	2	2 months
	3§	6 months	3	4 months
			4§	6 month (Pediarix) or 12–15 month (Comvax)
Negative	1*,**	Birth (before discharge)	1*,**	Birth (before discharge)
	2	1–2 months	2	2 months
	3§	6–18 months	3	4 months
			4§	6 month (Pediarix) or 12–15 month (Comvax)

* Recombivax HB or Engerix-B should be used for the birth dose. Comvax and Pediarix cannot be administered at birth or before age 6 weeks.

† Hepatitis B immune globulin (0.5 mL) administered intramuscularly in a separate site from vaccine.

§ The final dose in the vaccine series should not be administered before age 24 weeks (164 days).

¶ Mothers should have blood drawn and tested for HBsAg as soon as possible after admission for delivery; if the mother is found to be HBsAg positive, the infant should receive HBIG as soon as possible but no later than age 7 days.

** On a case-by-case basis and only in rare circumstances, the first dose may be delayed until after hospital discharge for for an infant who weighs ≥2 000 g and whose mother is HBsAg negative, but only if a physician's order to withhold the birth does and a copy of the mother's original HBsAg-negative laboratory report are documented in the infant's medical record.

Treatment of HBV in pregnancy (Algorithm 5.5)

- Family planning should always be discussed with women of childbearing age before initiating HBV therapy. The woman should be informed about the safety data of the drugs on a possible pregnancy.
- There is a considerable body of safety data from the Antiretroviral Pregnancy Registry in pregnant HIV-positive women who have received tenofovir and/or lamivudine or emtricitabine. No increased risk of major birth defects including in non-live births was observed for pregnant women exposed to antivirals relevant to CHB treatment overall or to lamivudine or TDF compared with population-based controls. Continued safety and efficacy reporting on antivirals in pregnancy are essential to inform patients on their risks and benefits during pregnancy.
- In a woman of childbearing age without advanced fibrosis who plans a pregnancy in the near future, it may be prudent to delay therapy until the child is born. In a woman of childbearing age with advanced fibrosis or cirrhosis who agrees to a "planned pregnancy" in the future, PEG-IFN therapy may be tried as it is given for a finite duration. It should be noted that effective contraception is required during PEG-IFN therapy. If PEG-IFN is not possible or has failed, treatment with a nucleoside analog has to be initiated and maintained even during a future pregnancy and tenofovir represents the most reasonable choice.
- If female patients become unexpectedly pregnant during anti-HBV therapy, treatment indications should be re-evaluated. The same treatment indications apply to women who are first diagnosed to have CHB during pregnancy. Patients with advanced fibrosis or cirrhosis should definitely continue to be treated with a category B drug. If a pregnant woman remains untreated or anti-HBV therapy is discontinued during pregnancy or early after delivery for any reason, close monitoring of the patient is necessary, as there is a risk of hepatic flares, especially after delivery.

EASL 2012: Recommendations for HBV-infected women who desire pregnancy

- Women without advanced fibrosis.
- Pregnancy before treatment.
- Women with advanced fibrosis or cirrhosis.
- "Planned pregnancy" in the future.
- PEG-IFN therapy may be tried as it is given for a finite duration.
- If IFN is not possible or has failed, treatment with an oral antiviral agent has to be initiated and maintained even during a future pregnancy. TDF represents the most reasonable choice.
- Unexpected pregnancy during anti-HBV therapy.
- IFN therapy must be stopped and the patients should continue on an oral drug.
- FDA category C drugs, particularly adefovir and entecavir, should be changed to a FDA category B drug.
- Women with mild liver disease, HBeAg+, and HBV DNA $>0^6$ copies/mL.
- Standard immunoprophylaxis may not be effective to prevent HBV MTCT.
- Treat with LdT, lamivudine or TDF in the third trimester to prevent HBV MTCT.

Other populations
Treatment in compensated and decompensated cirrhosis

- All patients with decompensated cirrhosis regardless of HBV DNA levels or HBeAg status should be considered for treatment and referred for liver transplant evaluation. Treatment should not be based on ALT levels. Interferon may precipitate decompensation. Preferred first line treatment is with combination therapy with tenofovir and lamivudine or possibly entecavir

Algorithm 5.5 Proposed management of HBV infection during pregnancy

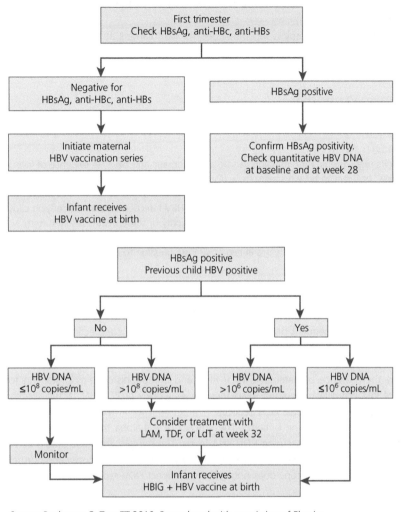

Source: Buchanan C, Tran TT 2010. Reproduced with permission of Elsevier.

or tenofovir monotherapy or tenofovir/ emtricitabine fixed dose (Truvada) and listing for transplantation.
- For those with compensated cirrhosis, treatment is based on DNA level rather then HBeAg status. Compensated patients with HBV DNA levels <2000 IU/mL may be treated or observed (preferred treatment is with either entecavir or tenofovir). Compensated patients with HBV DNA levels ≥2000 IU/mL long-term treatment is preferred with either entecavir or tenofovir. If lamividine exposured, tenofovir is preferred. Adjust entecavir and tenofovir per package insert for decreased GFR.

Prophylaxis in immunosuppression
- Reactivation of HBV replication with increase in serum HBV DNA and ALT levels has been reported in 20–50% of hepatitis B carriers undergoing immunosuppressive or chemotherapy.

- HBsAg and HB core antibody testing should be performed in all patients prior to receiving chemotherapy or immunosuppressive treatment (see Algorithm 5.1 for serum markers for hepatitis B).
- Prophylactic antiviral therapy is recommended for HBV carriers at the onset of immunosuppressive treatment.

Section 6: Prognosis

CLINICAL PEARLS
- Persons with chronic HBV infection can be asymptomatic and have no evidence of liver disease, or they can have a spectrum of disease, ranging from chronic hepatitis to cirrhosis or liver cancer.
- USA mortality data for 2000–2003 indicated that HBV infection was the underlying cause of an estimated 2000–4000 deaths annually. The majority of these deaths resulted from cirrhosis and liver cancer.
- Treatment of chronic hepatitis B is aimed at viral suppression to reduce hepatic damage and improve overall survival rate.

Hepatitis D (Delta) virus

Hepatitis D virus is dependent on HBV for its reproduction. HDV co-infection is associated with more severe disease with a higher incidence of cirrhosis, hepatic decompensation and HCC compared with those with chronic HBV infection alone. Active co-infection with HCV is confirmed by the presence of detectable HCV RNA and immunohistochemical staining for HCV antigen of IgM anti HDV. IFN-alpha 9MU three times weekly or PEG-IFN 180μg weekly is the only effective treatment against HDV replication. Treatment for at least 1 year appears to have long-term beneficial effects on patients. The efficacy of IFN-alpha therapy should be assessed throughout treatment by measuring HDV RNA levels. The primary endpoint should be suppression of HDV replication, decrease in necroinflammatory activity on liver biopsy and normalization of ALT. Nucleoside monotherapy does not appear to impact HDV replication.

Section 7: Reading List

Brown R, Verna EC, Pereira MR, et al. Hepatitis B virus and human immunodeficiency virus drugs in pregnancy: findings from the Antiretroviral Pregnancy Registry. J Hepatol 2012;57:953–9

Buchanan C, Tran TT. Management of chronic hepatitis B in pregnancy. Clin Liver Dis 2010;14:495–504

Centers for Disease Control and Prevention (CDC). The ABC's of Viral Hepatitis—fact sheet. Available at: http://www.cdc.gov/hepatitis/HBV/ProfResourcesB.htm#section1

European Association for the Study of the Liver. EASL Clinical Practice Guidelines: Management of Chronic Hepatitis B. J Hepatol 2009;50:227–42

Ghany MG, Doo EC. Antiviral resistance and hepatitis B therapy. Hepatology 2009; 49:S174–S184

Keeffe EB, Dieterich DT, Han SH, et al. A treatment algorithm for the management of chronic hepatitis B virus infection in the United States: 2008 update. Clin Gastroenterol Hepatol 2008;6:1315–41

Lee C, Gong Y, Brok J, Boxall EH, Gluud C. Effect of Hepatitis B immunization in newborn infants of mothers positive for hepatitis B surface antigen: systemic review and metanalysis. BMJ 2006;332:328–36

Lok ASF, McMahon BJ. Chronic hepatitis B. Hepatology 2007;45:507–39

Mast EE, Weinbaum CM, Fiore AE, et al. Advisory Committee on Immunization Practices (ACIP) Centers for Disease Control and Prevention (CDC): A comprehensive immunization strategy to eliminate transmission of hepatitis B virus infection in the United States: recommendations of the Advisory Committee on Immunization Practices (ACIP) Part II: immunization of adults. MMWR Recomm Rep 2006;55: 1–33; quiz CE1-4. (Published erratum in MMWR Morb Mortal Wkly Rep 2007;56:1114)

Pan CQ, Duan ZP, Bhamidimarri KR, et al. An algorithm for risk assessment and intervention of mother to child transmission of hepatitis B virus. Clin Gastroenterol Hepatol 2012;10:452–9

Wedemeyer H, Manns MP. Epidemiology, pathogenesis and management of hepatitis D: update and challenges ahead. Nat Rev Gastroenterol Hepatol 2010;7:31–40

Woo G, Tomlinson G, Nishikawa Y, et al. Tenofovir and entecavir are the most effective antiviral agents for chronic hepatitis B: a systematic review and Bayesian meta-analyses. Gastroenterology 2010;139: 1218–29

Zhang SL, Yue YF, Bai GQ, Shi L, Jiang H. Mechanism of intrauterine infection of hepatitis B virus. World J Gastroenterol 2004;10:437–8

Section 8: Guidelines
National society guidelines

Guideline title	Guideline source	Date
AASLD Practice Guideline update Chronic Hepatitis B	American Association for the Study of Liver Diseases (AASLD) http://www.aasld.org/practiceguidelines/Documents/Bookmarked%20 Practice%20Guidelines/Chronic_Hep_B_Update_2009%208_24_2009.pdf	2009

International society guidelines

Guideline title	Guideline source	Date
EASL Clinical Practice Guidelines: Management of Chronic hepatitis B	European Association for the Study of the Liver (EASL) http://www.easl.eu/assets/application/files/ef520780b91cf4f_file.pdf	2012
APASL Guidelines for HBV Management	Asian Pacific Association for the Study of the Liver (APASL) http://file.yynet.cn:8080/37fa75524fc47e0a68e909a2c415ee93/2012+APASL+HBV+guidelines.pdf	2008

Section 9: Evidence

See Guidelines listed in Section 8.

Section 10: Images

Not applicable for this topic.

Additional material for this chapter can be found online at:
www.mountsinaiexpertguides.com
This includes a case study, multiple choice questions, advice for patients and ICD codes

CHAPTER 6

Hepatitis C: Diagnosis, Management and Treatment

Alicia C. Stivala,[1] Deepti Dronamraju[2] and Douglas T. Dieterich[2]

[1]Division of Infectious Diseases, Icahn School of Medicine at Mount Sinai, New York, NY, USA
[2]Division of Liver Diseases, Icahn School of Medicine at Mount Sinai, New York, NY, USA

OVERALL BOTTOM LINE
- HCV is a major healthcare problem with an estimated 180 million people affected worldwide. It remains a leading cause for liver transplantation in the USA and accounts for roughly 8–13 000 deaths per year in this country.
- Spontaneous clearance of the virus is rare and 80–100% will become chronically infected.
- The primary goal of HCV treatment is cure, or eradication of the virus, which can be achieved successfully with currently approved combination therapies.
- Cure of HCV will prevent disease progression, reduce cirrhosis and its associated complications and decrease the risk of developing HCC.
- PEG-IFN and RBV remain the backbone of therapy for those eligible for treatment of HCV and the standard of care for genotypes other than 1.
- PIs BOC and TVR are recently approved drugs that can dramatically increase SVR when used in conjunction with current therapy. Their approval has changed the standard of care in chronic HCV treatment, for genotype 1 HCV, to include PEG-IFN, RBV and either of these two PIs.
- Treatment of acute HCV is nearly always successful when initiated early.

Section 1: Background
Definition of disease
- Hepatitis C is an inflammatory liver disease caused by the hepatitis C virus. Transmission of the disease is blood-borne and without treatment almost 50% will progress to liver cirrhosis.

Incidence/prevalence
- In the 2006 NHANES III study the prevalence of anti-HCV in the USA was 1.6%, equaling about 4.6 million people: 1.3% of the population was infected chronically.
- The WHO estimates that worldwide about 3% of the population has been infected with HCV and that almost 170 million people are chronically infected.
- Egypt has the highest worldwide prevalence with 9% of the country infected (up to 50% in rural areas).
- Incidence of the disease is difficult to evaluate given that the vast majority of newly infected individuals are completely asymptomatic.
- Genotypes 1, 2 and 3 have worldwide distribution. 1a and 1b comprise 70% of the HCV infections in the USA. Genotype 3 is seen in younger populations and in South Asia and geno-

---

Mount Sinai Expert Guides: Hepatology, First Edition. Edited by Jawad Ahmad, Scott L. Friedman, and Henryk Dancygier.
© 2014 John Wiley & Sons, Ltd. Published 2014 by John Wiley & Sons, Ltd.
Companion website: www.mountsinaiexpertguides.com

type 4 is common in Egypt. Genotype 5 is found predominantly in South Africa and genotype 6 in Southeast Asia.

Economic impact
- In 1998, the estimated cost burden of this disease was 1 billion dollars.
- This figure is expected to quadruple between 2010 and 2020.

Etiology
- The causative agent of hepatitis C is the hepatitis C virus.
- HCV is an enveloped single-stranded positive sense RNA virus.
- HCV belongs to the Flaviviradae family.
- There are six HCV virus genotypes based on genetic variations within virus isolates. Genotype and subtype are important in determining treatment duration.
- Transmission is blood-borne and usually transmitted via the sharing of infected needles. Transmission through sexual contact is rare compared with hepatitis B and HIV.

Pathology/pathogenesis
- After blood-borne inoculation, the virus is taken up by hepatocytes by means of one or multiple viral surface receptors. Once inside, the virus uncoats and releases its genome for mass replication.
- The HCV virus and its proteins have been shown to induce fibrosis directly through interference of cell activation pathways.
- Viral proteins may also lead to fibrosis secondarily through induction of liver steatosis. Implicated proteins include core and NS5A proteins.
- HCV genotype 3 has been suggested to be directly involved in steatosis as treatment of this genotype leads to complete resolution of steatosis.

Predictive/risk factors
- Risk factors for accelerated disease progression:
  - Older age at time of infection.
  - Male gender.
  - Presence of steatosis.
  - Other co-morbid illnesses.
  - Co-infection with HIV or HBV.
  - Persistence of ALT elevations.
  - Host genetics.
  - Heavy ETOH use.

Section 2: Prevention

CLINICAL PEARLS
- The key to preventing HCV infection is to educate patients about avoidance of exposure to infected blood and contaminated instruments, especially drug paraphernalia. Efforts are needed to educate high risk populations, including intravenous drug users, intranasal drug users and MSMs.

(Continued)

- Primary prevention interventions that have led to reductions in HIV incidence have not been as successful in reducing HCV incidence.
- There is observational data for needle exchange programs in reducing prevalence of HCV in IV drug users.

Counseling tips to reduce transmission of HCV

- Those who are HCV infected should avoid sharing toothbrushes, dental or shaving equipment and cover bleeding wounds.
- Counsel to stop using illicit drugs or not share works. Those who continue to inject drugs should be counseled to avoid reusing or sharing syringes, needles, straws, water, swabs and cotton, or other paraphernalia and to dispose safely of syringes and needles after use. Direct active users to needle exchange programs, where available.
- Latex condoms should always be used in HCV-positive persons who are not in long-term monogamous relationships.
- HCV-infected persons should be advised to not donate blood, body organs, other tissues or semen.

Screening

- History of ever having used illicit drugs via injection or intranasal route.
- Populations with HIV, on dialysis, and those with unexplained elevated liver enzymes.
- Transfusion of blood or blood products, or transplantation prior to 1992.
- Children born to HCV-infected mothers.
- Healthcare workers after needle stick injury to known HCV.
- Those born in high-risk endemic areas (Former Soviet Union, Pakistan, Mongolia and Egypt).
- Regardless of HCV risk factors, the CDC recommends one-time testing for all persons born between 1945 and 1965. This population has been shown to have a high prevalence of HCV infection and related disease.

Secondary prevention

- After SVR has been obtained with HCV treatment, patients can be re-infected. Always counsel patients to avoid high risk behaviors in order to avoid re-infection.
- Special attention should be paid to active drug users or prior drug users with high risk of relapse, and MSM who engage in unprotected sexual activity.

Section 3: Diagnosis (Algorithm 6.1)

CLINICAL PEARLS
- Generally patients with acute HCV are asymptomatic. They may have fatigue, nausea, malaise, occasional RUQ pain and rarely jaundice.
- Jaundice, hepatomegaly and RUQ tenderness may be noted on physical examination.
- Liver function tests, HCV antibody, quantitative HCV RNA should be sent for initially.
- HCV RNA can be detected as early as 2 weeks after exposure but antibody may not be detected until between 8 and 12 weeks. If HCV RNA is detected, HCV genotyping should be sent.

Algorithm 6.1 HCV diagnosis

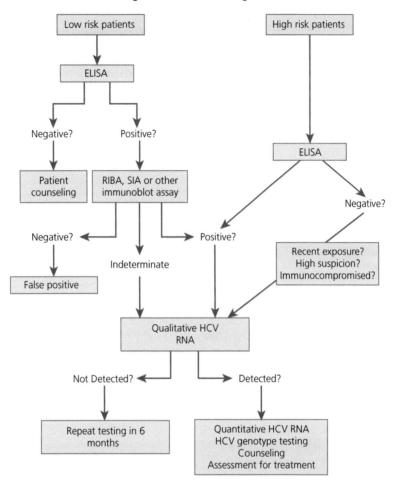

Differential diagnosis

Differential diagnosis	Features
Hepatitis B virus infection	Family history, from high endemic area, and positive hepatitis B serology
Alcoholic hepatitis	Drinking history, 2:1 AST/ALT ratio and negative hepatitis serologies
NASH (fatty liver)	Large body habitus or increased abdominal adiposity on physical examination. Negative hepatitis serologies
Wilson disease	Family history of disease, Kayser–Fleischer rings on physical examination. Check serum ceruloplasmin, 24 hour urine copper measurements

(Continued)

Differential diagnosis	Features
DILI	Presenting symptoms may be similar but hepatitis serologies will be negative. Temporal association with elevated LFTs and initiation of medication/s
Autoimmune hepatitis	ANA, SMA, anti-LKM may be positive on laboratory investigations. Affected population tends to be women with other autoimmune history or family history

Typical presentation

- Patients are usually asymptomatic from acute HCV infection. Those who present with symptoms usually have non-specific ones such as fatigue, nausea, malaise, occasionally RUQ pain and rarely jaundice. These symptoms are self-abating and last from 2 to 12 weeks. Chronic HCV infection is usually detected after abnormal LFTs are noted on routine screening by primary care physician. Most symptoms and complications associated from HCV are secondary to development of cirrhosis.

Clinical diagnosis

History

- Obtain an accurate and comprehensive history. History of the following exposures should be elicited:
  - History of ever having used illicit drugs via injection or intranasal route.
  - Populations with HIV, on dialysis, and those with elevated liver enzymes of still unclear etiology.
  - MSM.
  - Transfusion or transplantation prior to 1992.
  - Children born to HCV-infected mothers.
  - Needle stick injury to known HCV.
  - Born in high risk endemic areas (Former Soviet Union, Pakistan and Egypt).

Physical examination

- Inspect the patient's skin, sclera and tongue for evidence of jaundice. Also assess skin for findings of spider angiomata.
- Inspect abdomen for evidence of bulging flanks or caput medusa. Palpate abdomen and check for hepatosplenomegaly, RUQ tenderness and presence of ascites.
- Other physical examination findings one should look for include: alteration in mental status, palmar erythema, and lymphadenopathy.

Disease severity classification

- Liver biopsy is useful to determine degree of liver injury, but not a requirement.
- Typically a biopsy is not needed in genotypes 2 and 3, if the patient is willing to be treated.
- A number of serologic assays measure indirect markers of liver fibrosis, including Fibroscore, Hepascore, Fibrotest, FIB 4 and APRI. They are all remarkably comparable and can distinguish those with very minimal or advanced fibrosis with good sensitivity and specificity, but are less useful for patients with intermediate stages of fibrosis.

- Liver biopsy: the gold standard for determining degree of fibrosis. It is useful in chronic disease for prognosis, and the decision to treat in those with slow disease progression. The following staging methods are used to identify degree of fibrosis on liver biopsy: Metavir, Ishak, IASL and Batts-Ludwig. Among these, Metavir and Ishak are most widely used, and consist of four and six stages, respectively.
- Transient elastography (Fibroscan): a non-invasive method of determining liver stiffness is highly accurate in detecting cirrhosis in chronic HCV infection but slightly less specific for non-cirrhotic stages of fibrosis. It is approved for use in Europe and Canada.

Laboratory diagnosis
List of diagnostic tests
- HCV antibody – ferritin, iron/total iron binding capacity.
- Quantitative HCV – viral load ANA, AMA.
- HCV genotype – if positive viral load.
- PT and INR – thyroid function tests and thyroid antibody.
- CBC with differential – lipid panel.
- Comprehensive metabolic panel, including ALT, AST, GGT, total bilirubin and direct bilirubin – HBsAg, HBsAb, HBcAb, HAV Ab.
- AFP – HIVAb.

Available imaging techniques
- The main reasons for imaging in HCV are to exclude the existence of other liver diseases, assess severity of disease and to screen for HCC.
  - Liver US: in acute HCV there may be decreased liver echogenicity. In chronic HCV there often is increased liver echogenicity. Ultrasound is useful in evaluation of suspected ascites. Ultrasound is not as sensitive as CT and MRI and may not detect subcentimeter HCC.
  - CT abdomen: hepatomegaly, diffuse steatosis and gallbladder wall thickening may be noted in HCV infection. In chronic infection CT can aid evaluation for cirrhosis and HCC. Dual phase or triple phase contrast studies are most sensitive in evaluation of HCC.
  - MRI abdomen: in HCV may see periportal hyperintensity in T2-weighted images secondary to edema. In chronic infection can evaluate for cirrhosis and HCC – order with contrast.
  - Varices, splenomegaly or ascites seen on any imaging modality suggest cirrhosis with portal hypertension.

Interpretation of serologic and molecular assays

HCV antibody	HCV RNA	Interpretation
Negative	Negative	Negative for HCV infection. Tests should be repeated in 4–6 weeks if clinical suspicion is high
Negative	Positive	Acute exposure to HCV or immunosuppressed patient with HCV. Repeat screening at weeks 4 and 12
Positive	Positive	Chronic HCV infection. Consider treatment
Positive	Negative	Patient has been exposed but has cleared infection; no treatment necessary

Potential pitfalls/common errors made regarding diagnosis of disease

- If suspicion for acute HCV is high anti-HCV testing should be repeated even if initial testing is negative, as anti-HCV can be detected in 90% of patients 12 weeks after exposure.
- False-negative anti-HCV also occurs in populations with immunocompromised states such as transplant populations, HIV patients, dialysis patients and those with hypoglobulinemia. In these groups, if suspicion is high, quantitative HCV RNA should be performed.

Important abbreviations and definitions in HCV treatment	
RVR	Rapid virologic response; HCV RNA undetectable (UD) at week 4
EVR	Early virologic response; HCV RNA UD at week 12
eRVR	Extended rapid virological response; HCV RNA UD at weeks 4 and 12
pEVR	Partial early virological response; 2 Log drop in HCV RNA at week 12
cEVR	Complete early virological response; HCV RNA UD at week 12
SVR	Sustained virologic response; UD 24 weeks after treatment completion
PR	Partial non-response; >2 log decrease at week 12, but detectable at weeks 12 and 24
DVR	Delayed virologic response; >2 log decline but detectable at week 12 and UD at week 24
NR	Null response; <2 log decrease at week 12
BT	Breakthrough of HCV RNA any time after being UD
EOT	End of treatment
RGT	Response guided therapy
UD	Undetectable
DAA	Direct Acting Antiviral Agent
PI	Protease Inhibitor
LLOD	Lower limit of detection. The lowest limit of HCV concentration that can be detected with a 95% probability to determine presence or absence of HCV RNA. True non-detectability on treatment is demonstrated when the HCV RNA is below the LLOD
LLOQ	Lower limit of quantification. Smallest amount of HCV RNA that can be detected and accurately quantified

Section 4: Treatment
Treatment rationale

- The primary goal of HCV treatment is to eliminate permanently HCV infection. A SVR is evidenced by undetectable HCV RNA 24 weeks after completion of HCV treatment, and is the primary endpoint of therapy.
- In the non-cirrhotic patient, achievement of SVR typically results in complete resolution of liver disease and prevents progression to cirrhosis, ESLD and HCC. Moreover, an SVR at least 6 months after treatment is highly durable and less than 5% of patients will have evidence of HCV up to 10 years later.
- Treatment with PEG-IFN and RBV has been deemed cost effective across all stages of fibrosis. The severe sequela of untreated HCV are much more costly to treat than the infection itself.

Algorithm 6.2 HCV Genotype 1 treatment naive

Choose either triple therapy combination, based on patient characteristics and provider/patient discussion

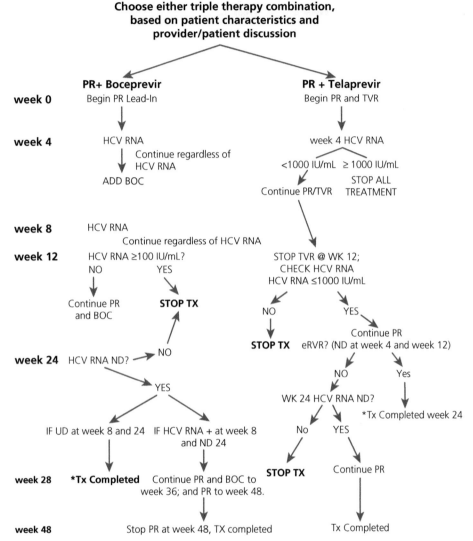

*All cirrhotics should be treated for 48 weeks if they meet stopping rules, regardless of having eRVR.
BOC, boceprevir; ND, nondetectable; PR, pegylated interferon and ribavirin; TVR, telaprevir.

Treatment of genotype 1 HCV (Algorithm 6.2)

- The first-line treatment of chronic hepatitis C in genotype 1 is the use of PEG-IFN administered weekly, subcutaneously and daily oral RBV, with the addition of a direct-acting HCV PI. Two PEG-IFN molecules, PEG-IFN-α-2a (180 μg once per week) and PEG-IFN- α-2b (1.5 μg/ kg once per week), can be used in combination with RBV and one direct acting agent: TVR or BOC.
- Treatment duration is determined by virologic response and stopping rules, which are detailed in the treatment tables: HCV treatment; HCV PI stop rules in treatment naïve/experienced genotype 1 HCV.

HCV PI stop rules in treatment naive genotype 1 HCV

PI	Week 0–4	Week 8	Week 12	Week 24–48
BOC	Lead-in with PR only Add BOC at end of week 4/start of week 5 No Stopping Rule	HCV RNA Continue PR/BOC No Stopping Rule	If HCV RNA <100 → continue PR and BOC If HCV RNA ≥100 IU/mL →STOP all treatment.	If HCV RNA UD at weeks 8, 12 and 24→stop all treatment at week 28 If HCV RNA + at week 8 and HCV UD at weeks 12 and 24 → continue BOC to week 36; continue PR through to week 48 If HCV RNA + at week 24, STOP all treatment If HCV RNA + after UD at any point,* STOP all treatment (all cirrhotics should be treated for 48 weeks, even if they have week 8 response)
TVR	Start PR/TVR If week 4 HCV RNA ≤1000 →continue PR/TVR If week 4 HCV RNA >1000 →STOP treatment	HCV RNA No Stopping Rule	HCV RNA All STOP TVR at week 12 If eRVR →continue PR to week 24 If HCV RNA ≤1000 continue PR→ If HCV RNA >1000→STOP Treatment*	If eRVR→stop treatment at week 24 If HCV RNA + at week 4 and 12 and UD at week 24 continue PR to week 48 If HCV RNA + after UD at any point*, STOP all treatment

* After confirming HCV RNA + with repeat assay; +, quantifiable or above the LLOD

Treatment of genotypes 2 and 3 HCV
- In Genotypes 2 and 3, first line therapy is PEG-IFN and RBV. Treatment duration is typically 24 weeks in HCV mono-infection.
- Response-guided therapy rules: if RVR, treat for 24 weeks; if EVR, treat for 48 weeks.
- Patients with risk factors for decreased SVR, including advance fibrosis and insulin resistance should also be treated for 48 weeks.

Treatment of genotypes 4, 5 and 6
- Standard of care remains PEG-IFN and RBV.
- Treatment duration is 48 weeks.

Options for "treatment-experienced" patients
- Genotype 1 treatment-experienced patients – see table: HCV PI stop rules in treatment naive genotype 1 HCV.
- Genotype 1 treatment-experienced patients who do not respond to triple therapy will need to await further progress or enroll in clinical trials with experimental treatments.
- Genotypes 2–6, who have not responded to PEG-IFN/RBV:

- Retreatment with PEG-IFN/RBV should be retried in patients who prematurely discontinued treatment or received suboptimal dosing.
- Await further data on retreatment with PIs in their genotypes or enroll in clinical trials.

HCV PI stop rules for treatment experienced genotype 1 HCV

PI	Week 0–4	Week 8	Week 12	Week 24–48
BOC	Lead-in with PR only	HCV RNA No Stopping Rule	Check HCV RNA If HCV RNA ≥100 IU/mL → stop all treatment. IF HCV RNA <100, continue BOC/PR.	If week 24 HCV RNA detectable, stop treatment
	Add BOC at end of week 4/start of week 5			If HCV RNA UD at week 8 and week 24→ continue all agents through to week 36
	No Stopping Rule			If week 8 HCV RNA + and week 24 HCV RNA UD →STOP BOC at week 36. Continue PR through week 48
				If HCV RNA + after UD at any point, * STOP all treatment
TVR	Start PR/ TVR	HCV RNA No Stopping Rule	HCV RNA STOP TVR IF HCV RNA ≤1000, continue PR. If HCV RNA >1000 →STOP treatment.	HCV RNA
	Week 4: HCV RNA			IF HCV RNA UD→continue PR to week 48
	If HCV RNA ≥1000 IU/mL, STOP treatment			If HCV RNA + after UD at any point, * STOP all treatment

* After confirming HCV RNA + with repeat assay; +, quantifiable or above the LLOD

Treatment monitoring, assessment and support

- Treatment monitoring should include assessment of treatment response at designated time points, assessing for side effects and providing supportive care by the medical team.
- Patients treated for HCV should be seen at weeks 1, 2 and 4 of treatment and at monthly intervals thereafter until completion of treatment. This will provide time sensitive opportunities to monitor the treatment efficacy, adherence and side effects.

Treatment efficacy

- The goal of treatment is SVR is defined as PCR negativity 6 months after stopping therapy.
- The best tool for monitoring response to treatment is real-time PCR-based assay, with a lower limit of detection of 10–50 IU/mL. The same assay should be used at different time points to ensure consistent results. A baseline HCV RNA should be drawn within 4 weeks prior to starting treatment.
- The EOT virological response is measured on the last day of treatment, which varies with RGT.
- According to current clinical guidelines, HCV RNA testing should be performed at 24 weeks after completion of treatment, which measures for SVR.
- In 2011, the FDA accepted SVR 12 as the endpoint for clinical trials because HCV relapse usually occurs within the first 12 weeks after the EOT. SVR 12 can be used with a 99.7 % positive predictive value for predicting SVR 24. SVR 24 should still be obtained as confirmation if the 12 week post-treatment assay is non-detectable.

Clinical side effects of treatment

- Patients should be advised of the risk of teratogenicity with RBV. Strict birth control should be required in patients of childbearing age treated with PEG-IFN and RBV during therapy and in the 6 months following treatment. Patients should be routinely counseled on this and asked about adherence to birth control during treatment. Baseline and monthly pregnancy tests are recommended in women of childbearing age while on treatment.
- Fatigue, depression, irritability, skin rashes, sleep disturbance and dyspnea are common side effects that should be assessed at each clinical follow-up.
- Patients should be taught how to prevent and manage common side effects using non-pharmacologic techniques, as well as antipyretics and analgesics.
- Antidepressants may be warranted given the high incidence of depression while on interferon, and consultation with a mental health provider should be considered in cases of severe depression, anxiety or psychosis. Initiating antidepressant therapy 1–2 months prior to the start of HCV therapy is appropriate in patients who have a history of depression.
- Severe reactions that require treatment discontinuation include autoimmune reactions, interstitial lung disease, neuroretinitis, bone marrow aplasia or idiopathic thrombocytopenia.

Hematological and biochemical side effects, including neutropenia, anemia, thrombocytopenia and TSH abnormalities

- CBC and LFTs should be assessed at each follow-up, beginning with week 2.
- In our clinical experience, anemia with the addition of HCV PIs has been more severe and more rapid than predicted by clinical trials. Follow CBCs very closely, starting at week 2 of treatment. If hemaglobin begins dropping, intervene and repeat weekly until stabilized by dose reduction, addition of growth factors or treatment discontinuation. Transfusion may be required.
- TSH should be monitored every 12 weeks because of the risk of autoimmune thyroiditis induced by interferon.

- The HCV PIs can inhibit hepatic drug-metabolizing enzymes such as cytochrome P450 2C (CYP2C), CYP3A4, or CYP1A. Before initiating treatment with BOC or TVR, check each of the patient's medications for possible drug–drug interactions.
- Use the package inserts of HCV PIs or the frequently updated website: http://www.hep-druginteractions.org.

- Baseline labs are crucial for denoting changes and monitoring response.
- CBC should be assessed at each follow-up, beginning with week 2.
- TSH and complete metabolic panel should be monitored every 12 weeks.
- HCV RNA should be checked at weeks 4, 8, 12, 24, 36 and EOT.
- Baseline and quarterly pregnancy tests are also recommended in women of child bearing age.

Treatment adherence, support and teaching

- Full adherence to PEG-IFN and RBV has been demonstrated to improve SVR rates. Adherence should be assessed at each follow-up, reinforced and encouraged. This becomes increasingly important with the use of DAAs, due to risks of resistance emergence.
- The Psychosocial Readiness Evaluation and Preparation for Hepatitis C Treatment (PREP-C) is a useful tool to provide an initial assessment of a patient's psychosocial readiness to begin HCV treatment. This questionnaire assesses for barriers to adherence, prior to treatment. https://prepc.org

Laboratory monitoring recommendations for patients on HCV treatment: Treatment ends at week 24 for genotypes 2 and 3; tailor to response-guided algorithms for patients on HCV PIs

	Baseline	Week 2	Week 4	Week 8	Week 12	Week 16	Week 20	Week 24 EOT for genotypes 2/3	Week 28	Week 32	Week 36	Week 48 EOT for all genotype 1 patients who do not achieve Ervr and all cirrhotics	24 weeks post -EOT†
CBC with diff	X	X	X	X	X	X	X	X	X	X	X	X	X
Hepatic function panel	X		X		X			X			X	X	X
Basic metabolic panel	X		X		X			X			X	X	X
TSH	X		X		X			X			X	X	X
HCV RNA	X	*	X	X	X			X			X	X	X
Pregnancy test, when applicable	X		X		X			X			X	X	X
Uric acid	X		X		X			X			X	X	X
PT/INR	X				X			X			X	X	

* For patients on HCV PIs, a 2 week HCV RNA may prove helpful to plot response and determine if true failure occurs at week 4

† As mentioned previously, 12 week SVR is now gaining wider acceptance, although current clinical guidelines recommend week 24 SVR assessment

IL28B

- IL28B genotyping may be ordered to assess genetic predisposition to respond to HCV treatment. A region in chromosome 19, the IL28B gene, codes for interferon responsiveness. Having the CC genotype at the SNP rs12979860 of IL28B gene is associated with a two- to threefold increase in SVR rates in genotype 1 patients treated with PEG-IFN and RBV. IL28B genotype has been shown to be the strongest baseline predictor of SVR in studies of patients treated with PEG-IFN and RBV.
- IL28 B has little impact on SVR rates in genotype 2 and 3 patients.
- IL28B geographic distribution may account for the differences seen in SVR between different racial groups.
- In Black people, roughly 20% have been shown to have type CC; in East Asians approximately 80%, while White people and Hispanics fall in between.
- With TVR and BOC, patients with IL28B CC genotype have increased SVR compared with CT and TT genotypes although the difference is not as marked as with PEG-IFN and RBV alone.
- The clinical utility of IL28B testing is unclear. Having a CC result may encourage patients to be treated. A CT or TT genotype, however, is not a reason to deny a patient treatment or discourage them. With new DAAs, all IL28B genotypes will have an excellent chance of response to treatment.

When to hospitalize

- Any sign of hepatic decompensation: coagulopathy, encephalopathy or ascites.
- Severe anemia.
- Severe thrombocytopenia.
- Severe rash.
- Bleeding.
- Severe depression, suicidal ideation or psychosis.
- Severe dyspnea or chest pain.
- Edema.
- Change in mental status.

Table of treatment (Algorithms 6.3 and 6.4)

Treatment	Comment
Conservative treatment • CBC, LFTs and chemistries • Patients with evidence of advanced fibrosis/cirrhosis: screen for HCC every 6 months with CT or MRI with contrast; AFP; EGD for esophageal varices	Recommend for patients with the following contraindications to HCV treatment: • Uncontrolled depression or psychosis • Uncontrolled epilepsy • Uncontrolled autoimmune diseases • Decompensated cirrhosis • Pregnant women, couples unwilling to comply with contraception • Poorly controlled hypertension, heart failure, poorly controlled diabetes, and chronic obstructive pulmonary disease Also use watchful waiting in: • Patients in which the risks outweigh benefits of treatment • Patients with minimal hepatic fibrosis and/or limited life expectancy • Patients who prefer to await not yet approved therapies

Treatment	Comment
Medical current standard of care *For genotype 1:* PEG-IFN-α-2a or PEG-IFN-α-2b plus RBV plus BOC or TVR *For genotypes 2 -6:* PEG-IFN-α-2a or PEG-IFN-α-2b plus RBV	Dosing and clinical pearls: • PEG-IFN-α-2a should be used at a dose of 180 µg once per week, whereas PEG-IFN-α-2b should be used at a weight-based dose of 1.5 µg/kg per week • The RBV dose depends on the HCV genotype. Patients infected with HCV genotypes 1 and 4–6 should receive weight-based dose of RBV. It can be dosed at 1000 mg/day if weight ≤75 kg or 1200 mg/day if weight >75 kg; or 15 mg/kg body weight. However, many experts use weight-based RBV for all genotypes • TVR – dosed at 750 mg by mouth every 8 hours with food containing 20 g of fat. • BOC – dosed at 800 mg by mouth every 7–9 hours with food. Capsules are available in 200 mg; total pill burden is 12 caps daily. Strong inhibitor of CYP3A 4/5. Check prescribing information for complete list of potential drug–drug interactions • Neither BOC nor TVR should be given as monotherapy • If PEG-IFN/RBV is discontinued, PI should also be stopped • In the genotype 2 or 3 patient, RBV dose is 800 mg/day. Patients with genotypes 2 and 3 with baseline factors predictive of poor response (insulin resistance, metabolic syndrome, severe fibrosis or cirrhosis, older age) should receive weight-based RBV. Many experts use weight-based RBV for all genotypes (see tables for sequencing and stop rules in genotype 1)
Complementary therapy • Milk thistle/silymarin decreased transaminases in four small studies. Unclear if this has any clinical significance	• Silymarin trials have been limited by small numbers and often lacked control arms • Silymarin is generally well tolerated, but not recommended during HCV treatment • No clinical trials have investigated the effects of alternative therapies when used in conjunction with PEG-IFN/RBV or the newer HCV PIS • St John's Wort should be avoided in patients on HCV treatment, as it may reduce treatment efficacy
Vitamin supplementation • The 25(OH)D level of all HCV-positive patients should be measured • Prescribe vitamin D3 supplements for patients with 25(OH)D levels below 20–25 ng/mL • The goal of supplementation is to raise the 25(OH)D level into the range of 25–50 ng/ml	• 1000–4000 IU/day of vitamin D3 is recommended • Repeat testing of levels after 3 months to assess the response • Low bone density is highly prevalent in HCV-positive patients • Among HCV-positive patients, vitamin D deficiency is associated with more advanced fibrosis, greater necroinflammation, and poorer response to HCV treatment

Prevention/management of complications

• Anemia – anemia rates increase with regimens containing BOC or TVR. When the hemoglobin falls below 10 g/dL, or if hemoglobin has dropped >3 g from baseline and patient is symptomatic, reduce RBV dose or add erythropoietin. In the case of a precipitous drop, consider both interventions. Hemoglobin should be reassessed every 1–2 weeks thereafter. RBV can be

Algorithm 6.3 HCV treatment

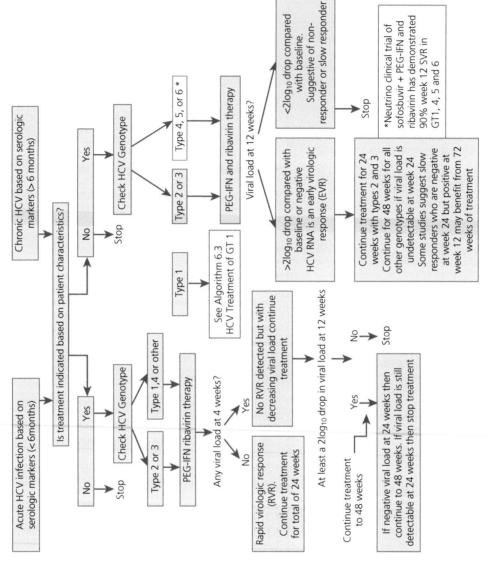

Algorithm 6.4 Management of chronic HCV genotype 2 and 3 with PEG-IFN/RBV

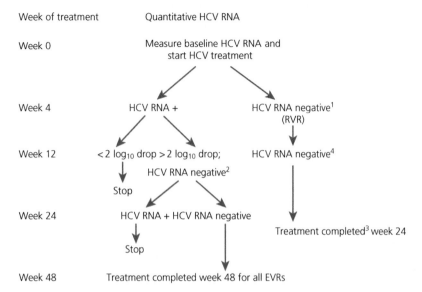

Week of treatment   Quantitative HCV RNA

Week 0   Measure baseline HCV RNA and
                            start HCV treatment

Week 4   HCV RNA +   HCV RNA negative[1]
                                                  (RVR)

Week 12   < 2 log$_{10}$ drop > 2 log$_{10}$ drop;   HCV RNA negative[4]
                            HCV RNA negative[2]

                Stop

Week 24   HCV RNA + HCV RNA negative

                                            Treatment completed[3] week 24
                Stop

Week 48   Treatment completed week 48 for all EVRs

[1] HCV RNA under the limit of detection at week 4 is termed RVR and its positive predictive value for achieving SVR is around 90%.
[2] HCV RNA under the limit of detection at week 12 is termed cEVR.
[3] In RGT may truncate treatment to 12–16 weeks if low HCV RNA and RVR, but is marginally less effective, specifically in genotype 3 with high baseline HCV RNA.
[4] If HCV RNA becomes positive after being RVR, assess adherence, recheck for laboratory error and direct patient according to Week 12 rules as if not RVR achieved.

titrated down until hemoglobin >10. If hemoglobin <8, RBV should be held and transfusion should be considered. RBV dose reduction in studies of TVR and BOC has demonstrated that early RBV dose reduction to ≤600 mg does not negatively impact SVR rates. Hold erythropoietin when hemoglobin >12 g/dL.

- Thrombocytopenia – for platelets <50000/mm^3 PEG-IFN dose should be reduced, and stopped for platelets <25000.
- Neutropenia – severe infections are uncommon from treatment-associated neutropenia. However granulocyte colony-stimulating factor may be used in cirrhotic patients or in patients with absolute neutrophil count <500 mm^3.
- Depression – refer patients to a psychiatrist or psychologist if mood changes, irritability, or anxiety are noted. Support with psychiatric medications may be needed for the duration of therapy. Complaints of severe depression, psychosis, suicidal or homicidal ideation call for prompt psychiatric admission.
- Rash – rashes and pruritus may occur with all currently used treatment combinations in HCV. However, the rates are higher in patients using TVR with PEG/IFN RBV. Use of oral antihistamines, topical steroids and/or systemic corticosteroids can help reduce and resolve most rashes associated with treatment. Less than 1% of patients in TVR trials experienced Stevens–Johnson Syndrome or drug-related eruption with systemic symptoms. BOC use is not associated with increased rash.

- Resistance to DAAs – encouraging optimal adherence prior to and during treatment is key to reducing rates of resistance, as is strict following of PI stopping rules. Of patients who did not obtain SVR with BOC, 53% developed one or more post-baseline treatment emergent protease domain amino acid substitution. Most reduce BOC activity. Two mutations within the viral sequences (T54S and R155K) were the most common substitutions remaining detectable after 2.5 years of follow up in clinical trials. Similar patterns of resistance were apparent in TVR trials, of which 89% disappeared at 2 year follow-up. The long-term clinical impact of these substitutions is unclear.

Section 5: Special Populations
Pregnancy
- HCV treatment should not be offered in pregnancy or to patients trying to conceive, due to the well-established teratogenic effects of RBV or for 6 months after stopping RBV.

Children
- Treatment of HCV-infected children with PEG-IFN and RBV is safe and FDA approved.
- Children aged 2–17 years who are infected with HCV can be considered appropriate candidates for treatment using the same criteria as that used for adults.
- Treat with PEG-IFN-α-2b, 60 μg/m^2 weekly in combination with RBV, 15 mg/kg daily for duration of 48 weeks.

Others
- Patients with CKD and hemodialysis patients: HCV treatment should be considered in all patients with CKD. Persons with CKD stages 1–2 (GFR 60–90 mL/minute), can be treated with PEG-IFN/RBV. For patients with worsening kidney function who are still pre-hemodialysis, in CKD stages 3–5 (GFR <60 mL/minute), data is limited. Cautious use of PEG-IFN can be adjusted to the level of kidney dysfunction. Doses for this group are PEG-IFN-α-2b, 1 μg/kg subcutaneously once weekly PEG-IFN- α-2a, 135 μg subcutaneously once weekly, and RBV, 200–800 mg per day in two divided doses. Start low and increase gradually, according to patient tolerance. Hemodialysis patients should be offered treatment when possible due to difficulties posed by treatment following renal transplant. PEG-IFN monotherapy has generally been recommended, due to RBVs renal clearance. Experienced clinicians may consider RBV 200 mg/day or every other day with close monitoring and support of growth factors, as needed.
- African-Americans: may have baseline neutropenia, which should not preclude treatment. African-Americans have lower SVR rates in clinical trials, across all genotypes, with both dual and triple therapy. They should be offered treatment using the most optimal regimen tolerated in the context of their genotype.
- Cirrhotics: patients with HCV and compensated cirrhosis/ CTP Class A can be successfully treated. Due to higher rate of treatment-related adverse effects of treatment, cirrhotics require close monitoring.
- Decompensated cirrhotics: cirrhotics with ascites, encephalopathy, variceal bleeding, and/or declining hepatic synthetic function should be referred for liver transplant evaluation prior to treatment. Treatment in this group can lead to life-threatening infection or rapid decompensation. PEG-IFN and RBV may be used in reduced doses, ideally in patients already deemed candidates for liver transplant, if closely monitored by experienced providers.

- Active substance users: treatment should be offered to all active substance users who demonstrate motivation to be treated and ability to adhere to treatment plan. Patients who abuse alcohol should not be denied treatment. Intensive counseling prior to and during treatment should be provided to encourage reduction or cessation of substance abuse and increase adherence. Ideally, an interdisciplinary team should manage and guide such patients, including mental health staff and substance abuse specialists.
- Patients with psychiatric disease: a thorough pre-treatment psychiatric evaluation and risk/benefit assessment should be implemented prior to treatment. Patients with psychiatric disease can be treated successfully with close multidisciplinary follow-up and management, and have similar SVR rates to those without pre-existing psychiatric diagnoses.
- Co-infection with HIV or HBV: see Chapter 7.
- Acute HCV: providers can delay treatment for up to 12 weeks after suspected onset of HCV to allow for spontaneous resolution, but should not wait longer to treat. Monotherapy with PEG-IFN is recommended by most expert panels, given that SVR rates of 90% and higher have been demonstrated with the single drug treatment. Addition of RBV should be considered when the diagnosis of acute vs chronic is uncertain, which is quite common, given the difficulties surrounding pinpoint and the actual timing of infection. Length of treatment should be 24 weeks.

Section 6: Prognosis

BOTTOM LINE
- Spontaneous clearance is rare and 80–100% remain HCV RNA positive.
- Many develop cirrhosis within 20 years and most complications of disease manifest at that time.
- Response to treatment varies by genotype with genotypes 2 and 3 having SVR rates of up to 80%.

Natural history of untreated disease
- Spontaneous clearance of HCV is rare and 80–100% remain HCV RNA positive while 60-80% continue to have elevated enzymes.
- Retrospective studies have shown that 17–55% develop cirrhosis within 20 years and most complications of disease manifest at that time.
- One such complication, HCC, develops in up to one-third of cirrhotics.

Prognosis for treated patients
- Predictors of SVR in those who are treated include genotype and pre-treatment viral load. Those with viral loads <400000 have been shown to have better response to treatment.
- Genotypes 2 and 3 have SVR rates of 80% with standard therapy. Genotypes 1 and 4 have less than 50% SVR with standard therapy.
- TVR and BOC are currently in phase III clinical trials. These drugs when combined with PEG-IFN and RBV dramatically increase SVR in patients with genotype 1 (see Table: Overall SVR rates in genotype 1).

Overall SVR rates in genotype 1		
Treatment combination	**Genotype 1 treatment naive**	**Genotype 1 treatment experienced**
PEG IFN/RBV	42–46%*	5–15%*
PEG-IFN/RBV/BOC	67%	59–66%
PEG-IFN/RBV/TVR	75%	51–66%; 88% in prior relapsers

*SVR rates varied amongst trials, populations studied and dosing

Follow-up tests and monitoring

- If in acute HCV infection, the HCV RNA becomes negative, repeating it several times is recommended since occasionally HCV will rise again after becoming negative, a clear indication for treatment. We recommend screening for HCV RNA every 3 months for the first year after obtaining negative serology.
- For those infected chronically, HCV infection is characterized by fluctuating LFTs. For those patients with the presence of anti-HCV but normal AST and ALT, the presence of liver inflammation should be assessed periodically over the course of a one year period laboratory testing.

Section 7: Reading list

Bedossa P, Poynard T. An algorithm for the grading of activity in chronic hepatitis C. The METAVIR Cooperative Study Group. Hepatology 1996;24:289–93

Berzigotti A, Abraldes JG, Tandon P, et al. Ultrasonographic evaluation of liver surface and transient elastography in clinically doubtful cirrhosis. J Hepatol 2010;52:846–53. doi: 10.1016/j.jhep.2009.12.031

Ghany, MG, Nelson DR, Strader, DB, Thomas, DL, Seef, LB. An Update on Treatment of Genotype 1 Chronic Hepatitis C Virus Infection: 2011 Practice Guideline by the American Association for the Study of Liver Diseases. Hepatology 2011;54:1433–44

Ghany MG, Strader DB, Thomas DL, Seeff LB. Diagnosis, management and treatment of Hepatitis C: an update. Hepatology 2009;49:1335–74

Hadziyannis SJ, SetteHJr, Morgan TR, et al. Peginterferon-alpha2a and RBV combination therapy in chronic hepatitis C: a randomized study of treatment duration and RBV dose. Ann Intern Med 2004;140: 346–55

Kwo, P, Lawitz, EJ, McCone, J, et al. HCV SPRINT-1 final results: SVR 24 from a phase 2 study of BOC plus PegIntron (Peginterferon alfa-2b)/RBV in treatment-naïve subjects with genotype 1 chronic Hepatitis C. Presented at the 44th Annual Meeting of the European Association for the Study of the Liver, Copenhagen, Denmark; April 22–26, 2009; abstract #4

Liang TJ, Rehermann B, Seeff LB, Hoofnagle JH. Pathogenesis, natural history, treatment, and prevention of hepatitis C. Ann Intern Med 2000;132:296-305

McHutchison JG, Everson GT, Gordon SC, et al. Telaprevir with peginterferon and RBV for chronic HCV genotype 1 infection. N Engl J Med 2009;360:1827–38

Sandrin L, Fourquet B, Hasquenoph JM, et al. Transient elastography: a new noninvasive method for assessment of hepatic fibrosis. Ultrasound Med Biol 2003;29:1705–13

Simmonds P, Bukh J, Combet C, et al. Consensus proposals for a unified system of nomenclature of hepatitis C virus genotypes. Hepatology 2005;42:962–73

Weiss JJ, Brau N, Stivala A, Swan T, Fishbein D. Review article: adherence to medication for chronic hepatitis C - building on the model of human immunodeficiency virus antiretroviral adherence research. Aliment Pharmacol Ther 2009;30:14–27

Section 8: Guidelines
National society guidelines

Guideline title	Guideline source	Date
Diagnosis, Management, and Treatment of Hepatitis C: An Update	American Association for the Study of Liver Diseases (AASLD) http://www.aasld.org/ practiceguidelines/Documents/Bookmarked%20 Practice%20Guidelines/Diagnosis_of_HEP_C_ Update.Aug%20_09pdf.pdf	April 2009
An Update on Treatment of Genotype 1 Chronic Hepatitis C Virus Infection	American Association for the Study of Liver Diseases (AASLD) http://www.aasld.org/ practiceguidelines/Documents/AASLDUpdateTreatm entGenotype1HCV11113.pdf	2011
American Gastroenterological Association Medical Position Statement on the Management of Hepatitis C	American Gastroenterological Association (AGA) http://www.gastrojournal.org/article/S0016-5085(05)02271-7/fulltext	2006

International society guidelines

Guideline title	Guideline source	Date
Practice Guidelines: Management of Hepatitis C Virus Infection.	European Association for the Study of the Liver (EASL) http://www.easl.eu/assets/application/ files/4a7bd873f9cccbf_file.pdf	2011

Section 9: Evidence

Type of evidence	Title, date	Comment
RCT	TVR with PEG-IFN and RBV for chronic HCV genotype 1 infection, April 2009	TVR-based regimen improved SVR in those with genotype 1.41% vs 67%.
RCT	Efficacy of BOC, an NS3 protease inhibitor, in combination with PEG-IFN-α-2b and RBV in treatment-naive patients with genotype 1 hepatitis C infection (SPRINT-1): an open-label, randomised, multicentre phase 2 trial, August 2010	Addition of BOC to standard treatment regimen in untreated genotype 1 patients after a 4 week lead-in period may increase SVR by 50%
Cross-sectional	The prevalence of hepatitis C virus infection in the United States, 1999 through 2002	Prevalence of HCV positive RNA individuals is increased in the 40–49 age group. Injection drug use is the strongest risk factor for infection

Section 10: Images

Not applicable for this topic.

Additional material for this chapter can be found online at:
www.mountsinaiexpertguides.com
This includes a case study, multiple choice questions, advice for patients and ICD codes

CHAPTER 7

HIV/HCV and HIV/HBV Co-infections

Marie-Louise C. Vachon,[1] Alicia C. Stivala[2] and Douglas T. Dieterich[1]
[1]Division of Liver Diseases, Icahn School of Medicine at Mount Sinai, New York, NY, USA
[2]Division of Infectious Diseases, Icahn School of Medicine at Mount Sinai, New York, NY, USA

OVERALL BOTTOM LINE
- HIV co-infection accelerates both hepatitis C and hepatitis B natural history leading to faster progression to and increased incidence of cirrhosis, HCC and death.
- HIV/HCV co-infected patients have twice the risk of developing cirrhosis and a sixfold increased risk of liver failure compared with those with HCV alone.
- Early diagnosis of viral hepatitis, accurate assessment of liver fibrosis, aggressive approach to hepatitis treatment and regular screening for HCC and EV can be life-saving in this high-risk population.
- HIV-infected individuals should all be tested for antibodies to HAV, HBV and HCV at least at the time of initial HIV diagnosis, and thereafter depending on ongoing risk factors.
- Susceptible individuals should be vaccinated according to the recommended schedule, ideally when CD4+ T-cells are above 200 cells/mm³.
- Outbreaks of HCV among HIV-infected MSM have been reported in Europe, Australia and the USA.
- Treatment of acute HCV is nearly always successful when initiated early.
- Effective treatment of HBV and HCV in HIV co-infected patients increases survival.
- New DAAs have revolutionized the treatment of HCV in HIV-infected patients.

Section 1: Background
Definition of disease
- Chronic hepatitis B and C (chronic viral hepatitis) are defined as persistent infections of the liver lasting for at least 6 months and leading to hepatocellular necrosis and inflammation, with or without associated fibrosis.
- In HIV co-infected patients, chronic viral hepatitis is associated with accelerated liver fibrosis progression compared with HCV-infected patients without HIV.

Disease classification
- Hepatitis B and C can be acute or chronic.
- Acute infection is defined as infection during the first 6 months following exposure.
- Chronic infection is defined as infection persisting more than 6 months after exposure.

Incidence/prevalence
- The estimated prevalence of chronic HCV in HIV-infected individuals is around 25–30% in the USA.

Mount Sinai Expert Guides: Hepatology, First Edition. Edited by Jawad Ahmad, Scott L. Friedman, and Henryk Dancygier.
© 2014 John Wiley & Sons, Ltd. Published 2014 by John Wiley & Sons, Ltd.
Companion website: www.mountsinaiexpertguides.com

- The estimated prevalence of chronic HBV in HIV-infected individuals is around 7–10 % in the USA.
- HCV incidence has been rising in HIV-infected MSM from an estimated range of 5.5–8.1 per 1000 person-years in 1995 to 23.4–51.1 per 1000 person-years in 2007.

Economic impact
- For HCV, in the 10-year period from 2010 to 2019:
  - The direct medical cost of chronic HCV infection is projected to exceed $10.7 billion.
  - The societal cost of premature mortality attributed to HCV infection is projected to be $54.2 billion.
  - The cost of morbidity from disability associated with HCV infection is projected to be $21.3 billion.
- In a model of cost-effectiveness of HCV treatment in a cohort of 35-year-old HIV-co-infected patients with a mean $CD4^+$ T-cell count of 350 cells/μL and moderate HCV, the average discounted quality-adjusted life expectancy was 83.8 months, and lifetime costs were $139,000.
- CDC projects that each one million high-risk adults vaccinated against HBV could save up to $100 million in future direct medical costs by preventing 50 000 new hepatitis B infections, 1000 to 3000 chronic hepatitis B infections, and 150–450 deaths from cirrhosis and liver cancer.

Etiology
- Hepatitis C is caused by HCV, a small, enveloped, positive-sense, single-stranded RNA virus of the family Flaviviridae.
- Following acute HCV, HIV-infected patients have a significantly lower rate of spontaneous clearance compared with HIV-uninfected patients, with 10–15% clearance rate compared with 15–25%.
- Hepatitis B is caused by HBV, a small, enveloped virus of the family Hepadnaviridae. It is a virus with circular, partially double-stranded DNA, with two DNA strands of different lengths.
- Spontaneous clearance of HBV after infection in the adult age group is about 90% and is significantly lower in HIV-infected patients.

Pathology/pathogenesis
- HCV is spread primarily through contact with blood. HCV is not typically transmitted between heterosexual partners in regular relationships after controlling for other risk factors. However, underlying STIs and HIV may increase risk of heterosexual transmission.
- Sexual transmission among MSM is well described and is largely responsible for the acute HCV outbreaks in HIV-infected MSM. The presence of several activities and conditions that disrupt anal mucosal integrity (traumatic sex, sex with visible blood, genital ulcerative diseases, use of sex toys) were frequently noted in instances of assumed sexual transmission.
- HBV is transmitted primarily through sexual contact and contact with blood (IVDU) in countries of low prevalence. Vertical transmission is the main mode of transmission in countries of high prevalence. Chronic HCV results from an inefficient or unsustained HCV-specific $CD4^+$ and $CD8^+$ T-cell responses. HBV and HCV are not cytopathic viruses. Infected hepatocytes trigger host cellular immunologic responses that eventually lead to destruction and clearance of infected hepatocytes. Prolonged liver injury leads to fibrosis. Cirrhosis is the result of continuing liver injury and fibrosis. The risk of developing cirrhosis and complications such as HCC secondary to HCV or HBV is increased in HIV-nfected patients and is associated with low $CD4^+$ T-cell counts.

Predictive/risk factors

Risk factors for fibrosis progression in HIV/HCV co-infected patients
- Age at time of infection.
- Older age.
- Male sex.
- Low CD4$^+$ T-cell count (<200 cells/mm^3).
- Detectable HIV viral load.
- Hepatic steatosis.
- Insulin resistance/diabetes.
- Alcohol abuse.
- Co-infection with HBV.

Risk factors for fibrosis progression in HIV/HBV co-infected patients
- Hepatitis B e antigen (HBeAg) positive.
- Higher HBV DNA levels.
- Older age.
- Elevated ALT levels.
- Alcohol abuse.
- Co-infection with HCV.

Section 2: Prevention

> **CLINICAL PEARLS**
> - The key to prevention of HCV is avoidance of exposure to infected blood and blood products and protected sexual intercourse among MSM.
> - HBV can be prevented by vaccination, vaccination and immunoglobulin administration to babies born from infected mothers, and avoidance of exposure to infected blood and protected sexual intercourse.
> - HBV is 100 times more infectious than HIV and HCV is 10 times more infectious than HIV by direct blood-to-blood contact.

Screening
- Screening for HBV infection is mandatory in all HIV-infected patients because of shared routes of transmission. The presence of HBV infection also influences the decision of when to start ART, what ART to start and future HIV management decisions. Initial testing should include HBsAg, anti-HBs and anti-HBc (Algorithm 7.1).
- Screening for HCV infection is mandatory in all HIV-infected patients at least at the time of initial HIV diagnosis. The updated New York State Guidelines on HCV/HIV-co-infection recommend that HIV-infected patients with continued high-risk behaviors who are seronegative for HCV at baseline receive annual testing thereafter. Many clinicians measure HCV Ab as often as every 3 months in sexually active MSM. Initial testing includes anti-HCV antibody test and HCV RNA in those with positive antibody test. HCV antibody may be negative in the acute phase and HCV RNA may be required for diagnosis.

Primary prevention
- Primary prevention interventions that have led to reductions in HIV incidence have not been as successful in reducing HCV incidence.

Algorithm 7.1 Screening algorithm for HBV in HIV-infected patients: five scenarios

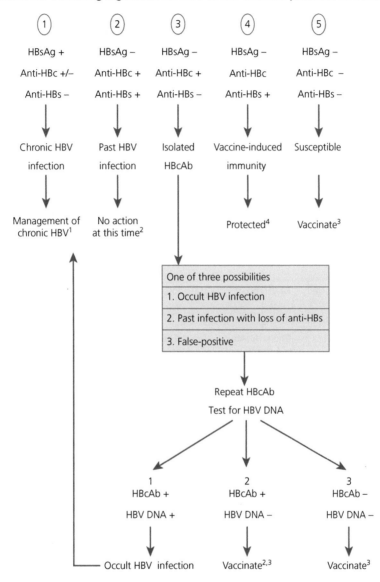

[1] See Algorithm 7.4.
[2] Keep in mind for future treatment decisions if immunosuppression state anticipated.
[3] See Algorithm 7.2.
[4] Follow-up HBsAb is warranted if high-risk behavior or immunosuppression.

- There is observational data for needle exchange programs in reducing prevalence of HCV in IV drug users.
- HBV vaccination of susceptible HIV-infected individuals is recommended (see Algorithm 7.2 – HBV vaccination of HIV-infected patients) as well as vaccination and administration of immunoglobulins to babies born to HIV/HBV-infected mothers who are more likely to vertically transmit HBV than HIV-uninfected mothers.

Algorithm 7.2 HBV vaccination of HIV-infected patients

Test result	HBsAg – HBsAb – HBcAc –	HBsAg – HBsAb +[3] HBcAc +/–	HBsAg – HBsAb – HBcAc +

HBV Status   Susceptible   Seroprotected   Isolated HBcAc

Vaccinate[1]   No vaccine needed[4]   1. HBV DNA
                                          (rule out occult HBV)

Negative   positive

Check HBsAb

titer 1 month post   2. One of two approaches[5]
3rd third dose[2]

Algorithm 7.4

HBsAb +[3]   HBsAb –   1   2

Seroprotected   Re-vaccinate[1]   One dose of vaccine[6]   Vaccinate[1]

Check HBsAb   Check HBsAb   HBsAb
titer 1 month post   titer 2 weeks post   titer 1 month
third dose   dose   post dose[2]

HBsAb +[3]   HBsAb –

Seroprotected   Vaccinate[1]

Check HBsAb
Titer 1 month post
dose[2]

[1] Vaccinate with 20 µg of either of the available anti-HBV vaccines at 0, 1 and 6 months. Some experts recommend using 40 µg.

[2] HIV-infected patients have decreased immune response to HBV vaccine and should have anti-HBs titer checked 1 month following the third dose of vaccine.

[3] HBsAb titer >10 IU/mL.

[4] Be mindful of HBcAb if immunosuppression state is anticipated, then HBV prophylaxis is recommended.

[5] Another approach would be to check for HBeAb. If positive, then no vaccination required.

[6] 20 µg of either available anti-HBV vaccines.

Secondary prevention

- Treatment of both HBV and HCV reduces liver-related complications and increases survival in HIV-infected individuals.
- Patients should be counseled to avoid high-risk behaviors after HCV clearance as re-infection can occur.

Algorithm 7.3 Diagnosis of HBV and HCV in HIV-infected patients

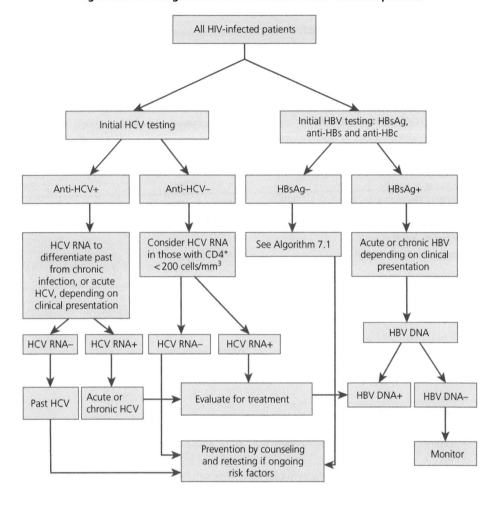

Section 3: Diagnosis (Algorithm 7.3)

BOTTOM LINE
- All HIV-infected patients are at risk for HBV and/or HCV co-infection because of shared routes of transmission.
- The physical examination is usually negative unless the patient has progressed to advanced liver disease.
- ALT and AST are highly elevated during acute HBV and HCV infections. In chronic infections, elevations of ALT above the upper limit of normal (19 IU/L for women and 30 IU/L for men) are frequent, but not universal, and the levels fluctuate.
- Diagnosis of both HBV and HCV in HIV-infected patients is done by the combination of serologic testing and nucleic acid testing (HCV RNA and HBV DNA)
- In HIV-infected patients, staging of fibrosis with liver biopsy is not mandatory to guide treatment decisions in any HCV genotype and should not be a barrier to HCV treatment.

Differential diagnosis

- Viral hepatitis B and C are straightforward to diagnose. They are often first suspected in patients who present with elevated liver enzymes.
- They can also co-exist with other liver diseases, especially non-alcoholic and alcoholic fatty liver disease. Antiretroviral liver toxicity is a diagnosis of exclusion.

Differential diagnosis	Features
Other viral hepatitides (A, B, C, D, E)	Serologic markers or nucleic acid testing
Hepatitis B can flare at time of discontinuation of HBV-active ART or because of HBV resistance	
Antiretroviral liver toxicity (four mechanisms) • Direct drug toxicity • Immune reconstitution (with co-existing HBV and/or HCV) • Hypersensitivity reaction • Mitochondrial toxicity	Temporal relationship with ART initiation, but may present late Diagnosis of exclusion Liver biopsy shows different features depending on mechanism of liver toxicity
Opportunistic liver infection	In AIDS patients with severe immunosuppression (<200 CD4$^+$ T-cells, usually <50 CD4$^+$ T-cells)
NASH	Associated or not with ART
Alcoholic steatohepatitis	History of alcohol abuse Liver biopsy shows centrilobular inflammatory infiltration and Mallory's hyaline
Autoimmune hepatitis	Positive autoimmune serum markers Liver biopsy shows plasma cell infiltration

Typical presentation

- Acute HCV and HBV infections in HIV-infected patients are usually asymptomatic. When symptomatic, patients may present with RUQ pain, nausea and vomiting with or without jaundice.
- Chronic HCV and HBV are usually asymptomatic. They can be associated with fatigue or they can present with symptoms and signs of ESLD including ascites, EV with or without bleeding, jaundice and encephalopathy. HCC may become symptomatic in the later stages.

Clinical diagnosis

History

- History of present illness should include identification of risk factors for transmission of HBV and HCV and potential timing of infection. The patient's symptoms are usually non-specific, the most common being fatigue. Signs and symptoms of extra-hepatic manifestations of HCV, cirrhosis and portal hypertension should be included in the history.

Physical examination

- Look for signs of cirrhosis and portal hypertension. Look at general appearance for anorexia, scleral icterus and temporal atrophy. Look for asterixis.
- Look specifically at the skin for jaundice, upper chest vascular spiders, abdomen vascular collaterals (caput medusa), and palmar erythema, and at the nails for Terry's nails and clubbing.
- Look for hepato/splenomegaly, hardening of the liver, presence of a mass and ascites at abdominal examination.
- Look for gynecomastia and testicular atrophy.

Laboratory diagnosis

List of laboratory tests to diagnose HCV
- HCV antibody (anti-HCV) test.
- HCV RNA.
- HCV genotype if positive HCV RNA.

List of laboratory tests to diagnose HBV
- HBsAg, HBsAb, and HBcAb.
- HBeAg, HBeAb and HBV DNA if HBsAg +.

List of laboratory tests to help assess disease severity
- CBC with differential and platelets.
- Comprehensive metabolic panel including GGT.
- PT/PTT and INR.
- AFP.

List of other laboratory tests useful at initial evaluation
- Anti-HAV.
- Ferritin, iron/TIBC.
- ANA, AMA.
- Ceruloplasmin.
- Thyroid function tests and thyroid antibodies.
- Lipid panel.
- Total insulin.

List of imaging techniques – US, CT or MRI
- The major purpose of imaging is to exclude other causes of liver disease, assess severity of disease, and screen for HCC.
- US – in acute hepatitis, there may be decreased liver echogenicity. In chronic HCV, there is usually increased liver echogenicity. Hepatomegaly and splenomegaly can be demonstrated.
- CT-SCAN and MRI – hepatomegaly and steatosis may be seen.
- Nodular liver may suggest cirrhosis.
- Varices, splenomegaly and ascites suggest portal hypertension.

Liver fibrosis assessment
- Liver biopsy is the gold standard for staging liver fibrosis in the USA. It shows necroinflammation and periportal fibrosis.
- Serologic biomarkers such as APRI and FIB-4 have been evaluated in HIV and can be useful in discriminating advanced fibrosis from no fibrosis, but are less accurate than liver biopsy, especially in the intermediate stages of fibrosis.
- Transient elastography (FibroScan®) is a promising non-invasive technique that has not been approved by the FDA, although it is standard in Europe and Canada.
- Liver biopsy is rarely indicated to evaluate the need for HBV treatment since chronic HBV infection is now an indication to start ART that covers both HIV and HBV, independently of the degree of fibrosis.
- In the rare cases where starting ART is not desirable, liver biopsy, or other methods of liver fibrosis assessment may guide the need to exclusively treat HBV.
- Liver biopsy can be helpful at ruling out other causes of liver diseases in these patients, such as steatosis and steatohepatitis.

Potential pitfalls/common errors in diagnosis

- All HIV-infected individuals should be screened for HCV and HBV at initial diagnosis of HIV and at regular intervals thereafter if they have continued high-risk behavior.
- Patients with positive anti-HCV must have HCV RNA testing performed to distinguish chronic (or acute) infection from cleared infection.
- Patients with negative anti-HCV and immunosuppression (CD4+ T-cell count <200 cells/mm^3) should have quantitative HCV RNA testing performed to rule out chronic HCV.
- Patients with negative anti-HCV and suspicion of acute HCV should have quantitative HCV RNA testing performed. Anti-HCV may become positive as long as 24 weeks after exposure whereas HCV RNA becomes positive within days of infection.
- Those who spontaneously cleared or cleared as a result of HCV treatment will usually remain anti-HCV positive indefinitely, and thus further anti-HCV testing is useless. Quantitative HCV RNA should be used to diagnose re-infection or relapse.
- Occult HBV infection must be ruled out in HIV patients with isolated HBcAb with HBV DNA testing.
- Staging of fibrosis with liver biopsy is not mandatory to diagnose HCV and to guide treatment decisions in any HCV genotype and should not be a barrier to HCV treatment.
- HIV/HCV and HIV/HBV-infected patients are at risk of developing HCC even in the absence of cirrhosis. Regular screening with ultrasound, CT or MRI is essential to make an early diagnosis that offers the possibility of effective treatment.

Section 4: Treatment (Algorithms 7.4, 7.5 and 7.6)

Treatment rationale

- In HIV/HCV co-infected patients, there is every reason to treat HCV of all genotypes including those with compensated (Child's A) cirrhosis. Patients who are willing to start therapy and who do not have contraindications to PEG-IFN and RBV should be encouraged to undergo treatment. SVR reduces liver-related morbidity and mortality in HIV/HCV co-infected patients. The indication for HCV treatment is clear in those with stage 2/4 and above on the METAVIR fibrosis scale. When the liver biopsy indicates fibrosis stage 0 or 1 and the decision is made to not undergo treatment, repeat fibrosis assessment and re-evaluation for treatment is recommended at 3-year intervals.
- At the time this is written, both TVR and BOC, recently approved HCV PI, have not been FDA approved for use in patient with HIV/HCV co-infection. However, available data demonstrate safety and improved SVR rates with the addition of DAAs, and consequently the US Department of Health and Human Services (DHHS) has updated its guidelines to recommend use of DAAs in HIV/HCV co-infection.
- Early on-treatment responses to TVR do not differ between HIV/HCV co-infected and HCV mono-infected patients (Mount Sinai Hospital Data).
- Higher SVR 12 rates were observed in chronic genotype 1 HCV/HIV co-infected patients treated with TVR combination treatment over PEG-IFN/RBV.
- SVR 12 rates increased from 45% with PEG-IFN/RBV to 74% with TVR/PEG-IFN/RBV in a phase II clinical trial.
- TVR exposures were comparable across specific ART regimens.
- In patients treated with TVR combination treatment, overall safety and tolerability profile was comparable to that previously observed in chronic genotype 1 HCV mono-infected patients.

Algorithm 7.4 Treatment algorithm for the management of chronic HBV in HIV-infected patients

1. Educate on risk factors for HBV transmission. Vaccinate susceptible contacts[1]
2. HIV treatment is desirable? Remember HBV co-infection is a reason to treat HIV

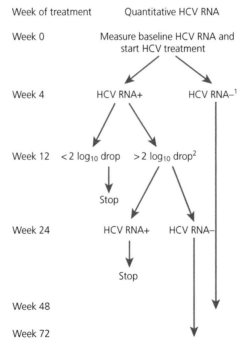

Yes (most cases)　　　　No

Treat both HIV and HBV　　3. Indication for HBV treatment?

Yes　　　　　　No

Treat HBV with drugs that　　Monitor both diseases
do not have activity　　and treat when
against HIV　　indicated

[1] Any susceptible contact base on risk factors for transmission, mostly household members and sexual partner(s).

Algorithm 7.5 Treatment algorithm for the management of chronic HCV genotype 1 and 4 in HIV-infected patients with PEG-IFN and RBV

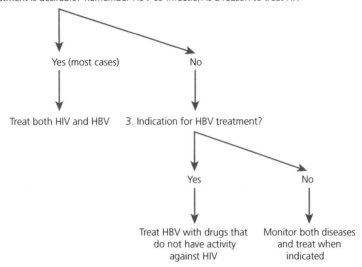

Week of treatment　　　　Quantitative HCV RNA

Week 0　　　　Measure baseline HCV RNA and start HCV treatment

Week 4　　　HCV RNA+　　　HCV RNA−[1]

Week 12　　<2 $\log_{10}$ drop　　>2 $\log_{10}$ drop[2]

Stop

Week 24　　　　HCV RNA+　　HCV RNA−

Stop

Week 48

Week 72

[1] HCV RNA under the limit of detection at week 4 is termed RVR and its positive predictive value for achieving SVR is approximately 90%.
[2] HCV RNA under the limit of detection at week 12 is termed cEVR. >2 $\log_{10}$ drop of HCV RNA at week 12 with HCV RNA that remains above the limit of detection is termed pEVR.

Algorithm 7.6 Treatment algorithm for the management of chronic HCV genotype 2 and 3 in HIV-infected patients

Week of treatment   *Quantitative HCV RNA*

Week 0   Measure baseline HCV RNA and
                          start HCV treatment

Week 4   HCV RNA+   HCV RNA–[1]

Week 12   < 2 $\log_{10}$ drop   > 2 $\log_{10}$ drop[2]

                          Stop

Week 24   HCV RNA+   HCV RNA–

                          Stop

Week 48

> Some evidence suggests that treatment may be discontinued at week 24 in those with low baseline viral load and mild liver fibrosis.

[1] HCV RNA under the limit of detection at week 4 is termed RVR and its positive predictive value for achieving SVR is around 90%.
[2] HCV RNA under the limit of detection at week 12 is termed cEVR. >2 $\log_{10}$ drop of HCV RNA at week 12 with HCV RNA that remains above the limit of detection is termed pEVR.

How to use HCV PI and avoid resistance

- Make sure your patients are taking all three doses of TVR and BOC.
- Don't continue the DAA if futility rules are met!
- Don't re-treat with the same or another protease with the same resistance pattern.
- Not every patient needs to be treated right away.
- Triage, and treat the sicker patients first, but the decompensated cirrhotics should not be treated unless listed for liver transplant first.
- There are other drugs pending approval soon that will be active against PI failures.

Treatment options for HIV/HCV genotype 1 patients: DHHS guidelines

Preliminary recommendations on use of BOC or TVR in HIV/HCV genotype 1 co-infected patients	
Patients not on ART:	Use either BOC or TVR
Patients receiving RAL + 2-NRTI:	Use either BOC or TVR
Patients receiving ATV/r + 2-NRTI:	Use TVR at standard dose. Do not use BOC
Patients receiving EFV + 2-NRTI:	Use TVR at increased dose of 1125 mg every 7–9 hours. Do not use BOC

Patients receiving other ARV regimens

- If HCV disease is minimal (i.e. no or mild portal fibrosis), consider deferring HCV treatment given rapidly evolving HCV drug development.
- If good prognostic factors for HCV treatment response are present – IL28B CC genotype or low HCV RNA level (<400 000 IU/mL) – consider use of PEG-IFN/RBV without HCV NS3/4A PI.
- On the basis of ART history and HIV genotype testing results, if possible, consider switching to the ART regimens in the DHSS guidelines to permit the use of BOC or TVR.
- For patients with complex ART history or resistance to multiple classes of ART, consultation with experts regarding the optimal strategy to minimize the risk of HIV breakthrough may be needed. In such patients, TVR may be the preferred HCV NS3/4A PI because its duration of use (12 weeks) is shorter than that of BOC (24–44 weeks in HIV/HCV co-infection).

- Until more data are available, there is no specific treatment algorithm for the use of HCV PIs in HIV co-infection. A conservative approach would include following early stopping rules described in the TVR and BOC respective package inserts. Treat all co-infected patients for 48 weeks if week 4, 12 and 24 rules for the specific PI are met.
- As new data are available, the guidelines will be updated. Check for updates at http://aidsinfo.nih.gov/guidelines/html/1/adult-and-adolescent-treatment-guidelines/26/hepatitis-c-hcv-hiv-coinfection

Five features of HCV treatment evaluation

1. Identify baseline factors associated with SVR (Table: Favorable baseline predictors of SVR).
2. Evaluate patient's motivation to undergo treatment.
3. Assess liver fibrosis if needed to evaluate treatment urgency.
4. Look for relative/absolute contra-indications to HCV treatment (see Chapter 6).
5. Optimize HIV management prior to starting HCV treatment:
   a. Start antiretroviral therapy (ART) if indicated, paying close attention to ARV drug–drug interactions with HCV DAA to be used. Select from DHHS recommended ARV combinations, whenever possible.
      i. Optimize CD4$^+$ T-cell count, but no minimum count recommended.
      ii. Achieve HIV RNA undetectability.
   b. Avoid zidovudine, didanosine, and stavudine to minimize side effects with HCV treatment. Abacavir may decrease SVR rates compared with tenofovir-containing ART.

Favorable baseline predictors of SVR
HCV genotype 2 or 3   **Low baseline HCV RNA (<400 000–800 000 IU/mL)**
Naïve to HCV treatment   Relapse to prior treatment with PEG-IFN/RBV   White race   IL28B CC genotype   Younger age   Female gender   Low-stage fibrosis   Absence of steatosis/steatohepatitis on liver biopsy   Absence of insulin resistance   Low BMI

- In HIV/HBV co-infected patients, any treatment decision for hepatitis B should take into account the possible impact on HIV and vice-versa. Recent evidence of a benefit for earlier initiation of ART in HIV-infected patients has led to a change in treatment recommendations issued by the DHHS. For HIV/HBV co-infected patients, initiation of ART with active anti-HBV coverage is now recommended at any CD4$^+$ T-cell count to reduce the risk of liver disease progression (Algorithm 7.4). Simultaneous treatment of HBV and HIV reduces the risk of immune reconstitution inflammatory syndrome that can be life-threatening. Likewise, if ART is changed, the new regimen must include active anti-HBV drugs to avoid HBV-related liver flare.
- The goals of HBV treatment are to prevent liver disease progression and reduce potential complications such as HCC development. In the rare cases where HIV treatment is not desirable, the antiviral used should have no anti-HIV activity. Some experts recommend treating HBeAg-positive and HBeAg-negative HBV at any HBV DNA level in all HIV-infected patients due to their accelerated liver disease progression.

When to hospitalize
- Hospitalize if signs of hepatic decompensation such as gastrointestinal bleeding, encephalopathy and coagulopathy.
- During HCV treatment, hospitalize if signs of hepatic decompensation, severe anemia or thrombocytopenia, severe depression, suicidal ideation or psychosis, severe dyspnea, and chest pain.

Managing the hospitalized patient
- Manage hepatic decompensation as in HIV-uninfected patients.
- Do not discontinue ART at admission unless it is indicated per patient's diagnosis.
- Consider infectious disease consultation.
- Hold HCV treatment according to clinical judgment.

Table of treatment

Treatment	Comment
Chronic HCV Conservative treatment Counsel on diet, exercise, avoidance of alcohol and achievement/maintenance of ideal weight • Optimally control HIV with liver-friendly ART • Screen for HCC every 6 months in those with bridging fibrosis and cirrhosis	Conservative treatment is suitable for those with • Absolute contraindications to HCV treatment (see Chapter 6) such as Child's B and C cirrhosis • Low stage fibrosis (stage 0–1) for which risks may outweigh benefits and/or if unwilling to undergo treatment • Prior failure to respond to optimal dosage of standard of care
Chronic HCV – treatment naive Standard of care HCV genotype 1 • PEG-IFN-α-2a 180 µg SC weekly or • PEG-IFN-α-2b 1.5 µg/kg SC weekly plus • TVR 750 mg PO tid with 20 g of fat per dose or BOC 800 mg tid with food	Clinical pearls • Although not demonstrated to be superior in a randomized controlled trial, many experts recommend RBV weight-based dosing for all HCV genotypes in HIV-infected patients • SVR is achieved in 14–38% of HIV/HCV genotype 1- and 4-infected patients with PEG-IFN and RBV

Treatment	Comment
Plus • Weight-based RBV HCV genotypes 4, 5 and 6 • PegIFN-α-2a 180 µg SC weekly or • PegIFN-α-2b 1.5 µg/kg SC weekly plus • Weight-based RBV HCV genotypes 2 and 3 • PegIFN-α-2a 180 µg SC weekly or • PegIFN-α-2b 1.5 µg/kg SC weekly plus 800 mg/day fixed-dose of RBV (divided in two) For 48 weeks for all genotypes	• SVR is achieved in 44–73% of HIV/HCV genotype 2- and 3-infected patients with PEG-IFN and RBV • New DAAs are being tested in HIV/HCV SVR is achieved in 60–74% of HIV/HCV genotype 1-infected patients with the use of BOC or TVR in clinical phase II trials
Chronic HCV – treatment experienced • Re-treatment decisions should be individualized • Same treatment and dosage are indicated for re-treatment • Longer treatment duration (72 weeks) can increase SVR in prior relapsers • DAAs will revolutionize re-treatment in HIV/HCV co-infected patients	• Patients who failed prior treatment are at increased risk of morbidity and mortality from liver disease compared to those who achieved SVR • Those who received a suboptimal treatment in the past or who modified host negative predictive factors of response should be re-treated adequately • Prior relapsers have higher SVR rates than non-responders at re-treatment • Overall, re-treatment leads to SVR in 15–30% of patients with PEG-IFN and RBV
Vitamin supplementation • We recommend measuring 25 (OH)D levels in all HIV/HCV co-infected patients • We recommend supplementing patients with levels below 25 ng/mL with vitamin D3 1000–4000 IU daily	• Among HCV-infected patients, vitamin D deficiency is frequent and has been associated with advanced fibrosis and decreased SVR • The optimal vitamin D3 supplementation regimen has not been determined in a RCT
Acute HCV Standard of care All HCV genotypes • PegIFN-α-2a 180 µg SC weekly or • PegIFN-α-2b 1.5 µg/kg SC weekly plus • Weight-based RBV • For 24 weeks in all genotypes if RVR • If no RVR, consider 48 weeks	• Treatment of HCV in the acute phase increases SVR rates • Following exposure, wait 12 weeks to allow spontaneous clearance to occur and frequently (2–4 weeks) monitor HCV RNA • If HCV viremia persists, treatment should be initiated early • Treatment of acute HCV in HIV-infected patients leads to SVR in up to 90% of patients
Chronic HBV Standard of care • The preferred regimen includes the combination of TDF 300 mg and emtricitabine 200 mg daily or • The combination of TDF 300 mg and lamivudine 300 mg daily	• The recommended ART regimen should include a combination of two anti-HBV-active agents to prevent emergence of resistance in HIV/HBV co-infected patients • Antivirals with activity against both HIV and HBV viruses should be used only when treatment of both diseases is indicated. They include:

(Continued)

Treatment	Comment
	• TDF • Emtricitabine (not FDA-approved for HBV treatment) • Lamivudine • Entecavir (not used to treat HIV but has activity against it and can induce resistance) • The antivirals with activity against HBV only are: • Adefovir 10 mg • Telbivudine 600 mg • Standard IFN-α and PEG-IFN-α.

Prevention/management of complications

- Treatment of HBV and HCV is aimed at reducing the risk of liver-related complications associated with HBV and HCV infection, namely cirrhosis and its complications including HCC.
- Treatment of HCV has led to liver decompensation, especially in those with baseline Child's B or C cirrhosis.
- Mitochondrial toxicity is increased with co-administration of RBV and NRTIs, especially didanosine and stavudine. They should not be used with RBV.

CLINICAL PEARLS

Tips to improve management of HIV/HCV co-infected patients
- Improve the CD4+ T-cell count to as high as possible.
- For acute HCV, diagnose early and treat early.
- Be aware of the effect of fat in the liver on response and treat it.
- Watch for drug–drug interactions: review all medications prior to treatment.
- Maximize dosage of RBV and PEG-IFN.
- Use a PI in combination with PEG-IFN and RBV to treat genotype 1 HCV.
- Growth factors are helpful to maintain maximal doses.
- Use longer treatment periods in HIV.
- Screen for HCC every 6 months in those with bridging fibrosis and cirrhosis.

Tips to improve management of HIV/HBV co-infected patients
- Initiate ART with active anti-HBV coverage at any CD4+ T-cell count.
- When ART is changed, make sure the new regimen covers HBV.
- Treat with a combination of two active anti-HBV antivirals with no overlapping resistance.
- Screen for HCC every 6 months independent of the presence of cirrhosis.
- Follow HBsAg, HBsAb, HBeAg at least yearly and HBV DNA at least three to four times yearly.

Section 5: Special Populations

Pregnancy

- HCV treatment is contraindicated during pregnancy and for 6 months after treatment discontinuation because of the teratogenic effects of RBV.
- Treatment of HBV during pregnancy is not contraindicated and depends on several factors including the mother's indications for ART at the time of pregnancy and the risk of HBV transmission to the fetus.
- Refer to Chapters 5 and 6.

Section 6: Prognosis

> **BOTTOM LINE**
> - Liver-related deaths are now the leading cause of non-AIDS-related deaths in HIV-infected patients.
> - HIV/HCV co-infected patients have twice the risk of developing cirrhosis and a sixfold increased risk of liver failure compared with those with HCV alone.
> - Successful treatment of HCV and HBV in HIV-infected patients reduces liver-related morbidity and mortality.
> - Regular screening for HCC can be life-saving and is mandatory in HIV-infected patients co-infected with HBV and/or HCV.

Natural history of untreated disease
- Spontaneous clearance of HCV is rare with rates of 10–15% in HIV-infected patients compared with 15–25% in HIV-uninfected patients.
- Cirrhosis develops in approximately 20% of patients with chronic HCV mono-infection within 20 years after acute infection and is estimated to double in HIV-infected patients.
- HIV/HCV co-infected patients with compensated cirrhosis have a 3-year survival of 85%. Those with decompensated liver cirrhosis have a 2-year survival of only 50%.

Prognosis for treated patients
- After a mean follow-up of about 2 years, HIV/HCV co-infected patients who achieved SVR were about six times less likely to die of all causes, seven times less likely to die of liver-related causes and 18 times less likely to develop hepatic decompensation compared with those who did not respond to therapy.
- Parameters of ESLD can substantially improve in patients with HIV/HBV-related cirrhosis successfully treated for HBV.

Follow-up tests and monitoring
- HIV/HCV co-infected patients with bridging fibrosis and cirrhosis should undergo HCC screening every 6 months. We recommend the same HCC screening intervals for patients who had cirrhosis at the beginning of HCV treatment and who achieved SVR. The risk of HCC still exists because of the underlying cirrhosis.
- HIV/HBV co-infected patients should undergo HCC screening every 6 months independent of the presence of cirrhosis.
- HIV/HCV and HIV/HBV patients should be seen every 3 months for follow-up at the outpatient clinic.

Section 7: Reading List

Berenguer J, Alvarez-Pellicer J, Martín PM, et al.; GESIDA3603/5607 Study Group. Sustained virological response to interferon plus ribavirin reduces liver-related complications and mortality in patients coinfected with human immunodeficiency virus and hepatitis C virus. Hepatology 2009;50:407–13

Chung RT, Andersen J, Volberding P, et al.; AIDS Clinical Trials Group A5071 Study Team. Peginterferon Alfa-2a plus ribavirin versus interferon alfa-2a plus ribavirin for chronic hepatitis C in HIV-coinfected persons. N Engl J Med 2004;351:451–9

Kuehne FC, Bethe U, Freedberg K, Goldie SJ. Treatment for hepatitis C virus in human immunodeficiency virus-infected patients: clinical benefits and cost-effectiveness. Arch Intern Med 2002;162:2545–56

López-Diéguez M, Montes ML, Pascual-Pareja JF, et al.; GESIDA 37/03-FIPSE 36465/03-NEAT IG5 Study Group. The natural history of liver cirrhosis in HIV-hepatitis C virus-coinfected patients. AIDS 2011;25:899–904

Matthews GV, Cooper DA, Dore GJ. Improvements in parameters of end-stage liver disease in patients with HIV/HBV-related cirrhosis treated with tenofovir. Antivir Ther 2007;12:119–22

Torriani FJ, Rodriguez-Torres M, Rockstroh JK, et al., APRICOT Study Group. Peginterferon Alfa-2a plus ribavirin for chronic hepatitis C virus infection in HIV-nfected patients. N Engl J Med 2004;351:438–50

Vachon ML, Dieterich DT. The HIV/HCV co-infected patient and new treatment options. Clin Liver Dis 2011;15:585–96

Van de Laar TJ, Matthews GV, Prins M, Danta M. Acute hepatitis C in HIV-infected men who have sex with men: an emerging sexually transmitted infection. AIDS 2010;24:1799–812

Van der Helm JJ, Prins M, Del Amo J, et al.; on behalf of the CASCADE Collaboration. The hepatitis C epidemic among HIV-positive MSM: incidence estimates from 1990 to 2007. AIDS 2011;25:1083–91

Wong JB, McQuillan GM, McHutchison JG, Poynard T. Estimating future hepatitis C morbidity, mortality, and costs in the United States. Am J Public Health 2000;90:1562–69

Useful websites

http://www.aidsinfo.nih.gov
http://www.hep-druginteractions.org/
https://prepc.org/

Section 8: Guidelines
National society guidelines

Guideline title	Guideline source	Date
HCV and HIV/HCV An Update of Treatment of Genotype 1 Chronic Hepatitis C Virus Infection	American Association for the Study of Liver Diseases (AASLD) http://www.aasld.org/practiceguidelines/Documents/AASLDUpdateTreatmentGenotype1HCV11113.pdf	2011
Diagnosis, Management, and Treatment of Hepatitis C: An Update	American Association for the Study of Liver Diseases (AASLD) http://www.aasld.org/practiceguidelines/Documents/Bookmarked%20Practice%20Guidelines/Diagnosis_of_HEP_C_Update.Aug%20_09pdf.pdf	2009
Updated New York State Guidelines on HCV/HIV-coinfection	New York State Department of Health AIDS Institute (NYS DOH/AI) http://www.aidsinfo.nih.gov/contentfiles/lvguidelines/glchunk/glchunk_26.pdf	2012
Guidelines for Prevention and Treatment of Opportunistic Infections in HIV-infected Adults and Adolescents	Centers for Disease Control and Prevention (CDC) http://aidsinfo.nih.gov/contentfiles/adult_oi.pdf	2013
HBV A treatment algorithm for the management of chronic hepatitis B virus infection in the United States	American Gastroenterological Association (AGA) http://download.journals.elsevierhealth.com/pdfs/journals/1542-3565/PIIS1542356508008537.pdf	2008
Chronic Hepatitis B: Update	American Association for the Study of Liver Diseases (AASLD) http://www.aasld.org/practiceguidelines/documents/bookmarked%20practice%20guidelines/chronic_hep_b_update_2009%208_24_2009.pdf	2009

Guideline title	Guideline source	Date
Guidelines for the use of antiretroviral agents in HIV-1-infected adults and adolescents	Department of Health and Human Services (DHHS) http://aidsinfo.nih.gov/contentfiles/lvguidelines/adultandadolescentgl.pdf	2013

International society guidelines

Guideline title	Guideline source	Date
Care of patients coinfected with HIV and hepatitis C virus: 2007 updated recommendations from the HCV-HIV international panel	HCV-HIV international panel http://ovidsp.tx.ovid.com/sp-3.10.0b/ovidweb.cgi?&S=MEJDFPMAOCDDBKMMNCNKOAOBEKMLAA00&Link+Set=S.sh.22.23.27.37%7c1%7csl_10	2007
Acute hepatitis C in HIV-infected individuals: recommendations from the European AIDS Treatment Network (NEAT) consensus conference	European AIDS Treatment Network (NEAT) http://ovidsp.tx.ovid.com/sp-3.10.0b/ovidweb.cgi?&S=MEJDFPMAOCDDBKMMNCNKOAOBEKMLAA00&Link+Set=S.sh.22.23.27.47%7c1%7csl_10	2011

Section 9: Evidence

See Guidelines listed in Section 8.

Section 10: Images

Not applicable for this topic.

Additional material for this chapter can be found online at:
www.mountsinaiexpertguides.com
This includes a case study, multiple choice questions, advice for patients and ICD codes

CHAPTER 8

Hepatic Abscess

Lawrence U. Liu

Division of Liver Diseases, Icahn School of Medicine at Mount Sinai, New York, NY, USA

AMEBIC LIVER ABSCESS

> **OVERALL BOTTOM LINE**
> - ALA is the most common manifestation of extraintestinal amebiasis.
> - Untreated amebic liver abscesses are not likely to resolve spontaneously, and will require specific treatment. Post-treatment prognosis is excellent.
> - Treatment is twofold and directed against both *Entamoeba histolytica* trophozoites and cysts to prevent infection relapses.
> - Abscess drainage is warranted when antimicrobial therapy is insufficient.

Section 1: Background
Definition of disease
- ALA is the most common manifestation of extraintestinal amebiasis.

Incidence/prevalence
- Amebic infection is estimated to be present in up to 50% of the tropical and subtropical population (e.g. Southeast Asia, India, Egypt, South Africa). Hepatic involvement, in the form of ALA, is noted in up to 1% of those with amebic infection.
- It is more common in men than in women (ratio of 10:1). The age group most commonly affected are those in the fourth and fifth decades of life.

Etiology
- Amebic infection can be caused by two protozoans, notably *E. histolytica* and *E. dispar*. However, hepatic amebiasis is caused solely by *E. histolytica* due to its invasive/pathogenic capacity.

Pathology/pathogenesis
- Ingestion of the *Entamoeba* cyst from fecally-contaminated food or water results in excystation and subsequent trophozoite formation. Through pathways that remain incompletely understood (and which may include genetic and immune mechanisms), the trophozoite can invade the intestinal mucosa and submucosa and thereby enter the superior mesenteric vein and portal venous system. Due to its increased portal venous drainage, the right hepatic lobe is more commonly the site of amebic abscess formation. The trophozoites cause areas of focal

Mount Sinai Expert Guides: Hepatology, First Edition. Edited by Jawad Ahmad, Scott L. Friedman, and Henryk Dancygier.
© 2014 John Wiley & Sons, Ltd. Published 2014 by John Wiley & Sons, Ltd.
Companion website: www.mountsinaiexpertguides.com

hepatic necrosis with continued amebic lysis of neutrophils at the edge of the lesion releasing mediators that then lead to hepatocyte death and further damage to distant hepatocytes. An increasing number of small necrotic lesions then coalesce to form a larger hepatic abscess.
- Complications from amebic liver abscess are curable but are at times life-threatening. Rupture of the abscess can occur in cephalad and caudad directions. Upward spread of infection can involve the diaphragm and thoracic cavity resulting in inflammation of the diaphragm, pleura, lungs and pericardium. Other thoracic complications include the formation of lung abscess and fistula (broncho-pleuro-hepatic type), and pericardial pathology such as pericarditis and cardiac tamponade. Downward extension of the abscess can result in peritonitis – which is the second most common complication of ALA, after pleuropulmonary disease.
- Left hepatic ALA, although much less common than right hepatic lesions, tend to be more life-threatening due to the development of multiple lesions and their closer proximity to the heart. These lesions are more likely to require invasive treatment strategies (e.g. aspiration, catheter drainage, surgery) – in addition to pharmacologic agents – compared with right hepatic abscesses.
- Culture of the lesion's material tends to be negative since the abscess is almost always sterile; however, collection at the abscess' edge can demonstrate the *Entamoeba* trophozoites.

Predictive/risk factors
- Risk factors for acquiring amebic infection include population overcrowding, poor hygiene and sanitation, and probably genetic and immune factors. Due to the protozoa life cycle, *Entamoeba* cysts are excreted in stool and thus transmitted to another human vector through the ingestion of fecally-contaminated food and water. Successful eradication of the infection in a person does not decrease the risk of another infection (i.e. the absence of immunologic protection) if the same risk factors remain present.
- Since the incidence of intestinal amebiasis does not demonstrate a sex predominance, male sex predisposes to ALA although the mechanism remains unclear.

Section 2: Prevention

CLINICAL PEARLS
- Prevention of overcrowding.
- Provision of adequate sanitation.
- Continued public health education.
- Proper diagnosis and prompt treatment of primary infection to prevent complications (e.g. extraintestinal amebiasis).

Screening
- Screening for amebic liver abscess is not practical since only up to 1% of people with amebic infections develop this complication. However, prompt diagnosis and treatment of amebic infection will significantly decrease the risk of ALA development.

Primary prevention
- Prevention of overcrowding.
- Provision of adequate sanitation.
- Continued public health education.

Secondary prevention
- Proper diagnosis and prompt treatment of primary infection to prevent extraintestinal complications (e.g. amebic liver abscess formation).

Section 3: Diagnosis

CLINICAL PEARLS
- Patients with ALA typically present with fever and RUQ pain. A prior history of a diarrheal illness is not always present although presentation is typically within 3–4 months of travel to an endemic area.
- Up to half of all patients have tender hepatomegaly on examination.
- All types of abdominal imaging demonstrate ALA.
- Serological testing of *E. histolytica* antibodies or antigens can be helpful in confirming the diagnosis.
- Aspiration of ALA can be done for therapeutic purposes but is usually not required for a diagnosis.

Differential diagnosis

Differential diagnosis	Features
Pyogenic liver abscess	Recent biliary disease and/or surgery
	Diabetes mellitus
	Positive culture growth in aspirate and/or blood
	Absent *E. histolytica* serology
	US may show multiple lesions and irregular (ill-defined) abscess wall
Echinococcal/hydatid cyst	More likely to be asymptomatic lesions
	Eosinophilia
	Imaging may demonstrate cyst calcification and/or presence of daughter cysts
	Note: secondary bacterial infection may occur

Typical presentation
- Patients with amebic liver abscess rarely recall having or have a recent history of gastrointestinal symptoms (e.g. abdominal pain, tenesmus, bloody diarrhea) despite requiring the prerequisite amebic infection – hence decreasing the success rate of ALA screening, if this is ever pursued.
- Travel to an endemic area is typically within the preceding 3–4 months but can be much longer in some cases.
- Signs/symptoms of ALA are generally of acute onset; these usually consist of fever, pain, and hepatomegaly.

Clinical diagnosis
History
- A patient is more likely to be suspected of having amebic liver abscess if living in or having recently resided in an endemic area.
  - Fever is commonly of a high temperature, continuous or intermittent, and accompanied by chills and significant sweating. The patient may also have non-specific constitutional symptoms such as malaise, anorexia, and weight loss.

Physical examination

- Physical examination can demonstrate the presence of fever, abdominal pain and an enlarged liver. Other constitutional signs and symptoms (e.g. malaise, nausea, weight loss) may be present. Dyspnea may be noted due to diaphragmatic compression from the enlarging abscess. The patient often finds symptomatic relief when turning to the opposite side of the lesion while lying supine.
  - The site of abdominal pain tends to correspond with the abscess location. With right hepatic lesions, pain is described in the right abdomen and may radiate to the right shoulder and the right back region. Pain from left hepatic lesions will be located in the epigastrium and left abdomen, and can radiate to the left back and scapula.
  - The degree of hepatomegaly varies with the side and site of the abscess. Large lesions may be palpated. Patients may note breathing difficulty due to diaphragmatic compression of the enlarging abscess.
- Jaundice is not a typical feature; if present, it corresponds to biliary pathology and may predict a worse prognosis.

Useful clinical decision rules and calculators

- A patient is more likely to be suspected of having amebic liver abscess if living in or having recently resided at an endemic area.
- Microbial and imaging studies have a higher diagnostic yield when compared with basic studies such as a CBC and biochemical tests.

Disease severity classification

- Disease severity is higher among these scenarios:
  - Left hepatic abscesses.
  - Jaundice and other signs of biliary disease.
  - Persistent symptoms (e.g. fever, abdominal pain) despite receiving adequate and appropriate antimicrobial treatment.
  - Large right hepatic abscess – which increases the risk of rupture.
  - Pulmonary complications from ALA.

Laboratory diagnosis
List of diagnostic tests

- Demonstration of *E. histolytica* cysts and/or trophozoites in the feces strengthens the suspicion for ALA. However, it should be noted that it may be difficult to distinguish *E. histolytica* from *E. dispar* (a non-invasive and non-pathogenic agent) from stool samples. Furthermore, up to 70% of patients with ALA will not have detectable *E. histolytica* in the stool.
- Due to the low yield of fecal sample testing, serologic tests have become a valuable tool for making a diagnosis. These tests detect specific circulating antibodies against *E. histolytica* and can therefore distinguish it from *E. dispar* and agents causing pyogenic abscesses.
  - Examples of these serologic tests include IHA, antigen-based ELISA kits specific for *E. histolytica*, and PCR testing. Unfortunately, these tests, although highly sensitive when compared with other tests, are not widely available due to their high cost and complicated process.
- A CBC is non-specific and may demonstrate mild–moderate leukocytosis and mild anemia that may be normochromic.
- Liver chemistries also yield non-specific findings.

List of imaging techniques
- A chest X-ray can demonstrate elevation of the right/left hemidiaphragm (depending on the location of the abscess), if present.
- Abdomen US is the most widely-used initial imaging study due to its easier access and lower cost. The amebic liver abscess is most commonly seen as round/oval, hypoechoic, and having well-defined margins. Abdominal CT scans have greater sensitivity and better resolution in detecting ALA, especially the smaller lesions and are thus useful for making an early diagnosis; lesions characteristically appear as a round shape with low density and well-defined margins.

Potential pitfalls/common errors made regarding diagnosis of disease
- The diagnosis of ALA can be missed since it can take up to 7 days for anti-amebic antibodies to become detectable. Although the antibody does not distinguish past from current infection, its specificity becomes more significant when the patient comes from a non-endemic area.
- With increasing global travel, precautions while traveling through endemic areas for amebiasis may be overlooked and thereby increasing the person's risk for acquiring this infection. A pertinent travel history also needs to be included when interviewing a patient, even if it appears to be unrelated to the person's symptoms.

Section 4: Treatment
Treatment rationale
- Uncomplicated amebic liver abscess is treated in a twofold manner. The first step involves trophozoite eradication utilizing a nitroimidazole derivative (metronidazole, tinidazole or secnidazole); these agents are given through the oral route.
- Among these agents, metronidazole is the oldest and most studied. Due to its excellent bioavailability as an oral agent, favorable pharmacokinetics and widespread distribution in the intestine and other tissues, it is the drug of choice for treating amebic liver abscess and invasive intestinal amebiasis.
  - Metronidazole is given at an oral dose regimen of 750 mg three times daily for 7–10 days.
  - Critically-ill patients, and those with large and/or multiple abscesses are given the agent intravenously at 500 mg every 8 hours for 5–10 days.
- In the absence of complications, cure rate with metronidazole therapy alone has been reported in more than 90% of cases; clinical improvement is noted after 3–4 days of treatment. Upon completion of treatment, the hepatic abscesses may take up to 3–12 months to heal and is monitored through imaging studies (e.g. US).
- Caveats for metronidazole therapy are noted as follows:
  - Common adverse effects include nausea and abdominal pain. A particular side-effect is a metallic taste sensation.
  - Metronidazole is found in breast milk.
  - Metronidazole has disulfiram-like properties; hence, alcohol ingestion during use of this agent must be avoided.
- Both tinidazole and secnidazole are relatively newer agents; although they have been found to be effective against intestinal amebiasis, they are not yet recommended for the treatment of ALA.
- Chloroquine is also effective against amebic liver abscess although it has no activity against intestinal disease. It has excellent tissue distribution and has high concentrations in the hepatic parenchyma. It is still not recommended as the primary treatment of ALA, and serves as adjunct

therapy to metronidazole for those with large and multiple abscesses and those with poor response to metronidazole monotherapy.
  • The chloroquine dose regimen against ALA is 300 mg every 12 hours followed by 300 mg once daily for 21 days.
• Since the nitroimidazole derivatives remain only in the intestine for a short period, infection relapses may occur. Similar to the treatment of intestinal amebiasis, further therapy with a luminal amebicidal agent – to eradicate *Entamoeba* cysts – is required after trophozoite eradication.
  • Paramomycin is given at a dose regimen of 30 mg/kg/day three times daily for 7 days. Its major adverse effects are abdominal pain, nausea/vomiting, and headache.
  • The second-line agent, diloxanide furoate, is given as 500 mg three times daily for 10 days. Its adverse effects include abdominal discomfort, flatulence and nausea.
  • In countries where it is available, etofamide is given as 500 mg three times daily for 3 days; adverse effects are abdominal discomfort, nausea/vomiting and dizziness.

When to hospitalize
• The decision to hospitalize patients for further management of amebic liver abscess can include:
  • Inability to tolerate oral therapy.
  • Need for supportive treatment, e.g. intravenous hydration.
  • Worsening of clinical symptoms, e.g. enlarging abscess, development of multiple lesions, spread to contiguous structures.
  • Development of complications, e.g. cardiopulmonary disease, peritonitis.

Managing the hospitalized patient
• Depending on the clinical scenario, further management of the hospitalized patient can include:
  • Intravenous hydration.
  • Enteral feeding.
  • Intravenous antibiotics using metronidazole and/or broad-spectrum agents. *E. coli* and *Klebsiella* are most commonly found to cause secondary bacterial infections.
  • Abscess drainage.
• Abscess drainage can be performed using either aspiration or catheter placement.
• Drainage is indicated in:
  • Lack of clinical improvement despite receiving adequate antimicrobial therapy for 48–72 hours.
  • Large right lobe abscess at risk of rupture (e.g. <10 mm rim of liver tissue surrounding the abscess).
  • Left lobe abscesses (due to the increased risk of being multiple, and more proximal to the pericardial space).
  • Pregnant patients for whom metronidazole is a contraindication.
  • Abscesses with contiguous spread and complications.
• Studies have not reported a distinct advantage of using either aspiration or catheter placement in the treatment of complicated ALA.
• Open surgical drainage is rarely indicated and the mortality rate is very high, largely contributed by the degree of clinical decompensation and exhaustion of less invasive methods by the time of its consideration.

Table of treatment

Treatment	Comment
Conservative treatment	Not applicable; all amebic liver abscesses must be treated promptly
Medical	Twofold treatment (discussed in "Treatment rationale")
Surgical	Rarely indicated; mortality rate is very high
Radiological	Use of imaging studies (e.g. US, CT scan) is warranted for localization if abscess drainage is performed
Psychological	Generally not applicable
Complementary	Supportive treatment (e.g. management of dehydration and inadequate oral intake) may be necessary

Prevention/management of complications
See "Treatment rationale."

> **CLINICAL PEARLS**
> - Untreated amebic liver abscesses are unlikely to resolve spontaneously, and will require specific treatment. Post-treatment prognosis is excellent.
> - Treatment is twofold and directed against both *E. histolytica* trophozoites and cysts to prevent infection relapses.
> - Abscess drainage is warranted when antimicrobial therapy is insufficient.

Section 5: Special Populations
Pregnancy
- Abscess drainage may be considered earlier in this population due to contraindication of metronidazole therapy.

Children
- Similar treatment strategies are offered to children as outlined in "Treatment rationale." However, the pharmacologic agents will need to be dosed according to the pediatric patient's body weight.
  - Metronidazole 50 mg/kg/day (in three doses) for 10 days.
  - Paramomycin 25 mg/kg/day (in three doses) for 7 days.
  - Diloxanide furoate 20 mg/kg/day (in three doses) for 10 days.
  - Etofamide 200 mg three times daily for 3 days.

Elderly
- Although elderly patients remain eligible for the same management strategy of ALA, they need to be monitored more closely due to their risk for poor tolerance of disease and treatment complications.

Section 6: Prognosis

> **CLINICAL PEARLS**
> - Untreated amebic liver abscesses are not likely to resolve spontaneously, and will require specific treatment. Post-treatment prognosis is excellent when treatment against both *E. histolytica* trophozoites and cysts are given.
> - Abscess drainage is warranted when antimicrobial therapy is insufficient.

Natural history of untreated disease
- Untreated amebic liver abscesses are not likely to resolve spontaneously, and will require specific treatment.

Prognosis for treated patients
- Prognosis during and after treatment of ALA is excellent. Metronidazole therapy results in more than a 90% cure rate. An increased chance of therapy success can occur if subsequent cyst eradication is performed and post-therapy monitoring with imaging studies is conducted.

Follow-up tests and monitoring
- Cyst eradication with paromomycin, diloxanide furoate or etofamide.
- Post-treatment abscess monitoring with imaging study (e.g. US).
- Abscess drainage (see "Managing the hospitalized patient") may be required.

Section 7: Reading List

Akgun Y, Tacyildiz IH, Celik Y. Amebic liver abscess: changing trends over 20 years. World J Surg 1999;23:102–6

Ayeh Kumi PF, Petri WA Jr. Diagnosis and management of amebiasis. Infect Med 2002;19:375–85

Jha AK, Das G, Maitra S, Sengupta TK, Sen S. Management of large amoebic liver abscess – a comparative study of needle aspiration and catheter drainage. J Indian Med Assoc 2012;110:13–15

Khanna S, Chaudhary D, Kumar A, Vij JC. Experience with aspiration in cases of amebic liver abscess in an endemic area. Eur J Clin Microbiol Infect Dis 2005;24:428–30

Salles JM, Moraes LA, Salles MJ. Hepatic amebiasis. Braz J Infect Dis 2003;7:96–110

Singh O, Gupta S, Moses S, Jain DK. Comparative study of catheter drainage and needle aspiration in management of large liver abscesses. Indian J Gastroenterol 2009;28:88–92

Section 8: Guidelines

Not applicable for this topic.

Section 9: Evidence

- Due to the need to treat all patients with amebic liver abscess, there are no RCTs for this population.

Section 10: Images

Not applicable for this topic.

PYOGENIC LIVER ABSCESS

> **OVERALL BOTTOM LINE**
> - Biliary tract disease is currently the most common cause for pyogenic liver abscess.
> - Pyogenic liver abscess is uniformly fatal when untreated.
> - Treated patients have a mortality rate ranging from <5 to 30%.
> - Treatment strategy includes the use of antibiotics with/without abscess drainage.

Section 1: Background
Definition of disease
- Pyogenic liver abscess is a purulent collection caused by bacteria. Biliary tract disease is now the most common cause for its development.

Incidence/prevalence
- In contrast to amebic liver abscess, pyogenic abscesses make up nearly 80% of all liver abscesses in the developed countries. However, it remains a rare condition, with a reported incidence of 0.5–0.8% in the western world and a frequency of 20 per 100 000 hospitalizations.

Etiology
- Bacterial infections are the cause of pyogenic liver abscesses; these include *Escherichia coli* and *Klebsiella pneumoniae* (currently the most common cause in Asia).
- Biliary tract disease has replaced acute appendicitis as the most common source for abscess development; examples are cholelithiasis, choledocholithiasis, tumors, strictures, congenital biliary tree anomalies, and biliary tree instrumentation. Due to improvement of conditions, other common causes of pyogenic liver abscesses such as diverticulitis, pylephlebitis, and other intra-abdominal infections have decreased in their incidence.

Pathology/pathogenesis
- Biliary tract obstruction can result in bile stasis and bacterial proliferation, which then cause seeding and abscess formation in the liver.
- Another mechanism for the development of pyogenic liver abscess is septic embolization from an intra-abdominal infection.

Predictive/risk factors
- Diabetes mellitus is a known risk factor for the development of pyogenic liver abscess and may be related to the person's decreased immune system.
- Older age (i.e. >65 years) may be related with atypical presentations.
- Reports of increased biliary and colon cancer incidence have been seen in those with pyogenic liver abscess.

Section 2: Prevention

> **CLINICAL PEARLS**
> - Treatment of intra-abdominal infections.
> - Management of biliary tract disease.
> - Adequate control of diabetes mellitus.

Screening
- Similar to amebic liver abscess, screening for pyogenic liver abscess is not practical – in the absence of strong and specific risk factors – due to its rare incidence. However, this condition should be strongly considered in patients with biliary disease and/or intra-abdominal infections who do not demonstrate clinical improvement with adequate therapy.

Primary prevention
- Treatment of intra-abdominal infections.
- Management of biliary tract disease.
- Adequate control of diabetes mellitus.

Secondary prevention
- Prompt treatment of biliary disease and/or primary intra-abdominal infection can prevent or decrease the development of pyogenic liver abscess.

Section 3: Diagnosis

CLINICAL PEARLS
- Patients with pyogenic liver abscess typically present with fever and RUQ pain.
- Up to half of all patients have findings on examination including hepatomegaly, RUQ tenderness and occasionally jaundice.
- Blood cultures are positive in up to half of cases.
- All types of abdominal imaging demonstrate pyogenic liver abscess.
- Aspiration of abscess material should be tested for Gram stain and culture.

Differential diagnosis

Differential diagnosis	Features
Amebic liver abscess	Residence or recent stay/travel in endemic areas for amebiasis
	E. histolytica trophozoites/cysts in feces (present only in <30% of patients)
	Demonstration of abscess in imaging studies
	Serologic tests (e.g. IHA, ELISA, PCR)
Echinococcal/hydatid cyst	More likely to be asymptomatic lesions
	Eosinophilia
	Imaging may demonstrate cyst calcification and/or presence of daughter cysts
	Note: secondary bacterial infection may occur

Typical presentation
- Signs/symptoms of pyogenic liver abscess are non-specific and do not differ greatly from other hepatobiliary infections. Most patients will present with acute symptoms which can include fever/chills, nausea/vomiting, anorexia and weight loss, malaise, and RUQ pain. Older patients (those older than 65 years of age) can also present with respiratory symptoms that may be a manifestation of sepsis.

Clinical diagnosis
History
- The most common complaint in the history is fever. Non-specific gastrointestinal symptoms are common.
- A suspicion for the development of pyogenic liver abscess is raised when there is a lack of or inadequate clinical improvement – with adequate treatment – in patients with biliary tract disease and/or intra-abdominal infection.

Physical examination
- Physical examination can demonstrate the presence of fever, chills, weight loss, malaise and RUQ pain. Features of sepsis such as tachycardia, hypotension and tachypnea may be present.
- Jaundice is not a typical presentation although it may be noted by the clinician.

Useful clinical decision rules and calculators
- Similar to amebic liver abscess, imaging and microbial studies have a higher diagnostic yield when compared with basic studies such as a CBC and biochemical tests.

Disease severity classification
- Untreated pyogenic liver abscess is fatal due to complications from sepsis. With adequate therapy, the current mortality rates are lower but range from <5 to 30%.

Laboratory diagnosis
List of diagnostic tests
- A CBC can demonstrate leukocytosis and nomochromic normocytic anemia. Liver chemistries generally yield non-specific findings although an elevated alkaline phosphatase level can be seen in nearly 90% of cases.
- Cultures from blood and/or the hepatic collection can be positive; common micro-organisms include *E. coli*, *Klebsiella pneumoniae* and Gram-positive bacteria but culture growth can also be polymicrobial.

List of imaging techniques
- Common imaging studies used to evaluate pyogenic liver abscess include US and CT scan.
- US is less costly and more easily available. However, the appearance of pyogenic liver abscess using this modality can differ according to its stage. In the initial phase, the abscess may appear hyperechoic and non-distinct. With disease progression and abscess growth, the lesion becomes hyperechoic with a distinct margin.
- Abdomen contrast CT scan is more accurate than US. Peripheral enhancement of the abscess wall is generally diagnostic; CT scan may also demonstrate the cause of the abscess formation in ~70% of cases.
- Abdomen MRI generally does not provide an advantage over CT scan but it can provide better imaging of the biliary system – which can be important in determining the abscess source.

Potential pitfalls/common errors made regarding diagnosis of disease
- Patients suffering from biliary tract disease and/or intra-abdominal infection, who fail to make adequate clinical improvement, should be investigated thoroughly due to the high mortality rate of untreated pyogenic liver abscess.

Section 4: Treatment
Treatment rationale
- Treatment strategies of pyogenic liver abscess include the use of broad-spectrum antibiotics and possible abscess drainage.
- Parenteral antibiotics are given for 2–3 weeks, or until there is a significant clinical response. Broad-spectrum antibiotics (covering abdominal flora and Gram-positive bacteria) are initially used while awaiting culture identification and susceptibility studies. These agents are then converted to oral formulation and given for another 2–4 weeks, or until complete abscess resolution is confirmed with further studies.
- The use of antibiotic therapy alone may not be enough to treat the liver abscess successfully unless it is small (i.e. less than 3 cm). The additional therapy of routine drainage of abscesses measuring more than 3 cm is recommended.
- The performance of abscess aspiration instead of drainage catheter insertion has been shown to have higher failure rates and a longer average time to achieve a 50% size reduction.

When to hospitalize
- Initial treatment of pyogenic liver abscess is performed as an in-patient (with the use of parenteral antibiotics and possible abscess drainage) due to the high mortality rates associated with this diagnosis.
- Further hospitalization is required for patients with slow or absent clinical improvement.

Managing the hospitalized patient
- The patient is closely monitored during the initial treatment phase to help determine if more aggressive strategies (e.g. catheter drainage, abscess aspiration, surgery) is required.
- Certain negative predictive factors have been noted with percutaneous drainage:
  - Presence of gas in the abscess.
  - Abscess size greater than 7.3 cm.
  - Short length to the liver capsule of <0.25 cm.
- Surgical intervention may be required if the patient does not respond adequately to antibiotics and percutaneous abscess drainage. The morbidity rates are comparable for both surgery and percutaneous drainage, with the surgical approach requiring less secondary procedures.
- Indications for surgery can include:
  - Absence of clinical improvement after 4–7 days of catheter drainage.
  - Presence of multiple, large or loculated abscess.
  - Thick-walled abscess with viscous pus that cannot be drained adequately.
  - Other intra-abdominal surgical pathology present.

Table of treatment

Treatment	Comment
Conservative treatment	Not applicable; pyogenic liver abscess must be treated promptly
Medical	Broad-spectrum antibiotics initially while awaiting culture results; these are given parenterally for 2–3 weeks. Conversion to oral agent is performed when there is clinical improvement, and is given for 2–4 more weeks

(Continued)

Treatment	Comment
Surgical	Percutaneous drainage (catheter drainage has an advantage over abscess aspiration) if there is no significant clinical response with antibiotic therapy alone
	Surgical intervention may be required if percutaneous drainage is not sufficient treatment
Radiological	The use of US, CT scan, or MRI is performed for making the initial diagnosis, and for monitoring the patient's clinical status and confirmation of abscess resolution
Psychological	Generally not applicable
Complementary	Supportive treatment (e.g. intravenous fluids, analgesia) may be required during the initial treatment phase

Prevention/management of complications
See "Treatment rationale."

> **CLINICAL PEARLS**
> - All patients with pyogenic liver abscess need to be treated promptly due to its high mortality rate.
> - Treatment involves the use of antibiotics with/without abscess drainage.
> - Surgical management may be necessary when there is lack of clinical improvement despite adequate antibiotic therapy and percutaneous abscess drainage.

Section 5: Special Populations
Pregnancy
- There are no special treatment strategies for pregnant patients with pyogenic liver abscess. The choice of antibiotic agent will need to be determined in terms of teratogenicity risk. Abscess drainage may become difficult if the uterus size causes significant organ displacement; surgical drainage may become a contraindication due to the need for general anesthesia and the possible risk to the fetus.

Children
- Similar treatment strategies are offered to children as outlined in "Treatment rationale." The pharmacologic agent(s) will need to be dosed according to the pediatric patient's body weight.

Elderly
- Elderly patients may present with atypical symptoms (e.g. respiratory compromise) and will require even closer monitoring; this population may also be less likely to tolerate surgical management of the abscess.

Section 6: Prognosis

> **CLINICAL PEARLS**
> - Untreated pyogenic liver abscess is fatal due to complications from sepsis. With adequate therapy, the current mortality rates are lower but range from <5–30%.

Natural history of untreated disease
• Pyogenic liver abscess is uniformly fatal if left untreated.

Prognosis for treated patients
• The disease will generally resolve in patients who are treated promptly. It should be noted that current mortality rates, although significantly lower than those in untreated patients, ranges from <5 to 30%.

Follow-up tests and monitoring
• After completion of antibiotic therapy and, if applicable, percutaneous/surgical drainage, patients with pyogenic liver abscess undergo serial imaging studies to confirm resolution of the disease. There are currently no guidelines on the frequency and type of imaging, and will depend on the clinician's preference.

Section 7: Reading List

Alsaif HS, Venkatesh SK, Chan DS, Archuleta S. CT appearance of pyogenic liver abscesses caused by *Klebsiella pneumoniae*. Radiology 2011;260:129–38

Bertel CK, van Heerden JA, Sheedy PF. Treatment of pyogenic hepatic abscesses. Surgical vs percutaneous drainage. Arch Surg 1986;121:554–8

Chung YF, Tan YM, Lui HF, et al. Management of pyogenic liver abscesses – percutaneous or open drainage? Singapore Med J 2007;48:1158–65

Heneghan HM, Healy NA, Martin ST, et al. Modern management of pyogenic hepatic abscess: a case series and review of the literature. BMC Research Notes 2011;4:80

Huang WK, Chang JWC, See LC, et al. Higher rate of colorectal cancer among patients with pyogenic liver abscess with Klebsiella pneumonia than those without: an 11-year follow-up study. Colorectal Disease 2012;14:794–801

Krige JE, Beckingham IJ. ABC of diseases of liver, pancreas, and biliary system. BMJ 2001;322:537–40

Kao WY, Hwang CY, Chang YT, et al. Cancer risk in patients with pyogenic liver abscess: a nationwide cohort study. Aliment Pharmacol Ther 2012;36:467–76

Law S-T, Li KK. Older age as a poor prognostic sign in patients with pyogenic liver abscess. Int J Infect Dis 2012 (article in press) PMID: 23140946

Rajak CL, Gupta S, Jain S, Chawla Y, Gulati M, Suri S. Percutaneous treatment of liver abscesses: needle aspiration versus catheter drainage. Am J Roentgenol 1998;170:1035–9

Zerem E, Hadzic A. Sonographically guided percutaneous catheter drainage versus needle aspiration in the management of pyogenic liver abscess. Am J Roentgenol 2007;189:138–42

Section 8: Guidelines

Not applicable for this topic.

Section 9: Evidence

• Due to the need to treat all patients with pyogenic liver abscess, there are no RCTs for this population.

Section 10: Images

Not applicable for this topic.

Additional material for this chapter can be found online at:
www.mountsinaiexpertguides.com
This includes a case study, multiple choice questions and ICD codes

---

CHAPTER 9

Biliary Infections

Gopi Patel

Division of Infectious Diseases, Icahn School of Medicine at Mount Sinai, New York, NY, USA

OVERALL BOTTOM LINE
- Acute cholecystitis and cholangitis are potential infectious complications of cholelithiasis (gallstones). Antibiotics covering bowel flora such as Enterobacteriaceae should be promptly initiated while considering surgical or radiologic intervention.
- Charcot's triad of fever, jaundice and abdominal pain remains the clinical standard for the diagnosis of acute cholangitis.
- AIDS cholangiopathy refers to the rare syndrome of biliary strictures and obstruction associated with infections in patients with CD4 counts of <100/mm³.
- Endoscopic or radiologic treatment of the biliary strictures and highly active antiretroviral therapy play important roles in the treatment of AIDS cholangiopathy.

Section 1: Background
Definition of disease
- Biliary infections encompass a variety of clinical syndromes including acute cholecystitis, cholangitis and AIDS cholangiopathy.
- Cholecystitis is inflammation of the gall bladder and can further be defined as calculous, in which gallstones obstruct the cystic duct leading to distension and inflammation, or acalculous.
- Cholangitis is defined as bacterial infection in the setting of obstruction of the common bile duct and is usually secondary to choledocholithiasis.
- AIDS cholangiopathy is a rare condition described in patients with AIDS characterized by abnormalities in the bile ducts and often associated with parasitic infections or CMV.

Disease classification
- Acute cholecystitis is associated with the relatively abrupt onset of fevers and RUQ pain. Leukocytosis is common, but jaundice is rare.
- Chronic cholecystitis is classically a histopathologic diagnosis associated with fibrosis and thickening of the gall bladder in the setting of cholelithiasis and mechanical irritation in the setting of recurrent attacks of acute cholecystitis.
- Clinically "chronic" cholecystitis can refer to recurrent attacks of RUQ pain in a patient with a history of cholecystitis.
- Acalculous cholecystitis occurs in about 10–15% of patients presenting with acute cholecystitis. These patients are often hospitalized and severely debilitated.

Mount Sinai Expert Guides: Hepatology, First Edition. Edited by Jawad Ahmad, Scott L. Friedman, and Henryk Dancygier.

Incidence/prevalence
- Acute calculous cholecystitis affects about 20% of patients with untreated symptomatic biliary colic. Most patients are women but disease presentation tends to be more severe in men. Patients with cholelithiasis and underlying diabetes mellitus are more likely to develop cholecystitis and more likely to have complicated disease.
- Cholangitis occurs in <1% of symptomatic patients with radiologic evidence of choledocholithiasis.
- Prior to the advent of HAART, the incidence of AIDS cholangiopathy approached 26% in patients with AIDS and CD4 counts of <100/mm^3 during outbreaks of cryptosporidiosis.

Etiology
- The vast majority of cases of acute cholecystitis and cholangitis are associated with cholelithisasis and with obstruction of the cystic duct or the common bile duct respectively.
- Most reported cases of AIDS cholangiopathy are associated with intestinal infections with *Cryptosporidium parvum*, Microsporidium (e.g. *Encephalitozoon intestinalis*), or *Cyclospora cayetanensis*. CMV has also been associated with AIDS cholangiopathy.

Pathology/pathogenesis
- In patients with cholelithiasis, transient obstruction of the cystic duct may result in pain or biliary colic. Prolonged impaction, however, can result in distension and inflammation of the gall bladder or cholecystitis. This often begins as a sterile process but can progress to infection with enteric flora including Enterobacteriaceae (e.g. *Escherichia coli* and *Klebsiella pneumoniae*) as well as enterococci and anaerobes.
- With incompetence of the ampulla (e.g. after stone passage, sphincterotomy or cannulation of the biliary tree, i.e. after an ERCP) bacteria can enter the biliary system from the gut (ascending cholangitis). Impedance of the mechanical flow of bile can lead to acute cholangitis. Enteric organisms are the most common pathogens implicated in ascending cholangitis.
- The pathogenesis of AIDS cholangiopathy remains unclear. *C. parvum* appears to have a tropism for bile ducts. Histopathologic specimens often reveal non-specific inflammation and changes similar to those described with PSC are noted surrounding the portal tracts.

Section 2: Prevention

CLINICAL PEARLS
- In the setting of symptomatic cholelithiasis, cholecystectomy is commonly employed to prevent future episodes of cholecystitis and/or cholangitis.
- In patients with a history of HIV infection, compliance with antiretroviral therapy is essential in preventing opportunistic infections and AIDS cholangiopathy as this syndrome is rare in patients without low CD4 counts.

Screening
- Routine screening for cholelithiasis, choledocholithiasis, and AIDS cholangiopathy in asymptomatic patients is not recommended.

Primary prevention
- Prevention of both cholecystitis and cholangitis can be achieved by treating biliary obstruction. Cholecystectomy is recommended for prevention of cholecystitis in patients with symptomatic cholelithiasis.

- Initiation of and compliance with HAART may prevent AIDS cholangiopathy, since the disease entity is rare in patients with elevated CD4 counts.

Secondary prevention
- In patients with a history of cholangitis secondary to mechanical obstruction by gallstones, a cholecystectomy is recommended to prevent recurrent episodes.
- The incidence of ascending cholangitis post-ERCP can be decreased by appropriate disinfection, peri-procedural antimicrobial prophylaxis in patients with incomplete drainage, stent placement in patients with incomplete drainage, and timely stent exchange.
- In patients with choledocholithiasis and cholangitis who are not candidates for cholecystectomy, endoscopic sphincterotomy provides partial protection against recurrent disease.

Section 3: Diagnosis

CLINICAL PEARLS
- A detailed history regarding fevers and pain including onset, frequency and quality, as well as any recent procedures, aid in determining the etiology of a biliary infection.
- Charcot's triad (jaundice, RUQ pain and fever), initially described in 1877, remains the clinical standard for diagnosing ascending cholangitis. Confirmation of this diagnosis includes aspiration of purulent biliary fluid during an ERCP or percutaneous or surgical biliary decompression. ERCP in the case of cholangitis serves as both a diagnostic and therapeutic tool.
- Ultrasound and hepatobiliary scintigraphy (e.g. HIDA scan) are the most common imaging studies employed to diagnose acute cholecystitis.
- AIDS cholangiopathy should be considered in the appropriate patient (HIV infection with CD4 count <100/mm^3) with a history of right upper quadrant pain and diarrhea. ERCP is often diagnostic.

Typical presentation
- Acute cholecystitis usually presents with severe pain localizing to the RUQ. Fevers are frequent, but frank jaundice is rare. Jaundice, however, is a hallmark of cholangitis along with RUQ pain and fevers.
- AIDS cholangiopathy often presents in patients with low CD4 counts with non-specific abdominal discomfort, weight loss and diarrhea. Fevers and jaundice are much less common than with cholecystitis or cholangitis.

Clinical diagnosis
History
- Many patients presenting with acute cholecystitis report a history of symptoms consistent with biliary colic. This includes episodic pain localizing to the epigastrium or the RUQ. The pain frequently is exacerbated with food intake or at night. Commonly the pain will radiate to the back and be associated with nausea and vomiting. In a patient with acute cholecystitis the pain persists, is severe, and localizes to the RUQ. A history of biliary colic may also be present in patients presenting with cholangitis. Charcot's triad – the triumvirate of pain, fever and jaundice – still remains helpful clinically in diagnosing cholangitis. A history of a recent biliary intervention (e.g. sphincterotomy or ERCP) may also contribute to the diagnosis.
- AIDS cholangiopathy should be considered in patients with low CD4 counts complaining of non-specific GI symptoms.

Physical examination

- The physical examination should include evaluation for jaundice. Patients with acute cholecystitis often have profound RUQ tenderness with some associated guarding. Murphy's sign can be present and is defined as inspiratory arrest while palpating the RUQ during a deep breath. A palpable mass in the RUQ can be present later in the course but is rare early in disease.
- In the setting of gangrenous or emphysematous cholecystitis or cholangitis signs of SIRS or sepsis is not uncommon.
- Patients with AIDS cholangiopathy are often wasted in appearance and can have fevers or jaundice, but the examination is often non-specific.

Useful clinical decision rules and calculators

Tokyo Guidelines for the diagnosis of acute cholecystitis

A Local signs of inflammation (Murphy's sign or tenderness or a palpable mass in RUQ).

B Systemic evidence of inflammation (e.g. fever, leukocytosis, or an elevated C-reactive protein).

C Radiologic or endoscopic evidence of an etiology (e.g. cholelithiasis, stricture, stent).

Definite diagnosis of acute cholecystitis if patient has one local sign of inflammation (A) and evidence of systemic inflammation (B) with a confirmatory imaging test (C).

Tokyo Guidelines for diagnosis of acute cholangitis

A Clinical history and physical findings
  - History of biliary disease (e.g. cholelithiasis, presence of a biliary stent, prior biliary surgery)
  - Fevers
  - Jaundice
  - Abdominal pain

B Laboratory data
  - Evidence of inflammation (e.g. abnormal leukocyte count, elevated CRP)
  - Abnormal liver function tests (e.g. AP, GGT, ALT, AST)

C Imaging findings
  - Biliary dilatation or evidence of a specific etiology (e.g. choledocholithiasis, stricture, stent)

Definite diagnosis with Charcot's triad (fever, jaundice, abdominal pain) OR two or more clinical parameters (A) with laboratory evidence of inflammation (B) in addition to supportive imaging findings (C).

Disease severity classification

Tokyo Guidelines for the severity grading of cholecystitis

Severity	Criteria
Mild (Grade 1)	Mild gall bladder inflammation in an otherwise healthy patient without evidence of organ dysfunction
Moderate (Grade 2)	One or more of the following: • Leukocytosis ($>18\,000/mm^3$) • Palpable tender RUQ mass • Symptom duration >72 hours • Marked local inflammation (e.g. peritonitis, pericholecystic abscess, gangrenous or emphysematous cholecystitis)

Severity	Criteria
Severe (Grade 3)	One or more of the following: • Hypotension requiring pressor support • Altered mental status • Hypoxia • Renal dysfunction • Hepatic dysfunction • Hematologic dysfunction (e.g. platelet count <100000/mm^3)

Tokyo Guidelines for the severity grading of cholangitis

Severity	Criteria
Mild (Grade 1)	Inflammation without evidence of organ dysfunction that responds to supportive care and antimicrobials
Moderate (Grade 2)	Inflammation that does not respond to initial conservative medical treatment without evidence of organ dysfunction
Severe (Grade 3)	One or more of the following: • Hypotension requiring pressor support • Altered mental status • Hypoxia • Renal dysfunction • Hepatic dysfunction • Hematologic dysfunction (e.g. platelet count <100000/mm^3)

Laboratory diagnosis
List of diagnostic tests
- Routine laboratory tests may reveal an elevated WBC count and abnormal liver enzymes in the setting of biliary infections.
- Blood cultures should be performed on all patients with suspected cholecysitis or cholangitis.
- Cultures can also be obtained from bile and/or foreign bodies removed during ERCP.
- Both GGT and AP can be markedly elevated in the setting of AIDS cholangiopathy.

List of imaging techniques
- Cholecystitis: abdominal US and HIDA scan are the most commonly employed imaging modalities to evaluate for acute cholecystitis.
  - US is widely available and non-invasive. Evidence of gall bladder wall thickening (≥5mm), pericholecystic fluid or a sonographic Murphy's sign supports the diagnosis.
  - HIDA scans evaluate gall bladder filling time. The absence of filling within 60 minutes of administration of the technetium-labeled tracer indicates cystic duct obstruction.
- Cholangitis:
  - US looking for biliary dilatation and choledocholithiasis is recommended but may not be as sensitive as other techniques.
  - MRCP is non-invasive. It may not be as sensitive as more invasive modalities for small stones.
  - ERCP has therapeutic in addition to diagnostic potential.
  - Endoscopic US is helpful in evaluating extrinsic compression as the cause of the obstruction.

- AIDS cholangiopathy:
  - ERCP is the diagnostic modality of choice for AIDS cholangiopathy.
  - Typical findings can be divided into four categories which are listed in the order of frequency.
    - › combined papillary stenosis and sclerosing cholangitis
    - › combined intra and extrahepatic sclerosing cholangitis without papillary stenosis
    - › isolated papillary stenosis
    - › long extrahepatic stricture with or without intrahepatic sclerosing cholangitis

Section 4: Treatment
Treatment rationale
- Patients with acute cholecystitis and cholangitis mandate treatment. Conservative medical management is reserved for patients with mild disease and includes antimicrobials, analgesics and intravenous fluids.
- The mainstay for the treatment of cholecystitis is a cholecystectomy. It can be performed by laparotomy or by laparoscopy and either at time of presentation ("early") or after symptom resolution ("delayed"). Early laparoscopic cholecystectomy is preferred.
  - In patients with severe cholecystitis who are hemodynamically unstable or who are poor surgical candidates, a percutaneous cholecystostomy can be performed.
- Many patients with acute cholangitis can be managed conservatively. However, moderate to severe cases may require biliary drainage, which is best achieved using ERCP.
  - PTC can be employed in patients with distorted biliary anatomy (e.g. choledochojejunostomy) or who have failed ERCP.
- Antibiotics for cholecystitis and cholangitis should cover enteric flora including Enterobacteriaceae. Coverage of enterococci and anaerobes should be considered for moderate to severe disease.
  - Knowledge of institutional and community antimicrobial susceptibilities aids in choosing empiric antibiotics.
- Treatment directed toward the infections associated with AIDS cholangiopathy does little to alleviate symptoms. Initiation of HAART and symptom driven treatment of cholangiographic abnormalities (e.g. sphincteromy) is recommended.

When to hospitalize
- Rarely, there are patients with a known cholelithiasis or intrinsic or extrinsic biliary disease and frequent bouts of mild cholangitis that can be managed with oral antimicrobials and analgesics. In these uncommon cases, patients can be managed at home – however, close follow-up is mandatory.
- Most patients with acute cholecystitis and/or cholangitis require hospitalization.
- Patients with AIDS cholangiopathy do not require hospitalization unless they require electrolyte and/or advanced nutritional support or endoscopic intervention.

Managing the hospitalized patient
- Fluids, antimicrobials, and analgesics are essential for the management of patients with biliary infections.
- Monitoring for signs of complicated infections or impending sepsis is essential.
- Surgical consultation services should be aware and actively involved in the management of patients with acute cholecystitis.

- Since biliary drainage is vital to the treatment of moderate or severe cholangitis, the availability of a skilled endoscopist is crucial to the successful management of these infections.
- Patients with severe cholangitis are best managed in a critical care unit.

Table of treatment

Treatment	Comment
Conservative/ Medical: Treatment of cholecystitis and cholangitis	Conservative management without surgical or endoscopic/radiologic intervention should be reserved for patients with mild to moderate disease
	Antibiotics directed toward Enterobacteriaceae are appropriate for all grades of disease. Addition of anaerobic coverage is recommended for patients with more severe disease presentation
AIDS cholangiopathy	Patients with AIDS cholangiopathy should be offered HAART
Surgical: Cholecystectomy	Cholecystectomy is recommended for patients with acute calculous cholecystitis. Early laparoscopic cholecystectomy is preferred
Endoscopic/ Radiologic: Cholecystostomy	In patients who are poor surgical candidates for cholecystectomy, percutaneous cholecystostomy placement can be considered
ERCP	Decompression of the bile duct is recommended in the treatment of moderate to severe cholangitis. ERCP is both a diagnostic and therapeutic modality for patients with probable cholangitis
	ERCP also allows for diagnosis and treatment of patients with AIDS cholangiopathy
PTC	In patients with distorted biliary anatomy or who failed ERCP, PTC may be an option to urgently decompress the bile duct

CLINICAL PEARLS
- Antibiotics, analgesics, fluids and cholecystectomy are recommended for the treatment of acute cholecystitis.
- Antibiotics, analgesics, fluids and biliary drainage are recommended for the treatment of moderate to severe cholangitis.
- Initiation of HAART and cholangiography are recommended for the treatment of AIDS cholangiopathy.

Section 5: Special Populations

Not applicable for this topic.

Section 6: Prognosis

CLINICAL PEARLS
- With early recognition and expedited appropriate aggressive management, patients with mild to moderate cholecystitis and cholangitis in the setting of cholelithiasis do well.
- Offering HAART to patients with AIDS cholangiopathy improves overall survival.

Natural history of untreated disease

- Complications of untreated cholecystitis include ischemia, necrosis, gangrene and perforation of the gall bladder. Biliary peritonitis and septicemia often result.
- Untreated cholangitis can result in biliary peritonitis and septic shock.
- Patient survival in patients with AIDS cholangiopathy is primarily determined by their immune status and most observational studies performed prior to the advent of HAART note high mortality rates.

Prognosis for treated patients

- The overall mortality of an isolated attack of cholecystitis is <5%. A patient's risk of morbidity and mortality is related to their underlying health including the presence of comorbid conditions and their surgical risk.
- Patients with severe cholangitis still suffer from high rates of morbidity and mortality despite aggressive treatment.
- More recent surveys of patients with AIDS cholangiopathy suggests the median survival after diagnosis is closer to 3 years, which is substantially higher than previous reports suggesting that treating the underlying immunodeficiency by offering HAART is imperative to improving overall survival.

Section 7: Reading List

Chen XM, LaRusso NF. Cryptosporidiosis and the pathogenesis of AIDS-cholangiopathy. Semin Liver Dis 2002;22:277–89

Devarbhavi H, Sebastian T, Seetharamu SM, Karanth D. IV/AIDS cholangiopathy: clinical spectrum, cholangiographic features and outcome in 30 patients. J Gastroenterol Hepatol 2010;25:1656–60

Hirota M, Takada T, Kawarada Y, et al. Diagnostic criteria and severity assessment of acute cholecystitis: Tokyo Guidelines. J Hepatobiliary Pancreat Surg 2007;14:78–82

Lee JG. Diagnosis and management of acute cholangitis. Nat Rev Gastroenterol Hepatol 2009;6:533–41

Solomkin JS, Mazuski JE, Bradley JS, et al. Diagnosis and management of complicated intra-abdominal infection in adults and children: guidelines by the Surgical Infection Society and the Infectious Diseases Society of America. Clin Infect Dis 2010;50:133–64

Strasberg SM. Acute calculous cholecystitis. N Engl J Med 2008;358:2804–11

Vakil NB, Schwartz SM, Buggy BP, et al. Biliary cryptosporidiosis in HIV-infected people after the waterborne outbreak of cryptosporidiosis in Milwaukee. N Engl J Med 1996;334:19–23

Wada K, Takada T, Kawarada Y, et al. Diagnostic criteria and severity assessment of acute cholangitis: Tokyo Guidelines. J Hepatobiliary Pancreat Surg 2007;14:52–8

Yamashita Y, Takada T, Kawarada Y. Surgical treatment of patients with acute cholecystitis: Tokyo Guidelines. J Hepatobiliary Pancreat Surg 2007;14:91–7

Section 8: Guidelines
National society guidelines

Guideline title	Guideline source	Date	Summary
Diagnosis and management of complicated intra-abdominal infection in adults and children	Surgical Infection Society and the Infectious Diseases Society of America (IDSA) http://www.idsociety.org/uploadedFiles/IDSA/Guidelines-Patient_Care/PDF_Library/Intra-abdominal%20Infectin.pdf	2010	Offers empiric antibiotic selection choices for the management of biliary infections

International society guidelines

Guideline title	Guideline source	Date	Summary
Diagnostic criteria and severity assessment of acute cholecystitis	Tokyo Guidelines http://www.ncbi.nlm.nih.gov/pmc/articles/PMC2784516/	2007	First consensus recommendations for the diagnosis and severity grading for acute cholecystitis
Diagnostic criteria and severity assessment of acute cholangitis	Tokyo Guidelines http://www.ncbi.nlm.nih.gov/pmc/articles/PMC2784515/	2007	First consensus recommendations for the diagnosis and severity grading for acute cholangitis
Surgical treatment of patients with acute cholecystitis	Tokyo Guidelines http://www.ncbi.nlm.nih.gov/pmc/articles/PMC2784499/	2007	Early recommendations for the timing of cholecystectomy in the setting of acute cholecystitis

Section 9: Evidence

Not applicable for this topic.

Section 10: Images

Not applicable for this topic.

Additional material for this chapter can be found online at:
www.mountsinaiexpertguides.com
This includes a case study and multiple choice questions

CHAPTER 10

Alcoholic Hepatitis

Scott L. Friedman
Division of Liver Diseases, Icahn School of Medicine at Mount Sinai, New York, NY, USA

OVERALL BOTTOM LINE
- AH represents a clinicopathologic spectrum of liver disease, ranging from mild to a severe, life-threatening injury in patients who drink to excess.
- AH is typically characterized by fever, hepatomegaly, jaundice and characteristic laboratory abnormalities, including moderate elevations of AST and ALT (<500 U/L) with AST>ALT.
- The disease may present with liver failure in patients who already have cirrhosis.
- Patients are at high risk for progressive liver injury, renal failure, infection and death.
- Corticosteroids may improve survival in appropriately selected patients.
- The key to long-term treatment success is abstinence from alcohol, usually require ongoing behavioral intervention or alcohol abuse counseling.

Section 1: Background
Definition of disease
- AH is a clinicopathologic syndrome of significant inflammatory liver disease in patients who have high-risk or excessive alcohol ingestion. The diagnosis can be strongly suspected based on clinical and laboratory features indicating liver injury in the setting of heavy ethanol use, with AST and ALT elevations (AST > ALT but both <500 U/L), and further established by liver biopsy demonstrating Mallory's hyaline, pericentral injury, steatosis and neutrophil infiltration.
- The disease may be classified in terms of severity based on a discriminant function formula or the MELD score (see Section 6).

Incidence/prevalence
- The overall prevalence of alcohol-related disorders has been estimated at 4.65% in the USA by the NIAAA 2001–2002 National Epidemiologic Survey on Alcohol and Related Conditions (NESARC) (see http://www.niaaa.nih.gov/Resources/DatabaseResources/QuickFacts/AlcoholDependence/Pages/abusdep1.aspx)
- Alcoholic liver disease accounts for up to 20% of all liver transplants in the USA, alone or in conjunction with HCV (www.unos.org).
- Up to 44% of all deaths from liver disease may be attributable to alcohol. Moreover, current prevalence data probably underestimate the true burden of disease.

Mount Sinai Expert Guides: Hepatology, First Edition. Edited by Jawad Ahmad, Scott L. Friedman, and Henryk Dancygier.
© 2014 John Wiley & Sons, Ltd. Published 2014 by John Wiley & Sons, Ltd.
Companion website: www.mountsinaiexpertguides.com

- In the European Union (see EU Alcohol and Health Forum http://ec.europa.eu/health/alcohol/forum/index_en.htm):
  - Fifty-five million adults are estimated to drink at harmful levels in the EU (more than 40 g of alcohol, i.e. four drinks per day for men and over 20 g, i.e. two drinks per day for women). Drinking more than this amount is known to carry a health risk.
  - Harmful alcohol consumption is estimated to account for approximately 195 000 deaths a year in the EU due to, e.g. accidents, liver disease, cancers, etc.
  - Harmful alcohol use is the third biggest cause of early death and illness in the EU, behind tobacco and high blood pressure.

Economic impact
- Alcoholic liver disease exacts a substantial cost exceeding $185 million/year in the USA.
- The cost of alcohol-related harm to the EU's economy has been estimated at €125 billion for 2003, equivalent to 1.3% of GDP. This estimate includes losses due to underperformance at work, work absenteeism and premature death.
- The actual spending on alcohol-related problems in the EU is estimated at about €66 billion, e.g. on crime, traffic accidents, health and disease treatment and prevention.

Etiology/pathogenesis
- Only about a third of patients with high-risk drinking histories will develop significant liver disease, but the reasons for this variable risk are not fully understood. In fact, the evidence for alcohol-induced liver disease is primarily epidemiologic, not biochemical.
- There are at least five potential pathogenic pathways that contribute to the development of AH:
  - LPS from leaky gut, with Kupffer cell activation – the intestinal wall becomes edematous and increased amounts of LPS from gut bacteria leak into the portal blood. Upon arrival in the liver LPS activates Kupffer cells, or resident macrophages, which secrete a number of inflammatory and fibrogenic cytokines including TNF-alpha, transforming growth factor beta 1 and interleukin 1. Direct activation of fibrogenic cells (activated stellate cells) by LPS via TLR4 also contributes to a fibrogenic response.
  - Centrilobular hypoxia – as ethanol is metabolized, oxygen is consumed, leading to relative hypoxemia in the region of the hepatic sinusoid furthest from oxygenated blood, which is the central vein. This hypoxemia is compounded by the fact that normally the blood that enters the liver is already hypo-oxygenated, since it is derived primarily from the portal vein.
  - Leukocyte infiltration – the infiltration of neutrophils is relatively unique to alcoholic liver disease and these inflammatory cells are a potent source of injurious enzymes and free radicals that damage cells in the liver.
  - Lipid peroxidation – alternate pathways of ETOH metabolism – chronic exposure of liver cells to ethanol induces a key alternative pathway to metabolize ethanol through cytochrome P450 2E1 (Cyp2E1). Unlike ethanol metabolism by ADH, Cyp2E1-mediated ethanol metabolism generates free radicals that are injurious to liver cells.
  - Acetaldehyde adduct formation – metabolism of ethanol to acetaldehyde allows this reactive metabolite to link with proteins on liver cells to generate neo-antigens. These neo-antigens elicit an immunologic reaction by antibodies and lymphocytes that may attack native proteins on resident liver cells.

Predictive/risk factors
- Amount and duration of intake.
- Gender: females > males.

- Concurrent liver disease: iron overload, HBV, HCV.
- Obesity.
- Genetic factors: determine both risk of alcoholism and likelihood of liver injury after heavy drinking (e.g. PNPLA3 gene variants).
- Family history of alcoholism.

Section 2: Prevention

> **BOTTOM LINE**
> - The key to prevention is abstinence:
>   - Abstinence is the single most important determinant of outcome in patients diagnosed with AH.
>   - Multiple studies indicate that in patients with alcoholic liver injury, continued alcohol ingestion guarantees that the disease will progress.
>   - A major responsibility of health professionals caring for patients with alcoholic liver disease is to encourage participation in alcohol abstinence programs.

Screening
- Screening strategies to identify individuals at risk for high-risk drinking and alcohol abuse are important complements to abstinence efforts in those already diagnosed with alcohol dependence disorders.
- The CAGE screening questions (see next section) are widely used in the USA.
- The AUDIT questionnaire is a more detailed questionnaire developed by the WHO that has 92% sensitivity and specificity of 94%.

Primary and secondary prevention
- Primary prevention is directed at identifying high risk drinking behavior before end-organ damage has occurred. In addition to the CAGE and AUDIT instruments, the National Institute of Alcohol Abuse and Alcoholism has a valuable web tool to educate the public in identifying such behaviors (see http://rethinkingdrinking.niaaa.nih.gov/).
- Enrolment in an alcohol rehabilitation program is an essential step in preventing continued alcohol abuse. Among these, Alcoholics Anonymous and related 12-step programs have the highest rate of long-term success (~ 50%).

Section 3: Diagnosis

> **BOTTOM LINE**
> - Patients with suspected alcoholic liver disease typically underestimate or may even deny alcohol consumption.
> - The presence of moderate elevations of AST and ALT (<500 U/L) in which AST > ALT should raise the concern for AH.
> - If AH is suspected based on history, yet AST and ALT greatly exceed 500 U/L, then additional etiologies must be considered, especially concurrent acetaminophen usage or viral hepatitis.
> - Liver biopsy may be necessary in cases where the diagnosis is in doubt or additional etiologies are suspected. Evidence of Mallory's hyaline, neutrophil infiltration and a centrizonal distribution of injury are consistent with alcoholic liver injury, but may also be seen in patients with NASH (see Differential diagnosis table that follows).

Differential diagnosis
• Although typical features of alcoholic liver injury are not difficult to identify, the disease may co-exist with other liver diseases, especially viral hepatitis or NAFLD.

Differential diagnosis	Features
NASH	This may be difficult to distinguish from alcoholic liver disease and both may co-exist. A formula (ALD/NAFLD Index – ANI) to distinguish the two may be useful: ANI Score = –58.5 + 0.637(MCV) + 3.91 (AST/ALT) – 0.406 (BMI) + 6.35 for male gender • ANI > 0 favors ALD • ANI < 0 favors NAFLD
Viral hepatitis	Evidence of serologic markers or viremia, consistent with viral liver disease Liver biopsy evidence of periportal, not pericentral, mononuclear leukocyte infiltration
Amiodarone hepatotoxicity	History of amiodarone use Liver biopsy with characteristic lamellar lysosomal inclusion bodies
Autoimmune hepatitis	Presence of serum autoimmune markers and elevated gamma globulin Liver biopsy with plasma cell infiltration and immune cells

Typical presentation
• The typical patient with alcoholic liver disease is asymptomatic for long periods despite sustained high-risk drinking behavior before coming to medical attention. In such a patient, the diagnosis only becomes apparent following review of standard liver chemistry studies demonstrating characteristic abnormalities. It is not unusual for patients to deny heavy alcohol use or underestimate their intake, which is why instruments such as the CAGE and AUDIT questions are so valuable.
• As liver disease becomes more symptomatic, patients may present with anorexia, RUQ discomfort, jaundice, coagulopathy, and stigmata of liver disease. Fever may be present, and infection must be excluded in such patients.

Clinical diagnosis
History
• It is essential to identify high risk drinking behavior in the patient with suspected alcoholic liver disease. Patient may complain of anorexia, malaise, weight loss, abdominal pain and/or low grade fevers.
• Two guidelines to identify high-risk drinking behaviour are listed here.

Low vs high risk drinking limits (Source: www.rethinkingdrinking.niaaa.nih.gov)

Low-risk drinking limit	Men	Women
On any single day:	No more than 4 drinks AND	No more than 3 drinks AND
Per week:	No more than 14 drinks	No more than 7 drinks

Screening for alcohol abuse – CAGE questionnaire

1. Have you ever felt you should **c**ut down on your drinking?
2. Have people **a**nnoyed you by criticizing your drinking?
3. Have you ever felt bad or **g**uilty about your drinking?
4. Have you ever had a drink first thing in the morning to steady your nerves or get rid of a hangover (**e**ye-opener)?

   Score ≥2 "Yes" answers: clinically significant drinking

Physical examination

- Fever.
- Hepatomegaly.
- Ascites.
- Encephalopathy.
- Gastrointestinal bleeding.
- Jaundice.

Useful clinical decision rules and calculators

See Algorithm 10.1.

Disease severity classification

- See Section 4, Treatment. Two systems are widely used to define disease severity, the Maddrey Discriminant Function score and the MELD. In addition, the Lille score is valuable in incorporating the response to corticosteroids as a prognostic element.

Laboratory diagnosis

List of diagnostic tests

- CBC.
- Anemia, with macrocytosis (e.g. elevated MCV).
- Leukocytosis, with elevated neutrophil count.
- Elevated AST > ALT. However, both AST and ALT <500 U/L.
- Elevated bilirubin, AP, GGT.
- Increased INR, decreased albumin.

Pathologic features on liver biopsy

- Liver biopsy is not indicated in every case if the history, clinical and laboratory features are all consistent with the diagnosis of alcoholic liver disease.
- However, other causes can be excluded by liver biopsy if the diagnosis is not clear, including drug-induced liver disease, Wilson disease, NAFLD and autoimmune liver injury.
  - Obligatory:
    - ➤ liver cell damage ranging from ballooning to cell death (apoptosis, necrosis).
    - ➤ PMNs.
    - ➤ Perivenular distribution.
  - Common:
    - ➤ bridging necrosis.
    - ➤ Mallory-Denk bodies.
    - ➤ fatty change.
    - ➤ bile duct proliferation.
    - ➤ cholestasis.

> perivenular fibrosis (sclerosing hyaline necrosis).
> giant mitochondria.

List of imaging techniques
- US, CT or MRI (none are specific for AH).
- Fatty, enlarged liver, with or without features of portal hypertension, may be apparent by ultrasound, CT or MRI.
- The major purpose of imaging is to exclude other causes of liver disease, vascular abnormalities (e.g. hepatic or portal vein obstruction), biliary obstruction or focal lesions or masses.
- Nodular liver may be suggestive of cirrhosis.
- Presence of varices and splenomegaly indicates likely portal hypertension.
- Features suggestive of alcoholic liver disease when present:
  - Higher caudate lobe volume.
  - More frequent visualization of right posterior hepatic notch.
  - Fewer regenerative nodules.

Algorithm 10.1 Diagnosis of AH

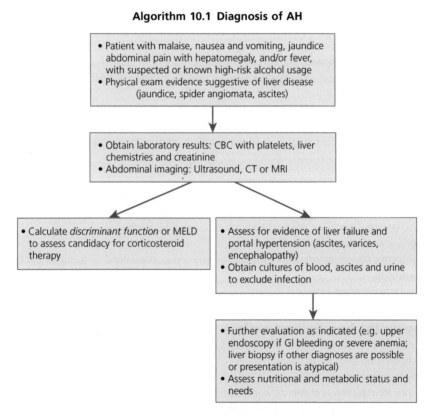

Source: O'Shea, et al. 2010. Reproduced with permission of John Wiley & Sons Ltd.

Potential pitfalls/common errors in diagnosis
- Patients typically underestimate or may deny alcohol abuse. If so, consider checking urinary alcohol concentrations or obtaining additional history from next-of-kin or health care proxy, and review all prior medical records.

- AH is not restricted to any socioeconomic level, race, level of education, intelligence or employment status, and must always be suspected when the diagnostic tests are compatible with this illness.
- If alcohol ingestion has been recent, patients must be monitored for evidence of withdrawal or delirium tremens and monitored or treated appropriately.
- Although fever can be caused by AH, infection must always be excluded first, especially since some patients will subsequently be treated with corticosteroids. This includes paracentesis or thoracentesis to exclude infection when ascites or pleural fluid is present.
- AH may complicate other liver diseases, especially viral hepatitis, so all additional causes of liver injury must be excluded with appropriate serologies.
- Patients with alcoholic cirrhosis are at risk for hepatocellular carcinoma, and regular imaging with ultrasound, CT or MRI is essential to make an early diagnosis that offers the possibility of effective treatment or cure.

Section 4: Treatment
Treatment rationale
- The primary goals for treatment are to preserve nutrition and hydration, remain vigilant for infections, and treat complications of end stage liver disease when present. In some patients, corticosteroids are indicated, based on accumulated data from dozens of clinical trials. Much more limited data suggest that pentoxyphylline may be effective as well.
- Abstinence:
  - Whether or not the patient stops drinking is the single most important predictor of outcome in alcoholic liver disease.
  - Progression and worsening of liver disease is virtually certain if the patient continues to drink alcohol.

When to hospitalize
- Evidence of altered mental status indicating either alcohol withdrawal, delirium tremens, hepatic encephalopathy or the possibility of intracranial hemorrhage.
- Rising liver tests, especially INR.
- Suspicion or evidence of infection, especially urinary sepsis, pneumonia or spontaneous bacterial peritonitis.
- Active gastrointestinal bleeding.

Managing the hospitalized patient
- Vigilance for delirium tremens or withdrawal symptoms and treatment when patient has been actively drinking prior to admission.
- Fluids, multivitamins.
- Vigilance for infection and hepatic encephalopathy.
- High calorie, low sodium diet and supplements. Do not restrict protein unless hepatic encephalopathy is present. Frequent interval feedings emphasizing a night time snack and morning feeding to improve nitrogen balance.
- Two related formulae, the Maddrey Discriminant Function or the MELD score are used to identify more severe cases of acute alcoholic liver disease in order to determine if treatment with corticosteroids is indicated (see "Table of treatment" and Algorithm 10.2):

- Maddrey Discriminant Function:
  DF = [4.6(prothrombin time − control)$_{sec}$] + bilirubin$_{mg/mL}$
- MELD score:
  MELD = 3.8 × log (e) (bilirubin mg/dL) + 11.2 × log (e) (INR) + 9.6 log (e) (creatinine mg/dL)
- A MELD of 21 portends a similar prognosis as a Maddrey Discriminant Function score of 32.

Table of treatment

Treatment	Comment
Medical:	
Corticosteroids: • If Maddrey score ≥32 or MELD ≥18–21 → prednisolone 32 mg/day × 4 weeks, then 4 week taper • BUT: those with creatinine >2.3 mg/dL or GI bleed do not benefit	Recent meta-analyses of individual patient data confirm that corticosteroids improve short-term survival in patients with severe AH
Pentoxiphylline	A single randomized trial (400 mg PO tid × 28 days) showed a survival benefit in patients with Maddrey Score >32, due to reduced development of hepatorenal syndrome
	A large multicenter trial of pentoxyphylline in advanced alcoholic cirrhosis had no impact on survival but reduced the complications
Surgical:	
Liver transplantation	Liver transplantation is a viable option for patients with advanced AH with good outcomes. However, most programs in the USA require 6 months of abstinence before patients will be evaluated
	Survival after liver transplantation for alcoholic liver disease is excellent, and comparable with other etiologies of liver failure.
	Liver transplantation for patients with AH who fail corticosteroids can be safely performed with acceptable outcomes, but is highly controversial because of concern that patients will not remain abstinent

Prevention/management of complications
- Alcohol withdrawal. Physicians must be vigilant for evidence of alcohol withdrawal manifested as increased autonomic activity and risk of hallucinosis in the recently hospitalized patient. Treatment with benzodiazepines and close observation is essential to prevent further deterioration and risk of delirium tremens or cardiovascular instability.
- Infection is always a persistent concern in the patients with AH, and a low threshold for culturing blood and body fluids must be preserved and treatment with appropriate antibiotics where indicated.
- Evidence of renal failure in the absence of dehydration may indicate impending hepatorenal syndrome, an ominous sign that portends a poor prognosis for which there are no specific treatments.

Algorithm 10.2 Therapeutic algorithm for the management of AH

```
                    ┌─────────────────────────┐
                    │ Establish disease severity │
                    └─────────────────────────┘
                        /                \
                       /                  \
┌──────────────────────────────┐   ┌──────────────────────────────┐
│          Low risk:           │   │          High risk:          │
│ MDF < 32 and 1st week decrease│   │ MDF ≥ 32, presence of HE, or │
│ in bilirubin, or MELD < 18 and│   │        MELD ≥ 18             │
│ 1st week decrease in MELD by  │   │                              │
│         2 points             │   │                              │
└──────────────────────────────┘   └──────────────────────────────┘
              │                                   │
              ▼                                   ▼
┌──────────────────────────────┐   ┌──────────────────────────────┐
│ Nutritional assessment/       │   │ Nutritional assessment/       │
│ Intervention                 │   │ Intervention                 │
└──────────────────────────────┘   └──────────────────────────────┘
              │                                   │
              ▼                                   ▼
┌──────────────────────────────┐   ┌──────────────────────────────┐
│ Supportive care and close     │   │ Consider liver biopsy if     │
│ follow-up                    │   │ diagnosis is uncertain       │
└──────────────────────────────┘   └──────────────────────────────┘
                                            │              \
                                            │               \
                                            │          *If steroid*
                                            │       *contraindications*
                                            │       *or early renal*
                                            │          *failure*
                                            ▼               ▼
                                    ┌──────────────┐  ┌──────────────┐
                                    │ Prednisolone │  │ Pentoxifylline│
                                    └──────────────┘  └──────────────┘
```

Source: O'Shea, et al. 2010. Reproduced with permission of John Wiley & Sons Ltd.

CLINICAL PEARLS

- Concurrent use of acetaminophen-containing products may precipitate severe liver injury even when ingested within the therapeutic range, because alcohol usage amplifies the hepatotoxicity of acetaminophen. This should be suspected if AST, ALT > 500 U/L. If acetaminophen toxicity is present or likely, use of N-acetyl cysteine is essential.
- As noted, while the decision to initiate treatment with steroids is difficult, if there is no improvement in bilirubin within 7 days (i.e. bilirubin not improved compared with first day of treatment), then they are not likely to improve survival and should be discontinued.
- In patients who fail to respond to corticosteroids, switching to pentoxiphylline offers no additional benefit.

Section 5: Special Populations
Pregnancy
- Acute liver disease of any type, in particular AH, significantly increases the risk of fetal demise or complications. Moreover, heavy ethanol use during pregnancy is associated with risk of fetal alcohol syndrome.

Others
- Concurrent liver disease from hepatitis C or other causes including NAFLD substantially increases the risk of fibrosis and decompensation.

Section 6: Prognosis

CLINICAL PEARLS
- Short-term (28 day) mortality of AH is extremely high and may exceed 35% in patients with severe disease.
- Both the Maddrey Discriminant Function and MELD scores accurately stratify patient risk prior to treatment with corticosteroids. The Lille Score additionally refines prognostic predictions by incorporating whether patients have responded to corticosteroids (http://www.lillemodel.com/score.asp).
- Despite abstinence after hospitalization, a smoldering, slowly deteriorating course is not unusual, associated with progressive and severe cholestasis, renal failure and ultimately death.
- Other factors that may contribute to long-term outcomes apart from those in the Maddrey, MELD or Lille scores include the extent of perivenular fibrosis and severe inflammation on liver biopsy, and whether there is co-existent liver disease from other causes.

Natural history of untreated disease
- For severe AH, controlled studies suggest that the control (untreated) patients have a 35% 28-day mortality. Long-term outcomes depend on whether the patients remain abstinent, and whether cirrhosis is already present.

Prognosis for treated patients
- Treatment with corticosteroids in responsive patients improves the 28-day survival to ~80%.

Follow-up tests and monitoring
Monitoring of patients who have survived an episode of AH must include vigilance for continued alcohol use, and insistence on participation in an alcohol rehabilitation program (e.g. Alcoholics Anonymous). Assessment of liver function with serum enzymes, albumin, INR and imaging is recommended at least every 6 months if the patient is otherwise medically stable.

Section 7: Reading List

Akriviadis E, Botla R, Briggs W, Han S, Reynolds T, Shakil O. Pentoxifylline improves short-term survival in serve acute alcoholic hepatitis: a double-blind, placebo-controlled trial. Gastroenterology 2000;119: 1637–48

Babor TF, Higgins-Biddle JC, Saunders JB, Monteiro MG. The Alcohol Use Disorders Identification Test, Guidelines for Use in Primary Care, Second Edition, Department of Mental Health and Substance Dependence, World Health Organization

Dunn W, Angulo P, Sanderson S, et al. Utility of a new model to diagnose an alcohol basis for steatohepatitis. Gastroenterology 2006;131:1057–63

Dunn W, Jamil LH, Brown LS, et al. MELD accurately predicts mortality in patients with alcoholic hepatitis. Hepatology 2005;41:353–8

Kamath PS, Wiesner RH, Malinchoc M, et al. A model to predict survival in patients with end-stage liver disease. Hepatology 2001;33:464–70

Lebrec D, Thabut D, Oberti F, et al. Pentoxifylline does not decrease short-term mortality but does reduce complications in patients with advanced cirrhosis. Gastroenterology 2010;138:1755–62

Lucey MR. Liver transplantation for alcoholic liver disease. Clin Liver Dis 2007;11:283–9

Lucey MR, Mathurin P, Morgan TR. Alcoholic hepatitis. N Engl J Med 2009; 360:2758–69

Mathurin P, Abdelnour M, Ramond MJ, et al. Early change in bilirubin levels is an important prognostic factor in severe alcoholic hepatitis treated with prednisolone. Hepatology 2003;38:1363–9

Mathurin P, Mendenhall CL, Carithers RL, Jr, et al. Corticosteroids improve short-term survival in patients with severe alcoholic hepatitis (AH): individual data analysis of the last three randomized placebo controlled double blind trials of corticosteroids in severe AH. J Hepatol 2002;36:480–7

Mathurin P, Moreno C, Samuel D, et al. Early liver transplantation for severe alcoholic hepatitis. N Engl J Med 2011;365:1790–800

Mathurin P, O'Grady J, Carithers RL, et al. Corticosteroids improve short-term survival in patients with severe alcoholic hepatitis: meta-analysis of individual patient data. Gut 2011;60:255–60

O'Shea RS, Dasarathy S, McCullough AJ. AASLD Practice Guidelines: alcoholic liver disease. Hepatology 2010;51:307–28

Section 8: Guidelines
National society guidelines

Guideline title	Guideline source
American Association for the Study of Liver Diseases Guidelines	American Association for the Study of Liver Diseases (AASLD) http://www.aasld.org/ practiceguidelines/Pages/SortablePracticeGuidelinesAlpha.aspx

International society guidelines

Guideline title	Guideline source	Date
Clinical Practice Guidelines on the Management of Alcoholic Liver Disease	European Association for the Study of Liver (EASL) http://www.easl.eu/_clinical-practice-guideline/ issue-9-june-2012-clinical-practice-guidelines-on-the-management-of-alcoholic-liver-disease	2012

Section 9: Evidence

See AASLD Guidelines.

Section 10: Images

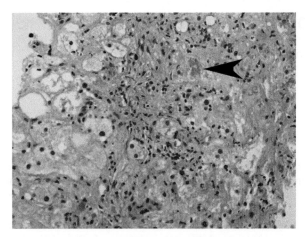

Figure 10.1 Pathologic features of AH. The photomicrograph shows Mallory-Denk bodies (arrow) with extensive ballooning degeneration of hepatocytes and scattered inflammatory cells (neutrophils and lymphocytes) in the lobules. H&E. Original magnification × 400. Source: Courtesy of Dr Isabel Fiel.

**Additional material for this chapter can be found online at:
www.mountsinaiexpertguides.com.
This includes a case study and multiple choice questions**

CHAPTER 11

Non-Alcoholic Fatty Liver Disease

Charissa Y. Chang

Division of Liver Diseases, Icahn School of Medicine at Mount Sinai, New York, NY, USA

OVERALL BOTTOM LINE

- NAFLD encompasses a spectrum of disease conditions ranging from simple steatosis to NASH which may progress to cirrhosis and hepatocellular carcinoma. Many patients who previously were labeled as having cryptogenic cirrhosis actually have NAFLD-induced cirrhosis.
- Pathogenesis of NAFLD is closely associated with metabolic syndrome and insulin resistance.
- NASH is characterized histologically by steatosis, features of cellular injury (hepatocyte ballooning, necrosis, apoptosis, Mallory-Denk bodies), inflammation, and variable degrees of fibrosis.
- Liver biopsy is the only investigation at this time that can differentiate NASH from bland steatosis.
- The mainstay of treatment is lifestyle modification (diet, exercise, weight loss). No widely approved pharmacologic treatment exists to date.

Section 1: Background
Definition of disease

- NAFLD refers to a spectrum of liver diseases that resemble/mimic alcohol-induced liver injury in patients who do not consume significant amounts of alcohol (women ≤20 g/day; men ≤40 g/day).

Disease classification

- Simple steatosis is defined by >5% of hepatocytes containing fat in the absence of histologic features of NASH.
- Definite NASH is defined by hepatic steatosis (macrovesicular > microvesicular) plus additional features of histologic liver injury (inflammation, Mallory-Denk bodies, ballooned hepatocytes) and fibrosis.
- Borderline NASH is defined by no hepatocyte ballooning, no Mallory-Denk bodies.

Incidence/prevalence

- NAFLD is the most common chronic liver disease in Western countries with a prevalence of about 30% in the adult population and 9% in children and adolescents. Approximately 55 million Americans have NAFLD.
- Prevalence of NASH in Western countries is estimated around 2.5%.

Mount Sinai Expert Guides: Hepatology, First Edition. Edited by Jawad Ahmad, Scott L. Friedman, and Henryk Dancygier.

Economic impact
- The economic impact of NAFLD is unknown. However, rising obesity trends will lead to continued importance of NAFLD as a major cause of chronic liver disease.

Etiology
- The exact etiology of NAFLD is unclear and remains an area of active investigation; however, there is a strong association with obesity, metabolic syndrome and insulin resistance.

Pathology/pathogenesis
Hepatic steatosis
- Hepatic steatosis may result from several factors including:
  - Increased circulating free fatty acids due to dietary fat.
  - Increased release of free fatty acids from adipose tissue due to increased stores found in obesity and insulin resistance.
  - Increased de novo lipogenesis in the liver.
  - Impaired fatty acid oxidation in the liver.
  - Decreased export of lipids from the liver as VLDL. Another theory is that hepatic steatosis is in fact a protective and adaptive mechanism in response to excess fat intake.

Steatohepatitis
- One theory is the "two hit" hypothesis which proposes a stepwise process where steatosis is the first "hit" and inflammation/fibrosis is the second "hit". Several possible mechanisms may be involved in the "second hit" that leads to additional features of liver injury found in NASH.
- Possible mediators of inflammation are:
  - Gut-derived endotoxin.
  - Proinflammatory cytokines TNF-α, IL-6 released by adipose tissue.
  - Endoplasmic reticulum stress.

Genetic predictors
- Genome wide association studies have found a single nucleotide polymorphism variant in the gene encoding PNPLA3 that is associated with NAFLD. PNPLA3 encodes a protein that belongs to the patatin-like phospholipase domain-containing family. Its function remains unclear; however, it appears to be involved in hydrolysis of triglycerides. Interestingly, the association between the PNPLA3 variant and NAFLD is independent of insulin resistance.

Predictive/risk factors

Risk factor	Odds ratio
Metabolic syndrome	4.68
Type 2 diabetes mellitus	3.37
Hypertension	2.21
Obesity	1.10–1.12
PNPLA3 rs738409 gene variant	3.26

Section 2: Prevention

- No specific interventions have been shown to prevent the development of the disease.

Screening

- No widely accepted screening methods exist. Prevalence rates of NAFLD are highest in patients with obesity, metabolic syndrome, type 2 diabetes mellitus, and dyslipidemia. Therefore, a targeted screening approach might be to screen these patients with ALT and/or ultrasound. This has not been studied and is not endorsed by guidelines.

Section 3: Diagnosis

CLINICAL PEARLS
- Careful history taking to exclude alcohol-associated liver disease is important in making the diagnosis, although some patients may have both alcoholic and non-alcoholic (metabolic/insulin resistance-associated) liver disease.
- Physical examination findings may include increased BMI, increased waist circumference, hypertension and acanthosis nigricans associated with insulin resistance.
- Laboratory findings are ALT > AST (usually 1–2 × ULN and are rarely >5 × ULN), elevated GGT, elevated ferritin (in approximately 50% of cases). AST and ALT can be normal even in cases of advanced fibrosis. Low titer ANA (≤1:320) can be found in up to 25% of patients with NAFLD.
- Abdominal imaging (US, CT scan or MRI) may demonstrate evidence of steatosis. US findings include increased echogenicity to detect 30% or more of fatty infiltration.
- There are no well-validated non-invasive biomarkers or imaging methods that can differentiate NASH from simple steatosis.

Differential diagnosis

Differential diagnosis	Features
Alcoholic liver disease	AST > ALT, elevated MCV, leukocytosis
	History of excessive alcohol intake (>40 g/day in men, >20 g/day in women)
Wilson disease	Low ceruloplasmin, elevated 24 hour urine copper, Kayser–Fleischer rings, neurologic symptoms
Viral hepatitis (HBV, HCV)	+HBsAg, +HCV Ab and RNA
Drug-induced liver injury	Recent new medications/herbal use
	Tamoxifen, amiodarone, valproic acid, antiretroviral agents and TPN have been associated with steatohepatitis on biopsy

Typical presentation

- Most patients are asymptomatic and present with incidentally noted liver enzyme elevation on routine blood tests or incidental fatty liver on imaging ordered for unrelated symptoms (such as abdominal US to rule out cholelithiasis). A subset of patients present with end stage complications of cirrhosis or hepatocellular carcinoma. This highlights the "silent nature" of NASH during the early stages of disease (much like chronic viral hepatitis).

Clinical diagnosis

History

- Careful assessment of alcohol intake is important in excluding alcoholic liver disease, which can cause identical or similar histologic findings to NASH.
- Assessment of a family history of metabolic syndrome is important in supporting a diagnosis of NASH. A review of systems assessment should include inquiry about associated conditions: diabetes mellitus, dyslipidemia, hypertension, obstructive sleep apnea, polycystic ovary syndrome, chronic hepatitis C. Medications associated with secondary NASH including amiodarone, TPN and antiretroviral drugs should be reviewed.
- The patient should be asked about weight gain and lifestyle factors including exercise and diet, with particular attention to intake of high fructose corn syrup containing foods and foods high in trans fats. Extreme degrees of rapid weight loss can also cause NASH. Therefore recent weight reduction surgery or other causes of weight loss may be revealed.

Physical examination

- Physical examination assessment should include anthropometric measurements (height, weight, waist circumference).
- In addition, the examination should include assessment for associated conditions: metabolic syndrome (blood pressure), insulin resistance (acanthosis nigricans), polycystic ovary syndrome (hirsutism) and obstructive sleep apnea. Lipodystrophy may be present in congenital associated causes of NASH or in NASH caused by antiretroviral therapy.

Useful clinical decision rules and calculators

- The HOMA (homeostasis model assessment) index can be used to estimate the presence of insulin resistance.

$$\frac{\text{fasting insulin (mIU/mL)} \times \text{fasting glucose (mmol/L)}}{22.5}$$

  - Convert glucose from mg/dL to mmol/L by multiplying by 0.0555.
  - HOMA >2.5 indicates insulin resistance.
- Metabolic syndrome definition (National Cholesterol Education Program Adult Treatment Panel III Guidelines). Three or more of the following criteria:
  1. Abdominal obesity (waist circumference: men >102 cm, women >88 cm*)
  2. Triglycerides ≥150 mg/dL
  3. Low HDL (men <40 mg/dL, women <50 mg/dL)
  4. Hypertension (BP ≥130/85 mmHg)
  5. Fasting glucose ≥100 mg/dL

*Note lower waist circumference threshold for Asians: men >90 cm, women >80 cm

Disease severity classification

- Histologic grading and staging of NASH is based on the Brunt classification criteria:
  - Grade 1: steatosis <33%, occasional ballooning, mild lobular inflammation, none or mild portal inflammation.
  - Grade 2: steatosis 33–66%, zone 3 ballooning, mild lobular inflammation, mild to moderate portal inflammation.

- Grade 3: steatosis >66%, marked ballooning (predominantly zone 3), acute and chronic lobular inflammation, mild to moderate portal inflammation.
  - Stage 1: zone 3 perivenular perisinusoidal/pericellular fibrosis.
  - Stage 2: periportal fibrosis.
  - Stage 3: bridging fibrosis.
  - Stage 4: cirrhosis.
- The NAS score was developed as a histologic scoring system for use in clinical trials to assess for improvement in histologic features of NASH on paired biopsy specimens before and after treatment intervention.
- NAS score = unweighted sum of:
  - Steatosis (0–3: <5%, 5–33%, 33–66%, >66%).
  - Lobular inflammation (0–3: none, mild, moderate, severe).
  - Ballooning (0–2: none, few, many).

Laboratory diagnosis

List of diagnostic tests
- While aminotransferase levels are often elevated in NAFLD, normal aminotransferases can be found in up to 50% of cases.
- Liver tests and non-invasive biomarkers cannot distinguish between simple steatosis and NASH.
- When elevated, the usual pattern associated with NASH is ALT > AST.
- AST and ALT elevations are rarely higher than 5–10 × ULN.
- GGT is often moderately elevated.
- Tests to exclude other causes of liver disease: HBsAg, hepatitis C antibody, autoimmune markers. Consider iron studies, alpha-1 antitrypsin phenotype and ceruloplasmin in select cases.

List of imaging techniques
- US can detect >30% steatosis with over 80% sensitivity.
- CT scan and MRI are more sensitive than US and should be considered over US in situations where hepatocellular carcinoma screening or detection is warranted (e.g. suspected cirrhosis, liver mass on ultrasound). Another alternative is contrast enhanced ultrasound, although this is not widely available in the USA.
- Magnetic resonance spectroscopy is an MRI technique which can directly measure hepatic triglyceride content with high levels of sensitivity. Its use at this time is limited to clinical trials.
- The diagnosis of NASH can only be made with liver biopsy. However, sampling variability may underestimate the severity of liver injury in up to 30% of patients.

Potential pitfalls/common errors made regarding diagnosis of disease

- Failure to obtain an accurate history of excessive alcohol intake. See Chapter 10 on alcoholic hepatitis for screening questionnaires to assess patients for significant alcohol intake.
- While a clinical diagnosis of presumed steatohepatitis can be made from history, laboratory tests and imaging, there are no available non-invasive tests to distinguish simple steatosis from steatohepatitis. Liver biopsy remains the gold standard for differentiating simple steatosis from

steatohepatitis. Biopsy may also be indicated to distinguish between autoimmune hepatitis and NAFLD in a patient with elevated ANA titers.

Section 4: Treatment
Treatment rationale

- NASH is a potentially progressive disease associated with a shortened life expectancy. Therefore, effective treatment options are needed. There are currently no approved pharmacologic treatments for NAFLD. Lifestyle modification and treatment of features of underlying metabolic syndrome remains the mainstay of management. No large trials comparing different diets exist; however, a diet low in saturated/trans fats and high fructose corn syrup containing products may be considered based on evidence linking these dietary factors with fatty liver. Exercise has been shown in one retrospective study to be associated with less disease severity of NASH. However specific exercise recommendations are lacking. Patients who are overweight or obese should target a goal weight loss of 10% over 3 months. Morbidly obese patients may benefit from weight reduction surgery, which has been shown to result in regression of fibrosis in patients with NASH. Bariatric surgery should not be performed in patients with decompensated NASH cirrhosis due to perioperative surgical risk associated with cirrhosis. There is no evidence to support the use of pharmacologic weight loss agents. Furthermore, over the counter herbal weight reduction products should be avoided in light of emerging case reports of hepatotoxicity and liver failure due to some of these agents.
- A prospective, randomized, placebo-controlled study called the PIVENS trial found a significant benefit from oral Vitamin E 800 IU daily compared with placebo in non-diabetic patients with NASH. However, only a minority of patients had histologic resolution of definite NASH and no improvement was found in fibrosis scores in any treatment arm.
- Insulin sensitizing agents such as thiazolidinediones and metformin have not been shown to clearly benefit patients with NASH; however, small pilot studies show short-term improvement in ALT and some histologic features (steatosis and inflammation but not fibrosis) with pioglitazone. It is reasonable to consider the use of these agents to treat diabetic patients with NASH. However, there is no data to support using these agents in the absence of diabetes.
- The potential beneficial effects of vitamin E and pioglitazone in NASH should be weighed against the increased mortality associated with vitamin E ($\geq$400 IU/day) and severe heart failure associated with pioglitazone. In addition, thiazolidinediones induce weight gain.

Table of treatment

Treatment	Comment
Conservative treatment	Weight loss in patients who are overweight or obese (10% over 3 months) Dietary modification in all patients Exercise in all patients
Medical	No effective pharmacological treatment available Consider thiazolidinediones or metformin in diabetic patients with NASH
Surgical	Bariatric surgery – morbidly obese patients, particularly with diabetes and/or other medical indications for weight loss surgery

Prevention/management of complications

- Rapid weight loss (>1.6 kg/week) associated with early bariatric surgery techniques that are no longer used should be avoided due to worsening of NASH.
- Screen for and manage metabolic syndrome: dyslipidemia, heart disease, diabetes mellitus.
- Screen for hepatocellular carcinoma in patients with NASH and cirrhosis.

Management/treatment

See Algorithm 11.1.

Algorithm 11.1 Diagnostic evaluation and treatment of patients with NAFLD

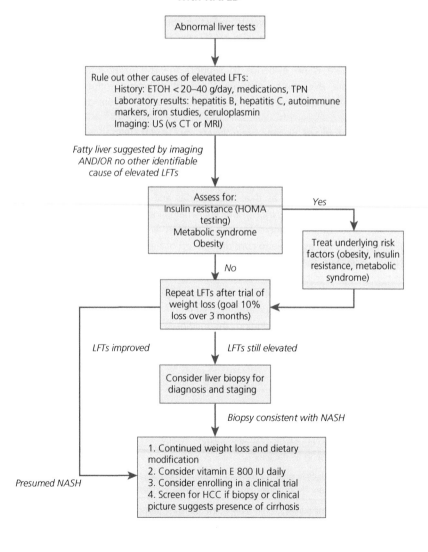

CLINICAL PEARLS
- There are currently no approved pharmacologic treatments for NAFLD.
- Lifestyle modification (weight loss, diet and exercise) and treatment of any features of underlying metabolic syndrome remains the mainstay of management.

Section 5: Special Populations

Not applicable for this topic.

Section 6: Prognosis

CLINICAL PEARLS
- Simple steatosis carries a benign prognosis.
- Prognosis of NASH is variable; natural history studies to date demonstrate that only a subset of patients with NASH (25–33%) develop progressive fibrosis over time. Predictive risk factors for disease progression are an area of active investigation. Some studies suggest that older age, diabetes mellitus and obesity may be factors that predict disease progression.
- Patients with NASH have decreased survival compared with the general population; comorbid cardiovascular disease accounts for a major cause of morbidity in patients with NASH.
- Rates of liver transplantation for NASH cirrhosis have been increasing.

Natural history of untreated disease
See "Clinical pearls" in this section.

Prognosis for treated patients
See Section 4: Treatment.

Follow-up tests and monitoring
- Patients with NASH cirrhosis should undergo regular surveillance imaging to screen for hepatocellular carcinoma.

Section 7: Reading List

Brunt E. Nonalcoholic steatohepatitis: definition and pathology. Semin Liver Dis 2001;21:3–16

Chalasani N, Younossi Z, Lavine J, et al. The diagnosis and management of non-alcoholic fatty liver disease: practice guideline by the American Association for the Study of Liver Diseases, American College of Gastroenterology, and the American Gastroenterological Association. Hepatology 2012;55:2005–23

Day CP, James OF. Steatohepatitis: a tale of two 'hits'? Gastroenterology 1998;114:842–5

Farrell GC, Chitturi S, Lau GK, et al. Guidelines for the assessment and management of non-alcoholic fatty liver disease in the Asia-Pacific region: executive summary. J Gastroenterol Hepatol 2007;22:775–7

Kleiner D, Brunt E, Van Natta M, et al. Design and validation of a histological scoring system for nonalcoholic fatty liver disease. Hepatology 2005;41:1313–21

Lazo M, Clark JM. The epidemiology of nonalcoholic fatty liver disease: a global perspective. Semin Liver Dis 2008;28:339–50

Ratziu V, Bellentani S, Cortez-Pinto H, Day C, Marchesini G. A position statement on NAFLD/NAS based on the EASL 2009 special conference. J Hepatol 2010;53:372–84

Sanyal A, Chalasani N, Kowdley K, et al. Pioglitazone, vitamin E, or placebo for nonalcoholic steatohepatitis. N Eng J Med 2010;362:1675–85

Wanless IR, Lentz JS. Fatty liver hepatitis (steatohepatitis) and obesity: an autopsy study with analysis of risk factors. Hepatology 1990;12:1106–10

Section 8: Guidelines
National society guidelines

Guideline title	Guideline source	Date
The diagnosis and management of non-alcoholic fatty liver disease: practice guideline by the American Association for the Study of Liver Diseases, American College of Gastroenterology, and the American Gastroenterological Association	American Association of Liver Diseases (AASLD), American College of Gastroenterology (ACG), and the American Gastroenterological Association (AGA) http://www.aasld.org/practiceguidelines/Documents/NonalcoholicFattyLiverDise ase2012_25762_ftp.pdf	2011

International society guidelines

Guideline title	Guideline source	Date
A position statement on NAFLD/NAS based on the EASL 2009 special conference	European Association for the Study of the Liver (EASL) http://f.i-md.com/medinfo/material/714/4e113707e4b02d0c1e8d2714/494B559E82E5F1F07D8015701B2ABFC6.pdf or http://ac.els-cdn.com/S0168827810004149/1-s2.0-S0168827810004149-main.pdf?_tid=064066cc-4ca0-11e3-bc27-00000aacb35e&acdnat=1384373773_4d82d3aa4d4148f7270c4da9eadc8eb0	2009
Guidelines for the assessment and management of non-alcoholic fatty liver disease in the Asia-Pacific region: executive summary	Asia Pacific Working Party for NAFLD http://onlinelibrary.wiley.com/doi/10.1111/j.1440-1746.2007.05002.x/pdf	2007

Section 9: Evidence

Type of evidence	Title, date	Comment
RCT	Pioglitazone, vitamin E or placebo for nonalcoholic steatohepatitis (2010)	Prospective, randomized placebo controlled trial comparing vitamin E 800IU daily vs pioglitazone 30mg daily vs placebo × 96 weeks for non-diabetic patients with NASH. 43% of patients in the vitamin E group showed significant improvement in histologic features of NASH compared with the placebo group. There was no significant improvement in the pioglitazone group compared with placebo

Section 10: Images

Not applicable for this topic.

Additional material for this chapter can be found online at:
www.mountsinaiexpertguides.com
This includes a case study and multiple choice questions

CHAPTER 12

Autoimmune Hepatitis and Overlap Syndromes

Joseph A. Odin

Division of Liver Diseases, Icahn School of Medicine at Mount Sinai, New York, NY, USA

OVERALL BOTTOM LINE
- AIH is characterized by immune-mediated destruction of hepatocytes leading to either acute liver failure or chronic liver disease.
- AIH is most often confused with drug-induced liver disease.
- The disease preferentially affects women under age 60 and typically responds well to treatment with immunosuppressive agents.
- Overlap syndromes exist in which features of both autoimmune hepatitis and cholestatic liver disease are present.

Section 1: Background
Definition of disease
- AIH is a chronic (>6 months) progressive immune-mediated inflammation of the liver, histologically most commonly characterized by an interface hepatitis, biochemically by a marked hypergammaglobulinemia, high titers of autoantibodies, elevated aminotransferases, and clinically by fatigue.
- AIH-overlap syndromes are characterized by the concomitant occurrence of AIH with PBC or PSC.

Disease classification
- Over time the classification of AIH has been changed multiple times. The current classifications are:

Type 1 AIH
- The most common form of AIH. It is distinguished by serum ANA or ASMA, elevated IgG levels and elevated aminotransferase levels.

Type 2 AIH
- Distinguished by anti-LKM autoantibodies in the presence of elevated aminotransferase levels. This form of AIH more often occurs in children and is more common in Europe than the USA.
- Of patients with the autoimmune polyglandular syndrome 1 10–15% also have type 2 AIH.

Type 3 AIH
- Characterized by antibodies against soluble antigen from liver and pancreas (anti-SLA/LP) in the presence of elevated aminotransferase levels.

Mount Sinai Expert Guides: Hepatology, First Edition. Edited by Jawad Ahmad, Scott L. Friedman, and Henryk Dancygier.
© 2014 John Wiley & Sons, Ltd. Published 2014 by John Wiley & Sons, Ltd.
Companion website: www.mountsinaiexpertguides.com

AIH–PBC overlap syndrome

- Infrequently individuals meet criteria for both AIH and PBC with both ANA and AMA present. Histology and significantly elevated aminotransferases consistent with AIH are usually required for this diagnosis beyond just the presence of ANA and AMA together.

AIH–PSC overlap syndrome

- In addition to meeting criteria for AIH, evidence of extra- or intra-hepatic bile duct stenosis/ dilatation is observed. This uncommon overlap is more frequent in children and may be a triad of disease that includes IBD.

Prevalence

- The overall disease prevalence is approximately 10 in 10000 and peak onset is typically in young or middle-aged individuals.
- The prevalence is threefold higher in women than men.

Economic impact

- Due to the limited number of affected individuals the overall economic impact of AIH is not very high; however, the costs for individual treatment can be high since lifelong treatment with immunosuppressive drugs and possibly liver transplantation may be necessary.
- According to UNOS a single liver transplant costs $314600 on average with annual follow up care costs averaging $21900.

Etiology

- Drug or environmental toxin exposures may trigger an autoimmune response directed against hepatocytes. A classic example is halothane exposure triggering AIH.

Pathophysiology

- The mechanism by which a drug or environmental toxin induces AIH is uncertain. There may be cross-reactivity with a self-antigen or exposure may lead to modification of a self-antigen making it immunogenic.
- Activation of autoreactive lymphocytes leads to primarily T-cell mediated destruction of hepatocytes, chiefly in zone 1 of the hepatic lobule bordering the portal tract (i.e. interface hepatitis).
- The disease activity may flare periodically with long quiescent periods or more rarely progress slowly to cirrhosis without any flares. In the latter group, aminotransferase levels may be relatively normal.

Risk factors

- Age (less than 60) and gender (female) are the primary risk factors.
- Those with other autoimmune diseases are more likely to develop AIH.
- Pregnancy is also a risk factor for disease onset and flares.
- Medications including minocycline and nitrofurantoin may cause a drug-induced AIH.

Section 2: Prevention

- Prevention of AIH is not generally considered feasible beyond avoidance of drugs and toxins known to induce AIH.

Screening

- Screening for AIH is not cost effective in any at risk group.

Primary prevention

- Avoid drugs or toxins known to induce AIH.

Secondary prevention

- Maintenance immunosuppressive therapy reduces the number of disease flares in individuals diagnosed with recurrent AIH.

Section 3: Diagnosis (Algorithm 12.1)

CLINICAL PEARLS
- AIH should be suspected in any person who presents with unexplained fatigue or jaundice and elevated aminotransferase levels, particularly younger women.
- ANA, ASMA, and anti-LKM levels should be checked.
- If these autoantibodies are absent in the presence of cryptogenic chronic hepatitis, anti-SLA/LP should be checked.
- A liver biopsy should be performed if AIH is suspected.
- The elevation in serum AST and ALT levels usually occurs at a 1:1 ratio.
- If AP or GGT levels are also significantly elevated, additional evaluation should be done to rule out alcoholic hepatitis or cholestatic liver disease (e.g. PBC, PSC).
- A validated scoring system has been developed by the IAIHG to aid in diagnosis since many features of autoimmune hepatitis are non-specific.
- Patients with type 3 AIH (anti-SLA/LP positive) do not differ from those with classic type 1 AIH with respect to age, gender and the response to immunosuppressive therapy. Antibodies against SLA/LP do not define a clinically discrete form of AIH, but they may be regarded as a specific diagnostic marker of AIH. The search for anti-SLA/LP attains special importance in patients with cryptogenic chronic hepatitis. Approximately 25% of these patients have anti-SLA/LP in serum, allowing for a change in diagnosis from cryptogenic hepatitis to AIH in which conventional autoantibodies are absent.

Simplified diagnostic criteria for AIH (Source: Hennes et al, 2008. Reproduced with permission of John Wiley & Sons Ltd.)

Variable	Cut-off	Points
ANA or SMA	≥1:40	1
ANA or SMA	≥1:80	2*
Or LKM	≥1:40	
Or SLA	Positive	
IgG	> ULN	1
	>1.1 × ULN	2
Liver histology	Compatible with AIH	1
	Typical AIH	2
Absence of viral hepatitis	Yes	2
		≥6 Probable AIH
		≥7 Definite AIH

*Addition of points achieved for all autoantibodies (maximum, 2 points)

Differential diagnosis

Differential diagnosis	Features
PBC	AMA and elevated AP levels are detectable along with intra-hepatic portal tract inflammation
PSC	Extra- and/or intra-hepatic abnormalities of the biliary tree are detectable on imaging. Atypical p-ANCA more likely present and associated with IBD
Viral hepatitis	Serological evidence of viral infection
Drug-induced liver injury	History of drug or toxin exposure. If LFT elevations persist after discontinuation of exposure, AIH may be present
Wilson disease	Kayser–Fleischer rings may be present. Low serum ceruloplasmin and high urinary copper level. Neurological or behavioral changes may be present

Typical presentation
- Asymptomatic or symptoms of fatigue, anorexia, nausea and abdominal pain.
- Although AIH is a chronic disease acute presentation occurs in 25% of patients.
- Elevated serum aminotransferase levels (three – 10-fold) above the upper limit of normal. Elevated serum IgG levels. Positive titers of autoantibodies.

Clinical diagnosis
History
- Individuals with AIH may complain of several weeks of fatigue, yellow eyes and jaundice along with RUQ pain.
- A careful history is required to rule out any potential hepatotoxic exposures or risk factors for viral hepatitis. A personal or family history of autoimmune disease makes the diagnosis of AIH more likely. A history of IBD raises the possibility of PSC or an overlap syndrome.
- A history of recent travel increases the likelihood of an infectious etiology.
- Complaints of confusion suggest a more severe episode of AIH.
- Others may present with symptoms of hepatic decompensation due to cirrhosis such as GI bleeding, ascites or confusion.

Physical examination
- General physical examination:
  - Normal or
  - Signs of chronic liver disease in those presenting with cirrhosis.
- Systemic examination:
  - Abdominal examination: hepatosplenomegaly, tenderness.
  - Eye examination: icteric sclerae.
  - Skin examination: jaundice.
Neurological examination: asterixis and confusion in those with acute liver failure or advanced cirrhosis.

Clinical decision rules
- AIH should be suspected in anyone presenting with liver disease without a known etiology.
- A liver biopsy is required for a definitive diagnosis of AIH.
- The response to treatment with glucocorticoids may aid in the diagnosis. Alternative diagnoses should be reviewed if there is minimal decrease in ALT/AST levels.

- Simplified criteria for the diagnosis of AIH may be useful in clinical practice but have yet to be prospectively validated (see Table: Simplified diagnostic criteria for AIH).

Disease severity classification
- Histological staging is required for evaluating disease severity in most cases. For those with acute liver failure, the King's College criteria are used for evaluating disease severity. The Child–Pugh score or MELD score is used for those with cirrhosis.

Laboratory diagnosis
- Serum LFTs: increased ALT and AST levels disproportionately greater than AP or GGT levels are observed. Usually the higher the elevation, the more severe the hepatitis. ALT/AST elevations over 1000 IU/L are not uncommon.
- Serological findings: positive ANA and ASMA titers are noted in type 1 AIH. Anti-LKM autoantibodies are observed in type 2 AIH. Anti-SLA /LP autoantibodies are present in both types, but do also occur alone in type 3 AIH. AMA are detected in AIH-PBC overlap syndrome. Atypical p-ANCA are more common in AIH-PSC overlap syndrome. Serum hypergammaglobulinemia (especially IgG) is associated with AIH.

Pathologic features on liver biopsy
- The liver biopsy features of AIH are non-specific and variable depending on the disease classification and stage.
  - Interface hepatitis.
  - A portal plasma cell infiltrate.
  - Bridging necrosis.
  - Biliary tree abnormalities may suggest overlap with PBC or PSC.

Imaging techniques
- US or CT abdomen: may show hepatomegaly or changes associated with cirrhosis depending on the stage of disease.
- MRCP or ERCP: beading or pruning of the biliary tree may be seen in PSC or AIH-PSC overlap syndrome.

Associated conditions
- Autoimmune thyroid disease.
- Type I diabetes.
- Ulcerative colitis.
- Synovitis.
- PBC, PSC.
- Autoimmune polyglandular syndrome 1.

Potential pitfalls/common errors in diagnosis
- Differentiating drug- or toxin-induced liver injury versus drug-induced autoimmune hepatitis may be difficult.
- A positive ANA or ASMA and elevated LFTs are most closely associated with AIH yet frequently occur (in low titer) in other liver diseases including NAFLD.
- Not to look for anti-SLA/LP in patients with cryptogenic hepatitis.
- In those diagnosed with PBC or PSC, a diagnosis of AIH overlap requires histological changes consistent with AIH along with characteristic serological abnormalities.
- In those presenting with cirrhosis, the diagnosis of AIH may be missed because of absent hepatic inflammation on liver biopsy (i.e. "burnt out AIH").

Algorithm 12.1 Diagnosis of autoimmune liver disease

Serological tests for AIH. The initial serological tests include ANA, SMA, antibodies LKM-1, and AMA. If one or more tests are positive, the diagnosis of AIH or PBC (AMA+) should be pursued. If these tests are negative, other serological assessments are appropriate, including tests for antibodies to actin (F-actin), SLA/LP, liver cytosol type 1 (LC-1), UDP-glucuronosyltransferases (LKM-3), the E2 subunits of the PDH complex (PDH-E2), pANCA. The results of these supplemental tests may suggest other diagnoses, including PSC, or cryptogenic chronic hepatitis.

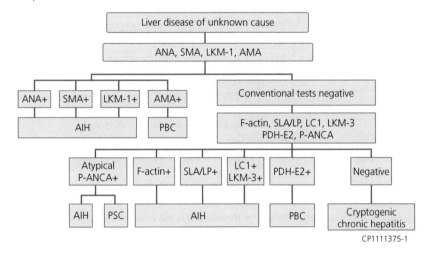

CP1111375-1

Source: Manns MP, et al. American Association for the Study of Liver Diseases. Diagnosis and management of autoimmune hepatitis. Hepatology. 2010 Jun;51(6):2193-213. Reproduced with permission of John Wiley & Sons Ltd.

Section 4: Treatment
Treatment rationale
- The basic treatment rationale is that reduced hepatic inflammation prevents AIH progression. Normalization of serum LFTs is employed as a marker of reduced hepatic inflammation. However, liver biopsy is recommended to confirm decreased hepatic inflammation.

Specific management for AIH patients
- Immunosuppression with glucocorticoids (prednisone, prednisilone, or budesonide) is the mainstay of treatment for those with active hepatitis. The initial dose and titration of glucocorticoids may be adjusted depending on the degree of hepatitis. Glucocorticoid treatment may be tapered off after 1 year if liver serum biochemistries have normalized.
- Maintenance therapy is typically started at the same time as glucocorticoids. Azathioprine is typically used for maintenance therapy and continued for 1–2 years after initial diagnosis.
- A liver biopsy should be performed after 1 year of therapy to guide further treatment.
- For those who do not completely respond to glucocorticoid treatment or have severe side-effects, alternative immunosuppressive medications (e.g. mycophenylate mofetil) may be administered.
- Hepatitis A and B vaccination if not already immune.

When to hospitalize
- Patients with a severe flare or fulminant liver failure should be hospitalized until LFTs begin to decline in response to treatment.
- Patients with severe complications of cirrhosis.

Table of treatment

Treatment	Comment
Medical: Initial episode or subsequent flare • Prednisone (up to 60 mg daily initially for 2–4 weeks followed by a slow taper to 5–10 mg daily for 6–24 months) and azathioprine (2–3 mg/kg daily) • Budesonide (3 mg tid or 9 mg qd) and azathioprine (2–3 mg/kg daily)	• Adjustments in dosage and length of treatment may be made depending on the degree of hepatitis and the response to treatment • Treatment with azathioprine alone may be effective after normalization of LFTs • A liver biopsy after one year of treatment is useful in guiding further therapy since LFTs may not reflect hepatic inflammation • Side effects due to systemic steroid treatment must be treated as needed • Azathioprine may cause cytopenias
Refractory AIH • Mycophenylate mofetil (500–1000 mg twice daily)	• Persistent elevated LFTs or hepatic inflammation on biopsy should prompt alternative immunosuppressive therapy • Diarrhea, rash, and anemia are common side effects of mycophenolate mofetil
Acute liver failure • Glucocorticoids and/or N-acetylcysteine depending on the status of the patient	• Hospitalization and evaluation for liver transplantation should be initiated
Maintenance therapy • Azathioprine (50–150 mg daily) (based on 2010 AASLD guidelines)	• It is recommended for those who have had a disease flare after completing treatment for their initial episode.
AIH cirrhosis • Immunosuppressive agents	• Initiation or continuation of immunosuppression may be beneficial in well compensated cirrhosis due to AIH
Overlap syndromes • Addition of ursodeoxycholic acid (13–15 mg/kg/day)	• Guidelines for the treatment of PBC and PSC should be incorporated into the treatment of AIH

Prevention/management of complications
- Those on systemic glucocorticoid therapy should be advised about complications associated with its use and an information brochure should be given that lists common side effects. It is recommended to use the least possible dose for the shortest duration.
- Glucocorticoid sparing agents should be used rather than maintaining patients on long-term, high-dose glucocorticoid treatment.
- Increased vigilance for hematological and skin cancers while on immunosuppressive agents is needed.

CLINICAL PEARLS
- Reliance solely on liver biochemistries and IgG levels to guide therapy may lead to undertreatment of AIH.
- Liver biochemistries may be normal while liver biopsy reveals significant inflammatory activity.
- Budesonide has proven more effective than prednisone in some recent clinical trials.
- Cirrhosis may develop early on (in up to 30% within a year).
- In cirrhosis due to AIH, liver biopsy may show few signs of prior inflammatory activity.

Section 5: Special Populations
Pregnancy
- AIH may present in late pregnancy or during the immediate post-partum period. It is safe to continue prednisone during pregnancy.

Children
- AIH-PSC overlap is as common as type 1 AIH in children. All children with a diagnosis of AIH should be screened for PSC.

Other
- Decompensated cirrhosis and fulminant liver failure: use of high-dose immunosuppressive medications may increase the risk of life-threatening infections and should be avoided in the immediate pre-transplant period.

Section 6: Prognosis

> **CLINICAL PEARLS**
> - A careful history is required to rule out drug or toxin-induced hepatitis.
> - A liver biopsy after one year of therapy is needed to guide management.
> - Steroid sparing agents such as azathioprine should be prescribed to avoid side effects from long-term glucocorticoid therapy.

Natural history of untreated disease
- If left untreated, AIH will lead to either fulminant liver failure or cirrhosis.

Prognosis for treated patients
- Ninety percent of patients have a complete response to immunosuppressive therapy upon their initial presentation.
- Of those who do not respond, liver transplantation is an option.
- Of those who have a complete response, 50–80% will have a recurrence within 5 years. Maintenance therapy is recommended after a recurrence resolves to prevent progression to cirrhosis.

Follow-up tests and monitoring
- Once in remission, repeat liver biochemistries every 6 months.
- For those on azathioprine, repeat complete blood count with platelets every 6 months.
- For those on glucocorticoid therapy, monitoring for diabetes, cataracts, glaucoma and osteoporosis should be performed regularly.
- For those with AIH cirrhosis, routine follow up for hepatic decompensation and screening for HCC is required.

Section 7: Reading List

Boberg KM, Chapman RW, Hirschfield GM, Lohse AW, Manns MP, Schrumpf E; International Autoimmune Hepatitis Group. Overlap syndromes: the International Autoimmune Hepatitis Group (IAIHG) position statement on a controversial issue. J Hepatol 2011;54:374–85

Hennes EM, Zeniya M, Czaja AJ, et al.; International Autoimmune Hepatitis Group. Simplified criteria for the diagnosis of autoimmune hepatitis. Hepatology 2008;48:169–76

Herkel J, Heidrich B, Nieraad N, et al. Fine specificity of autoantibodies to soluble liver antigen and liver/pancreas. Hepatology 2002;35: 403–8

Kanzler S, Weidemann C, Gerken G, et al. Clinical significance of autoantibodies to soluble liver antigen in autoimmune hepatitis. J Hepatol 1999;31: 635–40

Mieli-Vergani G, Vergani D. Autoimmune hepatitis in children: what is different from adult AIH? Semin Liver Dis 2009; 29:297–306

Section 8: Guidelines
National society guidelines

Guideline title	Guideline source	Date
Diagnosis and management of autoimmune hepatitis	American Association for the Study of Liver Diseases (AASLD) http://www.aasld.org/practiceguidelines/Documents/AIH2010.pdf	2010

Section 9: Evidence

See Guidelines listed in Section 8.

Section 10: Images

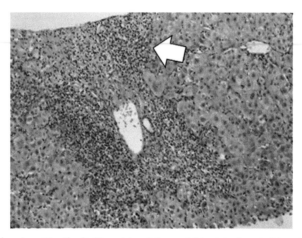

Figure 12.1 Interface hepatitis. The limiting plate of the portal tract is disrupted by a lymphoplasmacytic infiltrate (white arrow). H&E × 200. Source: Manns MP, et al. American Association for the Study of Liver Diseases. Diagnosis and management of autoimmune hepatitis. Hepatology. 2010 Jun;51(6):2193-213. Reproduced with permission of John Wiley & Sons Ltd.

Additional material for this chapter can be found online at:
www.mountsinaiexpertguides.com
This includes a case study and multiple choice questions

CHAPTER 13

Primary Biliary Cirrhosis

Nancy Bach and Joseph A. Odin
Division of Liver Diseases, Icahn School of Medicine at Mount Sinai, New York, NY, USA

OVERALL BOTTOM LINE
- PBC is a slowly progressive autoimmune liver disease that causes destruction to the small- and medium-sized intrahepatic bile ducts.
- Most patients with PBC are diagnosed after abnormal liver chemistries are noted on routine testing. However, some patients come to medical attention because of complaints of fatigue and pruritus.
- The cholestatic liver chemistries (AP and GGT) are elevated and more than 95% of patients have a positive AMA.
- Ursodeoxycholic acid (13–15 mg/kg/day) is considered the treatment standard of care.
- Though PBC can cause significant portal hypertension and other complications of ESLD including the rare development of HCC, the majority of patients do not die of liver disease.

Section 1: Background
Definition of disease
- PBC is a chronic disease of unknown cause in which the small- and medium-sized intrahepatic bile ducts are progressively destroyed.
- The first description of PBC may date back to the 1800s when cases of "xanthomatous cirrhosis" and "biliary cirrhosis without biliary obstruction" were described. The term "primary biliary cirrhosis" was first coined in 1950 and the first full description of the disease appeared in the *New England Journal of Medicine* in 1973.

Incidence/prevalence
- The incidence and prevalence of this disease varies worldwide; PBC is most common in Northeast Europe and Scandinavia. The prevalence decreases with decreasing latitude.
- In the USA the disease prevalence is estimated at about 40 cases per 100 000 and the incidence is around three cases per 100 000.
- The prevalence of AMA in the general population may be as high as one in 200 (0.5%).
- The incidence and prevalence of the disease appear to be rising.
- Relatives of patients with PBC have a 1–5% risk of developing/having the disease.
- The prevalence is ninefold higher in women compared to men.

Mount Sinai Expert Guides: Hepatology, First Edition. Edited by Jawad Ahmad, Scott L. Friedman, and Henryk Dancygier.
© 2014 John Wiley & Sons, Ltd. Published 2014 by John Wiley & Sons, Ltd.
Companion website: www.mountsinaiexpertguides.com

Etiology

- The exact etiology of PBC remains unknown but both genetic predisposition and environmental exposure are important.
- Significant associations between PBC and common genetic variants of the HLA Class II, IL12A and IL12RB2 loci suggest that the interleukin 12 immunoregulatory signaling axis is relevant to the pathophysiology of the disease. Thus, most individuals have a genetic predisposition to the disease.
- Several groups have shown an increased familial prevalence of the disease ranging from 1% to 5%.
- Exposure to various microbes and xenobiotics including tobacco smoke, have been associated with the disease.

Pathology/pathogenesis

- PBC is an autoimmune disease characterized by the presence of highly specific AMA and bile duct destruction mediated by autoreactive T cells. Loss of self-tolerance appears to be due to exposure either to a cross-reactive microbial or xenobiotic antigen and/or modification of self-antigens. Poor macrophage clearance of apoptotic biliary epithelial cells and autophagy may contribute to inappropriate cell surface presentation of mitochondrial self-antigens by healthy biliary epithelial cells. These cells are then targeted for destruction by autoreactive T cells.
- Eventually bile duct loss is significant enough to lead to cholestasis and possibly cirrhosis. For unknown reasons, portal hypertension and esophageal variceal bleeding may occur earlier than expected.

Risk factors

- Female gender.
- History of urinary tract infections.
- More likely to use nail polish.
- Likely to have smoked cigarettes.
- More likely to live or have lived near toxic waste site.
- More likely to have used reproductive hormone replacement therapy.

Section 2: Prevention

CLINICAL PEARLS
- No intervention has been demonstrated to prevent the development of the disease.

Section 3: Diagnosis (Algorithm 13.1)

- The diagnosis of PBC is based on finding two out of following three:
  - Elevated cholestatic liver biochemistries (AP and GGT).
  - AMA greater than 1:20.
  - Histologic findings consistent with primary biliary cirrhosis including florid duct lesions and non-caseating granulomas.
- The AMA is considered the hallmark of the disease and is highly sensitive and specific for the disease (present in >95% of patients).
- Serum IgM is typically increased.

Differential diagnosis

Differential diagnosis	Features
AIH	ANA, interface hepatitis on histology, and ALT/AST much greater than AP
Autoimmune cholangitis	Serum AMA negative, ANA positive in high titer, high IgG, liver biopsy consistent with PBC
Overlap AIH/PBC	Features of PBC and AIH. Higher ALT and IgG levels than in typical PBC. Bile duct damage and interface hepatitis on liver biopsy
PSC	Cholangiogram with biliary strictures and peribiliary fibrosis on histology
Extrahepatic biliary obstruction	Presence of secondary bile duct obstruction on imaging studies
Sarcoidosis	Absence of AMA; may be difficult to differentiate histologically from PBC
Drug-induced cholestasis	History reveals diagnosis
Idiopathic adulthood ductopenia	Bile duct loss without autoantibodies; no inflammation and fibrosis on histology

Typical presentation
- The typical PBC patient is a middle-aged woman; however, patients have presented as young as their teens and as late as the ninth decade of life.
- Most commonly the patient is asymptomatic but noted to have abnormal liver chemistries during routine blood tests. Other patients are symptomatic and come to medical attention with complaints of fatigue and pruritus.
- Less frequently a patient is diagnosed after presenting with evidence of portal hypertension or complications of cirrhosis.
- Abnormal cholestatic liver chemistries, a positive AMA and a confirmatory liver biopsy most commonly clinch the diagnosis.

Associated diseases
- Sjögren's syndrome.
- CREST syndrome (calcinosis cutis, Raynaud's phenomenon, esophageal dysfunction, sclerodactyly, telangiectasia).
- Other collagen vascular diseases.
- Autoimmune thyroiditis (20% of PBC patients).
- Celiac disease (6% of PBC patients).
- Autoimmune thrombocytopenia.
- Autoimmune hemolytic anemia.
- Interstitial lymphocytic pneumonitis.

Clinical diagnosis
History
- Most patients come to medical attention because they are found to have elevated liver biochemistries during routine testing.

- However, some patients are identified during the investigation of complaints of fatigue and/or pruritus.
- On rare occasions, a patient will present with signs and symptoms of ESLD and a diagnosis of PBC is subsequently made.

Physical examination
- About half the patients with PBC have an enlarged liver and up to a third will have splenomegaly upon presentation. Other physical findings may include xanthelasma, xanthomas and a butterfly pattern of hyperpigmentation on the patients back. Non-specific stigmata of chronic liver disease including spider angiomata, palmar erythema and Dupuytren's contracture may also be noted. Jaundice and/or ascites when present are late findings.

Useful clinical decision rules and calculators
- Treatment with UDCA is the standard of care for all patients with PBC though its benefits may be more profound in those with Stage I–II disease.
- Those without significant improvement in liver biochemistries after one year of treatment should be considered for treatment with novel agents or therapeutic trials.

Disease severity classification
- The Mayo Natural History Model utilizes the serum albumin, total bilirubin, prothrombin time and edema to calculate the estimated probability of short-term survival in PBC (http: www.mayoclinic.org/gi-rst/mayomodel1.html).
- The MELD score is a disease severity scoring system that utilizes the serum bilirubin, creatinine and INR and has been applied to PBC (http://optn.transplant.hrsa.gov/resources/MeldPeld Calculator.asp?index=98).

Laboratory diagnosis
List of diagnostic tests
- Elevated AP and GGT activity that is greater than the increase in ALT or AST activities.
- Elevated bilirubin seen in latter phases of disease.
- Positive AMA.
- Elevated immunoglobulin levels particularly IgM.
- Liver biopsy often performed to confirm diagnosis, assess stage of disease and identify co-existing diseases or overlap with AIH or PSC.
- Histologic features may include the "florid duct lesion" or chronic non-suppurative destruction of the bile ducts, bile ductular proliferation, bile duct loss, fibrosis or frank cirrhosis.

List of imaging techniques
- The following imaging techniques are not performed to diagnose PBC but primarily to exclude other cholestatic liver diseases.
  - Abdominal US to rule out intra- and/or extrahepatic bile duct dilatation, space-occupying lesions.
  - CT or MRI to rule out space-occupying lesions, e.g. HCC if cirrhosis is present or liver metastases.
  - MRCP (or ERCP) if the presence of PSC is uncertain.

Algorithm 13.1 Diagnosis of primary biliary cirrhosis

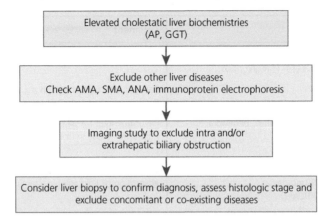

Elevated cholestatic liver biochemistries
(AP, GGT)

↓

Exclude other liver diseases
Check AMA, SMA, ANA, immunoprotein electrophoresis

↓

Imaging study to exclude intra and/or
extrahepatic biliary obstruction

↓

Consider liver biopsy to confirm diagnosis, assess histologic stage and
exclude concomitant or co-existing diseases

Potential pitfalls/common errors made regarding diagnosis of disease

- Though the majority of patients with PBC have a positive AMA (>95%), some patients are AMA negative. AMA negative PBC presents similarly to AMA positive PBC.
- Sarcoidosis and drug-induced liver injury may be difficult to distinguish from PBC.
- Men can have PBC.
- A positive AMA usually pre-dates the development of clinical signs of PBC.
- Family members of affected individuals may have AMA and never develop evidence of disease.
- The term PBC is a misnomer – not all patients have or will develop cirrhosis.

Section 4: Treatment (Algorithm 13.2)

Treatment rationale

- UDCA is the standard for treating PBC. It may be more effective when initiated at the earlier stages I–II of PBC, and should be continued indefinitely. Several randomized controlled trials have shown that UDCA improves biochemical parameters, delays histologic progression and improves transplant free survival. Additionally the number of individuals requiring transplant for PBC has decreased in the UDCA era though a controlled trial has not proven this observation. UDCA can improve or exacerbate pruritus and fatigue.
- Much of the therapy of PBC involves dealing with quality-of-life issues such as pruritus, fatigue, hypercholesterolemia and a "possible" increased risk of osteoporosis.

When to hospitalize

- Evidence of complications of ESLD including variceal bleeding, unmanageable hepatic encephalopathy, hepatorenal syndrome or suspicion of infections such as SBP.

Table of treatment

Treatment	Comment
Medical: Ursodeoxycholic acid (13–15 mg/kg/day)	Most beneficial in stages I–II
Surgical: Liver transplant	Patients with rising bilirubin Patients with uncontrolled complications of ESLD
Psychological (includes cognitive, behavioral therapies): Regular exercise	Recommended for all patients; particularly helpful for those with fatigue
Complementary: Calcium 1200–1500 mg/day Vitamin D 800–100 IU/day Multivitamin	Children's vitamins can be used to improve absorption of lipid soluble vitamins

Prevention/management of complications
- Screening for varices should occur in patients with platelet counts <200000.
- Early studies suggested accelerated bone loss in patients with PBC though more recent data has questioned a direct association of PBC and osteoporosis.
- Hypercholesterolemia is present in 75% of patients with PBC though it is unclear if this increases the risk of atherosclerotic disease in PBC patients.
- The prevalence of significant fatigue varies in different studies. Patients are encouraged to exercise and rest as needed. Small trials have found modafinil (100–200 mg daily) beneficial for those with severe fatigue.
- Pruritus is controlled by cholestyramine (up to 16 g/daily in four divided doses) in the majority of symptomatic patients. Rifampin (150–600 mg daily), naltrexone (12.5–50 mg daily) and sertraline (75–100 mg daily) have also been used with some success.

Algorithm 13.2 Management of primary biliary cirrhosis

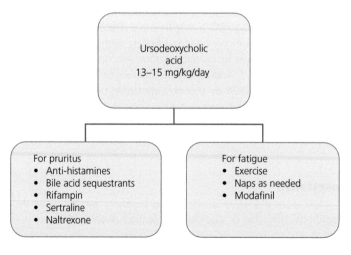

> **CLINICAL PEARLS**
> - UDCA dosing is for 24 hours. Dose can be taken daily or divided as per patients preference and is weight based (13–15 mg/kg/day).
> - UDCA is manufactured as pills or capsules. Patient preference may dictate what prescription is written. If bile acid sequestrants are used for pruritus, other medications including UDCA should not be taken for at least 2 hours before or after.
> - Bile acid sequestrants are most effective when given before and after breakfast.
> - Though pruritus is not histamine related, the sedative effect of antihistamines may be beneficial when given in the evening.

Section 5: Special Populations

Pregnancy

- PBC may present before, during or after pregnancy. Generally pregnant women and their infants do well. Pruritus may be exacerbated during pregnancy. Complications of portal hypertension including variceal bleeding have been reported because of the increased blood volume associated with pregnancy.
- Treatment with UDCA may continue during pregnancy.

Section 6: Prognosis

> **CLINICAL PEARLS**
> - The majority of patients with PBC suffer little morbidity and no mortality from their liver disease. However, a minority group will develop complications due to ESLD.
> - The rate of disease progression varies from patient to patient.
> - Liver transplant is a viable therapy in patients with ESLD with very favorable outcomes; PBC may recur in the transplanted liver but is rarely problematic.
> - Patients may present with complications of portal hypertension, including variceal bleeding even in the absence of cirrhosis.
> - HCC in PBC is rare. However, the risk is increased slightly and patients with long-standing disease should be screened accordingly.

Natural history of untreated disease

- Approximately 20% of those with PBC will develop cirrhosis if left untreated.
- The most common cause of death in those with PBC is cardiovascular disease.

Prognosis for treated patients

- Survival of non-cirrhotic patients with PBC who are treated with UDCA is comparable with that of an age- and sex-matched population.
- Survival of cirrhotic patients treated with UDCA is slightly worse than a matched population but better than that of untreated patients.

Section 7: Reading List

Combes B, Carithers RL Jr, Maddrey WC, et al. A randomized, double-blind, placebo-controlled trial of ursodeoxycholic acid in primary biliary cirrhosis. Hepatology 1995;22:759–66

Dickson ER, Grambsch PM, Fleming TR, Fisher LD, Langworthy A. Prognosis in primary biliary cirrhosis: model for decision making. Hepatology 1989;10:1–7

Gershwin ME, Selmi C, Worman HJ, et al. Risk factors and comorbidities in primary biliary cirrhosis: a controlled interview-based study of 1032 patients. Hepatology 2005;42:1194–202

Heathcote EJ, Cauch-Dudek K, Walker V, et al. The Canadian Multicenter Double-blind Randomized Controlled Trial of ursodeoxycholic acid in primary biliary cirrhosis. Hepatology 1994;19:1149–56

Hirschfield GM, Liu X, Chun XY, et al. Primary biliary cirrhosis associated with HLA IL12A and IL12RB2 variants. N Engl J Med 2009;306:2544–55

Invernizzi P, Crosignani A, Battezzati PM, et al. Comparison of the clinical features and clinical course of antimitochondrial antibody-positive and negative primary biliary cirrhosis. Hepatology 1997;25:1090–5

Kaplan MM, Gershwin ME. Primary biliary cirrhosis. N Engl J Med 2005;353:1261–73

Lindor KD, Therneau TM, Jorgensen RA, Malinchoc M, Dickson ER. Effects of ursodeoxycholic acid on survival in patients with primary biliary cirrhosis. Gastroenterology 1996;110:1515–18

Poupon RE, Bonnand AM, Chretien Y, Poupon R. Ten-year survival in ursodeoxycholic acid-treated patients with primary biliary cirrhosis. The UDCA-PBC Study Group. Hepatology 1999;29:1668–71

Poupon RE, Lindor KD, Cauch-Dudek K, Dickson ER, Poupon R, Heathcote EJ. Combined analysis of randomized controlled trials of ursodeoxycholic acid in primary biliary cirrhosis. Gastroenterology 1997;113:884–90

Poupon RE, Poupon R, Balkau B. Ursodiol for the long-term treatment of primary biliary cirrhosis. The UDCA-PBC Study Group. N Engl J Med 1994;330:1342–7

Suggested website
www.aasld.org/.../PrimaryBiliaryCirrhosis7-2009.pdf

Section 8: Guidelines
National society guidelines

Guideline title	Guideline source	Date	Summary
Primary Biliary Cirrhosis	AASLD Practice Guidelines http://www.aasld. org/practiceguidelines/Documents/ Bookmarked%20Practice%20Guidelines/ PrimaryBillaryCirrhosis7-2009.pdf	July 2009	Comprehensive review of the management of PBC

International society guidelines

Guideline title	Guideline Source	Date	Summary
Management of Cholestatic Liver Diseases	EASL Practice Guidelines http://www. easl.eu/assets/application/files/ b664961b2692dc2_file.pdf	June 2009	Comprehensive review of the management of PBC and other cholestatic liver diseases

Section 9: Evidence

Not applicable for this topic.

Section 10: Images

Not applicable for this topic.

Additional material for this chapter can be found online at:
www.mountsinaiexpertguides.com
This includes a case study and multiple choice questions

CHAPTER 14

Primary Sclerosing Cholangitis

Nancy Bach and Joseph A. Odin

Division of Liver Diseases, Icahn School of Medicine at Mount Sinai, New York, NY, USA

OVERALL BOTTOM LINE
- PSC is a cholestatic liver disease characterized by inflammation and fibrosis of the biliary system that can result in the formation of multifocal biliary strictures.
- Though the etiology of the disease remains elusive, evidence suggests the role of genetic and immunologic factors.
- Disease progression varies from patient to patient; the disease can result in complications of ESLD, portal hypertension, cholangitis and/or the development of cholangiocarcinoma.
- While the majority of patients with PSC have or develop IBD (70–90%; mainly ulcerative colitis), a minority of patients with IBD have or will develop PSC (2.4–7.5%).
- No specific therapy is of proven benefit and treatment is supportive. Liver transplantation is a viable option and should be considered early for those that have complications of their disease.

Section 1: Background
Definition of disease
- PSC is a chronic progressive fibro-obliterative bile duct inflammation that can involve any part of the biliary tree.

Disease classification
- PSC needs to be distinguished from secondary causes of sclerosing cholangitis.

Incidence/prevalence
- The incidence of the disease ranges from 0.5 to 1.25 cases/100 000.
- The prevalence of the disease ranges between six and 20 cases/100 000.
- Men are more likely to be affected (70%).
- Prevalence of PSC may be increased in first degree relatives of PSC patients.

Etiology
- The exact etiology of PSC remains unknown and multiple factors likely play a role.
- Immune-mediated injury to the bile ducts may be responsible.

Mount Sinai Expert Guides: Hepatology, First Edition. Edited by Jawad Ahmad, Scott L. Friedman, and Henryk Dancygier.
© 2014 John Wiley & Sons, Ltd. Published 2014 by John Wiley & Sons, Ltd.
Companion website: www.mountsinaiexpertguides.com

- Other factors including bacteria, viruses, toxic bile acids, ischemia or environmental factors may precipitate the occurrence of this disease in an otherwise genetically susceptible individual.

Pathology/pathogenesis

- The characteristic lesion seen on liver histology is an onion skin-type periductal fibrosis. The duct eventually degenerates and disappears leaving a bile duct scar. Depending on the disease severity, portal fibrosis becomes more pronounced and biliary cirrhosis develops.

Predictive/risk factors

Risk factor	Frequency amongst affected individuals
Male gender	70%
IBD (pancolitis > distal colitis)	70–90%
HLA B8	60–80%

Section 2: Prevention

- No medical intervention has been demonstrated to prevent the disease.
- The lifetime risk of developing cholangiocarcinoma is around 10%. Unfortunately lack of good surveillance tools limits early detection of cholangiocarcinoma.
- The increased risk of gall bladder cancer and colorectal tumors leads to the recommendation of annual US and periodic colonoscopies.

Screening

- Any patient with a repeatedly abnormal cholestatic pattern of liver chemistries should be evaluated. Likewise, patients with IBD and abnormal liver chemistries should be evaluated for PSC though only 2.4–7.5% will have or develop PSC.

Section 3: Diagnosis (Algorithm 14.1)

- Most patients with PSC present with abnormal liver chemistries in a cholestatic pattern though some will present with complaints of pruritus.
- Rarely patients will be diagnosed with PSC after a bout of cholangitis or after presenting with ESLD or cholangiocarcinoma.
- The physical examination findings of PSC are non-specific.
- The diagnosis is typically established using cholangiographic techniques to define the biliary tract anatomy.
- Rarely the diagnosis is made by finding characteristic "periductal" fibrosis on liver histology and normal cholangiography (i.e. small duct PSC).

Differential diagnosis

Differential diagnosis	Features
AIDS cholangiopathy	History of positive HIV antibody differentiates
Bile duct neoplasm	Can be difficult to distinguish. Brushings and biopsy of the bile duct make the diagnosis
Biliary tract surgery	History of prior biliary surgery
Choledocholithiasis	History of pain and differences in cholangiographic appearance
Congenital abnormalities	Cholangiography should be able to differentiate
Ischemic injury to the bile duct	History of ischemic injury
Caustic injury – excluding chemotherapy	History of caustic injury
IgG4 sclerosing cholangitis	Distinguished based on laboratory testing and history of pancreatitis

Typical presentation
- The majority (>75%) of patients with PSC have or will develop IBD.
- The disease is slightly more common in younger men.
- At the time of diagnosis, the typical patient is asymptomatic though pruritus may be noted in some.
- A small percentage of patients will present with jaundice, symptoms of cholangitis (fever, chills, RUQ pain, jaundice) or with evidence of ESLD.

Clinical diagnosis
History
- The physician should question the patient about symptoms of jaundice, pruritus and pain. Bouts of bacterial cholangitis (fever, pain and jaundice) though not usual, may occur. Symptoms of IBD, including bloody diarrhea may occur before, during or after the diagnosis of PSC.
- Family members of the patient may have other autoimmune diseases including IBD.
- The disease should be considered in anyone with a diagnosis of IBD and abnormal liver chemistries.

Physical examination
- The physical examination findings of PSC are non-specific.
- Hepatomegaly is common. Up to a third of patients may have splenomegaly on presentation.
- Excoriations from pruritus may be noted as well as other signs of chronic liver disease including spider angiomata, Dupuytren's contracture and palmar erythema. Jaundice may be present.
- Decompensated cirrhosis and/or development of cholangiocarcinoma can result in ascites and muscular atrophy.

Disease severity classification
- The Mayo Model can be used to help predict the probability of survival based on several parameters including bilirubin, AST, albumin, history of variceal bleeding and age of the patient (www.mayoclinic.org/girst/mayomodel3.html).

Laboratory diagnosis

List of diagnostic tests

- Elevated AP and GGT predominate.
- Serum aminotransferase levels are typically less than 200 IU/L
- Bilirubin may be elevated.
- Albumin is typically normal except in those with active IBD.
- Non-specific auto-antibodies including P-ANCA (30–80%), ANA (30%) and SMA (80%).
- Liver biopsy (may be contraindicated in patients with significant ductal dilatation).

List of imaging techniques

- MRC or if the diagnosis is still suspected and MRC is negative, consider ERC.
- Liver biopsy if typical cholangiographic findings not identified and disease is still suspected or in those with disproportionate elevation of aminotransferase levels.

Algorithm 14.1 Diagnosis of primary sclerosing cholangitis

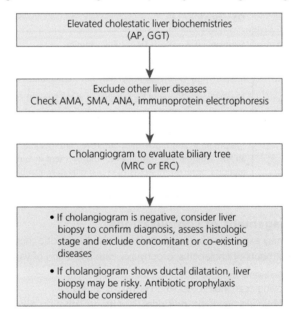

Potential pitfalls/common errors made regarding diagnosis of disease

- A normal US (no ductal dilatation) does not rule out the diagnosis of PSC.
- It is important to rule out IgG4-associated cholangitis because this entity may be steroid responsive.
- Differentiating strictures of PSC from ductal neoplasms can be difficult.
- The gall bladder and cystic duct may be involved and the risk of gall bladder cancer is increased in those with a mass.
- Majority (>85%) of patients have intra- and extrahepatic bile duct involvement. About 10% have intrahepatic biliary duct disease only.

Section 4: Treatment (Algorithm 14.2)

• UDCA (13–15 mg/kg/day) may reduce the serum levels of cholestic liver enzymes in some patients. However, a beneficial effect of UDCA on the natural course of PSC has not been proven.
• Repeated endoscopic (or percutaneous) dilatation of dominant bile duct strictures appears to slow the progression of PSC.
• Liver transplantation is the only life saving procedure for patients with PSC and cirrhosis.
• Treatment is aimed at the management of symptoms and treatment of complications that may be associated with the disease.

When to hospitalize
• Evidence or suspicion of bacterial cholangitis.
• Life-threatening complications of portal hypertension or cirrhosis.

Table of treatment

Treatment	Comment
Conservative treatment	Supplementation with fat soluble vitamins
Medical	Use of UDCA is very controversial and generally not recommended. High dose therapy (>18 mg/kg/day) may have a negative effect on prognosis
Surgical	Liver transplant should be considered early. Survival rates are excellent
Radiological	Successful endoscopic or radiologically guided balloon dilatation or placement of a stent across a dominant stricture may lead to symptomatic and biochemical improvement in some. Studies have not shown whether this translates to improvement in survival. Those with jaundice or recurrent bouts of cholangitis may also be candidates for such therapy

Prevention/management of complications
• Patients with PSC may experience bouts of cholangitis and antibiotic therapy is indicated. In those with recurrent bouts of cholangitis, prophylaxis with a rotation of various antibiotics has been used.
• Surveillance for cholangiocarcinoma (up to 30% risk) is difficult.
• The presence of cholangiocarcinoma precludes liver transplantation except under available research protocols.
• Screening for colonic and gall bladder cancer can lead to early detection and treatment.

CLINICAL PEARLS
• IgG4 sclerosing cholangitis, unlike PSC, may respond to steroid therapy. Therefore this condition needs to be differentiated from PSC.
• The diagnosis of cholangiocarcinoma can be very difficult. Its early diagnosis is essential for any chance of successful therapy.
• Most cases of cholangiocarcinoma are diagnosed within 10 years of the diagnosis of PSC.
• Patients with PSC and IBD have an increased risk of colorectal carcinoma.
• Evaluation for cholangiocarcinoma should ensue in any patient whose clinical course or laboratory values change.

Algorithm 14.2 Management of primary sclerosing cholangitis

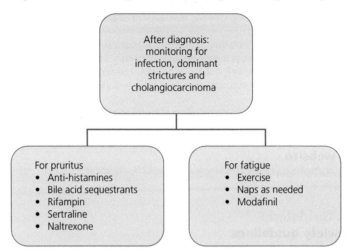

Section 5: Special Populations

Not applicable for this topic.

Section 6: Prognosis

CLINICAL PEARLS
- PSC is usually a progressive disease and can result in complications of ESLD, infection and cholangiocarcinoma.
- Median transplant free survival is 10–12 years from the time of diagnosis. However, a remarkable variation in the course of this disease exists amongst individuals.
- Factors at the time of diagnosis correlating with poor prognosis:
  - Symptoms.
  - Low serum albumin.
  - Persistent bilirubin elevation (>3 months; >4 times the upper limit of normal).
  - Hepatomegaly.
  - Splenomegaly.
  - Dominant bile duct stricture(s).
- The survival of patients with small duct PSC is similar to that of the general population.
- Patients with small duct PSC do not have an increased risk of cholangiocarcinoma.
- Few patients with small duct PSC may progress to large duct PSC.

Section 7: Reading List

Angulo P, Lindor KD. Primary sclerosing cholangitis. Hepatology 1999;30:332–924

Bambha K, Kim WR, Talwalkar J, Torgerson H, Benson JT, Therneau TM, et al. Incidence, clinical spectrum and outcomes of PSC in a US community. Gastroenterology 2003;125:1364–9

Berstad AE, Aabakken I, Smith HJ, Aasens S, Boberg KM, Schrumpf E. Diagnostic accuracy of magnetic resonance and endoscopic retrograde cholangiopancreatography in primary sclerosing cholangitis. Clin Gastroenterol Hepatol 2006;4:514–20

Card T, Solaymani-Dodaran M, West J. Incidence and mortality of primary sclerosing cholangitis in the UK: a population based cohort study. J Hepatol 2008;48:939–44

Chapman R, Fevery J, Kalloo A, et al. Diagnosis and management of primary sclerosing cholangitis. Hepatology 2010;51:660

Gluck M, Cantone NR, Brandabur JJ, Patterson DJ, Bredfedt JE, Kozarek RA. A twenty year experience with endoscopic therapy for symptomatic primary sclerosing cholangitis. J Clin Gastroenterol 2008;42:1032–9

Gotthardt DN, Rudolph G, Kloters-Plachky P, Kulaksiz H, Stiehl A. Endoscopic dilatation of dominant stenoses in primary sclerosing cholangitis: outcome after long-term treatment. Gastrointest Endosc 2010;71: 527–34

Tischendorf JJW, Hecker J, Kruger, et al. Characterization, outcome and prognosis in 273 patients with primary sclerosing cholangitis: a single center Study. Am J Gastroenterol 2007;102:107–14

Suggested website

http://www.aasld.org/practiceguidelines/Documents/Practice%20Guidelines/PSC_2-2010.pdf

Section 8: Guidelines
National society guidelines

Guideline title	Guideline source	Date	Summary
Diagnosis and Management of Primary Sclerosing Cholangitis	AASLD Practice Guidelines http://www.aasld.org/practiceguidelines/Documents/Practice%20Guidelines/PSC_2-2010.pdf	Published February/July 2010	Comprehensive review of the management of PSC

International society guidelines

Guideline title	Guideline source	Date	Summary
Management of Cholestatic Liver Diseases	EASL Practice Guidelines http://www.easl.eu/assets/application/files/b664961b2692dc2_file.pdf	June 2009	Comprehensive review of the management of PSC and other cholestatic liver diseases

Section 9: Evidence

Not applicable for this topic.

Section 10: Images

Not applicable for this topic.

Additional material for this chapter can be found online at:
www.mountsinaiexpertguides.com
This includes a case study and multiple choice questions

CHAPTER 15

Hereditary Hemochromatosis

Jawad Ahmad
Division of Liver Diseases, Icahn School of Medicine at Mount Sinai, New York, NY, USA

OVERALL BOTTOM LINE
- HH is an autosomal recessive disease caused by mutations in the HFE gene leading to increased iron absorption and deposition of iron in various organs, including the liver.
- It is the most common hereditary disorder in White people with a prevalence as high as 1 in 140 individuals in some studies although phenotypic expression is much less common.
- It typically presents as asymptomatic elevation in iron studies but can present in middle age with abnormal liver enzymes and hepatomegaly as well as arthralgias, loss of libido, diabetes and heart failure due to iron deposition in other organs.
- The diagnosis relies on demonstration of elevated body iron stores with a high iron saturation and ferritin. Testing for HFE gene mutations and hepatic iron content on liver biopsy can also be helpful.
- Treatment is based on depletion of iron through phlebotomy and improves survival and can even reverse cirrhosis in selected patients.

Section 1: Background
Definition of disease
- There is no universally accepted definition of HH but it is essentially an inherited condition leading to increased total body iron.

Disease classification
- The disease can be classified into stages:
  - Stage 1: patients with the genetic disorder (positive HFE gene test) but normal iron stores.
  - Stage 2: patients with the genetic disorder and elevated iron stores but no tissue/organ damage.
  - Stage 3: patients with the genetic disorder with iron overload and tissue/organ damage.
- In addition, iron overload can be classified according to whether it is an inherited disorder (as in HH) or one of the many causes of secondary iron overload.

Incidence/prevalence
- The prevalence of HH defined by HFE gene polymorphisms varies according to population but is as high as 1 in 140 for C282Y homozygosity in people of Northern European ancestry and 1 in 330 in a racially mixed population.

Mount Sinai Expert Guides: Hepatology, First Edition. Edited by Jawad Ahmad, Scott L. Friedman, and Henryk Dancygier.
© 2014 John Wiley & Sons, Ltd. Published 2014 by John Wiley & Sons, Ltd.
Companion website: www.mountsinaiexpertguides.com

- The frequency of the C282Y allele is as high as 12.5% in Ireland.
- C282Y homozygosity accounts for approximately 80% of inherited iron overload syndromes, with 5% accounted for by C282Y and H63D heterozygosity. The remaining 15% likely have mutations in other genes involved in iron absorption and metabolism.

Economic impact
- The economic impact of HH is unclear. Despite the high prevalence of the disorder, the low phenotypic expression and simplicity of treatment would suggest a minimal economic impact compared with other causes of chronic liver disease.

Etiology
- There are several genetic defects that have been identified in HH.
- The commonest genetic defect is closely linked to the HLA-A3 locus on the short arm of chromosome 6. In 1996, two missense mutations were identified on a candidate gene and termed the HLA-H or HFE gene.
- Substitution of tyrosine for cysteine at amino acid position 282 (C282Y) of the HFE gene product is the commonest with C282Y homozygotes accounting for 80–85% of all HH patients. Substitution of histidine for aspartate at position 63 (H63D) and serine substituted for cysteine at position 65 (S65C) make up the other two commonly identified mutations but are rarely seen in iron overload unless associated with C282Y in a compound heterozygote.
- Several other mutations in genes encoding for a variety of other proteins involved in iron regulation (hepcidin, ferroportin, hemojuvelin, and transferrin receptor 2, ceruloplasmin) probably play a role in HH in the absence of HFE gene mutations.

Pathology/pathogenesis
- In normal individuals, 1 mg of iron is lost daily through skin, sweat and the gastrointestinal tract and is replaced by 1 mg absorbed through duodenal enterocytes, a process regulated by iron stores.
- In HH, failure of this regulatory mechanism leads to absorption of several milligrams of iron daily which overcomes the normal iron loss. After the increased need for iron in childhood and adolescence abates, iron stores gradually increase at a rate of approximately 1 g a year (less in women due to menstruation, pregnancy and lactation). By middle age 20–30 g of excess iron has been deposited in several organs leading to the clinical manifestations.
- Liver damage in HH is thought to be related to iron-dependent oxidative processes which damage several cell functions initiating a cascade of cytokines that ultimately lead to fibrosis.
- The function of the HFE gene protein is still unclear but it is structurally similar to major histocompatibility complex class-1 proteins and can bind to transferrin receptors (1 and 2). The resulting complex may have a role in sensing iron on the hepatocyte cell membrane and/or affecting hepcidin expression, and may be involved in iron uptake by duodenal enterocytes.
- Hepcidin appears to be the most important peptide in iron regulation. It is made in hepatocytes and secreted into the circulation where it encounters ferroportin on macrophages and enterocytes. The hepcidin binds to ferroportin which is internalized and inhibits iron release. Excess iron induces hepcidin expression while iron deficiency decreases it.
- HFE gene mutations decrease hepcidin expression leading to up-regulation of ferroportin levels in enterocytes and an increase in intestinal iron absorption.

Section 2: Prevention

> **CLINICAL PEARLS**
> - No interventions have been demonstrated to prevent the development of the disease.
> - By definition, HH is a genetic disease so cannot be prevented. However, treatment ideally should be started in asymptomatic patients prior to clinical evidence of the disease.

Screening
- Screening tests for HH depend on the patient population being investigated.
- Despite the high prevalence of HFE gene mutations, the low disease penetrance means that routine screening of the general population is not recommended.
- Patients with abnormal liver enzymes or clinical evidence of liver disease should be screened for HH.
- Patients with a family history of HH should be screened.
- The initial screening test for HH should include serum iron studies: transferrin saturation and ferritin.
- If the transferrin saturation is greater than 45% or the ferritin is above the normal range, genetic testing for HFE mutations is recommended.
- In patients with a first degree relative with HH, iron studies and HFE genetic testing is recommended.

Section 3: Diagnosis

> **CLINICAL PEARLS**
> - Due to the increased awareness of HH and the availability of genetic testing, approximately 75% of patients are asymptomatic at presentation.
> - When present symptoms include generalized weakness and fatigue, skin changes (hyperpigmentation), loss of libido and arthralgias.
> - Examination findings can include cardiomegaly, hepatomegaly, testicular atrophy, skin pigmentation and arthritis.
> - Laboratory testing for HH is usually prompted by the finding of abnormal liver enzymes. The initial evaluation includes demonstration of elevated iron stores based on an iron saturation of greater than 45% and an elevated ferritin.
> - HFE gene testing is appropriate for patients with elevated iron studies.
> - Liver biopsy and hepatic iron content are helpful in certain cases where the diagnosis is in doubt and to assess the degree of fibrosis.
> - Imaging can be helpful if cirrhosis is suspected and newer MRI techniques can demonstrate increased hepatic iron content.

Differential diagnosis

Differential diagnosis	Features
Other causes of liver disease/cirrhosis	History and physical examination may be similar. Iron studies can be elevated in cirrhosis (particularly alcoholic liver disease). Genetic testing should differentiate from HH
Heart failure/congestive hepatopathy	History and physical examination may be similar. Iron studies and imaging should differentiate from HH

Typical presentation
- The typical presentation of HH is with elevated iron studies drawn because of abnormal liver tests or on routine screening.
- Occasionally, the patient presents for testing because of a family history of HH.
- Advanced disease with fatigue, arthralgias, loss of libido, diabetes, skin hyperpigmentation ("bronze diabetes"), and symptoms and signs of heart failure has become very uncommon.

Clinical diagnosis
History
- The typical patient with HH will be asymptomatic. However, it is important to enquire about fatigue, weakness, abdominal discomfort (particularly RUQ), arthralgias (particularly second and third metacarpophalangeal joints), impotence, loss of libido, skin changes and symptoms associated with heart failure and diabetes such as weight gain, ankle edema, chest pain and shortness of breath.

Physical examination
- The physical examination in HH should look for stigmata of chronic liver disease if cirrhosis is suspected. Clinical signs include hepatomegaly, testicular atrophy, arthritis and skin pigmentation.
- Patients can have heart failure with cardiomegaly, pulmonary edema and fluid overload. Conduction abnormalities such as sick sinus syndrome can rarely be seen.

Useful clinical decision rules and calculators
- The serum ferritin level is a useful test to exclude iron overload in HH and also can predict the degree of fibrosis or cirrhosis.
- A normal ferritin essentially excludes iron overload in HH.
- A level below 1000 µg/L usually excludes cirrhosis while a level greater than 1000 µg/L with elevated liver enzymes (ALT or AST) and platelets below 200×10^9/L strongly suggests cirrhosis (in C282Y homozygotes).

Laboratory diagnosis
List of diagnostic tests
- All patients suspected of having HH should have iron studies including a transferrin saturation and serum ferritin.
- The test can be repeated if only mildly elevated and ideally the patient should be fasting.
- If the transferrin saturation is >45% and/or the ferritin is abnormal (>300 µg/L in men, >200 µg/L in women), HFE genetic testing should be ordered.
- HFE genetic testing should be performed on first degree relatives of HH patients.
- Liver biopsy is not required to make the diagnosis but is helpful in determining the severity of liver disease.
- Some experts suggest that C282Y homozygous patients with normal ALT/AST, elevated transferrin saturation but ferritin <1000 µg/L do not require liver biopsy and should proceed directly to treatment.
- The HII and HIC were useful tests before the advent of HFE genetic testing. An HII of >71 µmol/g dry liver is indicative of hepatic iron overload. The HIC is the HII divided by the patient's age in years. An HIC ≥0.9 was taken as good evidence of phenotypic HH but at least 30–50% of C282Y homozygotes do not have elevated iron studies and hence will not have an elevated HIC. These tests should be reserved for situations where iron studies might indicate iron overload but genetic testing is negative.

List of imaging techniques
- Imaging is helpful in HH to assess for advanced fibrosis/cirrhosis.
- CT but particularly MRI scanning can document the hepatic iron content with some accuracy using T2-weighted or R2 (mean liver proton transverse relaxation rate) images.
- The risk of HCC in HH patients is approximately 3–4% per year in patients with cirrhosis. Hence, patients with HH and advanced fibrosis/cirrhosis should be screened every 6 months with imaging (US) and AFP. CT or MRI can be used to follow up in certain situations and to confirm findings on US.

Potential pitfalls/common errors made regarding diagnosis of disease
- Being C282Y homozygous does not necessarily lead to phenotypic HH. Hence, HFE genetic testing should only be performed in individuals with elevated iron studies or first degree relatives of HH patients.
- An elevated serum ferritin can be seen in many inflammatory conditions, particularly chronic liver diseases due to alcohol, viral hepatitis and fatty liver disease.

Section 4: Treatment
Treatment rationale
- Phlebotomy is the simplest and most effective method to remove excess iron in HH and is recommended for patients with homozygous HH and elevated iron stores irrespective of symptoms (Algorithm 15.1). In patients with symptoms phlebotomy may reduce disease progression and even in patients with advanced fibrosis or cirrhosis there is a possibility of some reversal of organ damage (although the risk of HCC remains in cirrhotic patients).
- Phlebotomy is performed intermittently (typically weekly) until total body iron stores are depleted. This can take several years in some patients and should be monitored by the serum ferritin level, with a target of 50–100 µg/L. Once this is achieved, maintenance phlebotomy may be required every few months.
- Iron chelation therapy is available as a subcutaneous infusion (deferoxamine) and also an oral form (deferasirox) but is seldom required in HH. However, it is the treatment of choice for secondary iron overload such as dyserythropoeisis syndromes (thalassemia, hemolytic anemia) where anemia prevents the use of phlebotomy.

Table of treatment

Treatment	Comment
Conservative treatment	Phlebotomy- suitable for all HH patients with iron overload
	One unit of blood (approximately 200–250 mg iron) should be removed weekly until ferritin drops to 50–100 µg/L
	Monitor hemoglobin prior to phlebotomy to avoid anemia (greater than 20% drop in hemoglobin)
	Once ferritin is below 50–100 µg/L may require maintenance phlebotomy intermittently
	The blood that is removed is suitable for transfusion purposes
	Vitamin C supplementation should be avoided as it increases iron mobilization.

(Continued)

Treatment	Comment
Medical (used in secondary iron overload conditions)	Deferoxamine: • Given as continuous subcutaneous infusion at 40 mg/kg/day for 8–12 hours for 5–7 days • Can monitor 24-hour urinary iron excretion or HIC on liver biopsy • Given orally at 20 mg/kg/day Deferasirox: • Adjust dose by 5 mg/kg/day depending on response

Prevention/management of complications

• Complications of phlebotomy include anemia but can be avoided by monitoring hemoglobin levels prior to each phlebotomy.

Algorithm 15.1 Diagnosis and management of HH

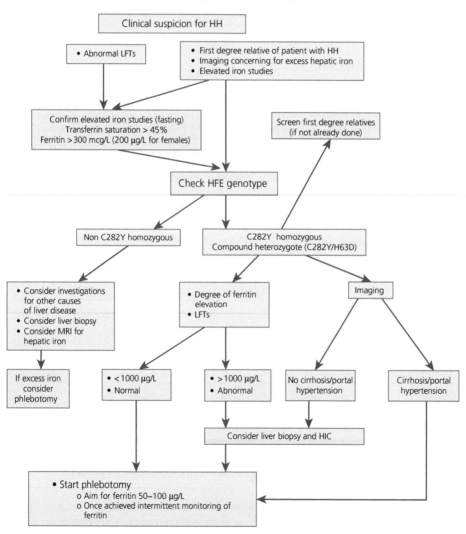

CLINICAL PEARLS
- Phlebotomy in patients with HH should be initiated prior to the onset of symptoms and before evidence of organ damage.
- In symptomatic patients, phlebotomy can be expected to improve fatigue, skin changes, insulin requirement in diabetics, cardiac function and reversal of fibrosis in some patients. It does not improve arthropathy or testicular atrophy.
- In HH patients without cirrhosis, removal of iron eliminates the risk of HCC.

Section 5: Special Populations

Pregnancy
- Although unusual, pregnancy can occur in patients with HH and can remove up to 1 g of iron. If iron overload is present, iron supplements should not be given during pregnancy. Treatment with phlebotomy should be deferred until after pregnancy.

Section 6: Prognosis

CLINICAL PEARLS
- Patients with HH and cirrhosis are at risk for decompensated liver disease and HCC.
- In patients with HH without cirrhosis, phlebotomy improves survival.
- Patients with cirrhosis are still at risk of HCC even after adequate phlebotomy.

Natural history of untreated disease
- Without treatment HH patients are at risk for decompensated cirrhosis and HCC although the actual risk is difficult to quantify due to lack of disease penetrance of C282Y homozygotes.
- HCC is a major cause of death in HH patients with cirrhosis.

Prognosis for treated patients
- Patients with HH who undergo phlebotomy prior to symptoms or cirrhosis have a normal life expectancy.

Follow-up tests and monitoring
- The serum ferritin level is used to monitor HH patients on treatment. A target level of 50–100 µg/L is optimal.
- Patients with HH and cirrhosis should undergo imaging every 6 months as surveillance for HCC.

Section 7: Reading List

Adams P, Brissot P, Powell L. EASL International Consensus Conference on Haemochromatosis. J Hepatol 2000;33:485–504

Adams P, Reboussin D, Barton J, et al. Hemochromatosis and iron-overload screening in a racially diverse population. N Eng J Med 2005;352:1769–78

Allen K, Gurrin L, Constantine C, et al. Iron-overload-related disease in HFE hereditary hemochromatosis. N Eng J Med 2008;358:221–30

Bacon B, Adams P, Kowdley K, et al. Diagnosis and Management of Hemochromatosis: 2011 Practice Guide-line by American Association for the Study of Liver Diseases. Hepatology 2011;54:328–43

EASL Clinical Practice Guidelines for HFE Hemochromatosis. J Hepatol 2010;53:3–22

Feder J, Gnirke A, Thomas W, et al. A novel MHC class I-like gene is mutated in patients with hereditary haemochromatosis. Nat Genet 1996;13:399

Pietrangelo P. Hereditary hemochromatosis: pathogenesis, diagnosis and treatment. Gastroenterology 2010;139:393–408

Suggested website

www.european-haemochromatosis.eu/index2.html

Section 8: Guidelines
National society guidelines

Guideline title	Guideline source	Date	Summary
Diagnosis and Management of Hemochromatosis: 2011 Practice Guideline by American Association for the Study of Liver Diseases	American Association for the Study of Liver Diseases (AASLD) http://www.aasld.org/practiceguidelines/Documents/Bookmarked%20Practice%20Guidelines/Hemochromatosis%202011.pdf	July 2011	Comprehensive review of disease and management
Screening for Hereditary Hemochromatosis: A Clinical Practice Guideline from the American College of Physicians	American College of Physicians (ACP) http://annals.org/article.aspx?articleid=718757	July 2005	Screening guidelines

International society guidelines

Guideline title	Guideline source	Date	Summary
EASL Clinical Practice Guidelines for HFE Hemochromatosis	European Association for the Study of the Liver (EASL) http://www.easl.eu/assets/application/files/03d32880931aac9_file.pdf	July 2010	Comprehensive review of disease and management

Section 9: Evidence

Type of evidence	Title, date	Comment
Cohort study	Long-term survival analysis in hereditary hemochromatosis. Gastroenterology 1991;101:368	Demonstrated that in HH with cirrhosis survival was poor. Phlebotomy prior to cirrhosis leads to long-term survival similar to the general population
Cohort study	Long-term survival in patients with hereditary hemochromatosis. Gastroenterology 1996;110:1107	Demonstrated that iron overload in HH is associated with worse outcome and phlebotomy essentially prevents this

Section 10: Images

Not applicable for this topic.

Additional material for this chapter can be fund online at:
www.mountsinaiexpertguides.com
This includes a case study and multiple choice questions

CHAPTER 16

Wilson Disease

Joseph A. Odin,[1] Nancy Bach[1] and Vivek Kesar[2]
[1]Division of Liver Diseases, Icahn School of Medicine at Mount Sinai, New York, NY, USA
[2]Lenox Hill Medical Center, New York, NY, USA

OVERALL BOTTOM LINE
- WD, also known as hepatolenticular degeneration, is a rare autosomal recessive systemic disorder caused by defective copper metabolism.
- It most commonly presents with isolated hepatic, neurological or psychiatric manifestations but multisystem involvement is not uncommon.
- Diagnosis of WD involves characteristic clinical, biochemical and molecular findings.
- Combined treatment with chelators, zinc and liver transplantation has proven lifesaving and even curative.
- Potential future therapies include isolated hepatocyte transplantation and gene therapy.

Section 1: Background
Definition of disease
- WD is an inherited rare autosomal recessive disease of copper metabolism characterized by copper accumulation in hepatocytes and in other extra hepatic organs.

Prevalence
- The prevalence of WD is estimated at three per 100 000.
- Siblings of a WD patient have a 1 in 4 risk of disease; children of a WD patient have one in 200 risk.
- The frequency of carriers of the ATP7B mutation is about 0.6–1%.
- Consanguinity increases prevalence in some regions (e.g. Crete, Sardinia, Japanese islands).

Economic impact
- Given the low prevalence of WD, its economic impact is not great.
- WD and alpha-1 antitrypsin deficiency disease combined account for less than 5% of liver transplant procedures in the USA according to Organ Procurement and Transplantation Network data.

Mount Sinai Expert Guides: Hepatology, First Edition. Edited by Jawad Ahmad, Scott L. Friedman, and Henryk Dancygier.
© 2014 John Wiley & Sons, Ltd. Published 2014 by John Wiley & Sons, Ltd.
Companion website: www.mountsinaiexpertguides.com

Etiology
- Homozygous or compound heterozygous mutations in the ATP7B gene (locus: 13q14.3-q21.1), which codes for an ATP-dependent copper export pump, are the cause of WD.
- Up to 300 mutations have been associated with WD.

Pathophysiology
- Copper is absorbed via the small intestine into the portal circulation. In the liver, hepatocytes take up copper and incorporate the copper into ceruloplasmin. Excess copper is bound to Apo metallothionein or secreted into bile.
- In WD due to mutations in the ATP7B gene, the incorporation of copper into ceruloplasmin and excretion of excess copper into bile is impaired.
- The excess copper is retained in the hepatocytes where it promotes free radical formation and oxidative damage to cellular lipids and proteins.
- As the hepatic copper burden increases further, copper is released into the circulation and deposited in other organs such as the nervous system.
- Secretion of ceruloplasmin into the circulation is dependent on copper incorporation. Hence serum ceruloplasmin levels are low in WD.
- Copper deposition in the cornea may manifest as Kayser–Fleischer (KF) rings.

Predictive/risk factors
- Inheritance of dual mutations in the ATP7B gene – nearly 100% penetrance.

Section 2: Prevention

- Low copper diet and zinc or chelation therapy may prevent disease onset.

Screening (Algorithm 16.1)
- Genetic, ophthalmologic and biochemical tests are used to screen for WD. It is not cost effective to screen the general population due to the large number of known mutations and the rarity of the disease. However, first degree relatives of any patient with WD should be screened since early treatment can prevent disease onset.
- Specific testing can be postponed until an abnormality develops on a regular check up or blood tests.
- For infants of affected families, a delay in achieving a developmental milestone should lead to testing.

Primary prevention
- Low copper diet and zinc or chelation therapy may prevent disease onset.

Secondary prevention
- Liver transplantation will prevent disease recurrence.

Algorithm 16.1 Screening algorithm for Wilson disease

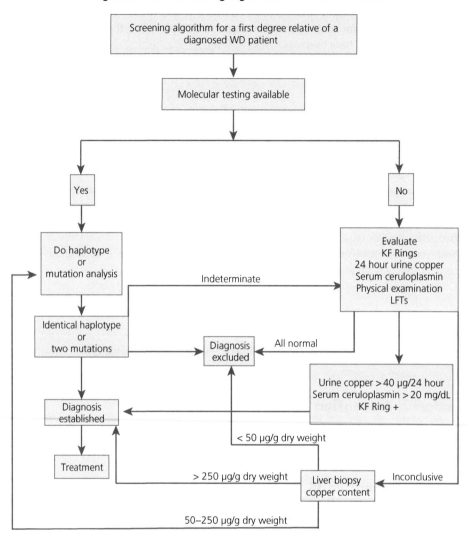

Section 3: Diagnosis (Algorithm 16.2)

CLINICAL PEARLS
- WD should always be considered in a patient <40 years of age who presents with unexplained liver, neurological or neuropsychiatric disease.
- Its clinical spectrum ranges from asymptomatic hepatomegaly or minor liver enzyme derangement to fulminant liver failure with neuropsychiatric symptoms.
- AP levels may be relatively low in WD.
- Presence of low serum ceruloplasmin levels, increased urine copper excretion and KF rings help in diagnosis of WD.
- If clinical and biochemical tests are inconclusive then confirmation can be performed by quantification of copper in the liver via liver biopsy or by molecular techniques such as haplotype or mutation analysis.

Differential diagnosis

Differential diagnosis	Features
Drug or toxin-induced hepatitis/liver failure	A thorough history is needed to rule out hepatotoxicity due to medications and toxin exposure. Be aware that multiple products contain acetaminophen
Viral hepatitis	History of travel, transfusion, needle sharing, or tattoos. Positive viral serological markers
AIH	Characterized by serum autoantibodies and interface hepatitis on the biopsy
NAFLD	Normal serum ceruloplasmin and urinary copper levels. No KF rings
Other psychiatric disorder	Normal serum ceruloplasmin and urinary copper levels. No KF rings. Diagnose by DSM IV

Typical presentation
- The most common age for presentation ranges from 5 to 40 years with hepatic features mostly preceding the neurological features except for those diagnosed in late second or third decade.
- The clinical spectrum of liver disease varies from asymptomatic liver enzyme elevation to chronic active hepatitis and cirrhosis or may present with acute liver failure with the most common initial presentation being cirrhosis. Those presenting with acute liver failure may also have hemolytic anemia and acute renal failure.
- Initial neurological manifestation is generally asymmetric tremors but other manifestations such as dysphagia, ataxia and mask-like facies are fairly common. About a third of patients manifest a neuropsychiatric finding: emotional liability, anxiety or even psychosis.

Clinical diagnosis
History
- It is important to enquire about symptoms of chronic liver disease and cirrhosis such as fatigue, confusion, GI bleeding, easy bruising and swelling.
- In fulminant liver failure cases, always exclude a history of drug intake (e.g. acetaminophen) and autoimmune hepatitis before diagnosing WD.
- Neuropsychiatric manifestations like tremors, mask-like facies, depression, mood swings should also be reviewed.
- New difficulties in school may presage WD onset in children.
- Always ask about risk factors (e.g. injection drug use or alcohol abuse) for other liver diseases and a family history of liver and neuropsychiatric disease.

Physical examination
- Evaluate for signs of chronic liver disease and cirrhosis.
- Refer to neurologist and ophthalmologist for detection of subtle neurological and ophthalmo-logical (i.e. KF rings) findings. KF rings are present in 44–62% of patients.

Psychiatric examination
- Consider psychiatric evaluation for those with behavioral or mood abnormalities.

Laboratory diagnosis
List of diagnostic tests
- Serum LFTs: generally increased ALT and AST levels are present in WD, but they are neither sensitive nor specific. A lower than expected AP is common. A decreased uric acid level is common. Those with severe disease may have a direct hyperbilirubinemia or an indirect hyperbilirubinemia if hemolysis is present.
- Serum ceruloplasmin: normal reference range 20–40 mg/dL. Serum ceruloplasmin is an acute phase reactant, which is decreased in patients with WD. A serum ceruloplasmin less than 20 mg/dL has been considered consistent with WD, and diagnostic if associated with KF rings. A low ceruloplasmin is present in 85% of cases. Use of serum ceruloplasmin alone as a diagnostic modality for WD is questionable as there are many clinical and normal physiological conditions that can alter the level of ceruloplasmin. A normal serum ceruloplasmin level does not exclude WD. The bottom line is that the lower the ceruloplasmin level (<20 mg/dL) the greater the suspicion of WD.
- Urine copper: 24-hour urine copper level should be obtained in all patients who are suspected of having WD. Typically a level above 100 μg/24 hours is observed in patients with WD but levels more than 40 μg/24 hours suggest further investigation for WD. Urine copper excretion is also used to monitor response to chelation therapy. Interpreting urine copper levels can be difficult because of overlap of results in other types of liver disease like acute liver injury, cholestatic conditions, autoimmune hepatitis and heterozygotes for ATP7B gene mutations.
- Hepatic parenchymal copper concentration: the normal concentration for hepatic copper is <55 μg/g dry weight. Determination of hepatic copper concentration requires a liver biopsy specimen and appropriate analytical equipment. It is only performed in those patients where other tests are suggestive but not diagnostic of WD. Levels >250 μg/g dry weight are diagnostic of WD and levels <50 μg/g dry weight almost always rule out WD. Levels between 60 and 240 μg/g dry weight are non-diagnostic and must be viewed in the context of other test results. Patients with cholestatic diseases and those heterozygous for ATP7B gene mutations may also present with increased hepatic parenchymal copper concentration.
- Genetic/molecular testing: genetic and molecular testing is now available. It may be helpful in difficult to diagnose cases. More than 95% of affected alleles may be determined. However, questions still remain about genotypic association with various phenotypes.

Pathologic features on liver biopsy
- The liver biopsy features of WD are non-specific. WD can easily be confused with the histologic features of either autoimmune hepatitis or NASH.
- Early findings may include micro- and macrovesicular steatosis, glycogenated nuclei and portal fibrosis. Mallory bodies may be present.
- Untreated, features may resemble autoimmune hepatitis and include piecemeal necrosis, periportal inflammation and lobular necrosis.
- Histologic stains for copper may show copper deposition in the liver, renal tubular cells and brain. However, copper staining is not reliable for making the diagnosis.
- Mallory bodies may be identified in up to 50% of biopsy specimens.

- Fulminant hepatitis may include parenchymal necrosis with significant collapse, ballooning of hepatocytes and features of cholestasis.
- Rate of pathologic change varies from individual to individual and may only include steatosis and fibrosis in earlier phases.

List of imaging techniques
- Radiological imaging using MRI should be considered in all patients who present with neuropsychiatric symptoms. MRI of the brain may show widespread lesions in putamen, globus pallidus, caudate and thalamus. These lesions show high signal intensity on T2-weighted images and low intensity on T1.

Algorithm 16.2 Diagnostic algorithm for Wilson disease

Associated conditions
- Coombs negative hemolytic anemia.
- Renal abnormalities including aminoaciduria and nephrolithiasis.
- Skeletal abnormalities including premature osteoporosis and arthritis.
- Cardiomyopathy.
- Pancreatitis.
- Hypoparathyroidism.
- Infertility or repeated miscarriages.

Potential pitfalls/common errors in diagnosis

- Harmful delays in the diagnosis of WD are common because patients may be asymptomatic with only mild laboratory abnormalities. A serum ceruloplasmin level should be part of the investigations for all patients with abnormal LFTs of unknown etiology.
- A normal serum ceruloplasmin level does not rule out WD.
- If a patient diagnosed with autoimmune hepatitis does not respond to steroids always keep WD in mind.
- Cholestasis of any etiology may cause low ceruloplasmin levels and increased urinary copper levels.

Section 4: Treatment (Algorithm 16.3)
Treatment rationale

- The primary goal of treatment is to produce a negative copper balance. Since treatment is lifelong and the clinical presentation is variable, therapy should be individualized to achieve this goal. Individualization also increases patient compliance and reduces adverse drug events.
- For patients who are asymptomatic without cirrhosis, zinc alone is the treatment of choice. Those who present with well-compensated cirrhosis should receive initial therapy with both zinc and a chelator (D-penicillamine or trientine hydrochloride) followed by long-term maintenance therapy with either low doses of a chelator or zinc once biochemical improvement is achieved. The same regimen can be tried for decompensated cirrhosis, but those who fail to improve should be referred for liver transplantation evaluation.
- Referral for liver transplantation should be immediate for those presenting with fulminant hepatic failure, development of coagulopathy and encephalopathy within less than 8 weeks from onset of illness. Until transplantation can be performed patients can be managed by dialysis, hemofiltration or plasmapheresis to prevent further renal or neurological complication.
- Patients who present with predominantly neurological features may be treated with ammonium tetrathiomolybdate where available, or zinc with a chelator is recommended. Few studies have compared D-penicillamine to trientine. However, based on the experience and observations of WD experts, AASLD guidelines suggest trientine may be better tolerated and have less adverse effects than trientine.

When to hospitalize

- Patients who present with fulminant hepatic failure should be quickly referred to a liver transplant center. Likewise patients with complications due to ESLD due to WD should be hospitalized and referred for transplant evaluation.

Table of treatment

Treatment	Comment
Conservative	• Dietary modifications: foods rich in copper like chocolate, shellfish, nuts should be avoided • Antioxidants: vitamin E
Medical: Chelators • D-penicillamine: 1000–1500 mg/day in 2–4 divided doses	• Adverse affects include: sensitivity reaction marked by rash, neutropenia, and lymphadenopathy; nephrotoxicity; bone marrow depression; and neurological deterioration • Starting with a low initial dosage of 250–500 mg/day and gradually increase over 4–6 weeks may limit adverse reactions • Take either 1 hour before or 2 hours after the meal • Pregnant women, children and the malnourished should take vitamin B6 supplements • Monitoring of urine protein and blood cell counts needs to be done regularly
• Trientine: Initiation phase: 750–1500 mg/day in 2–3 divided doses Maintenance dose: 750–1000 mg/day In 2–3 divided doses • Ammonium tetrathiomolybdate	• It should always be taken either 1 hour before or 2 hours after the meal • Efficacy similar to D-penicillamine but has the benefit of fewer side effects • Preferred for those with predominantly neurological symptoms where available
Non-chelator • Zinc: dosage of 150 mg is administered in adults and 75 mg in small children is administered in three divided doses Combination therapy • Zinc + chelator Dialysis, hemofiltration, or plasmapheresis	• Take either 1 hour before or 2 hours after the meal. • Adverse effects: immune suppression, pancreatitis • To check the efficacy of treatment, 24-hour urinary copper excretion is measured. The level should be high for chelator therapy and low for zinc therapy • There should be a 3–4 hour interval between doses • Emergency treatment for copper overload in fulminant liver failure
Surgical: • Liver transplantation	• For patients with fulminant liver failure or decompensated cirrhosis who fail to respond to medical therapy

Prevention/management of complications

- Complications are most common with D-penicillamine treatment as noted in the table. Starting with a low dose and titrating upward over a few weeks may reduce complications. If complications do develop, stop D-penicillamine and change to trientene or ammonium tetrathiomolybdate if neurological symptoms worsen.
- Zinc treatment is an option for those who are asymptomatic or cannot tolerate chelator therapy.

CLINICAL PEARLS
- Chelating agents may cause worsening of neurologic symptoms when therapy is initiated. Gradually increasing the dose of these agents may help in decreasing this problem.
- Asymptomatic individuals should be encouraged to continue zinc treatment lifelong.
- Those who become asymptomatic on treatment should not stop treatment, but can be switched to zinc alone. Zinc may be considered in patients who cannot tolerate first line agents or who have worsening of neuropsychiatric disease with the chelating agents.
- Urinary copper testing can be performed to detect suspected non-compliance with treatment.
- D-penicillamine inactivates pyridoxine so small doses of pyridoxine (25 mg/day) should be given with D-penicillamine.

Algorithm 16.3 Treatment of Wilson disease

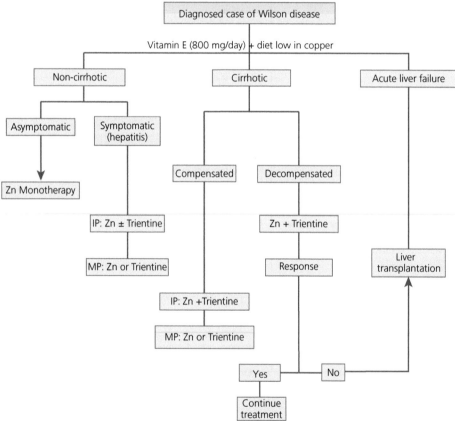

IP, initiation phase – initial acute phase of the disease. MP, maintenance phase – after the initial phase, when the patient stabilizes

Section 5: Special Populations
Pregnancy
- Treatment must be continued during the entire course of pregnancy. Both chelators and zinc have been associated with favorable outcome. However, due to the safety profile of zinc and

trientine, they are preferred over penicillamine. Chelators should be used at the lowest effective dose.

Children

- The treatment options remain the same although dose reductions are required. Zinc or trientine are the safer option.

Section 6: Prognosis

> **CLINICAL PEARLS**
> - Without treatment WD is inevitably fatal.
> - In general early onset disease is associated with a worse prognosis.
> - If the treatment is begun early enough symptomatic recovery is usually complete and a normal life expectancy can be expected.

Natural history of untreated disease

- Untreated WD leads to liver failure and progressive neuropsychiatric deterioration.

Prognosis for treated patients

- The prognosis for asymptomatic patients who undergo treatment is excellent. However, those with cirrhosis may progress to liver failure and need transplantation even with therapy. The prognosis after liver transplantation is excellent since the genetic defect is not present in the new liver.
- Neuropsychiatric manifestations should not progress after transplantation but improvement may be limited compared with hepatic improvement.

Follow-up tests and monitoring

- Perform a physical examination, 24-hour urinary copper excretion assay, CBC count, urinalysis, serum ceruloplasmin level and renal and liver function tests on a biweekly basis for first 2 months, followed by monthly visits for the next 2 or 3 months and after that every 6 months.
- In patients with a KF ring a yearly slit lamp examination should be performed.
- Patients should be told about warning symptoms of worsening liver or neurological disease.
- After dosage adjustment of a chelator, a 24-hour urinary copper measurement should be performed.
- If non-compliance with chelator therapy is suspected, measure the level of non-ceruloplasmin bound copper which will be increased in those who are non-compliant.

Section 7: Reading List

Ala A, Schilsky ML. Wilson disease: pathophysiology, diagnosis, treatment, and screening. Clin Liver Dis 2004;8:787–805

De Bie P, Muller P, Wijmenga C, Klomp LWJ. Molecular pathogenesis of Wilson and Menkes disease: correlation of mutations with molecular defects and disease phenotypes. J Med Genet 2007;44: 673–88

Huster D. Wilson Disease. Best Pract Res Clin Gastroenterol 2010;24:531–9

Lorincz MT. Review. Neurologic Wilson's disease. Ann NY Acad Sci 2010;1184:173–87

Section 8: Guidelines
National society guidelines

Guideline title	Guideline source	Date	Summary
AASLD	American Association for the Study of Liver Diseases (AASLD) http://www.aasld.org/ practiceguidelines/Documents/Bookmarked%20 Practice%20Guidelines/Diagnosis%20and%20 Treatment%20of%20Wilson%20Disease.pdf	2008	Data-supported approach to diagnosis and treatment

International society guidelines

Guideline title	Guideline source	Date	Summary
EASL clinical practice guidelines	European Association for the Study of the Liver (EASL) http://www.easl.eu/assets/application/files/ e793d591ec4de1c_file.pdf	2012	Guidelines for diagnosis and management

Section 9: Evidence

Not applicable for this topic.

Section 10: Images

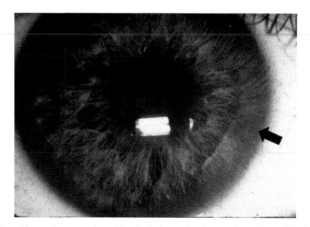

Figure 16.1 KF ring. Aberrant copper deposition in WD may be detected as a brownish ring (KF ring) in the limbus zone of the eye (black arrow). A slit-lamp examination may be needed to detect KF rings in early stage disease. Not all individuals with WD will have KF rings. Source: Courtesy of Dr Alan Friedman, Icahn School of Medicine at Mount Sinai, New York, NY, USA.

**Additional material for this chapter can be found online at:
www.mountsinaiexpertguides.com.
This includes a case study and multiple choice questions**

CHAPTER 17

Alpha-1 Antitrypsin Deficiency

Joseph A. Odin[1] and Vivek Kesar[2]
[1]Division of Liver Diseases, Icahn School of Medicine at Mount Sinai, New York, NY, USA
[2]Lenox Hill Medical Centre, New York, NY, USA

OVERALL BOTTOM LINE
- Alpha-1 antitrypsin (AAT) deficiency is an inherited disease primarily affecting the lungs and liver, which is most often due to a defect in the release of AAT from hepatocytes into the circulation.
- Diagnosis involves measurement of serum levels of AAT along with determination of the phenotype or genotype.
- Apart from liver transplantation, specific liver-related treatment is not available but enzyme replacement therapy is available for those with lung disease.

Section 1: Background
Definition of disease
- AAT deficiency is a rare autosomal codominant disorder due to mutation in the SERPINA1 gene.
- The most common manifestation is emphysema, which becomes evident by the third to fourth decade. Liver disease is a less common manifestation of the deficiency and may affect children and adults.

Disease classification
- At least 100 alleles of SERPINA1 have been identified. On the basis of plasma levels and function of AAT, alleles are classified into four basic groups.
  - Normal – normal allele (M type), phenotype (MM). It is associated with normal levels (>20 mol/L) and function of AAT.
  - Deficient – deficient alleles (Z type) and (S type), phenotype (ZZ) and (SS) respectively. The Z allele is carried by approximately 2–3% of the White population in the USA. The homozygous ZZ phenotype is associated with a high risk of both emphysema and liver disease. The S type, which is mainly found in the Mediterranean area, is not associated with liver disease.
  - Dysfunctional – dysfunctional alleles produce a normal quantity of AAT protein but the protein does not function properly. Liver disease is less common in this group.
  - Null – null alleles are associated with no detectable AAT protein in the plasma. Lung disease is the most severe in this group, but they do not develop liver disease.

Mount Sinai Expert Guides: Hepatology, First Edition. Edited by Jawad Ahmad, Scott L. Friedman, and Henryk Dancygier.

Prevalence
- In the USA approximately 100 000 individuals (1 in 2000 to 8000 population) are severely affected (phenotype ZZ, SZ). The overall prevalence of AAT deficiency may be as high as 1 in 300, but disease penetrance is less than 100%.
- AAT deficiency is equally common in men and women.
- White people are more commonly affected than other races.

Economic impact
- Due to the limited number of affected individuals the overall economic impact of AAT deficiency is not significant though the costs for individual treatment can be high.
- Most of the costs are due to repeated hospitalizations for those with emphysema.
- AAT protein replacement therapy is an expensive intervention ($30 000–$40 000 per patient annually).
- AAT deficiency and WD combined account for less than 5% of liver transplants each year.
- According to the UNOS each liver transplant costs $314 600 on average with annual follow-up care costs averaging $21 900.

Etiology
- AAT deficiency is an inherited autosomal codominant disease caused by mutation in the SERPINA1 gene (locus 14q32.1). Homozygosity for the Z allele is the most common disease phenotype.
- Environmental (e.g. smoking) and genetic cofactors affect disease penetrance.

Pathology/pathogenesis
- AAT is a serine proteinase (elastase) inhibitor and acute phase protein produced by hepatocytes.
- In patients homozygous for the Z type allele, the AAT polypeptide chain undergoes abnormal conformational changes resulting in polymerization and accumulation of AAT within the hepatocyte endoplasmic reticulum. This disrupts the normal cellular protein synthesis leading to oxidative stress and progressive liver injury.
- About 10% of newborn ZZ homozygotes develop liver disease that often leads to fatal childhood cirrhosis. However, overall only 12–15% of individuals with this phenotype develop liver disease, implying that other cofactors modulate protein accumulation and oxidative stress due to AAT polymerization.
- A lag in degradation of polymerized AAT may be specific for the development of liver disease in ZZ homozygotes.
- AAT deficiency causes unopposed activation of neutrophilic elastases in the lung, leading to progressive emphysema.
- Smoking and environmental or occupational toxin exposure is known to exacerbate lung damage due to AAT deficiency.

Predictive/risk factors
- SERPINA1 gene mutations – but disease penetrance is less than 100%.
- More common in people of northern European, North American and Iberian descent.

- Smoking and environmental and occupational toxin exposure increase progression of lung disease in AAT deficiency patients.
- Hepatic inflammation/oxidative stress worsen liver disease due to AAT deficiency.

Section 2: Prevention

- Avoid tobacco smoke and environmental/occupational toxin exposure.
- Avoid alcohol use.

Screening
- It is immensely important to screen patients for AAT deficiency since avoidance of risk factors can prevent progression of disease. It is not cost-effective to screen the general population. The AASLD and EASL have no practice guidelines for AAT deficiency. According to American and European Lung Societies, AAT screening is recommended in the following circumstances:
  - Early-onset pulmonary emphysema (regardless of smoking history).
  - Dyspnea and cough occurring in multiple family members in the same or different generations.
  - Family members of known AAT deficiency patients.
  - Liver disease of unknown cause.
  - All subjects with chronic obstructive pulmonary disease.
  - Adults with bronchiectasis without evident etiology.
  - Patients with asthma whose spirometry fails to return to normal with therapy.
  - Unexplained panniculitis and anti–proteinase-3 vasculitis.

Primary prevention
- Genetic counseling for couples may be helpful though no recommendations exist.
- For newborns with known ZZ phenotype, avoidance of oxidative stress limits liver damage.
- Onset of symptoms can be prevented by avoidance of smoking and environmental and occupational toxins.

Secondary prevention
- Recurrent symptoms can be minimized by avoidance of smoking and environmental and occupational toxins.

Section 3: Diagnosis (Algorithm 17.1)

CLINICAL PEARLS
- AAT deficiency should be suspected in any person who presents with unexplained liver or respiratory symptoms.
- The gold standard for diagnosis is AAT phenotype determination (e.g. MM, ZZ) by serum protein isoelectric focusing.
- Measurement of serum AAT activity is not diagnostic.
- SERPINA1 genetic analysis is rarely necessary.

Differential diagnosis

Differential diagnosis	Features
Bronchiectasis	History of chronic respiratory symptoms, such as a cough and viscous sputum production, along with CT findings such as bronchial wall thickening and luminal dilatation. AAT phenotype is normal
Chronic bronchitis	Cough with sputum production for at least 3 months a year in two consecutive years. AAT phenotype is normal
Viral hepatitis	History of travel, needle sharing, tattoo. Positive viral serological markers along with a normal AAT phenotype
AIH	More common in younger women. Positive serum ANA or ASMA and a normal AAT phenotype

Typical presentation
- The presentation depends on the type of mutation associated with the AAT deficiency. Only the ZZ phenotype presents with liver disease, which usually predates the development of respiratory disease.
- In children, liver disease associated with AAT deficiency presents with neonatal cholestatic jaundice, abnormal LFTs, hepatitis or even cirrhosis.
- Adults typically present in the third or fourth decade of life with chronic hepatitis, cirrhosis or liver cancer.
- Early onset emphysema associated with cough and/or dyspnea is the most common respiratory presentation.

Clinical diagnosis
History
- The presenting hepatic symptoms in children are variable and may include low grade fever, jaundice, dark urine and dull pain in the RUQ. In adults, symptoms of hepatic decompensation predominate along with weight loss for those with liver cancer. Respiratory symptoms may include shortness of breath and cough. These symptoms are initially intermittent and may be evident only with exertion.
- A complete family history is mandatory. Family members should be questioned about similar symptoms. Smoking and smoke exposure history are important as well as environmental and occupational exposures. The presence or absence of risk factors for other liver and lung diseases should also be identified.

Physical examination
- General physical examination – signs of respiratory distress and stigmata of chronic liver disease should be assessed as well as panniculitis.
- Systemic examination:
  - Abdominal examination – hepatomegaly can be seen.
  - Respiratory examination – wheezing, hyperresonance on percussion.

Clinical decision rules
- AAT deficiency should be expected in any person who presents with early onset emphysema irrespective of smoking history.
- Those who present with unexplained liver disease with or without respiratory symptoms should also be evaluated for AAT deficiency.

Laboratory diagnosis

- Serum LFTs: increases in bilirubin, AST, ALT are observed, but they are neither sensitive nor specific.
- Spirometry: it plays an important role in diagnosis of obstructive lung disease which is characterized by increased total lung capacity, reduced FEV1, reduced FCV and reduced FEV1/FVC ratio.
- Serum level of AAT: levels below 11 μmol/L are consistent with AAT deficiency, though diagnosis of AAT deficiency on serum levels alone is questionable. AAT is an acute phase protein, therefore its levels may be elevated in any inflammatory conditions. Hence AAT levels alone lack sensitivity and specificity necessary for diagnosis of the disease.
- Genotyping: DNA analysis is done to evaluate presence of a particular mutation. Methods and kits are available to detect the presence of the more prevalent and clinically relevant alleles.
- Phenotyping: according to the American Thoracic Society and the European Respiratory Society, phenotypic analysis using IEF is the classical method to determine the AAT "phenotype" and is considered the "gold standard" for diagnosis. Although analysis can determine both rare and common alleles it is time consuming and cannot determine homozygous deficient state from heterozygous with null allele.
- Pathologic features on liver biopsy. The liver biopsy features of AAT are non-specific and variable depending on the disease classification and stage:
  - A liver biopsy may show the presence of PAS-positive globules (Figure 17.1).
  - Due to poor sensitivity and specificity biopsy findings cannot replace IEF as a mode of diagnosis.
  - An incidental finding of PAS positive globules warrants further investigation for the presence of AAT.

Imaging techniques

- Chest X-ray: changes consistent with emphysema: hyperlucent lung fields, flattened diaphragm.
- High resolution CT chest: emphysema is characterized by the presence of abnormally low accentuation. In AAT deficiency, the classic finding is panacinar emphysema with predominantly lower lobe distribution.
- CT abdomen: it may show hepatomegaly or changes associated with cirrhosis or hepatocellular carcinoma.

Associated conditions

- Emphysema.
- Panniculitis.

Algorithm 17.1 Diagnosis of alpha-1 antitrypsin deficiency

Indications for further investigation for AAT
- Early-onset pulmonary emphysema (regardless of smoking history)
- Dyspnea and cough occurring in multiple family members in same or different generations
- Family members of known AAT-deficient patients
- Liver disease of unknown etiology
- All subjects with chronic obstructive pulmonary disease
- Adults with bronchiectasis without obvious etiology should be considered for testing
- Patients with asthma whose spirometry fails to return to normal with therapy
- Unexplained panniculitis and anti-proteinase-3 vasculitis

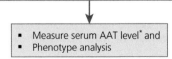

- Measure serum AAT level* and
- Phenotype analysis

* May be falsely elevated in those with AAT due to inflammation

Potential pitfalls/common errors in diagnosis
- AAT serum levels alone lack sensitivity and specificity necessary for diagnosis of the disease.
- Phenotype analysis should be ordered in those suspected of having the disease.
- Due to rarity and varied presentation, diagnosis of AAT deficiency is delayed until late stages when mortality and morbidity are significantly increased.

Section 4: Treatment (Algorithm 17.2)
Treatment rationale
- The basic treatment rationale is to maintain a normal serum level of AAT and prevent progression of lung disease (emphysema) along with therapies that will prevent complications associated with chronic liver disease. Every effort must be made to stop smoking tobacco since tobacco smoke exposure worsens both emphysema and liver fibrosis.

Liver disease
- The current approach is to prevent or manage complications of cirrhosis such as variceal bleeding, ascites, encephalopathy, and hepatocellular carcinoma. Specific details are addressed elsewhere in this manual.

Specific management for AAT deficient patients
- AAT augmentation therapy: enzyme supplementation is provided intravenously for those with a plasma level of AAT <11 μmol/L or severe pulmonary disease. Supplementation does not aid in the treatment of liver disease due to AAT.
- Some gene therapy studies have shown promising results in preliminary testing but further studies are required.

When to hospitalize
- Patients with acute exacerbation of COPD.
- Patient with COPD who develop upper respiratory infection, pneumonia that is severe enough to require admission.
- Patients with complications of cirrhosis.

Table of treatment
- There is no specific medical or surgical treatment for AAT liver disease. Liver transplantation is only recommended for those who develop decompensated cirrhosis.

Treatment	Comment
Conservative: Smoking cessation	It is regarded as the most effective strategy in preventing progression and onset of lung disease and slows liver disease progression. Hence it should be strongly recommended for all
Avoiding environmental and occupational pollutant exposure	It is recommended in all patients. If exposure is very frequent change of occupation may be warranted
Vaccination	Vaccination for influenza and pneumococcus has been recommended in all patients with AAT. Those patients with overt liver disease are advised to receive hepatitis A and B vaccination

Algorithm 17.2 Treatment of alpha-1 antitrypsin deficiency

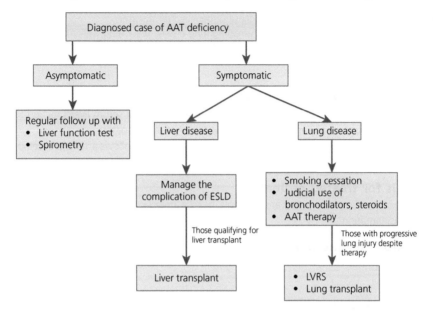

> **CLINICAL PEARLS**
> - Asymptomatic AAT patients should be monitored annually with history, physical examination, spirometry, and liver function tests.
> - Smoking cessation should be advised for all patients with AAT deficiency.
> - Those with symptomatic liver disease should be frequently monitored for onset of complications and managed accordingly.
> - Those fitting the criteria for AAT augmentation therapy should be evaluated and started on supplementation therapy which has been known to prevent progression and complications associated with lung disease.

Section 5: Special Populations
Pregnancy
- There is an increased risk of miscarriage and stillbirth in patients with AAT deficiency.
- It is advisable to augment the second stage of labor to prevent occurrence of lung-associated complications like pneumothorax.
- Use of steroids and antibiotics should be very judicious.

Children
- Management of children is essentially the same except that children with ESLD are prime candidates for liver transplantation.

Section 6: Prognosis

- Approximately one in five individuals homozygous for the Z allele will develop clinically significant liver disease.

> **CLINICAL PEARLS**
> - In children, AAT is the most common cause of genetic liver disease.
> - Enzyme supplementation is effective in treating lung disease associated with AAT, but it is not effective for liver disease.

Natural history of untreated liver disease
- The earliest sign of liver disease due to AAT is typically abnormal serum liver function tests.
- Cirrhosis may manifest as variceal bleeding, ascites or encephalopathy.
- Hepatocellular carcinoma affects a small percentage and usually follows after the development of cirrhosis.

Prognosis for treated patients
- Liver transplantation is curative and patients have a greater than 90% survival at 5 years post-transplantation.

Follow-up tests and monitoring
- Asymptomatic individuals with liver disease should have blood test monitoring every 6 months.

Section 7: Reading List

Ekeowa UI, Marciniak SJ, Lomas DA. α(1)-antitrypsin deficiency and inflammation. Expert Rev Clin.Immunol 2007;7:243–52

Eriksson S, Carlson J, Velez R. Risk of cirrhosis and primary liver cancer in alpha 1-antitrypsin deficiency. N Engl J Med 1986;314:736–9

Flotte TR, Mueller C. Gene therapy for alpha-1 antitrypsin deficiency patients. Hum Mol Genet 2011;20:R87–92

Hogarth DK, Rachelefsky G. Screening and familial testing of patients for alpha1-antitrypsin deficiency. Chest 2008;133;981–8

Fairbanks KD, Tavill AS. Liver disease in alpha 1-antitrypsin deficiency: a review. Am J Gastroenterol 2008;103:2136–41

Sveger T. Liver disease in alpha 1-antitrypsin deficiency detected by screening of 200,000 infants. N Eng J Med 1976;294:1316–21

Sveger T, Eriksson S. The liver in adolescents with alpha 1-antitrypsin deficiency. Hepatology 1995;22:514–7

Teckman JH, Lindblad D. Alpha-1-antitrypsin deficiency: diagnosis ,pathophysiology and management. Curr Gastroenterol Rep 2006;8:14–20

Teckman JH, Qu D, Perlmutter DH. Molecular pathogenesis of liver disease in alpha1-antitrypsin deficiency. Hepatology 1996;24:1504–16

Section 8: Guidelines

No liver society guidelines but American Thoracic Society/European Respiratory Society have a joint guideline for diagnosis and management of AAT deficiency (Am J Respir Crit Care Med 2003;168:818–900).

Section 9: Evidence

Not applicable for this topic.

Section 10: Images

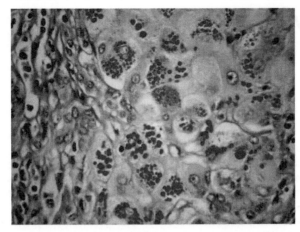

Figure 17.1 PAS-positive globules. Source: Courtesy of Dr Swan N. Thung, The Mount Sinai Medical Center, New York, NY, USA.

Additional material for this chapter can be found online at:
www.mountsinaiexpertguides.com
This includes a case study and multiple choice questions

CHAPTER 18

Portal Hypertensive Bleeding

Jawad Ahmad

Division of Liver Diseases, Icahn School of Medicine at Mount Sinai, New York, NY, USA

OVERALL BOTTOM LINE

- Bleeding due to portal hypertension remains a significant cause of morbidity and mortality in cirrhotic patients.
- Portal hypertension can lead to bleeding from esophageal varices, gastric varices, portal hypertensive gastropathy and ectopic varices.
- Several methods are employed to control active bleeding from portal hypertension including pharmacological, endoscopic, radiological and surgical.
- In most centers the initial approach to portal hypertensive bleeding should include adequate resuscitation, reduction of portal pressure using somatostatin analogues, and an attempt at endoscopic therapy.
- Primary and secondary prophylaxis of portal hypertensive bleeding are established treatment strategies to improve outcome.

Section 1: Background
Definition of disease

- Portal hypertensive bleeding is bleeding from porto-systemic collaterals that develop in patients with portal hypertension, most commonly in the setting of cirrhosis.
- The pressure gradient between the portal and hepatic veins needs to be above 12 mmHg for bleeding to occur from esophageal varices.

Disease classification

- There is no strict disease classification for portal hypertensive bleeding but it can be classified according to the cause of bleeding since management will differ.

Incidence/prevalence

- Variceal bleeding complicates cirrhosis in approximately one-third of cases.
- Despite improvements in management, mortality from an episode of variceal bleeding is 20–30% and the risk of rebleeding without treatment within the next year is 60–70%.

Economic impact

- The cost of managing variceal bleeding, particularly when there is failure to control the initial event and in patients with more severe liver disease, is high.

Mount Sinai Expert Guides: Hepatology, First Edition. Edited by Jawad Ahmad, Scott L. Friedman, and Henryk Dancygier.
© 2014 John Wiley & Sons, Ltd. Published 2014 by John Wiley & Sons, Ltd.
Companion website: www.mountsinaiexpertguides.com

• Average inpatient costs range from $15 000 to $25 000 and up to $45 000 when more than one procedure is required to control bleeding.

Etiology
• Bleeding from portal hypertension is due to esophageal varices, gastric varices, portal hypertensive gastropathy or ectopic varices.
• Acute upper gastrointestinal bleeding in the patient with portal hypertension is usually due to esophageal or gastric varices.
• Portal hypertensive gastropathy bleeding typically presents with more insidious bleeding with melena or anemia.
• Ectopic varices can present with occult gastrointestinal bleeding depending on the location or rectal bleeding if in the colon or rectum.

Pathology/pathogenesis
• The normal portal pressure is less than 5 mmHg. The portal system has the capacity to double the flow without an increase in pressure (as occurs after eating) but obstruction to flow leads to portal hypertension. This most commonly occurs at the sinusoidal level from cirrhosis but can occur pre-sinusoidal (portal vein thrombosis or portal fibrosis) or post-sinusoidal (Budd–Chiari syndrome or sinusoidal obstruction syndrome). An increase in portal inflow is also seen in cirrhosis due to splanchnic arteriolar vasodilation (and occasionally an arterio-portal fistula can lead to portal hypertension).
• The rise in portal pressure leads to the development of porto-systemic collaterals that decompress the portal system. These can occur in several locations but typically in the distal esophagus and proximal stomach.
• A pressure gradient of >12 mmHg between the portal and hepatic veins is required for the development of bleeding from esophageal varices.

Predictive/risk factors (for esophageal variceal bleeding)
• A prognostic risk index was developed using a combination of Child's class, variceal size and appearance that can predict the risk of initial variceal bleeding.

Risk factor	Comment
Size of varices	Increased risk correlates with increased size
Endoscopic appearance of varices	Red wale signs, cherry red spots and hematocystic spots increase the risk of bleeding
Severity of liver disease (Child's score)	Child's C have higher risk of bleeding
Variceal pressure	Not routinely measured but directly correlates with risk of bleeding
	No bleeding at pressure ≤12 mmHg

Section 2: Prevention

CLINICAL PEARLS
• Non-selective beta-blockers such as propranolol and nadolol decrease the risk of initial variceal bleeding compared with placebo.
• Endoscopic band ligation of esophageal varices (grade 2 or larger) is as effective as non-selective beta-blockers in preventing variceal bleeding.

Screening
- All patients with cirrhosis should undergo endoscopy to assess for portal hypertension and determine the severity and risk for bleeding.
- In patients with compensated cirrhosis without varices endoscopy should be repeated every 2–3 years.
- In patients with compensated cirrhosis and small varices without stigmata of high risk for bleeding (red wale signs, etc.), non-selective beta-blockers can be used although the benefit is not clear. If pharmacotherapy is not used, endoscopy should be repeated annually.
- In patients with compensated cirrhosis and medium/large (grade 2 or higher) varices, or small varices with stigmata of high risk for bleeding, non-selective beta-blockers should be used. Repeat endoscopy is not required. In patients intolerant of beta-blockers (or contra-indicated), band ligation of esophageal varices can be performed and continued until varices are eradicated and then annual endoscopy should be performed.
- In decompensated cirrhosis the presence of varices should lead to the use of non-selective beta-blockers and repeat endoscopy is unnecessary. In patients intolerant of beta-blockers (or contra-indicated), band ligation of esophageal varices can be performed and continued until varices are eradicated and then annual endoscopy should be performed.

Primary prevention
- Most of the studies examining primary prevention deal only with esophageal varices.
- Patients with cirrhosis and other causes of portal hypertension should undergo periodic endoscopy (every 2–3 years in Child's A patients, annually in Child's B or C patients) to be screened for the presence of varices.
- If significant varices are present (grade 2 or higher for esophageal varices), a non-selective beta blocker (propranolol, nadolol or carvedilol) should be used if no contra-indication to decrease the portal pressure. The dose should be titrated to achieve a resting heart rate of 55–60 beats/minute.
- Non-selective beta-blockers reduce the risk of first variceal hemorrhage by up to 50% although an overall survival benefit has not been consistently demonstrated.
- Non-selective beta-blockers do not prevent the formation of varices although they may reduce the risk of smaller varices progressing to larger varices.
- Several meta-analyses have demonstrated endoscopic therapy using band ligation is at least as effective as beta-blockers for prevention of first variceal bleed and can be used as an alternative in situations where beta-blockers are contra-indicated.

Secondary prevention
- After an initial episode of variceal bleeding, one third of patients will rebleed within the next 6 weeks.
- Endoscopic therapy using band ligation at periodic intervals (typically 1–6 weeks) until esophageal varices have been eradicated is effective in preventing rebleeding.
- Non-selective beta-blockers reduce the risk of recurrent variceal bleeding by 30–40% and reduce the risk of death by 20%.
- The combination of endoscopic band ligation and non-selective beta-blockers is more effective than either modality alone in preventing recurrent variceal bleeding.
- TIPS is effective at preventing recurrent variceal bleeding (decreasing the risk down to 10–20%) and can be used as salvage therapy when bleeding cannot be controlled with endoscopy. However, it is associated with the risk of hepatic encephalopathy.

- A recent study has suggested that early TIPS (within 72 hours) in patients with cirrhosis and acute variceal bleeding who were treated with endoscopic therapy had lower rebleeding rates and decreased mortality.
- Surgery (usually distal splenorenal shunt) reduces the risk of recurrent variceal bleeding compared with endoscopic sclerotherapy but is limited to well-compensated patients, does not improve survival, and needs an experienced surgeon, severely limiting its role.
- Liver transplantation is the definitive treatment to prevent recurrent variceal bleeding in appropriate cirrhotic patients.

Section 3: Diagnosis

CLINICAL PEARLS
- The patient presenting with portal hypertensive bleeding is typically not a diagnostic dilemma as the presentation is commonly with hematemesis or melena in a patient with underlying cirrhosis.
- Examination findings can confirm the presence of cirrhosis and portal hypertension with palmar erythema, spider nevi and splenomegaly among other stigmata of chronic liver disease.
- The initial investigations depend on the presentation. Patients with significant blood loss and hypotension need to be resuscitated, usually in an intensive care setting. Blood tests may show a low hematocrit, coagulopathy and thrombocytopenia. Emergent endoscopy can make the diagnosis and affords the opportunity to provide therapy.
- Other causes of portal hypertensive bleeding can present more insidiously with anemia in the case of portal hypertensive gastropathy, occult gastrointestinal bleeding for small bowel varices and rectal bleeding with rectal varices.

Differential diagnosis

Differential diagnosis	Features
Any other cause of gastrointestinal bleeding	History demonstrates no risk factors for chronic liver disease but might indicate risk factors for other causes, e.g. non-steroidal anti-inflammatory drug use leading to peptic ulceration
	Examination does not show stigmata of chronic liver disease
	Endoscopy should differentiate the cause of bleeding but some other causes are also common in patients with liver disease such as peptic ulceration
Non-cirrhotic portal hypertension can lead to identical causes of bleeding	History may not demonstrate risk factors for cirrhosis but there may be risk factors for non-cirrhotic portal hypertension such as ethnicity (for schistosomiasis)
	Examination may be similar with palmar erythema, spider nevi, ascites and splenomegaly
	Endoscopy will show the same features

Typical presentation

- The typical presentation of portal hypertensive bleeding from esophageal or gastric varices is with hematemesis or melena in a patient known to have underlying liver disease. Other causes of portal hypertensive bleeding can lead to a more insidious presentation with anemia in the case of portal hypertensive gastropathy, occult gastrointestinal bleeding with small bowel varices and rectal bleeding from rectal varices. Occasionally bleeding from stomal varices may be seen in patients with portal hypertension and prior stoma formation.
- Examination usually confirms cirrhosis and portal hypertension with stigmata of chronic liver disease such as palmar erythema, spider nevi and splenomegaly.

Clinical diagnosis

History

- The history in portal hypertensive bleeding is usually straightforward with hematemesis, coffee ground emesis or melena the presenting complaints.
- It is important to ask about risk factors for underlying liver disease such as alcohol and viral hepatitis.
- A prior history of variceal bleeding is common.
- Use of aspirin or other non-steroidal anti-inflammatory agents is important as peptic ulcer disease is common in cirrhotics and can present in a similar fashion.
- If the patient is unable to give a history due to being moribund then it is important to get these details from family or friends.

Physical examination

- During the physical examination it is important to look for stigmata of chronic liver disease if the diagnosis is not apparent from the history.
- This includes palmar erythema, spider nevi, scleral icterus, ascites and portal hypertension.
- A rectal examination with a stool guaiac test can confirm melena.

Disease severity classification

- Although there are no standard criteria of disease severity in variceal bleeding, certain parameters have been defined by a series of consensus conferences for the purposes of studies and clinical trials. The most recent is Baveno V that defines:
  - Failure to control initial bleeding: based on fresh blood in nasogastric aspirate, decrease in hemoglobin, transfusion requirement, development of hypovolemic shock, or death.
  - Failure of secondary prophylaxis: clinically significant re-bleeding resulting in hospital admission, blood transfusion, drop in hemoglobin or death within 6 weeks.

Laboratory diagnosis

List of diagnostic tests

- All patients presenting with suspected variceal bleeding should have the following laboratory tests sent:
  - Complete blood count.
  - Prothrombin time.
  - Chemistry panel.

List of imaging techniques

- In patients with upper gastrointestinal bleeding from suspected esophageal or gastric varices abdominal ultrasound with Doppler is sensible to determine hepatic vascular patency (particularly the portal vein) in case TIPS is required subsequently.
- If occult bleeding from portal hypertension is suspected, abdominal imaging with CT or MRI is not unreasonable and tagged red cell scan and angiogram may be required.

Potential pitfalls/common errors made regarding diagnosis of disease

- The diagnosis of portal hypertensive bleeding can be confused with bleeding from other causes, particularly if there is massive bleeding obscuring the endoscopic view.
- There can also be confusion in determining whether bleeding came from esophageal or gastric varices when both are present. This can lead to fear that banding esophageal varices may make gastric varices bleed although anecdotally this does not appear to be the case.

Section 4: Treatment
Treatment rationale

- The treatment for portal hypertensive bleeding depends on the cause but for all patients with significant bleeding the first step is resuscitation (Algorithm 18.1). This involves securing the airway with intubation if necessary, at least two large bore intravenous access catheters, starting intravenous fluids or colloid and blood and blood products as necessary. Patients should not be overtransfused and a hemoglobin of 8 g/dL is the goal.
- Intravenous somatostatin analogues such as octreotide and a proton pump inhibitor should be started and a dose of intravenous antibiotics such as ciprofloxacin should be given.
- Endoscopy should be performed after resuscitation, octreotide and antibiotics.
- Endoscopic therapy with band ligation for esophageal varices (or sclerotherapy with 5% sodium morrhuate or 5% ethanolamine if banding is not possible) or cyanoacrylate injection (if available) for gastric varices should be performed, with the airway secured if there is active bleeding.
- If bleeding is from esophageal or gastric varices and cannot be controlled endoscopically, balloon tamponade can be used (where a balloon is inserted nasally or orally into the proximal stomach and distal esophagus and inflated) temporarily.
- Radiologic therapy with TIPS (or other modalities particularly for gastric varices such as coil embolization or BRTO) can be used if endoscopic therapy is unsuccessful.

When to hospitalize

- All patients with portal hypertensive bleeding should be hospitalized.
- If facilities do not exist for endoscopic or radiological treatment the patient should be transferred to another center that provides these services after the patient has been resuscitated and stabilized.

Managing the hospitalized patient

- All of the management in portal hypertensive bleeding applies to the hospitalized patient.
- If facilities are available then the patient with active variceal bleeding should be managed in the intensive care unit setting.

Algorithm 18.1 Therapeutic algorithm for patient with known/suspected portal hypertensive bleeding

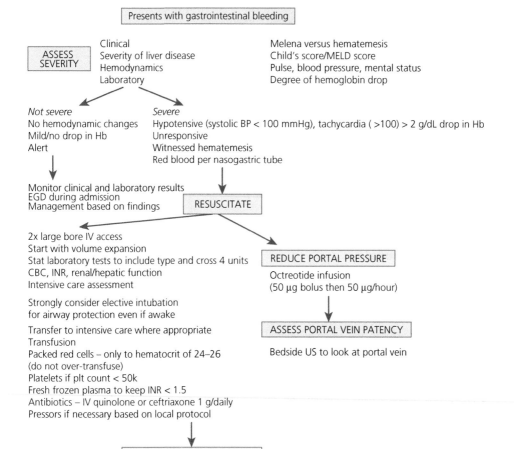

| Presents with gastrointestinal bleeding |

ASSESS SEVERITY

Clinical
Severity of liver disease
Hemodynamics
Laboratory

Melena versus hematemesis
Child's score/MELD score
Pulse, blood pressure, mental status
Degree of hemoglobin drop

Not severe
No hemodynamic changes
Mild/no drop in Hb
Alert

Severe
Hypotensive (systolic BP < 100 mmHg), tachycardia (>100) > 2 g/dL drop in Hb
Unresponsive
Witnessed hematemesis
Red blood per nasogastric tube

Monitor clinical and laboratory results
EGD during admission
Management based on findings

RESUSCITATE

2x large bore IV access
Start with volume expansion
Stat laboratory tests to include type and cross 4 units
CBC, INR, renal/hepatic function
Intensive care assessment

REDUCE PORTAL PRESSURE

Octreotide infusion
(50 μg bolus then 50 μg/hour)

Strongly consider elective intubation
for airway protection even if awake

Transfer to intensive care where appropriate
Transfusion
Packed red cells – only to hematocrit of 24–26
(do not over-transfuse)
Platelets if plt count < 50k
Fresh frozen plasma to keep INR < 1.5
Antibiotics – IV quinolone or ceftriaxone 1 g/daily
Pressors if necessary based on local protocol

ASSESS PORTAL VEIN PATENCY

Bedside US to look at portal vein

THERAPEUTIC ENDOSCOPY

Aim to get EGD within 3–4 hours of presentation but definitely within 12 hours
Blood, blood products and octreotide should have been given/started

Algorithm 18.1 (*Continued*)

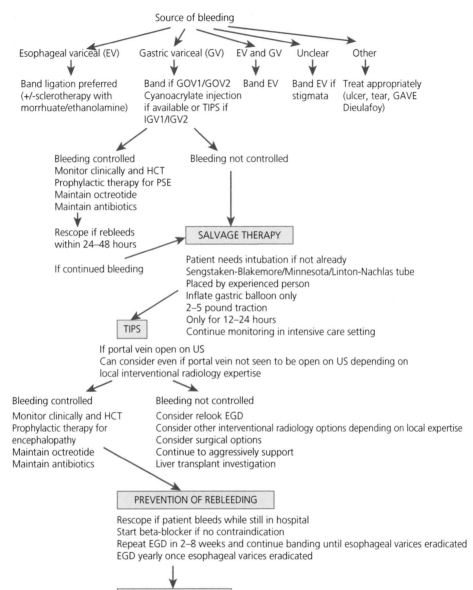

Source of bleeding

| Esophageal variceal (EV) | Gastric variceal (GV) | EV and GV | Unclear | Other |

Band ligation preferred (+/-sclerotherapy with morrhuate/ethanolamine)

Band if GOV1/GOV2 Cyanoacrylate injection if available or TIPS if IGV1/IGV2

Band EV

Band EV if stigmata

Treat appropriately (ulcer, tear, GAVE Dieulafoy)

Bleeding controlled
Monitor clinically and HCT
Prophylactic therapy for PSE
Maintain octreotide
Maintain antibiotics

Rescope if rebleeds within 24–48 hours

If continued bleeding

Bleeding not controlled

SALVAGE THERAPY

Patient needs intubation if not already
Sengstaken-Blakemore/Minnesota/Linton-Nachlas tube
Placed by experienced person
Inflate gastric balloon only
2–5 pound traction
Only for 12–24 hours
Continue monitoring in intensive care setting

TIPS

If portal vein open on US
Can consider even if portal vein not seen to be open on US depending on local interventional radiology expertise

Bleeding controlled

Monitor clinically and HCT
Prophylactic therapy for encephalopathy
Maintain octreotide
Maintain antibiotics

Bleeding not controlled

Consider relook EGD
Consider other interventional radiology options depending on local expertise
Consider surgical options
Continue to aggressively support
Liver transplant investigation

PREVENTION OF REBLEEDING

Rescope if patient bleeds while still in hospital
Start beta-blocker if no contraindication
Repeat EGD in 2–8 weeks and continue banding until esophageal varices eradicated
EGD yearly once esophageal varices eradicated

CONTINUED BLEEDING

If continued bleeding despite secondary prophylaxis measures
Consider TIPS
Consider distal spleno-renal (or other) shunt in Child's A and MELD < 10–12
Consider expeditious liver transplant investigation

Table of treatment

Treatment	Comment
Medical: Octreotide	Given as 50 µg bolus followed by 50 µg per hour for 3–5 days
Somatostatin (not available in USA)	Given as 250 µg bolus followed by 250 µg per hour for 3–5 days
Terlipressin (not available in USA)	Given 2 mg IV every 4 hours and decreased to 1 mg IV every 4 hours if bleeding controlled and given for 3–5 days
Balloon tamponade	Typically used as a temporary measure where bleeding cannot be controlled endoscopically and while arrangements are being made for TIPS. Patient should be intubated prior to insertion and less complications in experienced hands
Surgical: Endoscopic Band ligation	Use for esophageal and gastroesophageal varices. Not to be used for isolated gastric varices
Sclerotherapy (with morrhuate, ethanolamine)	Use for esophageal and gastroesophageal varices. Can be used for isolated gastric varices if no other options
Sclerotherapy with cyanoacrylate (very limited availability in USA) Surgery:	Use for gastric varices
Porto-systemic shunting, such as distal splenorenal or portacaval shunt	Can use in selected well-compensated patients after control of initial bleeding if local surgical expertise available
Radiological: TIPS	Can use for esophageal and gastric variceal bleeding if cannot control endoscopically. Can also use as secondary prophylaxis in selected patients where initial bleeding controlled and high risk for further bleeding
BRTO	Can use for selected cases of gastric variceal bleeding if local expertise available

Prevention/management of complications
- Balloon tamponade can lead to esophageal rupture during placement (particularly if placed by someone inexperienced with the technique). If the balloon is left inflated for >12–24 hours, pressure necrosis can occur.
- Rebleeding can occur when the balloon is deflated.
- Endoscopic therapy can be associated with several complications including bleeding from ulceration from the banding or sclerotherapy and the latter can lead to esophageal stricture formation. It can also worsen any bleeding from portal hypertensive gastropathy.
- Cyanoacrylate injection is relatively safe in experienced hands but can rarely lead to distant emboli (in less than 1% of cases).
- TIPS is associated with hepatic encephalopathy in up to a third of cases.

> **CLINICAL PEARLS**
> - The patient needs to be adequately resuscitated before any endoscopic or radiologic therapy.
> - Octreotide and antibiotics should be given before any endoscopic therapy to try and decrease the bleeding allowing for a better view.
> - If massive bleeding is noted before or during endoscopy, intubation for airway protection is essential.
> - Balloon tamponade should be readily available in the intensive care unit and someone who has placed a balloon before should be present.

Section 5: Special Populations
Pregnancy
- The literature on treating portal hypertensive bleeding in pregnancy is limited to case reports and does not differ significantly from typical cirrhotic patients.

Section 6: Prognosis

> **CLINICAL PEARLS**
> - Variceal bleeding still carries a high mortality.
> - The severity of liver disease impacts on survival.
> - Even in Child's A patients, variceal bleeding should prompt consideration for liver transplant evaluation.

Natural history of untreated disease
- The mortality for each episode of variceal bleeding is 20–30% but rises with more severe liver disease.
- Mortality in untreated patients is 60–70% at 2 years.

Prognosis for treated patients
- The prognosis for successfully treated patients will depend on the cause and the severity of the underlying liver disease.
- Child's B and C patients should undergo liver transplant evaluation if no contraindication.

Follow-up tests and monitoring
- In patients with variceal bleeding that has been controlled initially, follow up will depend on the cause of the bleeding and the severity of liver disease.
- For esophageal variceal bleeding, endoscopy should be repeated every few weeks (2–6 weeks) until the varices are eradicated and then annually afterwards.
- Non-selective beta-blockers should be started after the initial control of bleeding as tolerated.
- For gastric variceal bleeding, if endoscopic therapy with cyanoacrylate is available and successful, periodic surveillance endoscopy should continue.
- If TIPS is required periodic US with Doppler to assess patency is required and surveillance endoscopy can be performed.

Section 7: Reading List

Besson I, Ingrand P, Person B, et al. Sclerotherapy with or without octreotide for acute variceal bleeding. N Engl J Med 1995;333:555–60

Boyer TD, Haskal ZJ, American Association for the Study of Liver Diseases. The role of transjugular intrahepatic portosystemic shunt (TIPS) in the management of portal hypertension: update 2009. Hepatology 2010; 51:306

de Franchis R. Revising consensus in portal hypertension: report of the Baveno V consensus workshop on methodology of diagnosis and therapy in portal hypertension. J Hepatol 2010;53:762–8

D'Amico, G, De Franchis, R. Upper digestive bleeding in cirrhosis. Post-therapeutic outcome and prognostic indicators. Hepatology 2003; 38:599–612

Fernandez, J, Del Arbol, LR, Gomez, C, et al. Norfloxacin vs ceftriaxone in the prophylaxis of infections in patients with advanced cirrhosis and hemorrhage. Gastroenterology 2006; 131:1049–56

García-Pagán JC, Caca K, Bureau C, et al. Early use of TIPS in patients with cirrhosis and variceal bleeding. N Engl J Med 2010;362:2370–9

Garcia-Tsao G, Sanyal AJ, Grace ND, et al. Practice Guidelines Committee of the American Association for the Study of Liver Diseases, Practice Parameters Committee of the American College of Gastroenterology. Prevention and management of gastroesophageal varices and variceal hemorrhage in cirrhosis. Hepatology 2007;46:922–38

North Italian Endoscopic Club for the Study and Treatment of Esophageal Varices. Prediction of the first variceal hemorrhage in patients with cirrhosis of the liver and esophageal varices. A prospective multicenter study. N Engl J Med 1988;319:983–9

Sarin SK, Kumar A, Angus PW, et al. Diagnosis and management of acute variceal bleeding: Asian Pacific Association for Study of the Liver recommendations. Hepatol Int 2011;5:607–24

Stiegmann GV, Goff JS, Michaletz-Onody PA, et al. Endoscopic sclerotherapy as compared with endoscopic ligation for bleeding esophageal varices. N Engl J Med 1992;326:1527–32

Thabut D, Hammer M, Cai Y, et al. Cost of treatment of oesophageal variceal bleeding in patients with cirrhosis in France: results of a French survey. Eur J Gastroenterol Hepatol 2007;19:679–86

Suggested website

http://www.aasld.org/practiceguidelines/Documents/Bookmarked%20Practice%20Guidelines/Prevention%20and%20Management%20of%20Gastro%20Varices%20and%20Hemorrhage.pdf

Section 8: Guidelines
National society guidelines

Guideline title	Guideline source	Date
Prevention and management of gastroesophageal varices and variceal hemorrhage in cirrhosis	American Association for the Study of Liver Diseases (AASLD), American College of Gastroenterology (ACG) http://www.aasld.org/practiceguidelines/Documents/Bookmarked%20Practice%20Guidelines/Prevention%20and%20Management%20of%20Gastro%20Varices%20and%20Hemorrhage.pdf	2007
The role of transjugular intrahepatic portosystemic shunt (TIPS) in the management of portal hypertension: update 2009	American Association for the Study of Liver Diseases (AASLD) http://www.aasld.org/practiceguidelines/Documents/Bookmarked%20Practice%20Guidelines/TIPS%20Update%20Nov%202009.pdf	2009

International society guidelines

Guideline title	Guideline source	Date
Diagnosis and management of acute variceal bleeding: Asian Pacific Association for Study of the Liver recommendations.	Asia Pacific Association for Study of the Liver (APASL) http://www.ncbi.nlm.nih.gov/pmc/articles/PMC3090560/pdf/12072_2010_Article_9236.pdf	2011

Section 9: Evidence

Type of evidence	Title, date	Comment
RCT	Endoscopic sclerotherapy as compared with endoscopic ligation for bleeding esophageal varices. N Engl J Med 1992;326:1527	Demonstrated that band ligation was more effective and safer than sclerotherapy for bleeding esophageal varices
RCT	Sclerotherapy with or without octreotide for acute variceal bleeding. N Engl J Med 1995;333:555	Demonstrated that the combination of endoscopic therapy with sclerotherapy and octreotide was more effective than sclerotherapy alone in controlling acute variceal bleeding
RCT	Prospective randomised study of effect of octreotide on rebleeding from oesophageal varices after endoscopic ligation. Lancet 1995;346:1666	Demonstrated that octreotide significantly reduces recurrent bleeding and the need for balloon tamponade in patients with variceal haemorrhage treated by endoscopic variceal ligation
RCT	A prospective, randomized trial of butyl cyanoacrylate injection versus band ligation in the management of bleeding gastric varices. Hepatology 2001;33:1060	Demonstrated that cyanoacrylate more effective than band ligation for gastric variceal bleeding
RCT	Norfloxacin vs ceftriaxone in the prophylaxis of infections in patients with advanced cirrhosis and hemorrhage. Gastroenterology 2006;131:1049	Demonstrated that intravenous ceftriaxone was more effective than oral norfloxacin in the prophylaxis of bacterial infections in patients with advanced cirrhosis and hemorrhage

Section 10: Images

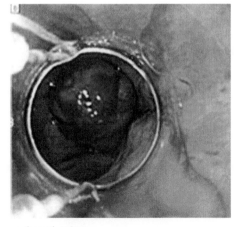

Figure 18.1 Band ligation esophageal varices.

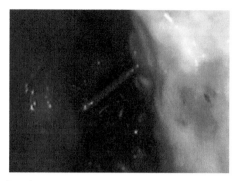

Figure 18.2 Bleeding gastric varix.

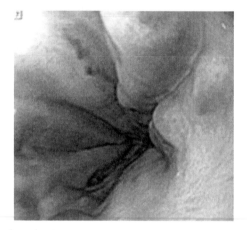

Figure 18.3 Medium esophageal varices.

Additional material for this chapter can be found online at:
www.mountsinaiexpertguides.com
This includes a case study and multiple choice questions

CHAPTER 19

Ascites

Henryk Dancygier

Departments of Medicine II and IV, Sana Klinikum Offenbach, Goethe University, Frankfurt am Main, Germany *and* Division of Liver Diseases, Icahn School of Medicine at Mount Sinai, New York, NY, USA

OVERALL BOTTOM LINE
- Ascites is the excessive accumulation of fluid in the peritoneal cavity.
- Eighty percent of cases are due to liver cirrhosis.
- Portal hypertension, reduced effective arterial blood volume, combined with impairment of renal Na^+ and water excretion are the main pathogenic mechanisms in cirrhotic ascites.
- Abdominal US is the imaging method of choice in demonstrating ascites.
- Diagnostic paracentesis with cell count and differential, determination of total protein concentration, serum-ascites albumin gradient and ascitic cultures are the essential initial procedures in the diagnostic investigations of a patient with ascites.
- In approximately 90% of patients ascites can be managed with diet and diuretics.
- The formation of grade 2 or 3 ascites is associated with a mortality of 50% and 80% within 2 and 5 years respectively after the first ascites episode.

Section 1: Background
Definition of disease
- Ascites denotes the pathologic accumulation of fluid in the peritoneal cavity.

Disease classification
- According to the amount of ascitic fluid grade 1–3 ascites may be distinguished:
  - Grade 1 ascites: mild ascites only detectable by US examination.
  - Grade 2 ascites: moderate ascites, manifest on physical examination by moderate symmetrical distension of the abdomen.
  - Grade 3 ascites: large, tense ascites or gross ascites with marked abdominal distension.
- May be classified depending on whether or not ascites can be managed successfully with dietary salt restriction and diuretics alone
- Uncomplicated ascites is differentiated from refractory (complicated) ascites (see Section 3).

Incidence/prevalence
- Approximately 25% of patients with compensated cirrhosis develop ascites during a follow up period of 10 years.

Mount Sinai Expert Guides: Hepatology, First Edition. Edited by Jawad Ahmad, Scott L. Friedman, and Henryk Dancygier.

Etiology

Causes of ascites

Cause	Frequency (%)
Parenchymal liver disease:	78
Cirrhosis	77
Fulminant liver failure	1
Malignancy:	12
Peritoneal carcinomatosis (gynecological tumors, gastric carcinoma, extensive liver metastases)	
Cardiovascular disease:	5
Congestive heart failure	
Constrictive or restrictive cardiomyopathy	
Thrombosis of inferior vena cava	
Budd–Chiari syndrome	
Veno-occlusive disease	
Infection:	2
Tuberculosis	
Fitz–Hugh–Curtis syndrome (chlamydiae, gonococci)	
Coccidioidomycosis	
Whipple's disease (*Tropheryma whipplei*)	
Renal:	1.5
Nephrotic syndrome	
Uremia	
Hemodialysis	
Pancreatic	1
Bacterial peritonitis	0.5
Other rare causes:	
Marked hypothyroidism	
Collagen vascular disease	
Familial Mediterranean fever	
Amyloidosis	
Hereditary angioneurotic edema	
Menetrier's disease and protein-losing enteropathy	
Starch peritonitis	
Trauma	
Arterioportal fistula after liver biopsy	
Pregnancy specific liver diseases	
Ovary overstimulation syndrome	

Causes of chylous ascites*

Neoplastic (e.g. lymphoma, carcinoid tumors, Kaposi's sarcoma)
Cirrhotic (common in adults)
Infectious:
Tuberculosis
Atypical mycobacteriosis (*Mycobacterium avium intracellulare*)
Filariasis (*Wuchereria bancrofti*)
Whipple's disease (*Tropheryma whipplei*)

Inflammatory:
Radiation
Pancreatitis
Constrictive pericarditis
Retroperitoneal fibrosis
Sarcoidosis
Celiac sprue
Retractile mesenteritis

Post-operative:
Abdominal aneurysm repair
Retroperitoneal node dissection
Catheter placement for peritoneal dialysis
Inferior vena cava resection

Traumatic:
Blunt abdominal trauma
Battered child syndrome

Congenital:
Primary lymphatic hypoplasia
Yellow nail syndrome
Klippel–Trenaunay syndrome
Primary lymphatic hyperplasia
Intestinal lymphangiectasia ("megalymphatics")

Other causes:
Right heart failure
Dilated cardiomyopathy
Nephrotic syndrome
Lymphangioleiomyomatosis (10% of cases show chylous ascites)

*Chylous ascites is a milky-appearing peritoneal fluid (lymph) that is rich in triglycerides (often greater than 1000 mg/dL).

Pathogenesis
- Portal hypertension is the main underlying pathogenetic factor in the development of ascites in patients with liver cirrhosis.
- Various mediators in portal hypertensive patients lead to peripheral and splanchnic vasodilation with reduction of the effective arterial blood volume, combined with an impairment of renal Na^+ and water excretion.
- In liver cirrhosis the balance between the extracellular fluid and Na^+-excretion is disrupted, i.e. despite an elevated extracellular fluid volume, Na^+ is inadequately retained (Algorithm 19.1).

Section 2: Prevention

- The key to prevention of ascites is prevention and treatment of the underlying disease(s).

Screening
- US is the most cost-effective imaging modality for the diagnosis of ascites. It detects as little as 100 mL ascites.
- CT and MRI are not superior to US in the diagnosis of ascites.

Algorithm 19.1 Pathogenetic factors responsible for increased Na⁺-retention in liver cirrhosis

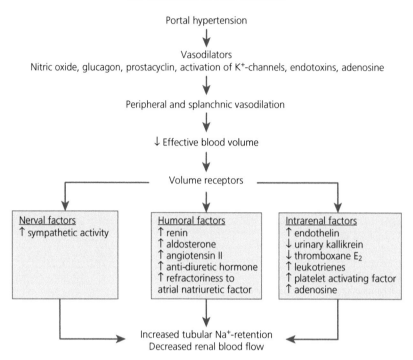

Portal hypertension
↓
Vasodilators
Nitric oxide, glucagon, prostacyclin, activation of K⁺-channels, endotoxins, adenosine
↓
Peripheral and splanchnic vasodilation
↓
↓ Effective blood volume
↓
Volume receptors
↓

Nerval factors	Humoral factors	Intrarenal factors
↑ sympathetic activity	↑ renin	↑ endothelin
	↑ aldosterone	↓ urinary kallikrein
	↑ angiotensin II	↓ thromboxane E₂
	↑ anti-diuretic hormone	↑ leukotrienes
	↑ refractoriness to	↑ platelet activating factor
	atrial natriuretic factor	↑ adenosine

Increased tubular Na⁺-retention
Decreased renal blood flow

- There is no evidence that screening for ascites improves the outcome of patients with liver cirrhosis.

Section 3: Diagnosis (Algorithm 19.2)

CLINICAL PEARLS
- A detailed history will provide the first clues to the presence and possible etiology of liver disease. Look for evidence of past hepatitis B (± D) or C, alcohol abuse, metabolic syndrome, autoimmune hepatitis.
- Physical examination is unreliable in diagnosing small amounts of ascites. The most informative examination finding is shifting dullness to percussion. However, eliciting this sign requires at least 750–1000 mL of ascites.
- Abdominal sonography is the imaging method of choice in demonstrating as little as 100 mL of ascites.
- US-guided paracentesis allows for obtaining ascitic fluid for further laboratory examinations, such as cell count and differential, SAAG, bacterial culture and cytology.

Differential diagnosis
- The differential diagnosis of ascites must include all the causes listed in the tables Causes of ascites/chylous ascites. Liver cirrhosis, malignancy and cardiovascular diseases account for 95% of all cases of ascites in Western countries.

Algorithm 19.2 Diagnostic approach to ascites

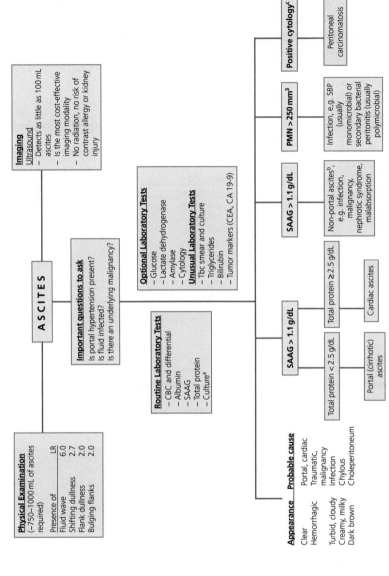

Physical Examination
(~750–1000 mL of ascites required)

Presence of	LR
Fluid wave	6.0
Shifting dullness	2.7
Flank dullness	2.0
Bulging flanks	2.0

A S C I T E S

Imaging
Ultrasound
– Detects as little as 100 mL ascites
– Is the most cost-effective imaging modality
– No radiation, no risk of contrast allergy or kidney injury

Important questions to ask
Is portal hypertension present?
Is fluid infected?
Is there an underlying malignancy?

Routine Laboratory Tests
– CBC and differential
– Albumin
– SAAG
– Total protein
– Culture[a]

Optional Laboratory Tests
– Glucose
– Lactate dehydrogenase
– Amylase
– Cytology
Unusual Laboratory Tests
– Tbc smear and culture
– Triglycerides
– Bilirubin
– Tumor markers ((CEA, CA 19-9)

SAAG > 1.1 g/dL

Total protein < 2.5 g/dL	Total protein ≥2.5 g/dL
Portal (cirrhotic) ascites	Cardiac ascites

SAAG > 1.1 g/dL

Non-portal ascites[b], e.g. infection, malignancy, nephrotic syndrome, malabsorption

PMN >250 mm³

Infection, e.g. SBP (usually monomicrobial) or secondary bacterial peritonitis (usually polymicrobial)

Positive cytology[c]

Peritoneal carcinomatosis

Appearance	Probable cause
Clear	Portal, cardiac
Hemorrhagic	Traumatic, malignancy
Turbid, cloudy	Infection
Creamy, milky	Chylous
Dark brown	Choleperitoneum

[a] Aerobic and anaerobic cultures should be obtained at the bedside
[b] Some patients with portal ascites have an SAAG < 1.1 g/dL. Think of infection. However, in the majority of these patients a specific cause for low SAAG cannot be found.
[c] Cytologic examination has a sensitivity of 96% in the diagnosis of peritoneal carcinomatosis, provided three samples are analyzed by an experienced examiner

- Four initial questions have to be answered when dealing with a patient with ascites:
  - What is the underlying cause? The diseases listed in the tables Causes of ascites/chylous ascites and the various etiologies of liver cirrhosis must be considered.
  - What is the SAAG and the total ascitic protein content?
  - Is ascites malignant?
  - Is ascites infected?

Causes of ascites based on the macroscopic appearance of ascitic fluid

Macroscopic appearance	Possible cause
Serous	Portal hypertensive
	Infectious
	Malignant
	Pancreatic
Hemorrhagic	Malignant
	Pancreatic
	Traumatic
Cloudy	Infectious (bacterial)
	Malignant
	Pancreatic
Chylous	Malignant
	Portal hypertensive

Causes of ascites based on serum-ascites albumin gradient

High gradient (≥1.1 g/dL)	Low gradient (<1.1 g/dL)
Cirrhosis	Peritoneal carcinomatosis
Alcoholic hepatitis	Tuberculous peritonitis
Cardiac failure	Pancreatic ascites
Massive liver metastases	Biliary ascites
Fulminant hepatic failure	Nephrotic syndrome
Budd–Chiari syndrome	Serositis
Veno-occlusive disease	Bowel infarction
Portal vein thrombosis	
Fatty liver of pregnancy	
Myxedema	

Typical presentation
- Cirrhotic ascites usually develops gradually, unnoticed by the patient and the physician. Often the patient complains of increasing meteorism before ascites becomes clinically manifest ("first the wind, and then the rain").
- Increasing abdominal girth and ankle edema are clinical evidence for the development of ascites in a cirrhotic patient.

Clinical diagnosis
History
- Enquire about past liver disease, potential risk factors associated with liver disease, such as intravenous drug use, promiscuity, previous viral infections, metabolic factors, e.g. obesity, type 2 diabetes mellitus.
- History of prior malignant disease.

Physical examination

- General appearance of the patient:
  - Facies alcoholica, alcoholic smell, fetor hepaticus (sweetish, ammoniacal, musty breath in patients with severe parenchymal liver disease).
  - Is the patient lethargic, confused?
  - Distended abdomen, umbilical hernia, penile or scrotal edema, generalized edema.
  - Cutaneous signs of chronic liver disease.
  - Gynecomastia.
- Physical examination is unreliable in diagnosing small amounts of ascites. The characteristic signs of ascites are bulging flanks in the supine position, tympany at the top of the abdominal wall (gas-filled small intestinal loops float on top of the fluid), shifting dullness when the patient turns to one side, and a fluid wave that may be elicited by tapping the patient's flank with a hand.
- The sensitivity and specificity of physical examination for the determination of ascites (equal clinical skills provided) depend primarily on the amount of peritoneal fluid present. The demonstration of shifting dullness is highly sensitive (up to 86%), while clear evidence of a fluid wave is highly specific (up to 82%) for the presence of ascites. However, eliciting these signs usually requires a minimum of approximately 750–1000 mL of ascites. If shifting dullness is absent, 750–1000 mL of ascites can be excluded with an accuracy of >90%.
  - Spider nevi, splenomegaly, dilated and prominent abdominal wall veins suggest cirrhosis.
  - Congested neck veins, systolic pulsations of jugular veins or of the liver may be observed in congestive right heart failure.
  - Pulsus paradoxus and a positive Kussmaul sign suggest constrictive pericarditis.
  - A pulsatile liver has been described in tricuspid regurgitation with pulmonary hypertension, and in constrictive pericarditis.
  - Visible veins on the patient's back suggest obstruction of the inferior vena cava.
  - Palpable abdominal masses, an immobile mass at the umbilicus (Sister Mary Joseph's nodule) or a coarse and nodular liver surface are highly suggestive of peritoneal carcinomatosis and metastatic liver disease.

Disease severity classification

See also Section 1.

Uncomplicated versus complicated ascites		
	Uncomplicated ascites	**Complicated ascites***
Ascites grade†	Grade 1 or 2	Grade 3
Encephalopathy	−	+
Na$^+$ in 24 hours urine	>20 mmol	<10 mmol
Serum Na$^+$	>130 mmol/L	<130 mmol/L
Serum K$^+$	3.6–4.9 mmol/L	<3.5 or >5 mmol/L
Serum creatinine	<1.5 mg/dL	>1.5 mg/dL
Serum albumin	>3.5 g/dL	<3.5 g/dL

* Spontaneous bacterial peritonitis may be present.
† See Section 1.

Refractory ascites

- Ascites refractory to therapy – either diuretic-resistant or diuretic-intractable ascites – occurs in 5–10 % of patients with cirrhotic ascites.

Diagnostic criteria of refractory ascites
Treatment duration: At least one week of intensive diuretic treatment (spironolactone 400 mg/day and furosemide 160 mg/day) accompanied by strict dietary Na$^+$-restriction of less than 90 mmol or 5.2 g of salt daily
Lack of response to therapy: Mean weight loss of <.8 kg over 4 days and 24 hours urinary Na$^+$-excretion less than oral sodium intake
Early ascites recurrence: Reaccumulation of grade 2 or 3 ascites within 4 weeks after initial mobilization
Diuretic-induced complications: *Hepatic encephalopathy*: development of encephalopathy in the absence of any other precipitating factor but diuretics *Renal insufficiency*: increase of serum creatinine by >100% to >2 mg/dL in patients with ascites responding to treatment *Hyponatremia*: decrease of serum Na$^+$ concentration by >10 mmol/L to <25 mmol/L. *Hypokalemia*: serum potassium concentration <3 mmol/L. *Hyperkalemia*: serum potassium concentration >6 mmol/L.

- Diuretic-resistant ascites refers to an ascites that despite maximal diuretic treatment (spironolactone 400 mg/day and furosemide 160 mg/day) of at least one week duration and strict dietary Na$^+$-restriction of (<90 mmol/day) cannot be mobilized or that recurs early despite intensive diuretic treatment and dietary compliance with fluid and Na$^+$-restriction. The intake of NSAIDs must be excluded, since NSAIDs blunt the response to diuretics.
- Diuretic-intractable ascites refers to an ascites that cannot be treated adequately with diuretics because diuretic-associated complications preclude the application of adequate doses of diuretics. Diuretic-induced complications are hepatic encephalopathy, renal insufficiency, hyponatremia and hypo- or hyperkalemia.

Laboratory diagnosis

Diagnostic tests

- Diagnostic paracentesis should be performed in all patients with new onset grade 2 or 3 ascites, and in all patients hospitalized for worsening ascites or any complication of ascites. Paracentesis (50–100 mL) allows further evaluation of ascites by biochemical, cytologic and bacteriologic techniques.

Evaluation of ascites obtained by diagnostic paracentesis	
	Comment
Gross inspection	See Table: Causes of ascites based on the macroscopic appearance of ascitic fluid
Cell count and differential	Cut off for spontaneous bacterial peritonitis is >250/mm^3 neutrophils (see Chapter 20)

	Comment
Total protein	Differentiates between a transudate (<3 g/L) and an exudate (>3 g/L)
Albumin, SAAG	The SAAG has largely replaced determination of total protein
	A SAAG greater than 1.1 g/dL is 97% accurate in the diagnosis of portal hypertension
	See Table: Causes of ascites based on serum-ascites albumin gradient
Amylase	Increased ascitic amylase levels are found in pancreatic ascites with levels greater than 20 000 IU/L suggesting a ruptured pancreatic duct or a leaking pseudocyst, while lower levels are seen in acute pancreatitis
Triglycerides	Chylous ascites has a milky or creamy appearance due to lymph in the abdominal cavity. Its triglyceride concentration exceeds that of plasma
LDH	Elevated in malignant and infectious ascites
Gram's and acid-fast stains	Very low diagnostic yield
Culture	10–20 mL of ascitic fluid should be inoculated into aerobic and anaerobic blood culture bottles *at the bedside*
	Ascitic mycobacterial cultures are 50% sensitive Perform also PCR for tuberculosis
Cytology	The sensitivity of cytology in differentiating between a benign and malignant ascites varies between 40% and 70%. The specificity and the positive predictive value reach >95% by experienced examiners, if at least three specimens are examined

Imaging techniques
- Abdominal US is the imaging method of choice in demonstrating as little as 100 mL of ascites. In addition, pleural and pericardial effusions may be demonstrated during the same examination, and the etiology of ascites (e.g. cirrhosis, portal vein thrombosis, liver tumors) may be determined in most cases.
- Provided US images are technically satisfactory, cost-intensive techniques such as CT and MRI are usually not mandatory.

Potential pitfalls/common errors in diagnosis
- Occasionally gaseous abdominal distension in marked obesity may mimic ascites on physical examination.
- Performing CT or MRI as the initial diagnostic imaging modality is not cost effective.
- Inoculation of ascitic fluid into culture bottles away from the bedside markedly reduces the sensitivity of ascites culture.

Section 4: Treatment (Algorithm 19.3)
When to hospitalize
- Every patient with grade 3 ascites or refractory ascites should be hospitalized.

Managing the hospitalized patient
- Cirrhotic ascites is managed by a stepped care approach (see Table "Stepped care approach to cirrhotic ascites").

Stepped care approach to cirrhotic ascites

Step	Action	Success rate
1	Bed rest and daily Na$^+$-restriction to 2 g Na$^+$ or 5.2 g dietary salt + Fluid restriction to 1–1.5 L/day	10–15%
2	In addition: spironolactone up to 400 mg PO/day	65%
3	In addition: loop diuretic, e.g. furosemide up to 160 mg PO or IV daily*	85–90%
4 (refractory ascites)	Paracentesis ≥ 5 L: albumin infusion 8 g/L of ascites removed Paracentesis < 5 L: albumin infusion 8 g/L ascites removed or consider infusion with synthetic colloidal plasma expander If not successful or intolerant of repeated large volume paracentesis: TIPS If not successful or complications: consider liver transplant	Nearly 100%

*Instead of a sequential treatment (start with spironolactone, then add a loop diuretic). A combined approach (spironolactone plus a loop diuretic from the start) may be practiced as step 2.

Bed rest
- The upright posture activates the sympathetic nervous system and the renin-angiotensin-aldosterone system.
- Bed rest may improve the response to diuretics in single cases. However, there have been no clinical studies to demonstrate increased efficacy of diuretics or shortened duration of hospitalization with bed rest.
- Bed rest is not recommended for the treatment of patients with uncomplicated ascites.

Diet
- Na$^+$-restriction to 90 mmol/day (corresponding to ~2 g Na$^+$/day or 5.2 g dietary salt/day) practiced as a no-added salt diet is advisable. A further reduction to ≤50 mmol/day (corresponding to ≤3 g dietary salt/day) is hardly practicable, since such an unpalatable diet will inevitably affect compliance with Na$^+$-restriction.
- Rigorous fluid restriction in patients with uncomplicated ascites is not warranted. In the presence of dilutional hyponatremia fluid should be restricted to 1 (–1.5) L/day (Note: no clinical trials available to assess the effect of water restriction on dilutional hyponatremia in patients with cirrhotic ascites; too rigorous water restriction may lead to central hypovolemia with consequent stimulation of ADH secretion and exacerbation of dilutional hyponatremia.)
- Protein restriction should only be carried out in the presence of clinical signs of hepatic encephalopathy.

Diuretics
- In 85–95% of patients ascites can be managed with diet and diuretics. The simplest way to control therapeutic response is by daily weighing.

- The main indications for the use of diuretics in patients with liver cirrhosis are:
  - Mild to moderate ascites.
  - Marked ascites that cannot be managed by large-volume paracentesis, e.g. because of peritoneal adhesions.
  - Patients with edema without ascites.
  - Prevention of recurrence of ascites after therapeutic paracentesis.

Diuretics used in the treatment of cirrhotic ascites				
	Dose (mg/day)	Onset of action after oral administration (hours)	Duration of action (hours)	$t_{1/2}$ (hours)
Loop diuretics				
Furosemide	40–160 PO or IV	0.5	4–6	1
Torsemide	5–40 PO	1–2	6–8	3
Bumetanide	0.5–2 mg/dose (maximum dose: 10 mg/day)	0.5–1	4–6	1–1.5
K⁺-sparing diuretics				
Spironolactone*	50–400 PO	1–2 days	3–5 days	1–1.5 (14–24)†
Eplerenone‡	25–50 PO	May take up to 4 weeks for full therapeutic effect		4–6
Amiloride§	5–10 (up to 30) PO	2	24	6–9

* Is transformed in the liver to the active metabolites canrenone and 7α-thiomethylspironolactone
† Due to active metabolites
‡ Not yet approved for the treatment of cirrhotic ascites. May be useful for patients intolerant of spironolactone
§ Not approved by the FDA for the treatment of cirrhotic ascites

Potassium-sparing diuretics

- Spironolactone is the diuretic of choice for the initial therapy of ascites due to cirrhosis. There is a lag of 3–5 days between the initiation of spironolactone therapy and the onset of natriuresis.
  - Start therapy with spironolactone 100 mg PO daily and increase progressively by 100 mg every 3–5 days if diuretic response is insufficient. The maximal daily dose is 400 mg, e.g. 200 mg twice daily.
  - Spironolactone alone is superior to loop diuretics used alone and may be used as monotherapy in the treatment of cirrhotic ascites. In patients intolerant to higher doses of spironolactone, the dose of spironolactone should be reduced and a loop diuretic added.
  - Adverse effects: antiandrogenic activity – painful gynecomastia, decreased libido, impotence; hyperkalemia; metabolic acidosis with or without hyperkalemia in patients with renal insufficiency.

- Triamterene does not cause gynecomastia. However, it is a relatively weak diuretic and inferior to spironolactone in mobilizing ascites. Dosage: initially, 50–100 mg PO twice daily. Maximum dosage is 300 mg PO daily.
- Amiloride 15–30 mg PO once a day; relatively weak diuretic action. Not approved by the FDA for the treatment of cirrhotic ascites.
- Eplerenone is a selective mineralcorticoid receptor antagonist with a lower incidence of endocrine-related side effects than spironolactone. It might become an alternative to spironolactone in patients with painful gynecomastia. Currently eplerenone is approved for the treatment of arterial hypertension and heart failure (not yet approved for cirrhotic ascites). Dosage: 25–50 mg PO once a day. Main adverse effect is hyperkalemia.

Loop diuretics

- Loop diuretics used alone have a significantly lower efficacy than spironolactone alone. A loop diuretic should not be used as the sole agent in patients with cirrhotic ascites, but be given as an adjunct to an aldosterone antagonist or to another potassium-sparing diuretic.
- Furosemide is the loop diuretic of choice in patients with cirrhotic ascites. It is administered initially, 20–40 mg PO or IV one to two times a day. Depending on the diuretic response dosage may be increased up to maximally 160 mg PO or IV daily.

  Adverse effects occur in up to 35% of patients: hypokalemia, hypochloremic metabolic alkalosis, hyponatremia, hypovolemia with prerenal azotemia, hepatorenal syndrome, hepatic encephalopathy, muscle cramps (often due to effective hypovolemia in ascitic patients). In patients with severe muscle cramps albumin, quinidine, quinine, zinc sulphate or magnesium may be tried.
- Torsemide has a longer half life than furosemide, but it is not superior to furosemide in the treatment of cirrhotic ascites. Initial dose 5–10 mg PO or IV once daily. If needed dose may be titrated upwards up to 40 mg PO or IV daily.
- Bumetanide is similar to furosemide. Initially, 1 mg PO or IV once daily. If necessary titrate upwards by doubling the dose. Maximum dose of bumetanide should not exceed 4–6 mg/day.

Practical approach to diuretic therapy

- Diuretics and dietary Na^+-restriction are the first line treatment of ascites.
- Do not be too aggressive in mobilizing ascites, do not overtreat. It is better to tolerate some ascites with normal renal function than to mobilize ascites rapidly and completely with the risk of potentially irreversible renal failure.
- A mild to moderate ascites may be treated initially solely with spironolactone 100 mg PO one to two times a day. Since the onset of action of spironolactone is gradual, 3–5 days should elapse before dosage is adjusted until diuresis is achieved.
- If the diuretic response is insufficient (weight loss <1 kg in the first week and <2 kg/week in subsequent weeks) a loop diuretic, preferentially furosemide 40 mg PO once a day is added (sequential therapy). The dosages are adjusted according to the clinical response (daily weight loss) while monitoring serum electrolytes and renal function. If serum creatinine rises to >1.5 mg/dL diuretics should be temporarily discontinued.
- Alternatively diuretic treatment can be started as a combination of spironolactone and furosemide at a ratio of 40 mg furosemide for every 100 mg of spironolactone (combined therapy).
- Do not treat patients with cirrhotic ascites with furosemide monotherapy.
- In hospitalized patients diuretic treatment may be monitored according to urinary Na^+-excretion.

- In the absence of renal insufficiency and with urinary Na$^+$-excretion >30 mEq/L, spironolactone may be used alone, at a daily dose of 100–200 mg PO. Increasing the dose to >400 mg once a day does not increase the diuretic efficacy.
- With a urinary Na$^+$-excretion of 10–30 mEq/L a loop diuretic is added to spironolactone, e.g. furosemide 40–160 mg PO or IV once a day or 20–80 mg PO two times a day. Thiazide diuretics, e.g. hydrochlorothiazide are rarely used.
- With a urinary Na$^+$-excretion < 10 mEq/L an additional large-volume therapeutic paracentesis is performed.
- The optimal daily weight loss in patients with peripheral edema is 1 kg, in those without peripheral edema 0.5 kg.
- More aggressive diuresis leads to intravascular hypovolemia, which may cause renal failure, electrolyte imbalances and precipitate hepatic encephalopathy.
- A urine Na$^+$-excretion of >80 mmol Na$^+$/24 hours, in patients whose ascites is not adequately mobilized and who do not lose weight, suggests dietary non-compliance with Na$^+$-restriction

Vasopressin receptor antagonists
- Vasopressin receptor antagonists specific for the V2 receptor, e.g. tolvaptan or satavaptan may be considered in the management of refractory hyponatremia. However, there are no data showing their clinical benefit in the long-term management of cirrhotic ascites, and their current cost is prohibitive.
- Tolvaptan is started at 15 mg PO once a day. The dose may be increased to 30–60 mg PO once a day titrating at 24-hour intervals to the desired serum sodium concentration. Tolvaptan is metabolized via the hepatic CYP3A4 system. Be aware of potential interactions with other drugs that are metabolized by CYP3A4.

Large volume paracentesis
- LVP is the initial treatment of choice in patients with tense (grade 3) and refractory ascites. Therapeutic paracentesis is the fastest method to mobilize ascites, it shortens the hospital stay and is associated with less complications than therapy with diuretics. In the absence of hepatic encephalopathy, gastrointestinal bleeding or a bacterial infection LVP may be performed in an outpatient setting.
- The goal of paracentesis is the complete removal of ascites. This can be attempted in one session. Single total paracentesis is as effective as and generally safer than repeated partial paracenteses.
- With paracentesis of ≥5 L acute reduction of effective blood volume with subsequent activation of the sympathetic nervous system and renin-angiotensin-aldosterone-system may lead to circulatory dysfunction with a fall in arterial blood pressure and increased cardiac output and complications, such as dilutional hyponatremia with rapid reappearance of ascites and renal dysfunction with irreversible renal failure in up to 20% of patients. The severity of post-paracentesis circulatory dysfunction correlates inversely with patient survival.
- To avoid hemodynamic changes and circulatory complications LVP of ≥5 L must be accompanied by plasma volume expansion, even in patients with peripheral edema. Albumin is the plasma volume expander of choice. Concomitant with LVP albumin is administered IV at a dose of 8 g/L ascites removed.
- Albumin is superior to synthetic plasma expanding solutions in preventing circulatory complications in patients with LVP ≥ 5 L. If less than 5 L of ascites is removed synthetic plasma expanding solutions may be used. The combination of midodrine and octreotide after LVP is not superior to albumin in preventing post-paracentesis circulatory dysfunction and recurrence of ascites.

Practical approach to paracentesis
- There is no evidence that spontaneous bacterial peritonitis, renal failure, hepatic encephalopathy or severe jaundice should be considered as contraindications for paracentesis.
- Caution is needed when performing paracentesis on patients with severe thrombocytopenia or an INR > 2.5, but mild coagulopathy does not need to be corrected with blood products prior to paracentesis. Renal insufficiency might be a risk factor for iatrogenic hemoperitoneum.
- Paracentesis should be performed preferably in a single session. This can be done over a period of 1–4 hours or much quicker by using vacuum-sealed containers which allow for removal of for example 8 L ascites in 30 minutes.
- Paracentesis < 5 L: cautious volume expansion with synthetic colloidal solutions or albumin monitoring pulse rate and blood pressure.
- Paracentesis ≥ 5 L: expansion of plasma volume with concomitant infusion of albumin at a dose of 8 g/L ascites removed.
- If following paracentesis diuretic therapy is not reinstituted, ascites will recur in >90% of patients. With diuretics the recurrence rate of ascites is 18%. Therefore, paracentesis has always to be followed by maintenance diuretic therapy and dietary sodium restriction to avoid recurrence of ascites.

Therapy of refractory ascites
- Serial LVP: Even in outpatients, LVP using strict aseptic techniques can be repeated safely every 10–14 days. The danger of bacterial peritonitis is low and there is no need to perform ascites cultures after each tap or to use antibiotics prophylactically. However, it is advisable to perform cell count and differential after each tap.
- PVS: PVS functions as a continuous paracentesis with venous reinfusion of ascitic fluid. Compared with LVP with albumin infusion PVS does not lead to any significant survival benefit but carries a considerable rate of up to 40% of serious complications, such as volume overload with congestive heart failure and pulmonary edema, variceal bleeding, myocardial infarction, bacterial peritonitis, septicemia, peritoneal fibrosis, disseminated intravascular coagulation, thrombosis of a central vein and/or thrombotic occlusion of the shunt. Therefore, there is little role, if any, for the use of PVS in the treatment of refractory ascites.
- TIPS:
  - TIPS is a method of portal decompression based on the non-surgical, radiologically controlled placement of an intrahepatic connection between the portal vein and the hepatic venous system.
  - TIPS corresponds functionally to a side-to-side portacaval shunt and has largely replaced surgically placed shunts.
  - TIPS is a highly effective treatment for refractory ascites and decreases the need for large-volume paracentesis in patients with refractory cirrhotic ascites. It leads to complete resolution of refractory ascites in up to 75% of cases.
  - The use of TIPS in patients with a MELD score greater than 18 runs the risk of worsening hepatic function.
  - TIPS should be considered as a treatment option for patients who need frequent LVP (>3 per month), who are intolerant of repeated LVP or in whom a LVP cannot be performed, e.g. because of extensive peritoneal adhesions. TIPS also resolves hepatic hydrothorax in 60–70% of patients.
  - TIPS leads to an increase in cardiac output, a rise in right atrial and pulmonary arterial pressure with a secondary fall of systemic vascular resistance, increase of pulmonary vascular resistance and of effective arterial blood volume, improvement of renal function and to an

increase in urinary Na$^+$-excretion. It is less effective in patients older than 60 years and in those with a pre-TIPS creatinine clearance of <40 L/minute.

- Acute complications: rupture of liver capsule with intra-abdominal bleeding.
- Long-term consequences: deterioration of liver function, increased incidence of hepatic encephalopathy (approximately in 30% of patients; the risk is higher in patients over the age of 60 years), TIPS-stenosis or occlusion (less frequent with expanded polytetrafluoroethylene-covered stents), hemolytic anemia, heart failure due to a rise in preload in patients with cardiac diseases. Therefore, determine the ejection fraction before placement of a TIPS.
- TIPS should be placed only in patients with an ejection fraction >55%.
- TIPS is an effective procedure to bridge the time to orthotopic liver transplantation.

Liver transplantation
- In any patient with cirrhosis who develops ascites, suitability for liver transplantation should be considered. In patients with refractory ascites liver transplant evaluation should be initiated, especially when complications, such as spontaneous bacterial peritonitis or hepatorenal syndrome occur.
- Patients with one or more of the following alterations should be regarded as candidates for liver transplantation:
  - Impaired free water clearance (urine volume <8 mL/minute after intravenous infusion of glucose 5% at a dose of 20 mL/kg body weight).
  - Dilutional hyponatremia (serum Na$^+$ < 130 mmol/L without diuretic therapy).
  - Arterial hypotension (mean arterial pressure <80 mmHg without diuretic therapy).
  - Diminished glomerular filtration rate (serum creatinine >1.2 mg/dL without diuretic therapy).
  - Marked Na$^+$-retention (urinary Na$^+$-excretion <10 mmol/24 hours with moderate dietary sodium restriction and without diuretic therapy).

Errors in the therapy of cirrhotic ascites
- Errors are summarized in the following table.

Errors in the treatment of cirrhotic ascites

Finding	Wrong action	Correct action
Marked hyponatremia (Na$^+$ ≤ 125 mmol/L)	Infusion of NaCl	Fluid restriction (however, rarely effective in complete correction of dilutional hyponatremia). Too vigorous fluid restriction may lead to renal impairment and to central hypovolemia with exacerbation of hyponatremia
		Consider reducing diuretic dose or interrupting diuretic therapy
		With elevated or rising serum creatinine stop diuretics and consider cautious volume expansion
		Serum Na$^+$ ≤ 120 mmol/L: stop diuretics
		Selective vasopressin 2 receptor antagonists (e.g. tolvaptan) are promising new agents that may become a rational choice in the future

(Continued)

Finding	Wrong action	Correct action
Impaired renal function (serum creatinine > 2 mg/dL; creatinine-clearance < 40 mL/min in the absence of prior renal disease)	Increase in dose of diuretics	Cautious volume expansion with synthetic colloid solutions or albumin (note: a 4.5% albumin solution contains a Na^+ concentration equivalent to normal saline!)
		Possibly vasopressin analogs, e.g. terlipressin (not approved by the FDA; available in Europe)
		In a few patients reversal of type 1 hepatorenal syndrome with the administration of midodrine, octreotide and albumin was reported
Marked, grade 3 ascites	Vigorous high dose diuretic therapy	Slow, stepwise increase in diuretic dosage attempting to achieve the desired daily weight loss of 0.5–1 kg. If not successful LVP, TIPS, or liver transplant

Algorithm 19.3 Treatment of patients with ascites

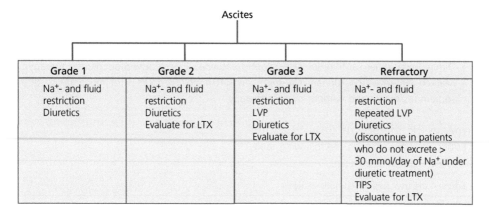

Grade 1	Grade 2	Grade 3	Refractory
Na^+- and fluid restriction Diuretics	Na^+- and fluid restriction Diuretics Evaluate for LTX	Na^+- and fluid restriction LVP Diuretics Evaluate for LTX	Na^+- and fluid restriction Repeated LVP Diuretics (discontinue in patients who do not excrete > 30 mmol/day of Na^+ under diuretic treatment) TIPS Evaluate for LTX

CLINICAL PEARLS
- Diuretics and dietary Na^+- restriction are the first line treatment of ascites.
- Do not be too aggressive in mobilizing ascites – do not overtreat.
- LVP is the initial treatment of choice in patients with tense (grade 3) and refractory ascites. Concomitant with LVP, albumin is administered IV at a dose of 8 g/L ascites removed.
- TIPS should be considered as a treatment option for patients who need frequent LVP (more than three per month), who are intolerant of repeated LVP or in whom a LVP cannot be performed.
- In any patient with cirrhosis who develops ascites suitability for liver transplantation should be considered.

Section 5: Special Populations

Not applicable for this topic.

Section 6: Prognosis

CLINICAL PEARLS
- No data exist on the natural history of grade 1 ascites, and it is not known how frequently patients with grade 1 ascites will develop grade 2 or 3 ascites.
- Predictors of an unfavourable prognosis in patients with cirrhotic ascites with still normal blood urea nitrogen and serum creatinine are:
  - Impaired free water clearance (water diuresis after a water load*).
  - Dilutional hyponatremia.
  - Marked Na$^+$-retention (diminished Na$^+$-excretion).
  - Reduction of glomerular filtration rate.
  - Increased plasma renin activity.
  - Increased plasma norepinephrine concentration.
  - Arterial hypotension.
  - Low cardiac output.
  - * Forty-five minutes infusion of glucose 5% at a dose of 20 mL/kg body weight. Fifteen minutes after the end of the infusion urine volume over 90 minutes is determined. Urine volume: >8 mL/min = normal water diuresis; 3–8 mL/min = moderate impairment of water diuresis; < 3 mL/min = strong impairment of water diuresis.
- The development of grade 2 or 3 ascites in patients with liver cirrhosis is associated with a mortality of 50% and 80% within 2 and 5 years respectively after the first ascites episode.
- Once refractory ascites develops, prognosis is extremely severe, with approximately 50% of patients dying within 6–12 months.
- Patients with refractory ascites undergoing liver transplantation have a 5 year survival probability of 70–80%.

Section 7: Reading List

Angeli P, Fasolato S, Mazza E, et al. Combined versus sequential diuretic treatment of ascites in non-azotaemic patients with cirrhosis:results of an open randomised clinical trial. Gut 2010;59:98–104

Arroyo V, Ginès P, Navasa M, et al. Renal failure in cirrhosis and liver transplantation. Transplant Proc 1993;25:1734–9

Bari K, Minano C, Shea M, et al. The combination of octreotide and midodrine is not superior to albumin in preventing recurrence of ascites after large-volume paracentesis. Clin Gastroenterol Hepatol 2012;10: 1169–75

Bernardi M, Caraceni P, Navickis RJ, et al. Albumin infusion in patients undergoing large-volume paracentesis: a meta-analysis of randomized trials. Hepatology 2012;55:1172–81

Cárdenas A, Chopra S. Chylous ascites. Am J Gastroenterol 2002;97:1896–900

Cardenas A, Gines P. Management of refractory ascites. Clin Gastroenterol Hepatol 2005;3:1187–91

Dancygier H. Clinical Hepatology. Principles and Practice of Hepatobiliary Diseases, 2010. Berlin: Springer

Fernández-Esparrach G, Sánchez-Fueyo A, Ginès P, et al. A prognostic model for predicting survival in cirrhosis with ascites. J Hepatol 2000;34:46–52

Ginès P, Arroyo V, Quintero E, et al. Comparison of paracentesis and diuretics in the treatment of cirrhotics with tense ascites:results of a randomised study. Gastroenterology 1987;93:234–41

Ginès P, Cardenas A, Arroyo V, et al. Management of cirrhosis and ascites. N Engl J Med 2004;350: 1646–54

Ginès A, Fernández-Esparrach, Monescillo A et al. Randomized trial comparing albumin, dextran 70, and polygeline in cirrhotic patients with ascites treated by paracentesis. Gastroenterology 1996;111:1002–10

Ginès P, Tito Ll, Arroyo V, et al. Randomized comparative study of therapeutic paracentesis with and without intravenous albumin in cirrhosis. Gastroenterology 1998;94:1493–502

Jaffe DL, Chung RT, Friedman LS Management of portal hypertension and its complications. Med Clin N Am 1996;80:1021–34

Krag A, Bendtsen F, Henriksen JH, et al. Low cardiac output predicts development of hepatorenal syndrome and survival in patients with cirrhosis and ascites. Gut 2010;59:105–10

Runyon BA. Paracentesis of ascitic fluid: a safe procedure. Arch Intern Med 1986;146:2259–61

Sansoé G, Ferrari A, Baraldi E, et al. Renal distal tubular handling of sodium in central fluid volume homeostasis in preascitic cirrhosis. Gut 1999;45:750–5

Wong F, Watson H, Gerbes A, et al. Satavaptan for the management of ascites in cirrhosis:efficacy and safety across the spectrum of ascites severity. Gut 2012;61:108–16

Section 8: Guidelines

Guideline title	Guideline source	Date
AASLD practice guidelines. The role of transjugular intrahepatic portosystemic shunt (TIPS) in the management of portal hypertension	American Association for the Study of Liver Disease (AASLD) http://www.aasld.org/practiceguidelines/Documents/Bookmarked%20Practice%20Guidelines/TIPS%20Update%20Nov%202009.pdf	2010
EASL clinical practice guidelines on the management of ascites, spontaneous bacterial peritonitis, and hepatorenal syndrome in cirrhosis	European Association for the Study of the Liver (EASL) http://www.easl.eu/assets/application/files/21e21971bf182e5_file.pdf	2010
AASLD practice guidelines. Management of adult patients with ascites due to cirrhosis: an update	American Association for the Study of Liver Disease (AASLD) http://www.aasld.org/practiceguidelines/Documents/ascitesupdate2013.pdf	2013

Section 9 Evidence

Not applicable for this topic.

Section 10: Images

Not applicable for this topic.

Additional material for this chapter can be found online at:
www.mountsinaiexpertguides.com
This includes a case study and multiple choice questions

CHAPTER 20

Spontaneous Bacterial Peritonitis

Henryk Dancygier

Departments of Medicine II and IV, Sana Klinikum Offenbach, Goethe University, Frankfurt am Main, Germany *and* Division of Liver Diseases, Icahn School of Medicine at Mount Sinai, New York, NY, USA

OVERALL BOTTOM LINE

- SBP is observed predominantly in patients with advanced cirrhosis.
- Gram-negative aerobic bacteria are causative in approximately 80% of patients, anaerobic bacteria occur in no more than 5% of patients, but the prevalence of multidrug resistant organisms is increasing.
- Diagnostic paracentesis with ascitic fluid analysis (PMN count and culture) is the cornerstone of diagnosis.
- Primary and secondary prophylaxis improves survival.
- Treatment (third generation cephalosporins are first line antibiotics) leads to resolution of SBP in 70–90% of patients.
- Early diagnosis and treatment have reduced in-hospital mortality from approximately 80% to 15–20%.

Section 1: Background

Definition

- SBP is a life-threatening infection of ascites in the absence of an intra-abdominal source of infection and with no obvious source of bacteria.

Epidemiology

- SBP is observed predominantly in patients with advanced cirrhosis.
- The prevalence of SBP in outpatients is 1.5–3.5% and approximately 15–20% in hospitalized patients.
- SBP occurs in between 25% and 65% of cirrhotic patients with acute GI bleeding.

Etiology

- Gram-negative aerobic bacteria is most common (80% of cases; *E. coli* > *Klebsiella* species).
- Gram-positive cocci, mainly *Streptococcus* species (*S. pneumoniae*) occur in 20% of cases.
- Anaerobic bacteria occur in <5% of patients.
- Ninety percent of all SBP cases are monomicrobial.
- Epidemiology of bacterial infections differs between community-acquired (Gram-negative infections predominate) and nosocomial infections (Gram-positive infections predominate).

Mount Sinai Expert Guides: Hepatology, First Edition. Edited by Jawad Ahmad, Scott L. Friedman, and Henryk Dancygier.
© 2014 John Wiley & Sons, Ltd. Published 2014 by John Wiley & Sons, Ltd.
Companion website: www.mountsinaiexpertguides.com

- Microbiology of SBP is changing with an increasing prevalence of MDR organisms. Suspect MDR organisms if:
  - SBP is nosocomial.
  - The patient was in hospital recently.
  - The patient had intestinal decontamination.

Pathogenesis
- Multifactorial, not well understood.
- Dysfunction of the immune system in cirrhosis.
- Activity of the RES-system (chemotaxis, phagocytosis, intracellular killing) impaired.
- Deficient phospholipase C activity in blood neutrophils.
- Increased intestinal permeability.
- Bacterial overgrowth and translocation of intestinal micro-organisms.
- Endotoxemia.
- Reduced levels of antibacterial substances in ascites (e.g. opsonins, complement components).

Risk factors
- The risk of SBP is increased in cirrhotic patients with the following conditions:
  - GI bleeding.
  - Low total protein concentration (<1–1.5 g/dL) in ascites.
  - Severe liver dysfunction.
  - History of previous SBP.
  - Use of proton pump inhibitors.

Section 2: Prevention

- Primary prophylaxis is restricted to patients with high risk of SBP.
- Third generation cephalosporins are first line antibiotics in patients with acute GI bleeding.
- Fluoroquinolones may be used in patients with low total protein content in ascites.
- Primary prophylaxis improves survival.
- Whether prophylaxis should be given intermittently or continuously remains unsettled.

Screening
- A diagnostic paracentesis should be performed:
  - In all cirrhotic patients with newly formed ascites.
  - In any patient with cirrhosis and ascites on hospital admission.
  - In patients with cirrhosis and ascites who develop compatible symptoms or signs of peritonitis (e.g. abdominal pain, fever).
  - In any patient with cirrhosis and ascites with worsening renal, liver or mental function/hepatic encephalopathy without an obvious cause (see Chapter 19).

Primary prevention
- Primary prophylaxis should be restricted to patients at high risk of SBP, i.e. those with:
  - Low total protein content in ascites (1–1.5 g/dL), and/or
  - Acute GI hemorrhage.

- Patients with acute GI bleeding and severe liver disease:
  - Ceftriaxone 1–2 g IV once a day for 3–4 days. May be switched to
  - Norfloxacin 400 mg PO twice a day after bleeding has been controlled.
- Patients with acute GI bleeding and less severe liver disease:
  - Norfloxacin 400 mg PO once to twice a day or
  - Ciprofloxacin 500 mg PO twice a day or 750 mg PO once weekly.
- Patients without GI bleeding with low total protein (<1–1.5 g/dL) in ascites:
  - Norfloxacin 400 mg PO once a day for 12 months.
- Whether prophylaxis should be given intermittently or continuously currently is unsettled.

Secondary prevention

- Patients recovering from one episode of SBP should receive long-term secondary prophylaxis with:
  - Norfloxacin 400 mg PO once a day (or another quinolone) or
  - Co-trimoxazole (TMP/SMX) 1 double-strength tablet PO once a day, 5 days per week.
- Secondary prophylaxis should be continued until the disappearance of ascites or until liver transplantation.
- Long-term secondary prophylaxis will result in a:
  - Change of bacterial spectrum towards Gram-positive cocci as well as
  - Emergence of quinolone resistant Gram-negative organisms.
- Patients who develop SBP on prophylactic quinolones respond as well to third generation cephalosporins as patients not on prophylaxis.

Section 3: Diagnosis

CLINICAL PEARLS
- Clinical findings are unreliable and may be misleading.
- The diagnosis of SBP is based on the results of ascitic fluid analysis:
  - Neutrophil cell count >250/mm^3 (>0.25 × 10^9/L).
  - Positive culture.

Differential diagnosis

Differential diagnosis	Features
Secondary bacterial peritonitis due to intestinal perforation	Suspect secondary bacterial peritonitis in patients with: • Polymicrobial ascites with very high ascitic PMN count (>5000 PMN/mm^3), and/or • High ascitic protein concentration or • Inadequate response to therapy (failure of neutrophil count to fall after 48 hours of antibiotic therapy)
Peritoneal tuberculosis	Culture-negative peritonitis; sensitivity of ascites smear for mycobacteria is 0%, that of ascites culture is approximately 50%
Peritoneal carcinomatosis	Culture-negative peritonitis; if three still warm ascites samples are examined without delay the sensitivity of cytological examination in diagnosing peritoneal carcinomatosis amounts to >90%

Typical presentation

- The clinical signs and symptoms of SBP may be subtle and range from:
  - Asymptomatic, to
  - Fever, abdominal pain, abdominal tenderness, altered mental status (50–60% of patients),
  - Diarrhea, paralytic ileus, hypotension, hypothermia (≤50% of patients).

Clinical diagnosis

History

- Enquire about the presence of chronic liver disease/liver cirrhosis, history of previous SBP and the use of proton pump inhibitors.

Physical examination

- The physical examination should be focused on signs and symptoms of liver cirrhosis (see Chapter 19).
- There are no specific physical signs of SBP. Look for signs and symptoms described in "Typical presentation."

Laboratory diagnosis

List of diagnostic tests

- Diagnostic paracentesis.
- Neutrophil cell count in ascites (results should be available 1–4 hours post-puncture).
- Ascites culture.

- A cut-off of 250 PMN/mm^3 ascites has the greatest sensitivity for the diagnosis of SBP. In patients with hemorrhagic ascites (in 30% underlying hepatocellular carcinoma, traumatic tap, in 50% no cause evident) with an erythrocyte count of >10 000/mm^3 ascites, subtraction of one PMN per 250 red blood cells should be made to adjust for the presence of blood in ascites.
- Ascitic fluid should be inoculated into two blood culture bottles (aerobic and anaerobic) at the bedside. Ascites culture is negative in as many as 60% of patients with clinical manifestations suggestive of SBP and increased ascites PMN count.
- Based on ascitic fluid analysis the following entities may be distinguished:
  - Culture-positive, neutrocytic ascites: positive culture result and a PMN cell count of >250/mm^3 (>0.25 × 10^9/L) ascites (typical of SBP).
  - Culture-negative, neutrocytic ascites: 250 PMN/mm^3 ascites with a negative culture result (culture negative SBP). With this combination of findings consider tuberculosis and peritoneal carcinomatosis as a diagnostic possibility.
  - Monomicrobial, non-neutrocytic bacterascites: culture positive for one pathogen with <250 PMN/mm^3 ascites.
  - Polymicrobial, non-neutrocytic bacterascites: several pathogens in ascitic fluid culture with <250 PMN/mm^3 ascites. This may be the result of inadvertent intestinal puncture during diagnostic paracentesis.
- A presumptive diagnosis of SBP is made with an ascites PMN cell count of >250/mm^3 – the definitive diagnosis is established by a positive culture result.
- Reagent strips designed for use in urine have a low diagnostic accuracy (false negative rate up to 55%) in SBP. Their use for the rapid diagnosis of SBP is not recommended.
- Detection of bacterial DNA in ascites by in situ hybridization may provide early and direct evidence of bacterial infection.
- Gram's stain of peritoneal fluid is not helpful in the diagnosis of SBP.

Imaging techniques

- Imaging techniques have no role in the diagnosis of SBP, but may help in excluding secondary peritonitis.

Potential pitfalls/common errors made regarding diagnosis of disease

- Not to perform a diagnostic paracentesis because the patient has no symptoms or signs suggestive of SBP.
- Not to inoculate culture bottles at the bedside.
- To use reagent strips for neutrophil count in ascites.
- To perform Gram's stain of peritoneal fluid.
- To discard the diagnosis of SBP because of negative ascites culture results.

Section 4: Treatment (Algorithm 20.1)

When to hospitalize

- Every patient with grade 2 or 3 ascites should be hospitalized (see Chapter 19).
- Every patient with the tentative diagnosis of SBP should be hospitalized.

Managing the hospitalized patient

- Upon clinical suspicion and/or PMN > 250/mm^3 ascites start empiric antibiotic treatment immediately after diagnostic tap, while awaiting the results of ascitic fluid culture. Antibiotic therapy is modified according to culture result.
- Patients who have culture-negative, neutrocytic ascites (culture negative SBP) and those who are symptomatic with monomicrobial, non-neutrocytic bacterascites are treated in the same way as patients with typical SBP.
- In asymptomatic patients with monomicrobial, non-neutrocytic ascites watchful waiting may be appropriate since in most of these patients ascites turns sterile without treatment.

Antibiotic treatment

- Third generation cephalosporins cover 95% of the flora isolated from ascitic fluid and are therefore the antibiotics of choice. Cefotaxime or amoxicillin/clavulanic acid are effective in patients who develop SBP while on norfloxacin prophylaxis.
- Start treatment with:
  - Ceftriaxone 2 g IV once a day or
  - Cefotaxime 2 g IV every 8–12 hours or
  - Ceftazidime 1 g IV every 12–24 hours.
- Alternative options:
  - Ampicillin/sulbactam 2 g/1 g IV every 6 hours or
  - Amoxicillin/clavulanic acid (IV preparation not available in the USA).
- Albumin 1.5 g/kg body weight IV at the time of diagnosis, followed by 1 g/kg on day 3 should be administered to patients with SBP at a high risk of developing renal dysfunction (serum bilirubin ≥68 μmol/L [4 mg/dL] or serum creatinine ≥88 μmol/L [1 mg/dL]).
- Repeat diagnostic paracentesis at day 2. A decrease of PMN cell count of less than 25% from baseline at day 2 suggests failure of antibiotic therapy (think of changing microbiology of SBP with an increasing prevalence of MDR). The use of extended spectrum antibiotics (e.g.

carbapenems, piperacillin/tazobactam) as initial empiric therapy should be considered in patients with nosocomial SBP because of the presence of MDR organisms.
- In asymptomatic patients and in those in whom ascites PMN count decreases by at least 25% from baseline at day 2, intravenous therapy can be switched to oral treatment:
  - Ofloxacin 400 mg PO twice a day or
  - Ciprofloxacin 500 mg PO twice a day or
  - Amoxicillin/clavulanic acid 1000/200 mg PO three times a day.
- Treatment is continued until complete resolution of all clinical signs of SBP and a decrease of PMN below 250/mm³. This takes usually 5–6 days.
- Immediately following successful treatment long-term secondary prophylaxis is begun.
- Patients on secondary prophylaxis for SBP should always be considered as potential candidates for liver transplantation.
- The performance of large-volume paracentesis should be delayed until after the resolution of SBP.

Algorithm 20.1 Management of SBP

CLINICAL PEARLS
- Upon clinical suspicion and/or PMN > 250/mm³ ascites start empiric antibiotic treatment immediately after diagnostic tap.
- Third generation cephalosporins are the antibiotics of choice.
- The use of extended spectrum antibiotics (e.g. carbapenems, piperacillin/tazobactam) as initial empiric therapy should be considered in patients with nosocomial SBP.
- Albumin at the time of diagnosis, and on day 3, should be administered to patients with SBP at a high risk of developing renal dysfunction.
- Immediately following successful treatment long-term secondary prophylaxis is begun.

Section 5: Special Populations

Not applicable for this topic.

Section 6: Prognosis

> **CLINICAL PEARLS**
> - Untreated SBP has an in-hospital mortality of up to 80%.
> - Early diagnosis and treatment have reduced early in-hospital mortality to 15–20%.
> - Renal dysfunction is one of the strongest predictors of mortality in patients with SBP.

Prognosis for treated patients
- The prognosis of SBP is poor with a recurrence rate of up to 60–70% within 1 year without adequate prophylaxis and a probability of survival at 1 year of 30–50% and 25–30% at 2 years.
- Primary prophylaxis significantly reduces the risk of development of the first episode of SBP, reduces the incidence of other severe infections, delays hepatorenal syndrome, and improves survival.
- Early diagnosis and prompt treatment have reduced early in-hospital mortality from approximately 80% to 15–20%.
- Success rate of antibiotic therapy of nosocomial SBP is only 40–50%.
- Pneumococcal peritonitis has a particularly poor prognosis.
- Renal dysfunction (creatinine >1.5mg/dL) is the most important independent predictor of mortality in patients with SBP. Serum bilirubin levels >4mg/dL and serum creatinine levels >1mg/dL at the time of diagnosis are significant risk factors for the adverse clinical outcome of patients with SBP. Albumin, but not hydroxyethyl starch, improves circulatory function and reduces risk of renal failure in patients with SBP. It reduces the rates of type 1 HRS from 30% to 10%, and improves in-hospital mortality and 3-month mortality from 29% to 10% compared with cefotaxime alone in patients at high risk for renal failure.

Section 7: Reading List

Andreu M, Sola R, Sitges-Serra A, et al. Risk factors for spontaneous bacterial peritonitis in cirrhotic patients with ascites. Gastroenterology 1993;104:1133–8

Bernard B, Grange JD, Khac EN, et al. Antibiotic prophylaxis for the prevention of bacterial infections in cirrhotic patients with gastrointestinal bleeding: a meta-analysis. Hepatology 1999;29:1655–61

Enomoto H, Inoue S, Matsuhisa A, et al. Development of a new in situ hybridization method for the detection of global bacterial DNA to provide early evidence of a bacterial infection in spontaneous bacterial peritonitis. J Hepatol 2012;56:85–94

Fernandez J, Acevedo J, Castro M, et al. Prevalence and risk factors of infections by multiresistant bacteria in cirrhosis: a prospective study. Hepatology 2012;55:1551–61

Fernandez J, Del Arbol LR, Gomez C, et al. Norfloxacin vs ceftriaxone in the prophylaxis of infections in patients with advanced cirrhosis and hemorrhage. Gastroenterology 2006;131:1049–56

Fernandez J, Monteagudo J, Bargallo X, et al. A randomized unblinded pilot study comparing albumin versus hydroxyethyl starch in spontaneous bacterial peritonitis. Hepatology 2005;42:627–34

Fernandez J, Navasa M, Garcia-Pagan JC, et al. Effect of intravenous albumin on systemic and hepatic hemodynamics and vasoactive neurohormonal systems in patients with cirrhosis and spontaneous bacterial peritonitis. J Hepatol 2004;41:384–90

Fernández J, Navasa M, Planas R, et al. Primary prophylaxis of spontaneous bacterial peritonitis delays hepatorenal syndrome and improves survival in cirrhosis. Gastroenterology 2007;133:818–24

Ginès P, Rimola A, Planas R, et al. Norfloxacin prevents spontaneous bacterial peritonitis recurrence in cirrhosis: results of a double blind, placebo-controlled trial. Hepatology 1990;12:716–24

Loomba R, Wesley R, Bain A, et al. Role of fluoroquinolones in the primary prophylaxis of spontaneous bacterial peritonitis: meta-analysis. Clin Gastroenterol Hepatol 2009;7:487–93

Rimola A, Garcia-Tsao G, Navasa M, et al. Diagnosis, treatment and prophylaxis of spontaneous bacterial peritonitis. A consensus document. J Hepatol 2000;32:142–53

Saab S, Hernandez JC, Chi AC, et al. Oral antibiotic prophylaxis reduces spontaneous bacterial peritonitis occurrence and improves short-term survival in cirrhosis:a meta-analysis. Am J Gastroenterol 2009;104:993–1001

Sort P, Navasa M, Arroyo V, et al. Effect of intravenous albumin on renal impairment and mortality in patients with cirrhosis and spontaneous bacterial peritonitis. N Engl J Med 1999;341:403–9

Tandon P, Garcia-Tsao G. Renal dysfunction is the most important independent predictor of mortality in cirrhotic patients with spontaneous bacterial peritonitis. Clin Gastroenterol Hepatol 2011;9:260–5

Suggested websites
www.aasld.org
www.easl.eu
www.bsg.org.uk

Section 8: Guidelines

Guideline title	Guideline source	Date
AASLD practice guidelines. Management of adult patients with ascites due to cirrhosis: an update	American Association for the Study of Liver Disease (AASLD) http://www.aasld.org/practiceguidelines/Documents/ascitesupdate2013.pdf	2013
EASL clinical practice guidelines on the management of ascites, spontaneous bacterial peritonitis, and hepatorenal syndrome in cirrhosis	European Association for the Study of the Liver (EASL) http://www.easl.eu/assets/application/files/21e21971bf182e5_file.pdf	2010

Section 9: Evidence

Not applicable for this topic.

Section 10: Images

Not applicable for this topic.

Additional material for this chapter can be found online at:
www.mountsinaiexpertguides.com
This includes a case study and multiple choice questions

CHAPTER 21

Hepatic Encephalopathy

Priya Grewal
Division of Liver Diseases, Icahn School of Medicine at Mount Sinai, New York, NY, USA

OVERALL BOTTOM LINE
- HE is a myriad of complex neuropsychiatric symptoms occurring in patients with significant liver dysfunction.
- It occurs most commonly in patients with cirrhosis, but can be a manifestation of ALF or major portosystemic shunts in the absence of cirrhosis.
- HE is an independent predictor of mortality in patients with cirrhosis, with 58% of the patients dying at 1 year and 77% at 3 years.
- The diagnosis of HE is clinical and ammonia levels have limited value except in patient with ALF where it can be a prognostic.
- Treatment of underlying precipitating factors is crucial in the management of HE.
- Lactulose improves symptoms of HE but it is poorly tolerated leading to poor compliance.
- Rifaximin decreases HE-related hospitalizations by 50%.
- Minimal HE is present in 60–80% of patients with cirrhosis and one-third develop overt HE over time.

Section 1: Background
Definition of disease
- HE is a chronically incapacitating syndrome of neuropsychiatric symptoms, which can develop in patients with both acute and chronic liver dysfunction once other known brain diseases have been excluded.
- HE leads to deterioration in mental status, psychomotor dysfunction, impaired memory, increased reaction time, sensory abnormalities, poor concentration, disorientation and in severe forms coma.

Disease classification (Figure 21.1)
- HE can be classified based on the type of liver dysfunction:
  - Type A – acute liver failure.
  - Type B – porto-systemic bypass and no intrinsic hepatocellular disease.
  - Type C – cirrhosis and portal hypertension.
- Type C HE can be further classified based on the duration and neurological manifestations:
  - Episodic HE: these episodes develop over a short period of time and fluctuate in severity. Episodic HE can be:
    - precipitated by an event such as GI hemorrhage or uremia.
    - spontaneous, when there is no recognized precipitating factors.
    - recurrent encephalopathy, when two episodes of episodic HE occur within 1 year.

Mount Sinai Expert Guides: Hepatology, First Edition. Edited by Jawad Ahmad, Scott L. Friedman, and Henryk Dancygier.
© 2014 John Wiley & Sons, Ltd. Published 2014 by John Wiley & Sons, Ltd.
Companion website: www.mountsinaiexpertguides.com

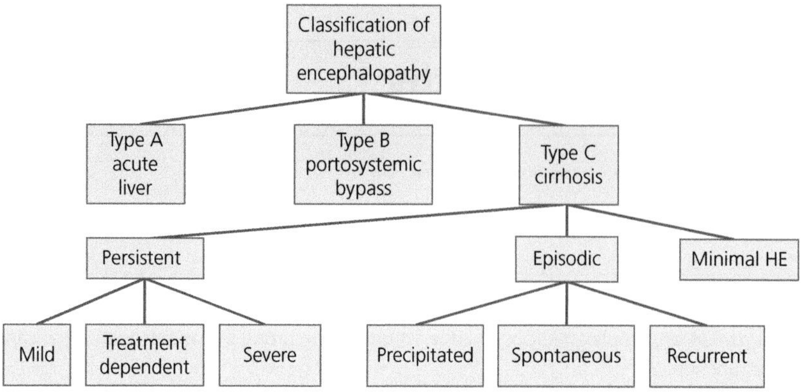

Figure 21.1 Classification of HE

- Persistent HE: this includes persistent cognitive deficits that impact negatively on social and occupational functioning of the patient:
  - mild (HE grade 1)
  - severe (HE grades 2–4)
- MHE: patients with MHE have no recognizable clinical symptoms of HE but do have mild cognitive and psychomotor deficits that are manifested by impairment in specialized testing of cognitive functioning.

Incidence/prevalence
- Cirrhosis affects about 5.5 million people in the USA and 30–45% of these patients will develop HE.
- HE also develops in 10–50% undergoing TIPS.

Economic impact
- Chronic HE is a common and expensive complication of liver failure, requiring more than 55 000 hospitalizations annually, and costing over $1.2 billion per year in 2003 in the USA alone.

Etiology
- The etiology of HE is primarily due to the accumulation of toxins in the serum due to liver dysfunction.
- The major factors leading to HE are the reduction in the hepatic function and mass accompanied by the development of porto-systemic collaterals which lead to the circulatory bypass of the liver.
- Ammonia is the toxin most frequently implicated in pathogenesis of HE.

Pathology/pathogenesis
- Nitrogenous substances derived from the gut adversely affect brain function. These compounds gain access to the systemic circulation as a result of decreased hepatic function or portal-systemic shunts. Once in brain tissue, they produce alterations of neurotransmission that affect consciousness and behavior, leading to motor dysfunction and extrapyramidal symptoms exhibited in HE.

- The principal neuro-inhibitory neurotransmitter GABA is also increased in the CSF of patients with encephalopathy. Other toxins identified in the CNS include increased levels of endogenous benzodiazepine-like compounds, manganese, oxygen free radicals, circulation opioid peptides and nitric oxide.

Predictive/risk factors
- Increased nitrogen load due GI bleeding, azotemia, infection especially SBP, electrolyte imbalance, blood transfusions, constipation, dehydration and non-compliance with lactulose.
- Decreased toxins clearance due to porto-systemic shunts, spontaneous, surgical, TIPS.
- Altered neurotransmission due to inadvertent use of benzodiazepines or psychoactive drugs.
- Hepatocellular damage with decrease in functional hepatic mass due to continued alcohol abuse, hepatocellular carcinoma or its treatment with TACE and acute portal vein thrombosis.

Section 2: Prevention
Screening

The West Haven Criteria (WHC)

Grade 1
Trivial lack of awareness
Euphoria or anxiety
Shortened attention span
Impaired performance of addition

Grade 2
Lethargy or apathy
Minimal disorientation for time or place
Subtle personality change
Inappropriate behavior
Impaired performance of subtraction

Grade 3
Somnolence to semistupor, responsive to verbal stimuli
Confusion
Gross disorientation

Grade 4
Coma (unresponsive to verbal or noxious stimuli)

Primary prevention
- Pre-emptive use of lactulose after TIPS as one third of patients may develop HE.
- Avoidance of constipation, psychoactive drugs, excessive diuretics.
- Prophylaxis against variceal bleeding and spontaneous bacterial peritonitis that can precipitate HE.

Secondary prevention
- Compliance with lactulose to ensure two to three bowel movements a day.
- Avoidance of sedatives and hypnotics in a hospitalized patient.
- Avoidance of dehydration due to overzealous use of diuretics or lactulose.

- Prompt diagnosis and treatment of GI bleeding or infection.
- Prompt correction of any electrolyte abnormalities.

Section 3: Diagnosis

- The diagnosis of HE is a clinical one based on symptoms reported by patients and more often their caregivers. These include a history of confusion, lethargy, memory loss, disorientation, slowness to respond, personality change with increased aggression or a reversal of day and night sleep pattern.
- In patients with recurrent admissions for HE a history of poor compliance with lactulose or overconsumption of proteins is often elicited.
- In a comatose patient, the presence of clonus may be a sign of HE though it is non-specific.

Differential diagnosis

Differential diagnosis	Features
Metabolic encephalopathies – hypoxia, hyponatremia, azotemia, diabetic coma	Blood gas, clinical chemistry, pulmonary evaluation, urinalysis based on indication
Intracranial disorders – tumors, hemorrhage, hematoma, meningitis, seizure disorder, dementia	Neurological imaging, lumbar puncture, EEG based on clinical suspicion, rapid plasma regain, vitamin B12 serum level
Toxins – alcohol, drugs, hypnotics, tranquilizers, analgesics, heavy metals	Urine and blood toxin screen, blood alcohol level

Typical presentation
- Patients may complain about increase in forgetfulness, memory loss or reversal of day and night sleep pattern. Patients may have trouble falling asleep or complain of early morning awakenings accompanied by increased day time sleepiness.
- Patient or family members may notice changes in hand writing, personal hygiene or the ability to concentrate and focus on any given task or activity. These symptoms may parallel a subtle worsening in the underlying liver disease.

Clinical diagnosis
History
- It is essential to identify recent changes in the patient's behavior or personality. Problems at work may surface due to lack of focus and concentration. Patient may also be at risk for increased or new traffic violations.
- In a hospitalized comatose patient flumazenil, a benzodiazepine-receptor antagonist can be used if the diagnosis of HE is suspected. The patient has to be monitored closely as this lowers the seizure threshold and can precipitate a seizure.

Physical examination
- Patient may have stigmata of chronic liver disease, such as jaundice, muscle wasting, gynecomastia, ascites, spider angioma, leg edema or splenomegaly.

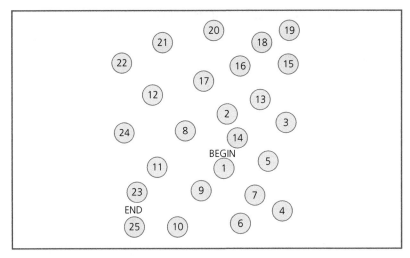

Figure 21.2 Sample number connection test

- Fetor hepaticus is a peculiar musty smell of the breath in patients with HE, caused by gut-derived methanethiol.
- Asterixis denotes hyperactive deep tendon reflexes which is a manifestation of stage 2HE.
- A number connection test or a mini-mental status examination can be performed when the diagnosis of HE is suspected. It tests the individual's orientation, attention, calculation, recall, language and motor skills (Figure 21.2).

Disease severity classification
- The West Haven Criteria (see "Screening").

Laboratory diagnosis
- The diagnosis of HE is a clinical one and though an ammonia level is routinely checked it has limited value in the absence of symptoms of HE. HE increases the blood–brain barrier's permeability to ammonia and hence correlation between ammonia level and mental state is poor.
- In acute liver failure, the ammonia level greater than 100 μmol/L was a risk factor for the development of severe HE and intracranial hypertension.

List of diagnostic tests
- The diagnosis of MHE involves a battery of neuropyschological tests including number connection test, figure connection test and three performance subtests of the Wechsler Adult Intelligence Scale – digit symbol test, picture completion test and block design test. The diagnosis of MHE is made if any two of the neuropsychological tests are impaired beyond 2 standard deviations of known control values.
- The critical flicker frequency, a neurophysiological test, is a highly objective and sensitive measure of minimal hepatic encephalopathy. "Triphasic waves" and a generalized slowing of the EEG supports the diagnosis of encephalopathy.

Algorithm 21.1 Treatment of HE in a hospitalized patient

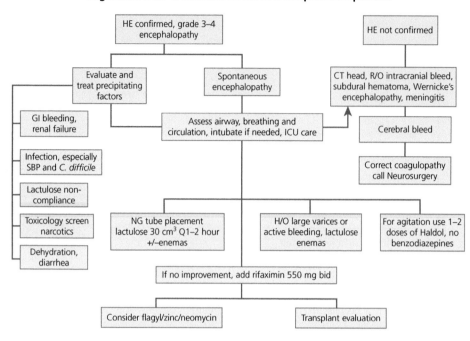

Potential pitfalls/common errors made regarding diagnosis of disease

- Onset of HE can be insidious and subtle – personality or behavior changes may go unnoticed by the clinician. Vigilance is crucial.
- Hospitalized cirrhotic patients with agitation due to HE are given sedatives precipitating lethargy and sometimes coma.
- Fetor hepaticus may be mistaken for recent alcohol consumption.
- High ammonia levels are not diagnostic for HE if symptoms are absent.
- *Clostridium difficile* is common in hospitalized cirrhotic patients even if they are on lactulose.

Section 4: Treatment (Algorithms 21.1, 21.2)
Treatment rationale

- Lactulose is a non-absorbable disaccharide first line drug for the treatment of HE. However its daily use is fraught with significant side effects including abdominal cramping, diarrhea, flatulence and bloating. This leads to non-compliance among patients and poor control of HE. Patients who have an aversion to the taste of lactulose can be switched to Kristalose, which is a tasteless powder.
- Rifaximin is the second line treatment for HE and has been approved for treatment of refractory encephalopathy. Rifaximin has a broad spectrum of antibacterial activity against both aerobic and anaerobic Gram-positive and Gram-negative organisms and minimal absorption. It can also be used instead of lactulose in patients intolerant of lactulose.

- Neomycin and metronidazole had been used in patients refractory or intolerant to lactulose. Rifaximin is now preferred in this setting. Their toxicity also limits their use in patents awaiting transplantation.

When to hospitalize
- The patient is becoming more lethargic in spite of lactulose or is unable to take lactulose at home.
- The threshold of hospitalizing a patient with decompensated cirrhosis and new HE or worsening HE should be low as the HE event is usually a manifestation of an underlying infection, bleeding, renal failure, hepatocellular carcinoma or portal vein thrombosis.

Managing the hospitalized patient (Algorithm 21.1)
- Ensure airway, breathing, and circulation.
- Intubate for airway protection if indicated.
- Evaluate for infection, bleeding or renal failure and treat appropriately.
- Correct electrolyte abnormalities, consider empiric antibiotics.
- Urine toxicology screen and blood alcohol level should be checked.
- CT head to rule out bleeding in patient with focal neurological signs.
- Lumbar puncture is a risky procedure in these coagulopathic patients and should be done only if clinical suspicion for meningitis is strong.
- Place NG tube and administer lactulose 30 cm³ every 1–2 hours until patient has a bowel movement.
- Haloperidol can be used to calm an agitated patient.
- Lactulose enemas can be used in patients who are bleeding or have a history of large varices.
- Monitor closely for hypernatremia which develops due to excessive lactulose use.
- Rifaximin can be added if the patient fails to improve on lactulose.

Table of treatment

Treatment	Comment
Conservative treatment	Adequate caloric (35–45 kcal/kg/day) and protein intake, 1–1.5 g protein/kg of bodyweight Vegetable protein may be superior to animal protein High fiber diet encouraged
Medical	Lactulose 15–30 cm³ q4–6 hours to ensure 2–3 bowel movements/day Rifaximin 550 mg PO bid
Complementary	Probiotics Yogurt
Surgical	Embolization of large porto-systemic collaterals in patient with spontaneous chronic incapacitating encephalopathy Liver transplantation

Prevention/management of complications

- Overzealous use of lactulose, e.g. every 1–2 hours via an NG tube, in a comatose hospitalized patient, can lead to life-threatening hypernatremia and worsening of mental status.
- Abdominal distension can worsen on lactulose and therefore abdominal examination should be performed frequently. If liver transplantation is imminent lactulose should be stopped as it can complicate surgery.

Algorithm 21.2 Treatment of HE in an outpatient setting

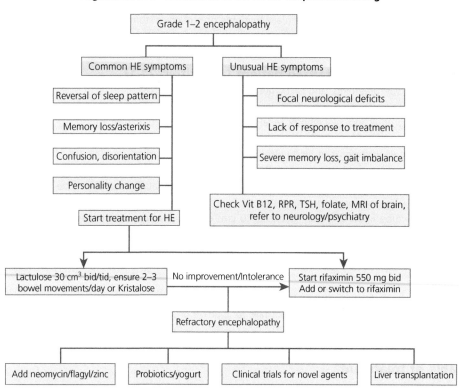

CLINICAL PEARLS
- Lactulose is effective but often poorly tolerated.
- Rifaximin can be used in addition or instead of lactulose in refractory cases.
- Protein restriction is not recommended as improved muscle mass is an important source of ammonia elimination.
- Probiotics and yogurt promote growth of non-urease-producing bacteria and decrease ammonia production.
- TIPS downsizing can be considered in patients who develop refractory HE after TIPS.
- Hospitalized patients often develop HE due to inadvertent use of sedatives to calm the "sun downing" patient.
- Patients should be closely monitored to prevent falls, fractures and other bodily injury.

Section 5: Special Populations
Elderly
- The elderly patient is particularly prone to diarrhea and tolerates lactulose poorly. Rifaximin should be considered first line in this population.
- They are at additional risk of falls from the HE standpoint.
- They also are at higher risk for HE after TIPS and therefore the indications for TIPS must be thought through carefully.

Section 6: Prognosis

> **CLINICAL PEARLS**
> - Onset of HE marks worsening of underlying liver disease and predicts increased mortality at 1 and 3 years.
> - Patients with HE should be evaluated for a liver transplantation.
> - Refractory HE may be the sole indication for liver transplantation in a small group of patients.
> - Patients with MHE are at increased risk for driving accidents and should not be allowed to drive.
> - The care of these patients can pose a significant burden, both economic and psychosocial, on the caregivers.
> - Some cognitive defects can persist even after liver transplantation.

Prognosis for treated patients
- With good response to treatment with lactulose and rifaximin patients with HE have a marked improvement in their quality of life.
- However as liver disease advances and portal hypertension worsens patients continue to have bouts of HE precipitated by bleeding, infection or azotemia. Such patients are best served by a timely liver transplantation.
- Within the current MELD allocation system there is no priority for refractory HE. Patients with refractory HE should be informed about the living donor liver transplantation option.

Section 7: Reading List

Bajaj JS, Riggio O. Drug therapy: rifaximin. Hepatology 2010;52:1484–8

Bajaj JS, Sanyal AJ, Bell D, Gilles H, Heuman DM. Predictors of the recurrence of hepatic encephalopathy in lactulose-treated patients. Aliment Pharmacol Ther 2010;31:1012–7

Bass NM, Mullen KD, Sanyal A, et al. Rifaximin treatment in hepatic encephalopathy. N Engl J Med 2010;362:1071–81

Bustamante J, Rimola A, Ventura PJ, et al. Prognostic significance of hepatic encephalopathy in patients with cirrhosis. J Hepatol 1999;30:890–5

Ferenci P, Lockwood A, Mullen K, Tarter R, Weissenborn K, Blei AT. Hepatic encephalopathy – definition, nomenclature, diagnosis, and quantification: final report of the working party at the 11th World Congress of Gastroenterology, Vienna, 1998. Hepatology 2002;35:716–21

Leevy CB, Phillips JA. Hospitalizations during the use of rifaximin versus lactulose for the treatment of hepatic encephalopathy. Dig Dis Sci 2007;52:737–41

Poordad FF. The burden of hepatic encephalopathy. Aliment Pharmacol Ther 2007;25 (Suppl 1):3–9

Prasad S, Dhiman, RK, Duseja A, et al. Lactulose improves cognitive functions and health-related quality of life in patients with cirrhosis who have minimal hepatic encephalopathy. Hepatology 2007;45:549–59

Sidhu SS, Goyal O, Mishra BP, et al. Rifaximin improves psychometric performance and health-related quality of life in patients with minimal hepatic encephalopathy (the RIME Trial). Am J Gastroenterol 2011;106: 307–16

Stewart CA, Malinchoc M, Kim WR, Kamath PS. Hepatic encephalopathy as a predictor of survival in patients with endstage liver disease. Liver Transpl 2007;13:1366–71

Section 8: Guidelines

Guideline title	Guideline source	Date
Practice Guideline: Hepatic encephalopathy	American College of Gastroenterology http://s3.gi.org/ physicians/guidelines/HepaticEncephalopathy.pdf	2001

Section 9: Evidence

Not applicable for this topic.

Section 10: Images

Not applicable for this topic.

CHAPTER 22

Hepatorenal Syndrome

Henryk Dancygier

Departments of Medicine II and IV, Sana Klinikum Offenbach, Goethe University, Frankfurt am Main, Germany *and* Division of Liver Diseases, Icahn School of Medicine at Mount Sinai, New York, NY, USA

OVERALL BOTTOM LINE

- HRS is a potentially reversible functional renal insufficiency in patients with cirrhosis, advanced liver failure and portal hypertension.
- There is no specific diagnostic test for HRS. The diagnosis is based on monitoring and interpreting renal function in a patient with liver insufficiency.
- Type 1 HRS is defined by doubling of the initial serum creatinine level to >2.5 mg/dL or 50% reduction of the initial 24-hour creatinine clearance to <20 mL/minute in less than 2 weeks.
- Type 2 HRS is characterized by impairment in renal function leading to serum creatinine level >1.5 mg/dL that does not meet the criteria for type 1 HRS.
- Without appropriate therapy the prognosis is extremely poor with a median survival time from the time of diagnosis of approximately 2 weeks for patients with type 1 HRS and 6 months for patients with type 2 HRS.
- Drug therapy is based on systemic arterial vasoconstrictors combined with volume expansion.
- Liver transplantation is the best treatment option with a 3-year survival rate of approximately 70%.

Section 1: Background
Definition of disease

- HRS is a potentially reversible functional renal insufficiency in patients with cirrhosis, advanced liver failure and portal hypertension in the absence of shock or an intrinsic parenchymal kidney disease.

Epidemiology

- Eighteen percent of patients with decompensated cirrhosis develop HRS within 1 year of decompensation and 39% within 5 years.
- The incidence of HRS in patients with liver cirrhosis who are admitted to the hospital because of ascites formation is 7–15%.
- In acute hepatic failure due to alcoholic hepatitis HRS occurs in approximately 27% of patients.

Etiology

- HRS most often occurs in patients with advanced cirrhosis, but may also complicate acute liver failure.

Mount Sinai Expert Guides: Hepatology, First Edition. Edited by Jawad Ahmad, Scott L. Friedman, and Henryk Dancygier.
© 2014 John Wiley & Sons, Ltd. Published 2014 by John Wiley & Sons, Ltd.
Companion website: www.mountsinaiexpertguides.com

- Most cases of type 1 HRS are elicited by precipitating factors, such as:
  - Infections (SBP is the most common infection precipitating HRS).
  - Viral, alcoholic, toxic or ischemic hepatitis superimposed on cirrhosis.
  - Major surgical procedures.
  - Gastrointestinal bleeding, intensive treatment with diuretics and diarrheal disease may elicit HRS, but more often cause prerenal insufficiency.

Pathogenesis

- Changes in endogenous vasoactive systems with marked renal vasoconstriction while at the same time extrarenal arteriolar vasodilatation, decreased systemic resistance and arterial hypotension predominate (Algorithm 22.1).
- The most important pathophysiologic change in HRS is a marked intrarenal arterial vasoconstriction with reduced renal perfusion and reduced glomerular filtration rate.

Algorithm 22.1 Pathogenesis of hepatorenal syndrome

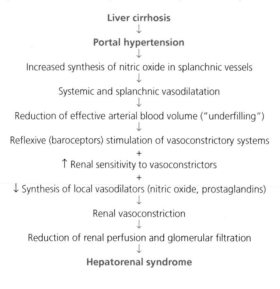

Liver cirrhosis
↓
Portal hypertension
↓
Increased synthesis of nitric oxide in splanchnic vessels
↓
Systemic and splanchnic vasodilatation
↓
Reduction of effective arterial blood volume ("underfilling")
↓
Reflexive (baroceptors) stimulation of vasoconstrictory systems
+
↑ Renal sensitivity to vasoconstrictors
+
↓ Synthesis of local vasodilators (nitric oxide, prostaglandins)
↓
Renal vasoconstriction
↓
Reduction of renal perfusion and glomerular filtration
↓
Hepatorenal syndrome

Predictive factors

- Predictive factors for the development of HRS in non-azotemic patients with liver cirrhosis and ascites:
  - Previous episodes of ascites.
  - Absence of hepatomegaly.
  - Poor nutritional status.
  - Moderately reduced glomerular filtration rate (>50 mL/minute).
  - Moderately increased BUN (<30 mg/dL).
  - Moderately increased serum creatinine (≤1.5 mg/dL).
  - Low serum Na^+.
  - High serum K^+.
  - Low urinary Na^+-excretion.
  - Low plasma osmolality.
  - High urine osmolality.

- High plasma renin activity.
- Low arterial pressure.
- Reduced free water clearance following a water load.
- Increased plasma norepinephrine.
- Esophageal varices.

Section 2: Prevention

Screening
- Every patient with liver cirrhosis admitted to the hospital should have serial determinations of serum creatinine levels and/or creatinine clearance.

Prevention
- Avoid and/or eliminate precipitating factors (see "Etiology" in Section 1).
- Patients with spontaneous bacterial peritonitis should be treated with albumin IV since this has been shown to decrease the incidence of HRS and improve survival.
- Pentoxifylline (400 mg PO three times a day for 28 days) has been shown to reduce the incidence of HRS in patients with severe (Maddrey Score >32) alcoholic hepatitis (only one randomized trial).

Section 3: Diagnosis

CLINICAL PEARLS
- There are no specific laboratory tests or imaging methods for the diagnosis of HRS.
- Diagnostic criteria for HRS have been developed by the International Ascites Club (see "Diagnostic criteria (International Ascites Club)".
- The diagnosis is based on interpreting serial serum creatinine levels and/or creatinine clearance in patients with severe hepatic insufficiency.
- HRS that does not meet the criteria of type 1 HRS is classified as type 2 HRS.

Differential diagnosis
- Most cases of renal dysfunction in cirrhosis are functional in nature. The differential diagnosis encompasses functional circulatory disturbances, obstructive lesions and pre-existing structural changes in the kidneys (acute-on-chronic kidney disease).
  - Pre-renal failure:
    - ➤ volume deficiency (e.g. vomiting, diarrhea, excessive administration of diuretics).
  - Acute tubular necrosis:
    - ➤ circulatory shock, severe bacterial infections, nephrotoxic drugs (NSAIDS, aminoglycosides).
  - Post-renal failure
    - ➤ urinary tract obstruction (e.g. stones, tumors).
- Monitoring renal function after withdrawal of diuretic treatment with subsequent intravenous volume expansion allows for important diagnostic conclusions. In pre-renal failure, renal function rapidly improves, while in HRS this measure remains without effect.

Differential diagnostic criteria for kidney dysfunction in cirrhosis

Diagnosis	Definition
Acute kidney injury	Rise in serum creatinine of >50% from baseline or a rise in serum creatinine by ≥26.4 µmol/L (≥0.3 mg/dL) in less than 48 hours
	HRS type 1 is a specific form of acute kidney injury
Chronic renal disease	Estimated glomerular filtration rate of <60 mL/minutes for more than 3 months calculated using the Modification of Diet in Renal Disease 6 (MDRD6) formula
	HRS type 2 is a specific form of chronic kidney disease
Acute-on-chronic kidney disease	Rise in serum creatinine of >50% from baseline or a rise in serum creatinine by ≥26.4 µmol/L (≥0.3 mg/dL) in less than 48 hours in a patient with cirrhosis whose glomerular filtration rate is <60 mL/minute for more than 3 months calculated using the MDRD6 formula

Differential diagnostic parameters in patients with cirrhosis, ascites and renal insufficiency (serum creatinine >3 mg%)*

Parameter	Hepatorenal syndrome	Pre-renal kidney failure	Acute tubular necrosis
Na^+-concentration in 24 hour urine (mEq/L)	<10	<10	>30
Urine-to-plasma osmolality ratio	>1	>1	<1
Urine-to-serum creatinine ratio	>30	<30	<20
Urinary sediment	Normal	Normal	Cylinders, epithelia
Improvement after volume expansion	No	Yes	No

*The parameters traditionally used to differentiate acute tubular necrosis from functional renal failure (urinary sodium excretion and urine: plasma osmolality ratio) are of very limited value in patients with cirrhosis and ascites. Possibly, urinary levels of β_2-microglobulin are markers of tubular damage in cirrhosis.

Typical presentation
- The presentation is that of a patient with advanced liver cirrhosis (see Chapter 19).
- Most patients have:
  - Diuretic resistant ascites.
  - Circulation which is hyperdynamic with high cardiac output and reduced total vascular resistance.

Clinical diagnosis
History
See Chapter 19.

Physical examination
- See Chapter 19.
- The clinical picture of patients with HRS mirrors:
  - Renal insufficiency.
  - Cardiocirculatory dysfunction.
  - Liver failure.

Disease severity classification

- Type 1 HRS is defined by doubling of the initial serum creatinine level to >2.5 mg/dL or 50% reduction of the initial 24-hour creatinine clearance to <20 mL/minute in less than 2 weeks.
- Type 2 HRS is characterized by impairment in renal function leading to a serum creatinine level >1.5 mg/dL that does not meet the criteria for type 1 HRS.
- Type 1 HRS is rapidly progressive, while in type 2 HRS renal insufficiency progresses more slowly, the decline of glomerular filtration rate is less dramatic, and renal function is more stable.

Laboratory diagnosis

Diagnostic tests

- There are no specific tests.
- The diagnosis of HRS is based on monitoring renal function, the demonstration of a reduced glomerular filtration rate in a patient with liver cirrhosis and ascites and on the exclusion of other disorders that can cause renal failure in cirrhosis (see "Diagnostic criteria (International Ascites Club)").

List of imaging techniques

- US is the most cost-effective imaging tool in visualizing the kidneys. It may demonstrate pre-existing structural changes and can rapidly exclude post-renal failure.
- The intrarenal hemodynamics in patients with liver cirrhosis and ascites may be assessed with Doppler-Duplex-sonography.
- If US images are unsatisfactory MRI may be performed.
- CT scanning is of limited use in patients with renal failure (do not apply contrast medium!).

Diagnostic criteria (International Ascites Club)

- Cirrhosis with ascites.
- Serum creatinine >133 mmol/L (>1.5 mg/dL).
- No improvement of serum creatinine (decrease to a level of ≤133 mmol/L or 1.5 mg/dL) after at least 2 days of diuretic withdrawal and volume expansion with albumin; the recommended dose of albumin is 1 g/kg body weight/day up to a maximum of 100 g daily.
- Absence of shock.
- No current or recent treatment with nephrotoxic drugs.
- Absence of parenchymal kidney disease as indicated by proteinuria >500 mg/day, microhematuria (>50 red blood cells/high-power field), and/or abnormal renal ultrasonography.

Potential pitfalls/common errors made regarding diagnosis of disease

- The most common diagnostic error in a cirrhotic patient with renal dysfunction is to overlook pre-renal or toxic factors, and/or underlying chronic kidney disease as the cause of rising serum creatinine, and to attribute the changes instead to HRS.

Section 4: Treatment

- HRS is a severe complication of advanced cirrhosis with a poor prognosis if left untreated. Current treatments are effective in up to 40% of patients. However, the available evidence is based on few studies with a small number of patients.

When to hospitalize
- Every patient with type 1 HRS must be hospitalized.

Managing the hospitalized patient
- Patients with type 1 HRS should be monitored carefully in an intensive care or semi-intensive care unit:
  - Urine output.
  - Fluid balance.
  - Arterial pressure.
  - Standard vital signs.
- Bacterial infections should be identified early and treated with antibiotics.
- There are no data whether it is better to stop or continue with beta-blockers in patients with type 1 HRS who are taking these drugs for prophylaxis against variceal bleeding.
- If patients have tense ascites, large-volume paracentesis with albumin is useful in relieving discomfort.
- All diuretics should be stopped in patients at the initial evaluation and the diagnosis of HRS. However, furosemide may be useful to maintain urine output and treat central volume overload if present.
- Spironolactone is contraindicated because of the high risk of life-threatening hyperkalemia.

Pharmacological therapy
- Drug therapy aims at correcting hypovolemia as well as reversing splanchnic vasodilation and renal vasoconstriction.
- Systemic arterial vasoconstrictor therapy combined with volume expansion is the current pharmacological approach to HRS.
- Adequate intravasal volume expansion with albumin is essential for vasopressors to be effective.
- Monotherapy with a vasoconstrictor or with octreotide is not effective.
- Hemodialysis and MARS are ineffective in patients with HRS.

Midodrine and octreotide
- Midodrine (a selective alpha-1 adrenergic agonist) is a systemic vasoconstrictor and octreotide (a somatostatin analog) is an inhibitor of endogenous vasodilator release.
  - Midodrine, initially 2.5–7.5 mg PO three times a day, increasing slowly to 12.5–15 mg PO three times a day, in combination with
  - Octreotide, initially 100 μg SC three times a day, increasing slowly to 200 μg SC three times a day and
  - Albumin 50–100 g IV per day.
- Noradrenaline (0.1–0.7 μg/kg/minute) combined with albumin may be as effective and safe as terlipressin in improving renal function in patients with HRS.
- Be aware that there is very limited information with respect to the use of midodrine, octreotide and noradrenaline in patients with type 1 HRS.

Terlipressin
- Terlipressin (a vasopressin analog; not available in the USA) decreases hepatic and renal arterial resistance in patients with cirrhosis. Combined with albumin it improves renal function and has been shown to prolong short-term survival in type 1 HRS.

- Terlipressin 0.5–1 mg IV bolus every 4 hours or as a continuous IV infusion 2–12 mg/day in combination with
  - Albumin 1 g/kg IV on day 1, thereafter 40 g IV once a day.
- Only approximately 30% of patients with type 1 HRS respond to treatment with terlipressin and albumin and a significant number of initial responders relapse after terlipressin withdrawal.
- Predictive factors of response to terlipressin and albumin therapy are baseline serum bilirubin (cut-off level of 10 mg/dL), baseline serum creatinine (<5.0 mg/dL) and a sustained rise in mean arterial pressure of ≥5 mmHg by day 3 of treatment.
- If serum creatinine does not decrease at least 25% from baseline after 3 days, escalate dose of terlipressin in a stepwise manner every 3 days up to a maximum of 2 mg every 4 hours.
- Discontinue treatment within 14 days in patients without complete response.
- Patients treated with terlipressin may show severe cardiovascular complications, e.g. ventricular fibrillation (torsade de pointes).
- Terlipressin plus albumin is effective in 60–70% of patients with type 2 HRS. However, there are insufficient data on the impact of this treatment on long-term clinical outcomes.

TIPS
- In patients with HRS TIPS may improve renal function for a short period of time and reduce the activities of the renin-angiotensin-aldosterone and the sympathetic nervous system.
- Preliminary data in few patients with a Child-Pugh score <12 show a sustained improvement of renal function with the combined approach of oral midodrine plus subcutaneous octreotide plus intravenous albumin followed by TIPS. However, there are insufficient data to support the use of TIPS as a treatment of patients with type 1 HRS.

Liver transplantation
- Liver transplantation is the treatment of choice in both type 1 and type 2 HRS, with survival rates of approximately 65% in type 1 HRS.
- Evaluation for orthotopic liver transplantation should be part of the initial management of patients presenting with predictive factors (see "Predictive factors" in Section 1) or suspected of having type 1 HRS, even before a diagnosis of HRS is made.
- The duration of renal dysfunction is the main predictor of the outcome of renal function after transplantation.
- There seems to be no advantage in using combined liver-kidney transplantation versus liver transplantation alone in patients with HRS.
- A subgroup of patients with HRS who require prolonged (>12 weeks) renal support therapy may possibly benefit from combined transplantation of liver and kidneys.
- Drug treatment of HRS can bridge the time to liver transplantation and may improve outcome after transplantation.
- The reduction in serum creatinine after treatment and the related decrease in the MELD score should not change the decision to perform liver transplantation since the prognosis after recovering from type 1 HRS is still poor.

Section 5: Special Populations

Not applicable for this topic.

Section 6: Prognosis

> **CLINICAL PEARLS**
> - Every patient with type 1 HRS must be hospitalized.
> - Current treatments of HRS are effective in up to 40% of patients.
> - Systemic arterial vasoconstrictor therapy combined with volume expansion with albumin is the current pharmacological approach to HRS.
> - Liver transplantation is the treatment of choice in both type 1 and type 2 HRS, with survival rates of approximately 65% in type 1 HRS.
> - The presence of alcoholic hepatitis more than doubles the risk of death in type 1 HRS.

Natural history of untreated disease
- HRS is a life-threatening complication of decompensated liver disease.
- Without appropriate therapy the prognosis is extremely poor with a median survival time from the time of diagnosis of approximately 2 weeks for patients with type 1 HRS and 6 months for patients with type 2 HRS.
- The presence of SIRS, with or without infection, is a major independent prognostic factor in patients with cirrhosis and acute functional renal failure.
- The MELD score is a useful indicator allowing for estimation of the outcome of patients with cirrhosis and HRS. While practically all patients with type 1 HRS have a high MELD score (≥20) and an extremely poor outcome, patients with type 2 HRS may be stratified according to a MELD score >20 with a median survival of 3 months and those with a MELD score <20 with a median survival of 11 months.

Prognosis for treated patients
- Patients undergoing liver transplantation have a 3-year survival rate of approximately 60–70%.

Section 7: Reading List

Akriviadis E, Botla R, Briggs W, et al. Pentoxifylline improves short-term survival in serve acute alcoholic hepatitis: a double-blind, placebo-controlled trial. Gastroenterology 2000;119:1637–48

Alessandria C, Ozdogan O, Guevara M, et al. MELD score and clinical type predict prognosis in hepatorenal syndrome: relevance to liver transplantation. Hepatology 2005;41:1282–9

Alessandria C, Ottobrelli A, Debernardi-Venon W, et al. Noradrenalin vs terlipressin in patients with hepatorenal syndrome: a prospective, randomized, unblinded, pilot study. J Hepatol 2007;47:499–505

Angeli P, Volpin R, Gerunda G, et al. Reversal of type 1 hepatorenal syndrome with the administration of midodrine and octreotide. Hepatology 1999;29:1690–7

Arroyo V, Fernandéz L. Management of hepatorenal syndrome in patients with cirrhosis. Nat Rev Nephrol 2011;7:517–26

Boyer TD, Sanyal AJ, Garcia-Tsao G, et al. Predictors of response to terlipressin plus albumin in hepatorenal syndrome (HRS) type 1: relationship of serum creatinine to hemodynamics. J Hepatol 2011;55:315–21

Charlton MR, Wall WJ, Ojo AO, et al. International liver transplantation expert panel consensus conference on renal insufficiency in liver transplantation. Liver Transpl 2009;15:S1–3

Ginès A, Escorsell A, Ginès P, et al. Incidence, predictive factors, and prognosis of the hepatorenal syndrome in cirrhosis. Gastroenterology 1993;105:229–36

Gluud LL, Christensen K, Christensen E, et al. Systematic review of randomized trials on vasoconstrictor drugs for hepatorenal syndrome. Hepatology 2010;51:576–84

Gonwa TA, Klintmalm GB, Levy M, et al. Impact of pretransplant renal function on survival after liver transplantation. Transplantation 1995;59:361–5

Levey AS, Bosch JP, Lewis JB, et al. Modification of Diet in Renal Disease Study Group. A more accurate method to estimate glomerular filtration rate from serum creatinine: a new prediction equation. Ann Intern Med 1999;130:461–70

Martín-Llahí M, Pépin MN, Guevara M, et al. Terlipressin and albumin vs albumin in patients with cirrhosis and hepatorenal syndrome:a randomized study. Gastroenterology 2008;134:1352–9

Nazar A, Pereira GH, Guevara M, et al. Predictors of response to therapy with terlipressin and albumin in patients with cirrhosis and type 1 hepatorenal syndrome. Hepatology 2010;51:219–26

Ortega R, Ginès P, Uriz J, et al. Terlipressin therapy with and without albumin for patients with hepatorenal syndrome: results of a prospective, nonrandomized study. Hepatology 2002;36:941–8

Salerno F, Gerbes A, Ginès P, et al. Diagnosis, prevention and treatment of hepatorenal syndrome in cirrhosis. Gut 2007;56:1310–8

Sanyal AJ, Boyer T, Garcia-Tsao G, et al. A randomized, prospective, double-blind, placebo-controlled trial of terlipressin for type 1 hepatorenal syndrome. Gastroenterology 2008;134:1360–8

Singh V, Ghosh S, Singh B, et al. Noradrenaline vs terlipressin in the treatment of hepatorenal syndrome: a randomized study. J Hepatol 2012;56:1293–8

Solanki P, Chawla A, Garg R, et al. Beneficial effects of terlipressin in hepatorenal syndrome: a prospective, randomized placebo-controlled clinical trial. J Gastroenterol Hepatol 2003;18:152–6

Sort P, Navasa M, Arroyo V, et al. Effect of intravenous albumin on renal impairment and mortality in patients with cirrhosis and spontaneous bacterial peritonitis. N Engl J Med 1999;341:403–9

Wong F, Nadim MK, Kellum JA, et al. Working party proposal for a revised classification system of renal dysfunction in patients with cirrhosis. Gut 2011;60:702–9

Section 8:Guidelines
National society guidelines

Guideline title	Guideline source	Date
AASLD practice guidelines: the role of transjugular intrahepatic portosystemic (TIPS) shunt in the management of portal hypertension	American Association for the Study of Liver Disease (AASLD) http://www.aasld.org/practiceguidelines/Documents/Bookmarked%20Practice%20Guidelines/TIPS%20Update%20Nov%202009.pdf	2009

International society guidelines

Guideline title	Guideline source	Date
EASL clinical practice guidelines on the management of ascites, spontaneous bacterial peritonitis, and hepatorenal syndrome in cirrhosis	European Association for the Study of the Liver (EASL) http://www.easl.eu/assets/application/files/21e21971bf182e5_file.pdf	2010

Suggested websites
www.aasld.org
www.easl.eu
www.bsg.org.uk

Section 9: Evidence

Not applicable for this topic.

Section 10: Images

Not applicable for this topic.

<table>
<tr><td>

Additional material for this chapter can be found online at:
www.mountsinaiexpertguides.com
This includes a case study and multiple choice questions

</td><td></td></tr>
</table>

CHAPTER 23

Hepatopulmonary Syndrome

Jawad Ahmad

Division of Liver Diseases, Icahn School of Medicine at Mount Sinai, New York, NY, USA

OVERALL BOTTOM LINE
- HPS is defined by decreased arterial oxygenation due to right to left shunting in patients with liver disease in the absence of intrinsic lung disease.
- HPS is a relatively common disease that can present without symptoms and therefore is often under-diagnosed.
- The diagnosis of HPS can be suspected based on arterial blood gas measurement and is usually confirmed by contrast echocardiography.
- Medical treatment of HPS is limited and the disease is slowly progressive but liver transplantation can be curative in selected patients.

Section 1: Background
Definition of disease
- HPS is defined by an increased alveolar–arterial gradient on room air with evidence of IPVDs occurring in patients with liver disease and in the absence of intrinsic lung disease.

Incidence/prevalence
- Prevalence estimates for HPS are varied due to the difficulty in making a definitive diagnosis on clinical grounds and the different criteria used. Some series suggest that up to half of all cirrhotics have evidence of HPS based on arterial hypoxemia on room air.
- In a recent study of cirrhotic patients undergoing liver transplant evaluation, 32% were found to have HPS and in older studies of patients with cirrhosis, 24% had a diagnosis of HPS.
- Most studies would suggest that it is routinely under-diagnosed.

Economic impact
- There is no data on the economic impact of HPS.
- Since it occurs commonly in cirrhotic patients and is a cause of increased pre-transplant mortality, the economic impact should be considerable. In addition, the main treatment for HPS involves supplemental oxygen and frequent clinical monitoring.

Mount Sinai Expert Guides: Hepatology, First Edition. Edited by Jawad Ahmad, Scott L. Friedman, and Henryk Dancygier.
© 2014 John Wiley & Sons, Ltd. Published 2014 by John Wiley & Sons, Ltd.
Companion website: www.mountsinaiexpertguides.com

Etiology

- The reason why some cirrhotic patients develop HPS and others do not is unclear.
- The presence of cirrhosis is not essential for the development of HPS as it can occur in non-cirrhotic portal hypertension and in ischemic hepatitis (with reversal of intrapulmonary vasodilation with correction of the underlying ischemia).
- There is no correlation between the degree of arterial hypoxemia or amount of shunting and the severity of liver disease (as measured by the Child–Pugh score).

Pathology/pathogenesis

- IPVDs are thought to arise due to poor clearance or excess production of pulmonary vasodilators and inhibition of circulating vasoconstrictors by the cirrhotic liver likely mediated through nitric oxide.
- The resultant dilation of the pulmonary vasculature leads to a large right to left shunt, which is not a true anatomical shunt as it partially responds to increased inspired oxygen concentration.
- The mechanism for this observation is unclear but may be a consequence of the vasodilation. The red cells stay in the center of the capillary lumen relatively distant to the oxygen in the alveolus. By increasing the inspired oxygen concentration more oxygen diffuses to the center of the capillary leading to increased arterial oxygen saturation.
- The important role of nitric oxide is suggested by animal studies demonstrating upregulation of endothelial nitric oxide synthetase in the pulmonary vasculature in rat models of HPS.
- In humans, nitric oxide inhibitors such as methylene blue can improve oxygenation in patients with HPS.

Section 2: Prevention

No interventions have been demonstrated to prevent the development of the disease

Screening

- All cirrhotic patients undergoing liver transplant evaluation should be screened for HPS using arterial oxygen saturation on room air and then arterial blood gas testing if necessary.
- A room air pulse oximetry value of ≤94% detects all patients with a partial pressure of oxygen <60 mmHg with a specificity of 93%.

Section 3: Diagnosis (Algorithm 23.1)

BOTTOM LINE/CLINICAL PEARLS
- The majority of patients with HPS do not present with pulmonary type symptoms but rather with symptoms related to chronic liver disease.
- Dyspnea in patients with cirrhosis should raise the suspicion for HPS. Platypnea (worsening dyspnea in the upright position) can be seen.
- Examination findings in HPS reflect stigmata of chronic liver disease but spider nevi tend to be more common. There should be no abnormal lung findings.
- Routine investigations which suggest HPS include arterial oxygen desaturation to <80 mmHg and an increased alveolar-arterial oxygen gradient (>20 mmHg) on room air.
- IPVDs can be confirmed by contrast echocardiography, macro-aggregated albumin scan or pulmonary angiogram.

Differential diagnosis

Differential diagnosis	Features
Chronic lung disease: COPD	Abnormal lung examination, abnormal lung imaging
Recurrent pulmonary emboli	Abnormal lung imaging
Portopulmonary hypertension	Abnormal echocardiogram

Typical presentation

- The typical presentation of HPS is not based on pulmonary complaints but rather symptoms related to ESLD such as fatigue, ascites, HE and variceal bleeding. Dyspnea is noted in a minority of patients and some of these patients will describe worsening dyspnea when standing upright from a recumbent position (platypnea). Physical examination is usually unhelpful in making a diagnosis of HPS although spider nevi tend to be more numerous and there can be signs of a hyperdynamic circulation.
- Since there is a paucity of specific symptoms, there needs to be a high index of suspicion for HPS, particularly in patients being evaluated for liver transplantation.

Clinical diagnosis

History

- The history in patients with HPS is usually unrevealing. Since the diagnosis only occurs in those with underlying liver disease, most of the symptoms reflect this including fatigue, confusion, abdominal distension, ankle swelling and gastrointestinal bleeding.
- It is important to ask about shortness of breath, particularly if it is worsened by standing upright from a recumbent position.
- HPS can occur even if the liver disease does not appear to be so severe.

Physical examination

- The physical examination in HPS is usually only significant for stigmata of chronic liver disease.
- Typically, the heart and lung examination are normal without evidence of pulmonary edema, pleural effusion or heart failure as these could mimic the clinical presentation of HPS.
- Spider nevi are very common in cirrhosis but may be more numerous in HPS.
- Severe ascites can cause elevation of the diaphragm and impair ventilation and lead to tachypnea.
- If arterial oxygen saturation is very low, central cyanosis may be noted.

Useful clinical decision rules and calculators

- Room air oxygen saturation of <96% should prompt further investigation for HPS, particularly in patients undergoing liver transplant evaluation.
- Room air oxygen saturation of <94% reliably indicates a arterial oxygen tension of <60 mmHg.
- The degree of right to left shunting can be measured by the shunt fraction which is usually <5% in normal subjects. It is measured while the patient breathes 100% oxygen for 20 minutes. It can be calculated using the formula:

$$Qs/Qt = (0.003 \times (PAO_2 - PaO_2)) / ((0.003 \times (PAO_2 - PaO_2) + 5)$$

Where Qs is shunt flow, Qt is total flow, PAO_2 is the alveolar oxygen tension and PaO_2 is the arterial oxygen tension.

Disease severity classification

- In general the severity of HPS can be assessed based on selection criteria for liver transplantation.
- Patients with severe disease have poor outcome after transplant.
- Severe disease in this context can be described as:
  - Room air arterial oxygen tension (PaO_2) <50 mmHg
  - Shunt fraction >20%

Laboratory diagnosis

List of diagnostic tests

- The initial test for HPS should include arterial oxygen saturation on room air. A value <96%, and definitely <94% strongly suggests HPS in the absence of cardiopulmonary disease in cirrhotic patients.
- The next test should be to measure the arterial blood gas on room air. This should demonstrate hypoxemia (typically <80 mmHg) and also enable calculation of the alveolar–arterial oxygen gradient which should be elevated in HPS (usually >20 mmHg) due to the ventilation perfusion mismatch.
- The alveolar–arterial oxygen gradient is defined as $PAO_2 - PaO_2$.
- PaO_2 is determined by the arterial blood gas, while PAO_2 is calculated using the alveolar gas equation:

$$PAO_2 = (FiO_2 \times (P_{atm} - PH_2O)) - (PaCO_2 \div R)$$

where FiO_2 is 0.21 at room air, P_{atm} is the atmospheric pressure of 760 mmHg at sea level, PH_2O is the partial pressure of water (47 mmHg at body temperature), $PaCO_2$ is the arterial carbon dioxide tension, and R is the respiratory quotient of 0.8.

- The typical gradient varies by age but is approximated by the equation

$$2.5 + (0.21 \times age\ in\ years)$$

- Right to left shunt fraction as shown in "Useful clinical decision rules and calculators." The normal level is 5%. Anything above 20% suggests a very significant shunt and increased mortality after liver transplant.
- Pulmonary function tests are generally not useful in HPS as any abnormalities are non-specific. However, they can be useful to exclude other lung diseases.

List of imaging techniques

- The imaging studies to diagnose HPS rely on demonstration of IPVDs as well as exclusion of underlying cardiopulmonary disease.
- A chest X-ray is usually sufficient to exclude significant pulmonary disease or a pleural effusion.
- High resolution CT scan of the chest is useful in selected cases and can show dilated peripheral pulmonary vessels and an increased pulmonary artery to bronchus ratio.
- A contrast echocardiogram can demonstrate a right to left shunt. Typically agitated saline is used to produce microbubbles that should not cross the pulmonary capillary bed. (Various dyes can also be used instead of microbubbles such as indocyanine green.) In the presence of a right to left shunt the microbubbles appear in the right atrium or ventricle and then in the left atrium or ventricle. The time between the appearance of microbubbles in the right then left can be used to determine whether the shunt is intracardiac (within three beats) or intrapulmonary (three to six beats).

- Nuclear scanning using Technetium-labeled macroaggregated albumin can be used to demonstrate the right to left shunt since the labeled albumin should not cross the pulmonary bed.
- Pulmonary angiography can be used as a diagnostic tool but is invasive and there has been limited experience in HPS. It can be useful to exclude other conditions that can mimic HPS such as pulmonary embolization.

Algorithm 23.1 Diagnosis and management for HPS

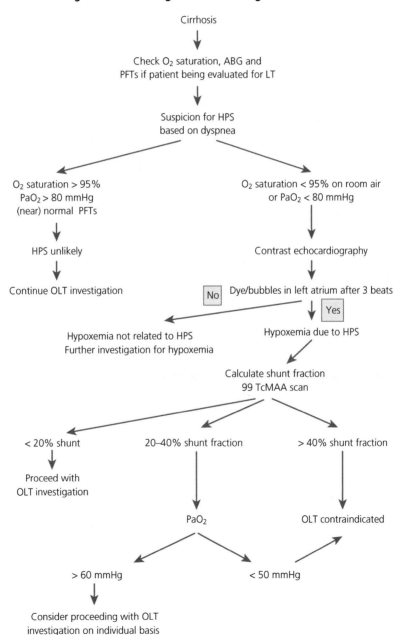

Potential pitfalls/common errors made regarding diagnosis of disease

- HPS is relatively frequent in cirrhosis and the diagnosis can easily be missed as the clinical findings are subtle.
- HPS can be masked by some of the complications of cirrhosis such as massive ascites causing elevated hemidiaphragms or a pleural effusion.
- HPS can be confused with portopulmonary hypertension (see Chapter 24).

Section 4: Treatment

Treatment rationale

- Multiple different agents have been tried as first line therapy for HPS but none have proved to be effective. Oxygen therapy can improve the arterial hypoxemia to a certain extent.
- In suitable patients, liver transplant provides the best opportunity to correct the underlying abnormalities in HPS and prevent the right to left shunting.
- Several series have shown acceptable outcome after liver transplantation for HPS but the results are lower than expected compared with patients without HPS (71% 1-year survival compared with 88–90%).
- Factors predictive of a poor outcome after transplant include a room air PaO_2 <50 mmHg and a shunt fraction >20%.

Table of treatment

Treatment	Comment
Conservative treatment	Oxygen can be used in all patients
Medical	None effective
Surgical	Liver transplant in patients with PaO_2 >55–60 mmHg and shunt fraction <20%

Prevention/management of complications

- HPS patients undergoing liver transplantation are at increased risk of early (within 3 months) mortality compared with non-HPS patients.
- Resolution of HPS after liver transplantation can occur quickly (over several days) but can also take several weeks or months.

> **CLINICAL PEARLS**
> - Liver transplant in selected patients is the only effective treatment for HPS.
> - Resolution of HPS after liver transplantation is not always immediate and can take several months to a year.

Section 5: Special Populations

Not applicable for this topic.

Section 6: Prognosis

> **BOTTOM LINE**
> * HPS is associated with significant mortality in patients with cirrhosis.
> * Without liver transplantation, arterial oxygenation levels steadily decrease in HPS.
> * Liver transplantation provides a survival benefit in HPS patients.

Natural history of untreated disease
* Without liver transplantation, there is a steady decline in arterial oxygenation levels by several mmHg per year.

Prognosis for treated patients
* With liver transplantation, 1 year survival in HPS is approximately 70%.
* Much of the mortality after liver transplantation in HPS occurs within the first 3 months.

Follow-up tests and monitoring
* There are no standardized guidelines to monitor HPS after liver transplantation but oxygen saturation and arterial blood gases do show improvement.

Section 7: Reading List

Arguedas MR, Singh H, Faulk DK, Fallon MB. Utility of pulse oximetry screening for hepatopulmonary syndrome. Clin Gastroenterol Hepatol 2007;5:749–54

Colle IO, Moreau R, Godinho E, et al. Diagnosis of portopulmonary hypertension in candidates for liver transplantation: a prospective study. Hepatology 2003;37:401–9

Hoeper, MM, Krowka, MJ, Strassburg, CP. Portopulmonary hypertension and hepatopulmonary syndrome. Lancet 2004;363:1461–8

Krowka, MJ, Mandell, MS, Ramsay, MA, et al. Hepatopulmonary syndrome and portopulmonary hypertension: a report of the multicenter liver transplant database. Liver Transpl 2004;10:174–82

Schenk P, Schniger-Hekele M, Fuhrmann V et al. Prognostic significance of the hepatopulmonary syndrome in patients with cirrhosis. Gastroenterol 2003;125:1042–52

Suggested website
http://www.aasld.org/practiceguidelines/Documents/Bookmarked%20Practice%20Guidelines/Liver%20Transplant.pdf

Section 8: Guidelines
National society guidelines

Guideline title	Guideline source	Date
AASLD practice guidelines: Evaluation of the patient for liver transplantation	AASLD http://www.aasld.org/practiceguidelines/ Documents/Bookmarked%20Practice%20Guidelines/ Liver%20Transplant.pdf	June 2005

Section 9: Evidence

Type of evidence	Title, date	Comment
Observational study	Resolution of gas exchange abnormalities and intrapulmonary shunting following liver transplantation. Hepatology 1997;25:1228	First large study to demonstrate that HPS patients could be successfully transplanted
Retrospective case series	Natural history of hepatopulmonary syndrome: impact of liver transplantation. Hepatology 2005;41:1122	Demonstrated survival benefit of liver transplantation over observation in patients with HPS

Section 10: Images

Not applicable for this topic.

Additional material for this chapter can be found online at:
www.mountsinaiexpertguides.com
This includes a case study and multiple choice questions

CHAPTER 24

Portopulmonary Hypertension

Jawad Ahmad

Division of Liver Diseases, Icahn School of Medicine at Mount Sinai, New York, NY, USA

OVERALL BOTTOM LINE
- PPHTN is the presence of pulmonary arterial hypertension in the setting of portal hypertension.
- The cause is unknown but appears to be related to cytokine-induced remodeling of the pulmonary arterial anatomy and possibly intravascular thromboses.
- The diagnosis is suspected on echocardiography and confirmed by right heart catheterization.
- Several medications can be used to treat PPHTN but need to be given for several months or years with periodic monitoring of pulmonary artery pressure.
- Liver transplantation is an option for selected patients with PPHTN and is associated with improvement of pulmonary arterial hypertension.

Section 1: Background
Definition of disease
- PPHTN is defined by pulmonary arterial hypertension in the setting of portal hypertension in the absence of other causes of pulmonary hypertension.

Disease classification
- There is no standard disease classification for PPHTN although it can be useful to separate the disease into mild (30–44 mmHg), moderate (45–59 mmHg) and severe (60 mmHg and over) based on the degree of pulmonary arterial hypertension.

Incidence/prevalence
- The prevalence of PPHTN ranges from less than 1% up to 16%.
- The prevalence appears to be higher in patients with more severe liver disease.
- The highest prevalence has been seen in patients being evaluated for liver transplantation.

Etiology
- The cause of the disease is unknown.
- PPHTN only occurs in the setting of portal hypertension.
- This is typically due to cirrhosis but can also occur in non-cirrhotic portal hypertension.

Pathology/pathogenesis
- The pathogenesis of PPHTN is unclear but may occur on the background of genetic susceptibility as there are cases of familial pulmonary hypertension related to dysfunction of the bone morphogenetic protein receptor type II.

Mount Sinai Expert Guides: Hepatology, First Edition. Edited by Jawad Ahmad, Scott L. Friedman, and Henryk Dancygier.

© 2014 John Wiley & Sons, Ltd. Published 2014 by John Wiley & Sons, Ltd.

Companion website: www.mountsinaiexpertguides.com

- Some studies suggest that the underlying portal hypertension leads to porto-systemic collaterals and substances that normally would be metabolized in the liver mediate the pulmonary hypertension. Multiple cytokines and hormones have been implicated including serotonin, IL-1, vasoactive intestinal peptide, glucagon, endothelin-1 and thromboxane B2.
- The hyperdynamic circulation seen in cirrhosis and chronic thromboembolism may also play a role.
- Pulmonary histology in PPHTN demonstrates *in situ* thrombosis, pulmonary arteriopathy and vasoconstriction.

Section 2: Prevention

> **BOTTOM LINE/CLINICAL PEARLS**
> - No interventions have been demonstrated to prevent the development of the disease.

Screening
- Typically PPHTN is found in patients with cirrhosis undergoing liver transplant evaluation during pre-operative cardiac testing.
- The clinical presentation of PPHTN can mimic other conditions seen in cirrhosis such as hepatopulmonary syndrome and ascites (with or without a pleural effusion). Hence cirrhotic patients presenting with dyspnea on exertion without an obvious cause should be screened for PPHTN.

Section 3: Diagnosis (Algorithm 24.1)

> **BOTTOM LINE/CLINICAL PEARLS**
> - Patients with PPHTN can present without symptoms but typically complain of shortness of breath on exertion. Other symptoms can include chest pain, fainting or dizziness.
> - Physical examination findings in PPHTN can be limited to signs of portal hypertension but a loud pulmonary component of the second heart sound, a pansystolic murmur heard at the left sternal border in the fourth intercostal space (from tricuspid regurgitation) that increases during inspiration, a parasternal heave and ankle edema can sometimes be appreciated.
> - The diagnosis can be suspected by echocardiography and is confirmed by right heart catheterization.

Differential diagnosis

Differential diagnosis	Features
Hepatopulmonary syndrome	History can be similar but usually no unique physical findings except for those of portal hypertension. Investigations show a low arterial oxygen saturation and normal right-sided pressures on echocardiography and right heart catheterization
Tense ascites and/or a pleural effusion	History of shortness of breath on exertion is usual. Physical findings demonstrate a fluid thrill or shifting dullness or decreased air entry (typically at the right lung base) with a stony dull percussion note. Ascites and effusions are readily seen on abdominal or chest imaging. Echocardiography and right heart catheterization should be normal

Typical presentation

- The typical patient with PPHTN is first diagnosed during investigation for liver transplantation. The diagnosis of portal hypertension is usually already apparent in a cirrhotic patient with complaints including abdominal distension, ankle edema and fatigue and physical examination demonstrating spider nevi, ascites and splenomegaly. Patients can present with symptoms of PPHTN including dyspnea on exertion, orthopnea and occasionally unexplained syncope or light-headedness. An abnormal cardiac examination with a pansystolic murmur at the left sternal edge and a loud pulmonary component of the second heart sound can be suggestive of PPHTN. During the transplant evaluation process, an echocardiogram can demonstrate high right-sided pressure which then leads to confirmatory testing.

Clinical diagnosis

History

- The history in PPHTN is notable for shortness of breath on exertion in most patients. It is important to ask about breathing difficulties when lying down (orthopnea) and any symptoms that might suggest right heart failure including chest pain, hemoptysis, ankle swelling and syncopal episodes.
- Abdominal distension from ascites is a feature but can obviously be seen in cirrhotic patients without PPHTN.

Physical examination

- On physical examination, signs of portal hypertension are invariably present including spider nevi, ascites splenomegaly and lower extremity edema.
- Examination findings specific to PPHTN include those seen in right heart failure such as a loud pulmonary component to the second heart sound, a pansystolic murmur due to tricuspid valve regurgitation, and a right ventricular heave. With higher right-sided pressures the physiological splitting of the second heart sound increases and an early diastolic flow murmur of pulmonary regurgitation can be heard. All of these cardiac auscultatory findings are accentuated by inspiration which increases flow through the right-sided cardiac chambers.

Disease severity classification

- There is no definitive disease severity classification system in PPHTN but other types of pulmonary hypertension have been classified using the WHO functional classification which has four levels:
  - Level 1 – no limitation in physical activity.
  - Level 2 – Comfortable at rest but symptoms from ordinary physical activity.
  - Level 3 – Comfortable at rest but symptoms from less than ordinary physical activity.
  - Level 4 – Symptoms at rest and with inability to carry out any physical activity without symptoms.

Laboratory diagnosis

List of diagnostic tests

- The initial diagnostic investigation for PPHTN is usually extensive as it occurs in the setting of liver transplant evaluation. Blood tests are usually unhelpful in making a diagnosis.
- Oxygen saturation is usually normal.

- Electrocardiographic changes are very common and reflect right heart failure or right heart strain. The cardiac axis is deviated to the right, the R waves are taller in the right-sided leads due to right ventricular hypertrophy and a right bundle branch block pattern can be seen. Occasionally P pulmonale is noted (increased P wave in lead II from right atrial enlargement).
- Pulmonary function tests can be used if intrinsic lung disease is a diagnostic concern.

List of imaging techniques
- Although not specific in making a diagnosis, a chest X-ray can show changes suggestive of pulmonary arterial hypertension including prominent pulmonary artery markings and cardiomegaly and right atrial enlargement from right-sided heart failure.
- Doppler echocardiogram is the initial screening test for PPHTN and is part of the routine investigations in liver transplant. PASP and right ventricular pressure and function can be estimated although the Doppler technique relies on a calculation based on significant tricuspid regurgitation. If this is absent the PASP is not accurate. This can lead to differences in pressure measurement >10 mmHg compared with right heart catheterization. Hence there should be a low threshold to proceed with more invasive investigation even with a mildly elevated PASP on echocardiogram.
- Right heart catheterization is the gold standard test in PPHTN and a MPAP of >25 mmHg at rest confirms the diagnosis. In addition the PCWP should be <15 mmHg, excluding left heart failure as a cause, and there is an increased PVR. The transpulmonary gradient can also be calculated and is the difference between the pulmonary artery diastolic pressure and the PCWP, and this should be increased in PPHTN.

Potential pitfalls/common errors made regarding diagnosis of disease
- It is important to differentiate between PPHTN and hepatopulmonary syndrome but this should be readily apparent on echocardiogram.
- Other causes of pulmonary hypertension need to be excluded before a diagnosis of PPHTN can be made confidently.

Section 4: Treatment
Treatment rationale
- Treatment for PPHTN is not standardized and no randomized trials have been conducted.
- In symptomatic patients or those with high PASP as a contraindication for liver transplant, several vasodilatory agents have been tried.
- The choice of treatment depends on local expertise and preference.
- Medical therapy is given for several months with periodic assessment of response based on exercise capacity and right heart catheterization measurements.
- In patients with PPHTN who are candidates for liver transplantation, medical therapy has been used to decrease the PASP to near normal levels prior to transplant.
- Although the data is limited, liver transplantation offers the possibility of reversal of the underlying abnormalities in PPHTN with acceptable perioperative morbidity in selected patients.
- It remains to be determined if pre-transplant medical therapy in PPHTN is associated with acceptable outcome after liver transplantation.

Algorithm 24.1 Diagnosis and management of PPHTN

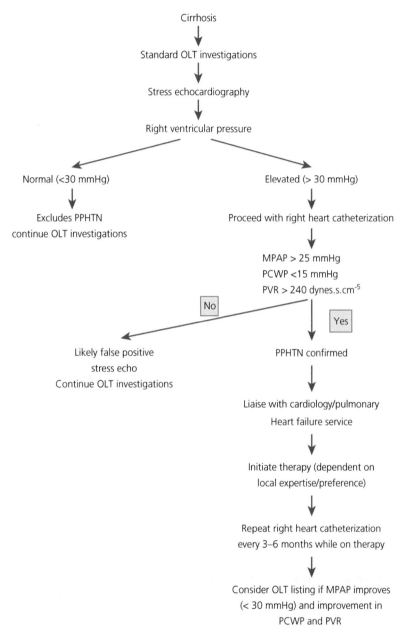

Cirrhosis

Standard OLT investigations

Stress echocardiography

Right ventricular pressure

Normal (<30 mmHg)

Excludes PPHTN
continue OLT investigations

Elevated (> 30 mmHg)

Proceed with right heart catheterization

MPAP > 25 mmHg
PCWP <15 mmHg
PVR > 240 dynes.s.cm^{-5}

No

Yes

Likely false positive
stress echo
Continue OLT investigations

PPHTN confirmed

Liaise with cardiology/pulmonary
Heart failure service

Initiate therapy (dependent on
local expertise/preference)

Repeat right heart catheterization
every 3–6 months while on therapy

Consider OLT listing if MPAP improves
(< 30 mmHg) and improvement in
PCWP and PVR

Table of treatment

Treatment	Comments
Conservative treatment	Only suitable for asymptomatic patients who are not transplant candidates
Medical: Epoprostenol (Flolan)	• Naturally occurring prostaglandin which inhibits platelet aggregation as well as being a potent vasodilator • Given as chronic intravenous infusion (using a permanent indwelling central venous catheter) starting at 2 ng/kg/minute and increased in increments of 2 ng/kg/minute as tolerated. Typical mean dose achieved is 12 ng/kg/minute • Monitor response based on 6 minute walk and hemodynamics at right heart catheterization
Iloprost (Ventavis)	• Prostacyclin analogue • Given as an inhaler starting at 2.5 µg and increased to 5.0 µg 6–9 times a day up to a maximum of 45 µg daily. • Side effects include flushing, headache, syncope and cough • Monitor response based on 6 minute walk and hemodynamics at right heart catheterization
Bosentan (Tracleer)	• Endothelin receptor antagonist • Given orally at starting dose of 62.5 mg twice daily for 4 weeks and increased to maintenance dose of 125 mg twice daily • LFTs need to be monitored • Monitor response based on 6 minute walk and hemodynamics at right heart catheterization.
Ambrisentan (Letairis)	• Selective endothelin type-A receptor antagonist • Given orally starting at 5 mg daily and increased to a maximum dose of 10 mg daily as tolerated • LFTs need to be monitored • Monitor response based on 6 minute walk and hemodynamics at right heart catheterization
Sildenafil (Revatio)	• Phosphodiesterase inhibitor • Can be given IV (10 mg three times daily) or orally 20 mg three times daily • Monitor response based on 6 minute walk and hemodynamics at right heart catheterization
Surgical: Liver transplantation	• Selected patients can show reversal of pulmonary hypertension after liver transplantation • Severe PPHTN (mean systolic PAP >60 mmHg) is probably a contraindication for liver transplantation

Prevention/management of complications
• Epoprostenol therapy has been associated with increased risk of death during one small study.
• Bosentan and Ambrisentan therapy can cause hepatotoxicity and liver enzymes should be monitored on a monthly basis during therapy.

CLINICAL PEARLS
• Treatment for PPHTN depends on local expertise and experience as there are no comparative trials.
• Most of the medical therapies lead to vasodilation and need to be given for months/years with intermittent monitoring of PAP by echocardiogram and right-heart catheterization.
• Liver transplantation offers the hope of reversal of PPHTN in selected patients with mild or moderate disease.

Section 5: Special Populations

Not applicable for this topic.

Section 6: Prognosis

> **BOTTOM LINE/CLINICAL PEARLS**
> * The prognosis of PPHTN is dependent on the severity of cirrhosis with mortality as high as 50% at 6 months.
> * Medical therapy appears to improve outcome in PPHTN.
> * Liver transplantation improves outcome in PPHTN.

Natural history of untreated disease
* Survival rates of untreated disease can approach 70% at 5 years.
* Patients with more advanced liver disease have poorer outcomes.

Prognosis for treated patients
* The prognosis for treated patients is dependent on the type of treatment.
* Bosentan therapy has been associated with 90% 3 year survival in a small case series.

Follow-up tests and monitoring
* Patients with PPHTN on therapy can be monitored clinically and with invasive tests. Exercise capacity as determined by NYHA or WHO functional class can be assessed before and during therapy, including 6 minute walking distance.
* Laboratory investigation with periodic LFTs and echocardiogram are important but mean PAP and PVR as measured at right-heart catheterization remain the gold standard to assess response to treatment.

Section 7: Reading List

Colle, IO, Moreau, R, Godinho, E, et al. Diagnosis of portopulmonary hypertension in candidates for liver transplantation: a prospective study. Hepatology 2003;37:401–9

Hadengue A, Benhayoun MK, Lebrec D, Benhamou JP. Pulmonary hypertension complicating portal hypertension: prevalence and relation to splanchnic hemodynamics. Gastroenterology 1991;100:520–8

Hoeper MM, Krowka MJ, Strassburg CP. Portopulmonary hypertension and hepatopulmonary syndrome. Lancet 2004;363:1461–8

Krowka, MJ, Mandell, MS, Ramsay, MA, et al. Hepatopulmonary syndrome and portopulmonary hypertension: a report of the multicenter liver transplant database. Liver Transpl 2004;10:174–82

Le Pavec J, Souza R, Herve P, et al. Portopulmonary hypertension: survival and prognostic factors. Am J Respir Crit Care Med 2008;178:637–43

Section 8: Guidelines

Not applicable for this topic.

Section 9: Evidence

Type of evidence	Title, date	Comment
Prospective study	Pulmonary hypertension complicating portal hypertension: prevalence and relation to splanchnic hemodynamics. Gastroenterology 1991;100:520	First large study demonstrating that PPHTN is more common than originally thought
Prospective randomized study	A comparison of continuous intravenous epoprostenol (prostacyclin) with conventional therapy for primary pulmonary hypertension. The Primary Pulmonary Hypertension Study Group. N Engl J Med. 1996;334:296	Demonstrated effectiveness of epoprostenol in primary pulmonary hypertension
Prospective multi-center study	Hepatopulmonary syndrome and portopulmonary hypertension: a report of the multicenter liver transplant database. Liver Transpl 2004;10:174	Demonstrated that PPHTN could be treated with liver transplant

Section 10: Images

Not applicable for this topic.

Additional material for this chapter can be found online at:
www.mountsinaiexpertguides.com
This includes a case study and multiple choice questions

CHAPTER 25

Pregnancy-Related Liver Disease

Priya Grewal

Division of Liver Diseases, Icahn School of Medicine at Mount Sinai, New York, NY, USA

OVERALL BOTTOM LINE

- Pregnancy-specific liver diseases are the most common cause of abnormal liver tests in pregnancy.
- It is imperative to evaluate for pre-existing or newly acquired liver disease (viral hepatitis) in pregnant patients with liver dysfunction.
- Hypertension-related liver diseases in pregnancy (pre-eclampsia, eclampsia, HELLP syndrome and hepatic rupture) have overlapping symptoms and similar management.
- Acute fatty liver of pregnancy is a rare catastrophic disorder presenting late in pregnancy, and usually improves with prompt delivery.
- Most pregnancy-related liver diseases tend to recur in subsequent pregnancies.

Section 1: Background
Definition of disease

- Liver dysfunction during pregnancy is encountered in 3–5% of patients. It can be caused by conditions that are specific to pregnancy or by liver diseases that coexist in pregnancy.
- Normal physiological changes in pregnancy include a low serum albumin (plasma volume expansion), increased alkaline phosphatase (placental secretion).
- The hyperestrogenic state of pregnancy can lead to spider angiomas and palmar erythema.

Disease classification

- Pregnancy-related liver diseases:
  - Hyperemesis gravidarum (HG).
  - Intrahepatic cholestasis of pregnancy (ICP).
  - Pre-eclampsia and eclampsia.
  - HELLP syndrome.
  - Acute fatty liver of pregnancy (AFLP).
- Pregnancy-unrelated liver diseases: all liver diseases that may affect non-pregnant women may also occur during pregnancy. They may be pre-existing or be acquired during pregnancy.

Mount Sinai Expert Guides: Hepatology, First Edition. Edited by Jawad Ahmad, Scott L. Friedman, and Henryk Dancygier.
Companion website: www.mountsinaiexpertguides.com

Incidence/prevalence

- HG occurs in 0.3–2.0% of all pregnancies in the first trimester.
- ICP affects in 0.1–1.5% of pregnancies, with a much higher incidence in Scandinavia and South Africa.
- Pre-eclampsia affects 5–7% of all pregnancies, complicated by HELLP syndrome in 4–12% of these women.
- AFLP occurs in the third trimester in 1 : 10 000–15 000 pregnancies.

Etiology

- ICP is related to abnormal biliary transport across the canalicular membrane due to mutations in the bile salt export pump – specifically the multidrug resistance protein 3 (MDR3).
- Pre-eclampsia is caused by placental ischemia leading to endothelial dysfunction and coagulation activation. An imbalance of prostacyclin and thromboxane has also been implicated.
- AFLP results from an abnormality in mitochondrial beta oxidation of fatty acids due to a deficiency in the LCHAD in the fetus.

Pathology/pathogenesis

- The pathogenesis of AFLP has been well elucidated. The LCHAD deficiency in the fetus leads to long-chain fatty acid accumulation which return to the maternal circulation, depositing in the liver causing microvesicular steatosis, diffuse cytoplasmic ballooning sparing the periportal hepatocytes and resultant AFLP.
- In pre-eclampsia/HELLP syndrome, liver injury is precipitated by intravascular fibrin deposition, hypovolemia, and increased sinusoidal pressure leading to sinusoidal fibrin thrombi, hemorrhage and hepatocellular necrosis in the periportal areas.

Predictive/risk factors

- HG: increased BMI, psychiatric illness, molar pregnancy, diabetes mellitus, multiple pregnancies, hyperthyroidism.
- Intrahepatic cholestasis: history of cholestasis on oral contraceptive pill, family history, ICP in previous pregnancy.
- Pre-eclampsia: extremes of maternal age, primiparity, pre-existing hypertension, family history and occurrence in previous pregnancy.
- HELLP: advanced maternal age, multiparity and white ethnicity.
- AFLP: low BMI, nulliparity, twin pregnancy.

Section 2: Prevention

> Regular pre-natal visits and screening for pre-eclampsia/ICH lead to early diagnosis and treatment especially in high risk patients and those with a family history

Section 3: Diagnosis (Algorithm 25.1)

> **CLINICAL PEARLS**
> - Patients with HG present in the first trimester with intractable vomiting resulting in dehydration, ketosis and weight loss of 5% or more. Symptoms typically resolve by week 18. Liver enzymes can be 20 times the ULN, along with renal failure.
> - ICP occurs in the second half of pregnancy usually after 25 weeks and resolves with delivery. The onset of disease is marked by pruritus of palms and soles followed rarely by jaundice in 2–4 weeks. Liver enzymes may be markedly increased and a fasting serum bile acid concentration >10 μmol/L is diagnostic.
> - Pre-eclampsia is characterized by hypertension and proteinuria (>300 mg in 24 hours) after 20 weeks of gestation and/or within 48 hours of delivery. Liver enzymes may be elevated to 10 times ULN; jaundice is uncommon.
> - HELLP syndrome is a combination of hemolysis with a micro-angiopathic blood smear, increased liver enzymes and low platelets; it develops in the second or third trimester or after delivery.
> - AFLP occurs in the third trimester and remains a medical and obstetric emergency due to liver failure and high fetal mortality. Hypertension, vomiting, hypoglycemia, lactic acidosis and hyperammonemia are the hallmarks of this condition.

Differential diagnosis

Differential diagnosis	Features
Cirrhosis with portal hypertension	History of pre-existing liver disease, ascites, abnormal liver synthetic function
Hepatitis A/Hepatitis E	History of travel to endemic areas, positive serology, marked elevation of liver enzymes, 16% mortality in acute HEV infection
AIH	Flares likely post-partum, azathioprine is safe
Wilson disease	Undiagnosed Wilson, presenting with liver failure and hemolytic anemia can be misinterpreted as HELLP. Check ceruloplasmin level
PBC	May present for first time with protracted pruritus post-delivery and misinterpreted as ICP. AMA positive in PBC
Biliary disease (gallstones)	More common in pregnancy due to lithogenic bile
Budd–Chiari syndrome	Prothrombotic state of pregnancy predisposes to syndrome presenting with RUQ pain, jaundice and ascites. Doppler US is diagnostic
Thrombotic thrombocytopenic purpura/hemolytic uremic syndrome	Renal failure, neurological symptoms, skin rash

Typical presentation
- HG presents in the first trimester with intractable vomiting, dehydration and weight loss and resolves at 18 weeks.
- ICP leads to pruritus with elevated serum bile acids in the second half of pregnancy and resolves after delivery.

- Hypertension-related liver disease defined by a blood pressure >140/90 mmHg on at least two occasions, presents after 20 weeks of gestation and/or within 48 hours of delivery. Most patients have RUQ pain, headache, nausea, vomiting, abnormal LFTs (10 × ULN) and near normal bilirubin.
- Presence of seizures makes the diagnosis of eclampsia.
- Atypical pre-eclampsia denotes absence of hypertension and proteinuria, but an otherwise typical presentation.
- HELLP syndrome is accompanied by hemolysis and thrombocytopenia and its presence defines severe pre-eclampsia.
- Hepatic hematoma, infarction and rupture can complicate HELLP/ pre-eclampsia/ AFLP and present with severe pain, fever, liver enzymes >3000 IU/L, leucocytosis and anemia.
- AFLP leads to liver failure in the second half of pregnancy – usually in the third trimester.

Clinical diagnosis
History
- History of intractable vomiting suggests HG, while severe pruritus heralds the onset of ICP.
- Hypertension, proteinuria, RUQ pain and vomiting in the latter half of pregnancy are characteristic of hypertension-related pregnancy disorders.
- AFLP leads to nausea, vomiting, abdominal pain, anorexia and jaundice. Signs of pre-eclampsia and liver failure, especially altered mental status suggestive of encephalopathy, can also be present.

Physical examination
- Signs of dehydration, weight loss and mild jaundice are seen in HG.
- Presence of excoriation and absence of jaundice is characteristic of ICP.
- Hypertension, RUQ pain and mild jaundice points toward hypertension-related liver disease in pregnancy while patients with AFLP are much sicker with more jaundice and possibly encephalopathy due to liver failure.
- Patients with hepatic hematoma/infarction or rupture are gravely ill with severe pain, respiratory distress and hypovolemic shock.

Useful clinical decision rules and calculators
- Classification systems used in HELLP syndrome:
  - Tennessee system
    - AST >70 IU/L.
    - LDH >600 IU/L.
    - Platelets <100 × 10^9/L.
  - Mississippi system
    - AST >40 IU/L and LDH >600 IU/L and:
    - Class I: platelets <50 × 10^9/L.
    - Class II: platelets 50–100 × 10^9/L.
    - Class III: platelets 100–150 × 10^9/L.

Disease severity classification
- Swansea diagnostic criteria for diagnosis of acute fatty liver of pregnancy. Six or more of the following features in the absence of another explanation:
  - Vomiting.
  - Abdominal pain.
  - Polydipsia/polyuria.

- Encephalopathy.
- High bilirubin (>14 μmol/L).
- Hypoglycemia (<4 mmol/L).
- High uric acid (>340 μmol/L).
- Leucocytosis (>11 × 10^6/L).
- Ascites or bright liver on US scan.
- High AST/ALT (>42 IU/L).
- High ammonia (>47 μmol/L).
  - ➤ Renal impairment (creatinine >50 μmol/L).
  - ➤ Coagulopathy (PT >4 seconds or APTT >34 seconds).
  - ➤ Microvesicular steatosis on liver biopsy.

Laboratory diagnosis
List of diagnostic tests
- Fasting serum bile acid concentration for ICP, levels below 40 μmol/L correlate with good fetal outcome.
- Lactate dehydrogenase, haptoglobin, platelet count and serum uric acid to evaluate for hemolysis and thrombocytopenia in HELLP syndrome. A serum uric acid level >464 μmol/L is a poor prognostic sign predicting high maternal and fetal mortality.
- Hepatitis A, B, C and E, viral serologies and autoimmune markers to rule out pre-existing or newly acquired liver disease.
- Liver biopsy is not recommended due to high risk and low likelihood of changing management.

List of imaging techniques
- US is safe in pregnancy to evaluate for gallstone disease, hepatic hematoma.
- MRI without contrast can be used for more detailed imaging when indicated.

Algorithm 25.1 Diagnostic algorithm for pregnancy-related liver disease.
↑ = increase. ↓ = decrease

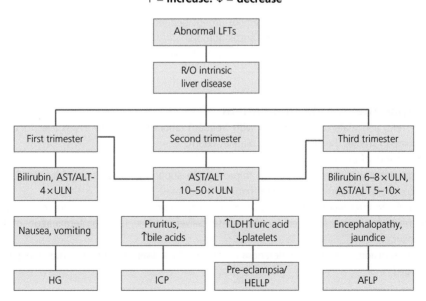

Potential pitfalls/common errors made regarding diagnosis of disease

- Pregnant patients are at increased risk (10%) of developing gallstones and present with pain, nausea and abnormal liver tests. Laparoscopic cholecystectomy can be performed in the second trimester if clinically warranted.
- Patient with pre-eclampsia/HELLP have marked elevation in AST and ALT (10–50 × ULN) compared with AFLP (5–10 × ULN).
- Jaundice in the third trimester is most marked in patients with AFLP.
- Patients with severe HG or ICP in the first half of pregnancy can have jaundice.
- In patients with recent travel to endemic areas, acute HEV hepatitis can lead to fulminant liver failure.
- HELLP syndrome resolves after delivery but laboratory tests can continue to worsen.

Section 4: Treatment (Algorithm 25.2)
Treatment rationale

- HG: supportive treatment with IV hydration, anti-emetics and vitamin supplementation especially thiamine to prevent Wernicke's encephalopathy.
- ICP: ursodeoxycholic acid (10–15 mg/kg bodyweight) relieves pruritus, improves liver tests. Cholestyramine can be used but is not very effective.
- Pre-eclampsia/HELLP: stringent blood pressure control with labetalol, hydralazine and nifedipine. Diuretics are avoided as they decrease placental flow. Urgent delivery is indicated in patients who deteriorate clinically in spite of supportive care.

When to hospitalize

- Patients with hypertension-related liver disease need to be hospitalized for supportive care, blood pressure control, and prompt delivery and possibly transferred to a transplant center if liver failure develops in spite of delivery.
- Hepatic hematoma or rupture may require urgent hepatic arteriography with embolization, surgery and in rare instances a liver transplantation.
- To prevent dehydration and ketosis in patients with HG.

Managing the hospitalized patient

- Close fetal and maternal monitoring with frequent laboratory tests to assess liver function, coagulation studies, hemoglobin and platelet count.
- Tight control of blood pressure.
- Prompt delivery if symptoms do not improve with supportive care after administration of corticosteroids to promote fetal lung maturity if indicated.
- In AFLP, hospitalization for stabilization of hypertension and DIC, seizure prophylaxis, and fetal monitoring followed by immediate delivery of the fetus or termination of the pregnancy.
- If liver functions continue to deteriorate transfer to a liver transplant center should be arranged.

Table of treatment

Treatment	Comment
Medical:	
HG	IV hydration
	Anti-emetics
	Vitamin supplementation
ICP	Ursodeoxycholic acid (10–15 mg/kg)
	Labetalol, hydralazine
Surgical:	
Pre-eclampsia/HELLP	Liver transplantation
AFLP with liver failure	
Radiological:	
Hepatic hematoma with ongoing bleeding	Hepatic arteriography with embolization

Algorithm 25.2 Management/treatment of HELLP syndrome and hepatic hematoma

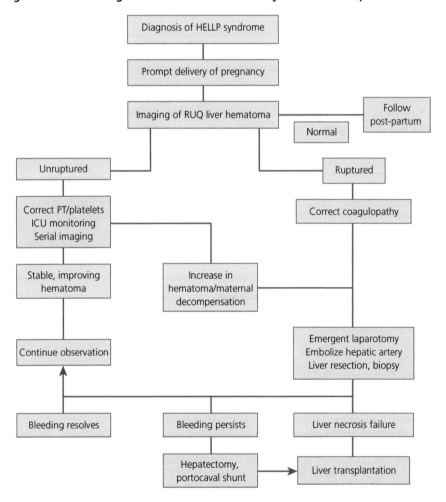

> **CLINICAL PEARLS**
> - Prompt diagnosis, close monitoring and supportive care are crucial in improving maternal and fetal outcomes in pregnancy-related liver disease.
> - In patients with progressive liver dysfunction in spite of delivery, timely transfer to a liver transplant center is crucial.
> - Pre-existing liver disease should be treated adequately during pregnancy, i.e. lamivudine/tenofovir in mothers with hepatitis B with significant viremia in third trimester. Women with AIH should be on stable immunosuppression throughout pregnancy.

Section 5: Special Populations

Not applicable for this topic.

Section 6: Prognosis

> **CLINICAL PEARLS**
> - HG resolves by 18 weeks of gestation and ICP after delivery. However, ICP can lead to fetal prematurity and anoxia and therefore delivery should be considered after fetal maturity has been achieved in refractory cases.
> - Counseling regarding recurrence in subsequent pregnancies is indicated.
> - ICP in rare familial forms can be a predictor of future biliary disease and cirrhosis.
> - Liver tests usually normalize within 2 weeks of delivery in hypertension-related disorders of pregnancy.
> - Hepatic hematoma/rupture resulting from HELLP/AFLP/thrombotic thrombocytopenic purpura or hemolytic uremic syndrome carries a 50% maternal mortality rate.
> - Fortunately, AFLP is very rare but associated with 1–20% maternal and fetal mortality. Majority of the deliveries are by cesarean section within 24 hours of presentation. Women who are carriers of the LCHAD mutation have a 20–70% risk of recurrence of AFLP in subsequent pregnancies.
> - Liver transplantation when indicated is associated with an excellent 5-year survival of 88%.

Natural history of untreated disease
- Pre-eclampsia/HELLP lead to maternal and fetal mortality due to liver failure, renal failure, and ultimately multisystem organ failure.

Section 7: Reading List

Bhatia V, Singhal A, Panda SK, Acharya SK. A 20-year single-center experience with acute liver failure during pregnancy: is the prognosis really worse? Hepatology 2008;48: 1577–85

Ch'ng CL, Morgan M, Hainsworth I, Kingham JG. Prospective study of liver dysfunction in pregnancy in Southwest Wales. Gut 2002;51:876–80

Glantz A, Marschall HU, Lammert F, Mattsson LA. Intrahepatic cholestasis of pregnancy: a randomized controlled trial comparing dexamethasone and ursodeoxycholic acid. Hepatology 2005;42:1399–405

Glantz A, Marschall HU, Mattsson LA. Intrahepatic cholestasis of pregnancy: relationships between bile acid levels and fetal complication rates. Hepatology 2004;40:467–74

Hay JE. Liver disease in pregnancy. Hepatology 2008;47:1067–76

Joshi D, James A, Quaglia A, Westbrook RH, Heneghan MA. Liver disease in pregnancy. Lancet 2010;375: 594–605

Pan C, Perumalswami PV. Pregnancy-related liver diseases. Clin Liver Dis 2011;15:199–208

Pathak B, Sheibani L, Lee RH. Cholestasis of pregnancy. Obstet Gynecol Clin North Am 2010;37:269–82

Shames BD, Fernandez LA, Sollinger HW, et al. Liver transplantation for HELLP syndrome. Liver Transpl 2005;11:224–28

Section 8: Guidelines

Not applicable for this topic.

Section 9: Evidence

Not applicable for this topic.

Section 10: Images

Not applicable for this topic.

Additional material for this chapter can be found online at:
www.mountsinaiexpertguides.com
This includes case studies and multiple choices questions

CHAPTER 26

Acute Liver Failure

Meena B. Bansal

Division of Liver Diseases, Icahn School of Medicine at Mount Sinai, New York, NY, USA

OVERALL BOTTOM LINE
- ALF is a rare disorder that occurs mostly in young adults and is associated with high mortality and resource cost. Severe hepatic injury results in rapid deterioration of liver function resulting in altered mental status and coagulopathy (INR ≥1.5) in a patient with no pre-existing liver disease.
- The diagnosis must be made early so that patients can be transferred to a Liver Transplant Center in a timely fashion before complications arise which would prohibit safe transfer.
- History taking is critical. Disease-specific therapy should be initiated where appropriate. If history is unavailable or any suspicion of acetaminophen toxicity, NAC therapy should be initiated.
- ALF results in multi-organ failure and requires a multidisciplinary approach for successful patient outcomes.
- With liver transplantation, one year patient survival approaches 65%.

Section 1: Background
Definition of disease
- ALF is a rare condition in which severe hepatic injury leads to rapid deterioration in liver function resulting in altered mental status and coagulopathy (INR ≥1.5) in a patient with no pre-existing liver disease.
- The illness is considered acute if less than 26 weeks in duration.

Disease classification
- ALF can be further divided into subgroups based on the length of illness: hyperacute (<7 days); acute (7–21 days); subacute (>21 days and <26 weeks).

Incidence
- ALF is rare. In the USA, there are about 2000 cases/year.
- Overall global incidence in developed countries is between one and five cases per million people every year.

Economic impact
- Based on the ALF Study Group database, the average age of presentation for ALF in the USA is between 37 and 40 years.

Mount Sinai Expert Guides: Hepatology, First Edition. Edited by Jawad Ahmad, Scott L. Friedman, and Henryk Dancygier.
© 2014 John Wiley & Sons, Ltd. Published 2014 by John Wiley & Sons, Ltd.
Companion website: www.mountsinaiexpertguides.com

- As this disease affects younger patients, there is a significant economic impact both by the early loss of life in those who don't survive and the cost of life-long immunosuppression in those who were successfully transplanted.

Etiology

- The most common cause of ALF in the USA and UK is acetaminophen poisoning, both intentional and unintentional. Idiosyncratic drug reactions are the next most common cause.
- In countries where viral hepatitis is endemic such as South East Asia, hepatitis viruses (hepatitis B±D, E and A) are the most common causes.
- Other causes of ALF are listed in the Table: etiologies of ALF.

Etiologies of ALF (Source: Sass DA and Shakil AO. Fulminant Hepatic Failure. Liver Transplantation, Vol 11, No 6, 2005: pp 594–605. Reproduced with permission of John Wiley & Sons Ltd.)

Viral
HAV, HBV ± HDV, HEV, HSV, CMV, EBV, herpes, varicella zoster virus, adenovirus, hemorrhagic fever viruses

Drugs and toxins
Dose-dependent: acetaminophen, carbon tetrachloride, yellow phosphorus, *Amanita phalloides*, *Bacillus cereus toxin*, sulfonamides, tetracycline, Ecstasy (methyldioxymethamphetamine), herbal remedies

Idiosyncratic: halothane, isoniazid, rifampin, valproic acid, NSAIDs, disulfiram

Vascular
Right heart failure, Budd–Chiari syndrome, veno-occlusive disease, shock liver (ischemic hepatitis), heat stroke

Metabolic
Acute fatty liver of pregnancy, Wilson disease, Reye's syndrome, galactosemia, hereditary fructose intolerance, tyrosinemia

Miscellaneous
Malignant infiltration (liver metastases, lymphoma), autoimmune hepatitis, sepsis

Indeterminate
Includes primary graft non-function in liver transplanted patients

---

Pathology/pathogenesis

- In ALF, there are two competing intrahepatic processes. On the one hand, there is overwhelming hepatocellular injury and on the other there is hepatocellular regeneration in an effort to compensate for the acute loss of hepatocyte function. The abrupt loss in hepatic metabolic and immunologic functions, leads to encephalopathy, coagulopathy, and in many cases results in multi-organ failure.
- While disease-specific etiologies have unique pathophysiologic features which require specific intervention, there are general features common to ALF regardless of the etiology and they are outlined here.
  - Cerebral edema and ICH:
    - ➤ Cerebral edema and ICH are the most serious complications of ALF.
    - ➤ The pathogenic mechanisms leading to cerebral edema and ICH are not completely understood but result from a combination of osmotic disturbances in the brain and increased cerebral blood flow due to loss of cerebrovascular autoregulation.

- Coagulopathy:
  - Loss of hepatocellular function results in decreased synthesis of Factor II, V, VII, IX, and X.
  - Abnormalities in platelet count, function, and morphology.
- Infection/sepsis:
  - Kupffer cell malfunction – resident macrophages in the liver provide an important function in the clearance of gut-derived bacteria and endotoxin. In FHF, impaired uptake has in part been ascribed to decreased fibronectin, an important co-factor made by the liver which is needed for opsonization.
  - Neutrophil malfunction – phagocytosis, opsonization and mobility are all decreased. May be related to decreased serum complement levels.
  - Cell-mediated immunity – defective lymphocyte function.
- Cardiovascular dysfunction and tissue oxygen debt:
  - Low systemic and pulmonary vascular resistance.
  - Compensatory increase in cardiac output.
  - Increased metabolic rate.
  - Abnormal oxygen transport and uptake.
  - Pathologic state is similar to that seen in septic shock.
- Renal failure:
  - Depending on the etiology of ALF, direct nephrotoxicity can be seen, such as the case for acetaminophen.
  - Hepatorenal syndrome can be seen which is due to intense renal vasoconstriction secondary to the systemic vasodilation. The etiology of specific hemodynamic changes is incompletely understood but renal function recovers fully after liver transplant.
  - Impaired hepatic urea production results in underestimation of renal impairment.
- Metabolic derangements:
  - Hypoglycemia is observed due to both defective gluconeogenesis and inadequate hepatic uptake of insulin.
  - Acidosis and alkalosis may both occur and should be managed by identifying and treating underlying cause.

Predictive/risk factors
- Since there are numerous etiologies for ALF, risk factors vary depending on the etiology.
- Acetaminophen poisoning: use of multiple medications containing acetaminophen, history of depression/suicidal behavior, chronic alcohol consumption, narcotic use.
- *Amanita phalloides* toxicity: ingestion of wild mushrooms.
- Fulminant hepatitis E: most common in women in third trimester of pregnancy. Limit travel to endemic areas during pregnancy.
- Reactivation of hepatitis B: chemotherapy or other immunosuppression.

Section 2: Prevention

CLINICAL PEARLS
- The key to prevention of acetaminophen-induced ALF is consumer education. Package insert for medications need to clearly delineate the dosage of acetaminophen. In the UK, bottles of acetaminophen are no longer sold. Consumers purchase limited amounts in blister packs.
- Avoidance of hepatotoxic drugs where possible.
- All patients scheduled to undergo chemotherapy should be evaluated for chronic hepatitis B. Virus reactivation is associated with greater risk of ALF then *de novo* infection. Reactivation of hepatitis B can be successfully averted with prophylactic treatment with anti-virals.

Screening
- Hepatitis B status in cancer patients to undergo chemotherapy or immunosuppressive therapy: check HBsAg and HBcAb. If either positive check HBeAg and HBV DNA levels.

Primary prevention
- Prophylactic oral nucleoside or nucleotide antiviral therapy should be administered to HBsAg-positive individuals several weeks before the onset of chemotherapy or immunosuppressive therapy. Antiviral therapy should be maintained for 6 months after completion of the chemotherapy or immunosuppressive therapy in patients with HBV DNA levels <2000 IU/mL. If HBV DNA >2000 IU/mL, continue antiviral therapy until HBV DNA is undetectable and ALT levels are normalized.
- Limiting availability of bulk acetaminophen: restriction in package size and use of blister packaging begun in 1998 in the UK to combat impulsive suicide overdose has had some benefit. Similar strategies are currently being considered by the FDA.

Secondary prevention
- Psychiatric assistance for those with depression and have attempted suicide.
- Patient education in those with accidental overdose.

Section 3: Diagnosis

- Taking an extensive history from the patient is critical to help identify etiology. If history cannot be obtained from a patient due to advanced encephalopathy, obtain from family members. The clinician needs to specifically ask about all medications and herbal preparations.
- On physical examination, the patient should not have stigmata of chronic liver disease (i.e. palmar erythema, spider angiomata, caput medusae, gynecomastia, testicular atrophy, ascites/portal hypertension). Signs of portal hypertension can occasionally be seen in cases of subfulminant liver failure such as autoimmune hepatitis but the presence of portal hypertension should raise the index of suspicion for an acute on chronic process. Inability to palpate the liver or inability to percuss a significant area of dullness over the liver can suggest loss of liver volume due to massive hepatocyte loss. An enlarged liver suggests etiologies for ALF such as malignant infiltration, Budd–Chiari syndrome, or CHF.
- If patient has a history of abnormal LFTs in the past, it suggests an acute on chronic process.

Differential diagnosis
- If there is evidence of acute hepatitis associated with INR >1.5 and altered mental status, the patient has ALF.
- Initially upon presentation before laboratory studies are available, the differential is broad to include anything that causes acute mental status changes such as drug overdose, psychosis, primary CNS pathology, sepsis, electrolyte/metabolic disturbances. Prior history and physical examination may help clarify differential.

Differential diagnosis	Features
Drug overdose	History of drug abuse. Physical examination may reveal track marks or nasal septum perforation. Laboratory studies will reveal positive toxicology screen with no evidence of acute hepatitis unless drug is causing ALF
Primary CNS pathology	Focal neurologic deficits. Head CT scan revealing primary CNS lesion

Typical presentation
- The typical patient with acute liver failure has no history of liver disease or abnormal liver tests. Patients are either brought in by family members due to acute change in mental status or the patient is noted to be jaundiced without obvious mental status changes. Jaundice is often but not always seen at presentation.
- The patient may also report RUQ tenderness, nausea and vomiting.
- For intentional acetaminophen overdose, the patient will often admit to family members that they took acetaminophen and are brought in prior to the development of either jaundice or acute mental status changes.

Clinical diagnosis
History
- It is essential to extensively review possible exposures to viral infection, drugs, or other toxins. In certain cases, treatment of specific etiologies can be life-saving. If the history cannot be obtained from the patient due to advanced encephalopathy, every effort must be made to obtain pertinent history from family members.
- The clinician needs to specifically ask about all prescribed and over the counter medications as well as herbal preparations.
- The clinician should ask about a history of abnormal LFTs. If previous abnormal liver tests are available, the index of suspicion increases for acute on chronic liver failure and the clinical course and management is different.
- Has the patient recently donated blood? If so, underlying viral hepatitis is unlikely as patient's blood is screened.
- The clinician should ask about alteration in sleep–wake cycle or subtle changes in cognitive function which reflect early grades of hepatic encephalopathy.

Physical examination
- On physical examination, the patient should not have stigmata of chronic liver disease (i.e. palmar erythema, spider angiomata, caput medusae, gynecomastia, testicular atrophy, ascites/portal hypertension). Signs of portal hypertension can occasionally be seen in cases of subfulminant liver failure such as autoimmune hepatitis but the presence of portal hypertension should raise the index of suspicion for an acute on chronic process.
- Inability to palpate the liver or inability to percuss a significant area of dullness over the liver can suggest loss of liver volume due to massive hepatocyte loss. An enlarged liver suggests etiologies for ALF such as malignant infiltration, Budd–Chiari syndrome or CHF.
- The presence of asterixis represents stage 3 hepatic encephalopathy. If the patient is unable to lift hands, one can ask the patient to squeeze your hand. Asterixis is failure to hold a sustained contraction and thus can be assessed in a variety of ways.

Useful clinical decision rules and calculators
- Once the diagnosis of ALF is suspected there are several decision points that must be quickly made while initiating etiology-specific therapy and providing supportive care.
- First, should the patient be admitted to the ICU? If not already at a transplant facility, treating clinicians need to know when to contact the local transplant facility. Finally, should the patient be listed for liver transplant (Algorithm 26.1)?

BOTTOM LINE
- Recognize early and refer

Disease severity classification

- On initial evaluation, determining the severity of hepatic encephalopathy is critical for the appropriate management of patients with ALF (see Table: grades of encephalopathy)
- If patient has grade I encephalopathy, contact local transplant center to arrange transfer.
- If grade II encephalopathy, admit to ICU.
- If grade III encephalopathy, consider intracranial pressure monitoring if institution has expertise.

Grades of encephalopathy	
I	Subtle changes in behavior with minimal change in level of consciousness
II	Obvious disorientation, drowsiness, inappropriate behavior, may have asterixis
III	Marked confusion, incoherent speech, sleeping most of the time but arousable to verbal stimuli, asterixis is present
IV	Obtunded, unresponsive to noxious stimuli, decerebrate or decorticate posturing (end-stage)

Laboratory diagnosis

List of diagnostic tests

- Complete blood count:
  - Leukocytosis: can be seen with acute hepatitis from any etiology but patients are at high risk for infection due to immunologic defects.
  - Thrombocytopenia: can be seen if patient in DIC but early in course – low platelets may suggest acute on chronic process.
  - Hemolytic anemia: Coombs negative hemolytic anemia classically seen in fulminant Wilson disease.
- Blood type and screen: two drawn independently needed for transplant evaluation. Patient may require blood products as part of supportive care.
- Serum chemistries:
  - Creatinine elevation either from direct nephrotoxic agent (excluding acetaminophen) or hepatorenal syndrome.
  - Evidence of acidosis.
  - AST, AST, AP: may provide clues to etiology of liver failure. Hepatocellular injury vs cholestatic. Low/normal AP in jaundiced young patient is suggestive of fulminant Wilson disease. AST or ALT >3500 IU/L should prompt suspicion of acetaminophen toxicity even if history is lacking.
  - Total bilirubin.
  - Phosphate: a low phosphate <1.1 is a good prognostic indicator of liver regeneration and should be repleted.
  - Glucose: hypoglycemia suggests loss in hepatic gluconeogenesis and may exacerbate encephalopathy. Begin 10% dextrose infusion and monitor closely.
- Arterial blood gas: acidosis is poor prognostic marker.
- Arterial lactate: elevated lactate is poor prognostic marker.
- Arterial ammonia: arterial ammonia >200 μg/dL is strongly associated with cerebral herniation.
- Toxicology screen: will provide insight into etiology of ALF and determine appropriateness of transplant candidacy. Active drug abusers are not candidates for transplant.
- Acetaminophen level: if timing of ingestion known can help provide prognostication on likelihood of survival without transplant though not routinely used anymore. NAC should be initiated before acetaminophen level is available if clinically indicated.

- Viral serologies: anti-HAV IgM, HBsAg, anti-HBc IGM, anti-HEV (if clinically suspected), anti-HCV (rules out underlying chronic HCV infection).
- Ceruloplasmin: low or normal consistent with Wilson disease. Levels may be normal since it is an acute phase reactant.
- Uric acid: if Wilson disease is suspected, levels may be low.
- Autoimmune markers: ANA, ASMA, IgG levels.
- Pregnancy test in females.
- HIV status.
- Amylase and lipase.
  List of imaging techniques
- Liver US with Doppler: can be done at bedside of sick patient.
- Abdominal CT scan with contrast or MRI with gadolinium if needed to evaluate further for malignant infiltration, Budd–Chiari syndrome, portal vein thrombosis.
- Non-contrast head CT to rule out other causes of changes in mental status. Not helpful to identify cerebral edema.

Algorithm 26.1 Diagnosis of ALF

- Patient presents acute mental status changes and no history of liver diseases
- Obtain extensive history regarding suicidal intent, drug use, mushroom ingestion, use of herbal remedies, history of abnormal LFTs
- Physical examination: no stigmata of chronic liver disease. May be jaundiced but not always

↓

Laboratory tests: CBC with platelets, comprehensive metabolic panel, INR, toxicology screen, ANA, ASMA, IgG levels, ceruloplasmin, arterial ammonia/lactate/pH, acetaminophen levels, hepatitis viral serologies, uric acid, HIV status, amylase/lipase, pregnancy test if appropriate, blood cultures
Abdominal imaging: evaluate for malignant infiltration, Budd–Chiari, portal vein thrombosis
Non-contrast head CT: rule out other causes of mental status changes

↓

- Begin disease specific therapy: if history unobtainable or any suspicion of acetaminophen toxicity, begin N-acetylcysteine
- Admit to ICU if ≥ grade 2 encephalopathy
- Activate multidisciplinary team: transplant hepatology and surgery, infectious diseases, neurology/neurosurgery, cardiology, social work, psychiatry, nephrology, and intensivist

Potential pitfalls/common errors made regarding diagnosis of disease

- False presumption of drug use in young patients presenting with acute mental status changes. Only when blood tests return do clinicians suspect ALF.
- Delay in contacting transplant center. The transplant center should be contacted immediately so that they can help expedite transfer while patient is stable. Once cerebral edema is advanced, transfer itself can result in cerebral herniation.

Section 4: Treatment (Algorithm 26.2)
General treatment principles for acute liver failure regardless of etiology
Hepatic encephalopathy/cerebral edema
- Patients with altered mental state should be admitted to ICU. Patients should be transferred to transplant center early (grade I–II encephalopathy) as risks involved with transfer may be prohibitive once patient reaches grade III/IV encephalopathy.
- Clinical signs are often unreliable and occur very late: Cushing reflex, decerebrate rigidity, disconjugate eye movements, loss of papillary reflexes.
- Intracranial pressure monitoring is suggested in patients with stage III encephalopathy or greater but local expertise in placement is critical. If an intracranial pressure monitor is placed, aggressive management to maintain cerebral perfusion pressure >50 mmHg. No controlled trials are available to demonstrate overall survival benefit.
- Neurological checks every 4 hours.
- Avoid narcotics and sedatives early in the course but if the patient is agitated it is more important to keep patient calm.
- NH_3 on admission >100 mmol/L may predict development of HE. In those with ALF and HE, NH_3 >200 mmol/L is predictive of ICH.
- Fluid status best managed with central pressure monitoring. While over-resuscitation can worsen cerebral edema, frequently patients are not adequately resuscitated and thus monitoring may be required to ensure adequate fluid resuscitation.
- Head of bed at 30 degrees.
- Quiet room with minimal suctioning/noxious stimuli.
- Mannitol (0.5 g/kg IV bolus; repeated 1–2 times as needed if serum osmolality <320 mosm/L). Mannitol is contraindicated in setting of renal failure.
- No role for hyperventilation.
- Experimental treatments include: controlled hypothermia, indomethacin, hypertonic saline.

Coagulopathy
- Overall management is expectant.
- No fresh frozen plasma unless active bleeding or need for invasive procedures. For latter, possible role of recombinant-activated Factor VII but expensive and carries risk of thrombosis in patients with ALF but not well studied.
- Prophylactic acid suppression with either H_2-blockers or PPIs is appropriate.

Infection/sepsis
- Surveillance cultures and low threshold to begin antibiotics if clinical change or positive cultures.
- Third generation cephalosporin + vancomycin. Diflucan if prolonged antibiotics or MICU stay, and if renal failure is present.

Cardiovascular dysfunction and tissue oxygen debt
- Maintenance of cardiac index >4.5 L/minute/m^2.
- Oxygen delivery >800 L/minute/m^2.
- Oxygen consumption >150 L/minute/m^2.
- Supplemental oxygen.
- Blood transfusions if needed to increase oxygen carrying capacity.

- Systemic vasopressor support with agents such as norepinephrine or dopamine to maintain MAP of 50–60 mmHg. Vasopressin should be avoided due to effects on increasing cerebral blood flow and intracranial hypertension.

Renal failure
- Avoidance of nephrotoxic agents. If IV contrast for imaging is needed, patients should be pretreated with NAC.
- CVVH – avoid heparin if possible.
- Hemodialysis if necessary. Continuous is preferred over intermittent to limit fluctuations in systemic pressure and therefore cerebral perfusion pressure.

Metabolic derangements
- Electrolytes such as phosphate, magnesium and potassium tend to be low and should be corrected as needed.
- Enteral feeding should be initiated early given the catabolic state of ALF. There is no need for severe protein restriction – 60 g of protein per day is appropriate.
- Acidosis and alkalosis may both occur and should be managed by identifying and treating the underlying cause

Etiology-specific treatments
Acetaminophen hepatotoxicity
- Dose-related toxin: most ingestions causing ALF exceed 10 g/day. One extra strength Tylenol contains 500 mg.
- If the patient presents within 4 hours of ingestion, administration of activated charcoal 1 g/kg slurry is indicated and does not interfere with NAC.
- If there is a history of acetaminophen ingestion or suspicion even without clear history, begin NAC. NAC may be given orally: 140 mg/kg by mouth or via nasogastric tube diluted to 5% solution, followed by 70 mg/kg by mouth every 4 hours × 17 doses. If the patient is not able to take oral medications, IV NAC with 150 mg/kg in 5% dextrose loading dose over 15 minutes, followed by 50 mg/kg over 4 hours and then 100 mg/kg over the next 16 hours.

Mushroom poisoning
- There are no serum tests to confirm mushroom poisoning so the history must be compatible with the onset of nausea, vomiting, diarrhea, abdominal cramping up to 24 hours after ingestion.
- If presentation is early, gastric lavage should be performed and activated charcoal administered.
- While liver transplantation is the only life-saving option for severe mushroom poisoning, penicillin G or silymarin can be administered.

Drug-induced hepatotoxicity
- Most drug reactions are idiosyncratic and occur within the first 6 months of drug initiation.
- The most common culprits include antibiotics, NSAIDs, and anti-seizure medications.
- Discontinue all non-essential medications when patient presents with ALF.

Viral hepatitis
- If herpes virus is suspected, begin acyclovir.
- If reactivation of hepatitis B, begin treatment (e.g. lamivudine, tenofovir).
- If acute hepatitis B, therapy is often started but no controlled trials exist to demonstrate impact on outcome.

Wilson disease

- Fulminant presentation of Wilson disease is death without transplant.
- Typical presentation includes abrupt onset of Coombs-negative hemolytic anemia with serum bilirubin >20 mg/dL, low serum ceruloplasmin (may be normal since acute phase reactant), high serum and urinary copper levels, high hepatic copper if liver biopsy performed, low AP and uric acid levels, renal injury due to direct toxicity of copper on renal tubular cells, Kayser–Fleischer rings on slit-lamp examination.
- While awaiting transplant, patients may benefit from plasmapheresis, plasma exchange or hemofiltration to lower copper levels.

Autoimmune hepatitis

- Biopsy to confirm diagnosis is indicated.
- Begin prednisone 40–60 mg/day but list for transplant as steroids may not be enough when presentation is fulminant.

AFLP/HELLP syndrome

- Generally occur in third trimester.
- Triad of jaundice, coagulopathy and low platelets. Features of pre-eclampsia such as hypertension and proteinuria are common.
- Oil Red O staining (do not fix in formaldehyde) if liver biopsy performed.
- Prompt delivery and transplant if mother continues to deteriorate.

Budd–Chiari syndrome

- Due to hepatic vein thrombosis.
- Triad of hepatomegaly, ascites and abdominal pain.
- Acute decompression may avert need for transplant.
- Need to evaluate etiology: hypercoagulation investigation, malignancy.
- Prognosis depends on underlying etiology of thrombosis.

Malignant infiltration

- Should be suspected if massive hepatomegaly and/or history of malignancy.
- Liver biopsy and imaging may be helpful.
- Not candidates for transplant.

When to hospitalize

- All patients with ALF should be hospitalized.
- Transfer to ICU for grade II encephalopathy or greater.
- Contact transplant center immediately and begin to coordinate transfer.

Prognosis and decision to proceed with liver transplantation

- UNOS Criteria for Status I Listing include:
  - Onset of any degree of encephalopathy within 8 weeks of onset of acute liver injury.
  - Absence of pre-existing liver disease.
  - Life expectancy with transplant <7 days.
  - In ICU requiring either mechanical ventilation, renal dialysis or INR >2.0.
- However, deciding to proceed to liver transplantation can be difficult. Given the shortage of donor organs, the lack of predictability as to when a donor organ will become available, and the potential complications of lifelong immunosuppression, the goal is to only transplant those

whose native liver will not recover. The ability to predict recovery before patients develop a complication that will prohibit transplantation is the challenge.

• While numerous prognostic criteria have been proposed, the most commonly utilized is King's College Criteria which takes into account etiology of disease as well as liver dysfunction. Other prognostic parameters that have been proposed include: pH, lactate, phosphate, Factor V, AFP, MELD score. However, because of the poor negative predictive values of such scoring systems, reliance entirely on scoring systems is not recommended and clinical judgment remains a critical element in determining the need to proceed with transplantation in patients with acute liver failure.

King's College criteria

Acetaminophen	Non-Acetaminophen
pH < 7.3	INR > 6.5
or	or
1. Grade III–IV encephalopathy 2. INR > 6.5 3. Serum creatinine > 3.4 (all three)	1. Age < 10 or > 40 2. Etiology (idiosyncratic drug, Wilson disease) 3. INR > 3.85 4. Serum bilirubin > 17 mg/dL 5. Period of jaundice to HE > 7 days (any three)

Algorithm 26.2 Management of acute liver failure

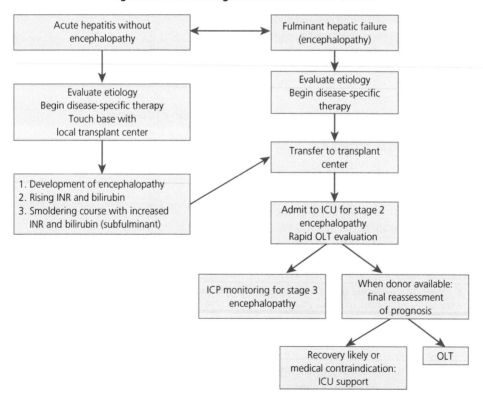

CLINICAL PEARLS
- If there is any suspicion of acetaminophen toxicity or history is unavailable, begin IV NAC. Best when started early.
- If fulminant Wilson disease is suspected, mortality is 100% without transplant – so list immediately.
- Early listing for transplant. Reassess hourly. You can always turn down a liver but need to be on the list to get the offer.
- Multi-organ failure requires a cohesive multidisciplinary team (transplant hepatology, ICU team, infectious diseases, nephrology, surgeon, neurology, social work, psychiatry, nursing staff).

Section 5: Special Populations

Pregnancy
- While the pregnant patient can suffer from any form of ALF, AFLP/HELLP syndrome are specific to the pregnant state. In addition, acute hepatitis E has a more fulminant course in pregnant women.
- If a pregnant patient presents with ALF, the goal is to safely deliver the baby as soon a possible. Steroids to promote fetal pulmonary maturity should be given immediately. US is the safest form of radiologic assessment.

Children
- In young children, clinical encephalopathy can be absent or occur very late in the disease process. Therefore, the definition of ALF does not depend on the presence of mental status changes in children and coagulopathy due to severe liver injury is sufficient.
- While living-related donation is not acceptable in adult patients, living-related donation (excluding mother to child) is an option for children with ALF. The PELD score and not the MELD score is used for children.

Elderly
- The management of ALF in the elderly is the same as in any other patient. Functional status of the patient is more important than chronologic age when assessing suitability for liver transplant.

Section 6: Prognosis

BOTTOM LINE/CLINICAL PEARLS
- Prognosis depends on etiology of ALF: acetaminophen toxicity carries the most favorable prognosis. Idiosyncratic drug reactions and Wilson disease carry the worst prognosis.
- Numerous studies have examined prognostic markers to assess mortality without transplant. The King's College criteria have been the most validated see "Prognosis and decision to proceed with liver transplantation" and divide prognostic factors into either acetaminophen-induced liver failure or non-acetaminophen-induced liver failure.

Natural history of untreated disease
- Prior to the advent of liver transplantation, ALF carried a 15% survival.

Prognosis for treated patients
- Overall short-term survival with transplantation is greater than 65%.

Follow-up tests and monitoring
- If the patient's native liver recovers from ALF, liver will be normal and the patient is not at an increased risk for liver disease in the future.

Section 7: Reading List

Bernal W, Auzinger G, Dhawan A, Wendon J. Acute liver failure. Lancet 2010;376:190–201

Bower WA, Johns M, Margolis HS, Williams IT, Bell BP. Population-based surveillance for acute liver failure. Am J Gastroenterol 2007;102:2459–63

Clemmesen JO, Larsen FS, Kondrup J, Hansen BA, Ott P. Cerebral herniation in patients with acute liver failure is correlated with arterial ammonia concentration. Hepatology 1999;29:648–53

Hawton K, Townsend E, Deeks J, et al. Effects of legislation restricting pack sizes of paracetamol and salicylate on self poisoning in the United Kingdom: before and after study. BMJ 2001;322:1203–7

Katz LH, Fraser A, Gafter-Gvili A, Leibovici L, Tur-Kaspa R. Lamivudine prevents reactivation of hepatitis B and reduces mortality in immunosuppressed patients: systematic review and meta-analysis. J Viral Hepat 2008;15:89–102

Keeffe EB, Dieterich DT, Han SH, et al. A treatment algorithm for the management of chronic hepatitis B virus infection in the United States: 2008 update. Clin Gastroenterol Hepatol 2008;6:1315–-41; quiz 1286

Mindikoglu AL, Regev A, Schiff ER. Hepatitis B virus reactivation after cytotoxic chemotherapy: the disease and its prevention. Clin Gastroenterol Hepatol 2006;4:1076–81

O'Grady JG, Alexander GJ, Hayllar KM, Williams R. Early indicators of prognosis in fulminant hepatic failure. Gastroenterology 1989;97:439–45

Polson J, Lee WM. AASLD position paper: the management of acute liver failure. Hepatology 2005;41: 1179–97

Sheen CL, Dillon JF, Bateman DN, Simpson KJ, MacDonald TM. Paracetamol pack size restriction: the impact on paracetamol poisoning and the over-the-counter supply of paracetamol, aspirin and ibuprofen. Pharmacoepidemiol Drug Saf 2002;11:329–31

Zimmerman HJ, Maddrey WC. Acetaminophen (paracetamol) hepatotoxicity with regular intake of alcohol: analysis of instances of therapeutic misadventure. Hepatology 1995;22:767–73

Section 8: Guidelines
National society guidelines

Guideline title	Guideline source	Date
AASLD Position Paper: The Management of Acute Liver Failure	AASLD http://www.aasld.org/practiceguidelines/Documents/AcuteLiverFailureUpdate2011.pdf	2011

Section 9: Evidence

Not applicable for this topic.

Section 10: Images

Not applicable for this topic.

Additional material for this chapter can be found online at:
www.mountsinaiexpertguides.com
This includes a case study, multiple choice questions and ICD codes

CHAPTER 27

Budd–Chiari Syndrome

Leona Kim-Schluger
Division of Liver Diseases, Icahn School of Medicine at Mount Sinai, New York, NY, USA

OVERALL BOTTOM LINE
- BCS is a vascular disorder of the liver causing outflow obstruction of blood flow.
- BCS can present as an acute fulminant hepatic failure with massive hepatic necrosis or as complications of cirrhosis and portal hypertension.
- The etiology is most commonly an underlying thrombotic condition leading to hepatic venous thrombosis and, rarely, a congenital web of hepatic vein/inferior vena cava.
- The medical management of BCS depends upon early diagnosis and treatment. In the acute presentation, thrombolysis should be considered. In patients with advanced cirrhosis and complications of portal hypertension, liver transplantation is an option.

Section 1: Background
Definition of disease
- BCS is a vascular disorder of the liver characterized by venous outflow obstruction that can occur at the level of the hepatic venules through to the right atrium leading to hepatic congestion. The most common causes of BCS are myeloproliferative disorders leading to a hypercoagulable predisposition. The presentation and management of BCS depends upon the acuity of the thrombosis.

Disease classification
- The presentation of BCS depends on whether the venous obstruction is acute or chronic, the extent of the thrombosis, the rapidity of onset, and whether there has been time for the development of collaterals.
- Acute BCS has features of acute hepatic ischemia and necrosis, presenting as fulminant hepatic failure.
- Chronic BCS has features of complications of portal hypertension.

Incidence/prevalence
- It is an uncommon disorder with an incidence of approximately 1 in 2.5 million persons per year.
- Published data from the Western countries include one from Denmark that gave an estimated incidence rate of 0.5 per million inhabitants and year. In Sweden, the incidence and prevalence rates are reported at 0.8 per million per year and 1.4 per million inhabitants, respectively.

Mount Sinai Expert Guides: Hepatology, First Edition. Edited by Jawad Ahmad, Scott L. Friedman, and Henryk Dancygier.
© 2014 John Wiley & Sons, Ltd. Published 2014 by John Wiley & Sons, Ltd.
Companion website: www.mountsinaiexpertguides.com

- Japan in 1989 reported an estimated incidence rate of 0.2 per million and a prevalence of rate of 2.4 per million inhabitants.

Etiology

- The etiology of BCS is most commonly an underlying thrombotic condition leading to thrombosis of the outflow vessels of the liver.
- Both inherited and acquired procoagulant disorders have been associated with BCS in about 75% of patients, with the presence of multiple causes in the same patient being more commonly recognized.
- The common inherited causes of hypercoagulable conditions include antithrombin III deficiency, protein C and S deficiencies, Factor V Leiden and prothrombin 20210 mutations.
- The common acquired causes of hypercoagulable conditions include myeloproliferative disorders, paroxysmal nocturnal hemoglobinuria, antiphospholipid syndrome, malignancies, pregnancy and oral contraceptives. Of these, myeloproliferative disorders are increasingly recognized as the most prevalent underlying condition leading to thrombosis, with the JAK2 V617F mutation occurring in about 40–50% of patients with BCS.
- Uncommon causes include congenital webs of the hepatic vein and inferior vena cava.

Pathology/pathogenesis

- The underlying pathogenesis of the clinical features of BCS is initiated by the blockage of venous outflow of the liver. The extent to which this blockage leads to hepatic damage is dependent upon the rapidity of the obstruction and the timeliness of the intervention.
- In the acute setting, there are minimal collateral vessels formation, and the end result is one of venous stasis and congestion, leading to hepatocyte hypoxia, hepatocyte necrosis, and liver failure, if the obstruction is not relieved. In this acute scenario, the features of fulminant hepatic failure are present, including encephalopathy and jaundice developing as a result of massive hepatocyte cell death.
- In the subacute and chronic forms of BCS, the thrombosis is more insidious, with the benefit of time for the development of collateral circulation, and the presentation is that of progressive damage leading to cirrhosis. In about 75% of patients, the underlying cause of the thrombosis can be identified.

Predictive/risk factors

Risk factor	Odds ratio
Oral contraceptives	2.37
Inherited: Factor V Leiden, prothrombin, protein C, S, and antithrombin deficiencies	N/A
Acquired: myeloproliferative disorders, antiphospholipid syndrome, paroxysmal nocturnal hemoglobinuria, pregnancy	N/A

Section 2: Prevention

- The key to prevention of the progression of disease is early identification and intervention with decompression/thrombolysis when the presentation is acute, and the initiation of anticoagulation in the subacute/chronic forms before the development of complications of portal hypertension.

• Despite these interventions, progression of disease may still occur.

Screening
• Since the majority of patients with BCS have an underlying hypercoagulable condition, anyone who presents with a history of venous thrombosis should be screened for inherited risk factors.

Section 3: Diagnosis (Algorithm 27.1)

• The diagnosis and clinical presentation will vary depending upon whether the thrombosis is acute or chronic.
• The history should include the rapidity of onset of symptoms, family history of hypercoagulable states and presence/absence of portal hypertensive complications.
• Examination should focus on stigmata of chronic liver disease (spider angiomata, muscle wasting, jaundice, asterixis, ascites) and fulminant hepatic failure specific to outflow obstruction (massive ascites, encephalopathy, jaundice).
• Diagnostic investigations should include comprehensive metabolic panel, coagulation profile, Doppler sonogram of the liver/hepatic vessels, MRI/MRV or CT scan with intravenous contrast to assess hepatic vasculature.
• Venogram of hepatic veins/inferior vena cava if the non-invasive testing is inconclusive.

Differential diagnosis

Differential diagnosis	Features
AIH	Autoimmune markers; liver biopsy with plasma cell infiltration
Viral hepatitis	Viral serologies. Liver biopsy histology with periportal abnormalities as compared with pericentral abnormalities and sinusoidal dilatation as seen in BCS

Typical presentation
• The typical presentation of an acute BCS is that of a fulminant picture with a rapid onset of massive intractable ascites. This acuity of hepatic necrosis is manifested with marked elevations of AST/ALT and in rare cases, the development of encephalopathy within 8 weeks of presentation of jaundice.
• The subacute and chronic forms of BCS are usually the presentations of complications of cirrhosis. These complications include variceal bleeding, progressive ascites, encephalopathy and muscle wasting.

Clinical diagnosis
History
• The history should include the time frame of the onset of symptoms. The symptoms to be queried include the degree of abdominal pain, history of jaundice, ascites and lower extremity edema and whether the patient had previous episodes of GI bleeding or encephalopathy.

- When querying medication, the query should include the use of oral contraceptives and pregnancy status in women.
- A detailed history of the potential presence of inflammatory conditions leading to a hyper-coagulable state such as inflammatory bowel disease, Behçet's syndrome and malignancies (hepatocellular carcinoma, renal cell carcinoma, adrenal carcinoma) should be done. A detailed history of previous thrombotic conditions (deep vein thrombosis, pulmonary emboli, multiple miscarriages) is important as well as a family history of hypercoagulable conditions.

Physical examination
- An assessment of nutritional status as determined by the presence of muscle wasting can provide an indication of the chronicity of the disease. Presence or absence of jaundice and spider angiomata should be noted. The degree of ascites and the presence of RUQ pain may provide information as to the rapidity of the onset of the disease. Hepatomegaly and spleno-megaly should be assessed.
- A full neurologic examination is important in determining the presence of encephalopathy.

Laboratory diagnosis
List of diagnostic tests
- Complete blood count: hemoglobin/hematocrit (polycythemia vera), platelet count (thrombocytosis).
- Comprehensive metabolic panel; degree of elevation of AST/ALT (usually five times the ULN in the acute forms of BCS, less so in the chronic forms).
- Elevated bilirubin, elevated AP, decreased albumin, elevated PT INR.
- Ascites evaluation for serum-ascitic fluid albumin gradient which is high (>1.1 g/dL) compatible with portal hypertension. The total protein in the ascitic fluid is also usually elevated to more than 2.5 g/dL (similar to that seen in patients with cardiac disease).

List of imaging techniques
- Conventional US and Doppler US of the liver (hypertrophy of the caudate lobe is a distinctive feature of BCS and is found in 80% of patients with occlusion of hepatic veins).
- Contrast-enhanced CT scanning.
- MRI (may provide a better image of the length of the IVC as compared with CT scan).

Algorithm 27.1 Diagnosis of Budd–Chiari syndrome

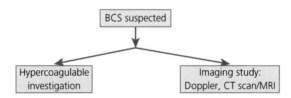

Potential pitfalls/common errors made regarding diagnosis of disease
- Patients who present with fulminant hepatic failure may be misdiagnosed with other causes such as viral, autoimmune or toxic/drug injury. A consideration for BCS is essential as early intervention with anti-coagulation and decompression may obviate the need for liver transplantation.

Section 4: Treatment (Algorithm 27.2)

- The medical management of BCS depends upon early diagnosis and treatment. If the patient already has end-stage cirrhosis with multiple complications of portal hypertension, the disease may be too advanced for anti-coagulation/decompression to change prognosis, and referral for liver transplantation is preferred. In patients with an acute BCS, or the chronic patient without complications of portal hypertension, early diagnosis, anti-coagulation therapy, and interventional/surgical decompression, may lead to stabilization of hepatic functioning and may avoid the need for liver transplantation.
- All patients with BCS should have an extensive hypercoagulable investigation and placed on anticoagulation if there are no obvious contraindications. In the acute presentation, thrombolysis should be considered as soon as the diagnosis is made. For thrombolysis to be effective, the thrombus must be recent and incompletely occluding the vessel. Thrombolysis can be achieved with urokinase (240 000 U per hour for 2 hours, followed by 60 000 U per hour) or tissue plasminogen activator (0.5–1.0 mg per hour) infused by a transfemoral or transjugular route.
- If thrombolysis is contraindicated, emergent decompression with either a TIPS or surgical shunt should be considered to prevent progression into fulminant hepatic failure and the need for emergent transplantation.

When to hospitalize
- Fulminant hepatic failure (King's College Criteria for prognostic indicators) with evidence of massive hepatic necrosis (marked elevation in AST/ALT), rising PT INR, encephalopathy, intractable ascites.
- Need for immediate thrombolysis (acute form) and decompression with either TIPS or surgical shunt.
- Decompensated cirrhosis with portal hypertensive complications requiring evaluation for liver transplantation.

Managing the hospitalized patient
- Appropriate and timely initiation of anti-coagulation.
- Careful monitoring of fluid status and renal function with diuresis.
- In acute form of BCS, avoid delay in decompression with TIPS or surgical shunt.

Table of treatment

Treatment	Comment
Conservative treatment	Initiate anti-coagulation
Medical	Anti-coagulation with heparin and conversion to coumadin to keep PT INR around 3. In acute form and incompletely occluding vessel, thrombolysis with urokinase or tissue plasminogen activator infused by transfemoral or transjugular route
Surgical	Surgical shunt
Radiological	TIPS procedure if there is incomplete thrombosis of the hepatic veins in acute form and in chronic, compensated cirrhosis
Other	Transplantation with cirrhosis and complications of portal hypertension

Prevention/management of complications
- Bleeding from over anti-coagulation: meticulous attention to dosing.
- Worsening of hepatic functioning after TIPS/surgical shunt with further ischemia: evaluation and listing for liver transplantation.

Algorithm 27.2 Management/treatment of Budd–Chiari syndrome

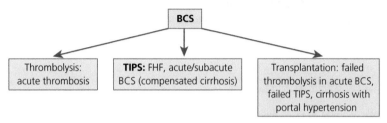

CLINICAL PEARLS
- If presentation is acute, thrombolysis and decompression with TIPS procedure must be considered in a timely fashion.
- When there is evidence of significant portal hypertensive complications (variceal bleeding, recurrent encephalopathy, decreased synthetic function–elevated INR/decreased albumin), TIPS may worsen liver disease and referral for liver transplantation is warranted. In the chronic BCS, MELD score should be used as a guide to decisions made with regards to potential risks and benefits of TIPS intervention.

Section 5: Special Populations
Pregnancy
- There is a known increased risk of the development of BCS during the pregnancy and peripartum state. Anti-coagulation with heparin should be considered and decompression remains a consideration in the acute form to avoid fulminant hepatic failure.

Section 6: Prognosis

CLINICAL PEARLS
- With early diagnosis and management with anticoagulation and/or TIPS, the prognosis of patients presenting with BCS has had significant improvement in the past few years.
- Liver transplantation is an option for fulminant hepatic failure and in patients with cirrhosis.
- The five-year survival post-transplantation remains excellent at >90%.

Natural history of untreated disease
- If left untreated, patients who present with massive hepatic necrosis and fulminant hepatic failure will have a poor prognosis without transplantation.

- In the subacute and chronic forms, patients will have progressive deterioration in hepatic functioning with the emergence of complications of portal hypertension such as varices, encephalopathy, and ascites.

Prognosis for treated patients

- Prognosis is excellent with early diagnosis, decompression and initiation of anti-coagulation.

Follow-up tests and monitoring

- Patients on anticoagulation therapy will need to be followed regularly for any signs of bleeding and for monitoring of PT INR for those on warfarin therapy.

Section 7: Reading List

Blum U, Rossle M, Haag K, et al. Budd-Chiari Syndrome: technical, hemodynamic, and clinical results of treatment with transjugular intrahepatic portosystemic shunt. Radiology 1995;197:805–11

Menon K, Shah V, Kamath P. The Budd-Chiari Syndrome. N Eng J Med 2004;350:578–85

Murad S, Plessier A, Henandez-Guerra M, et al. Etiology, management, and outcome of the Budd-Chiari syndrome. Ann Intern Med 2009;151:167–75

Rautou P, Plessier A, Bernuau J, Denninger M, Moucari R, Valla D. Pregnancy: a risk factor for Budd-Chiari syndrome? Gut 2009;58:606-8

Zimmerman M, Cameron A, Ghobrial R. Budd-Chiari Syndrome. Clin Liver Dis 2006;10:259–73

Section 8: Guidelines

Not applicable for this topic.

Section 9: Evidence

Not applicable for this topic.

Section 10: Images

Not applicable for this topic.

Additional material for this chapter can be found online at:
www.mountsinaiexpertguides.com
This includes a case study, multiple choice questions and advice for patients

CHAPTER 28

Portal Vein Thrombosis

Leona Kim-Schluger

Division of Liver Diseases, Icahn School of Medicine at Mount Sinai, New York, NY, USA

OVERALL BOTTOM LINE

- PVT can be divided into acute and chronic depending upon the rapidity and cause of the thrombosis.
- PVT is also commonly distinguished according to etiology: tumorous obstruction, that caused by cirrhosis, and hypercoagulable predisposition.
- In patients without cirrhosis, PVT may be the presenting symptom of a myeloproliferative disorder leading to a hypercoagulable state.
- Both local factors and systemic prothrombotic conditions are implicated in the formation of PVT. A local risk factor can be identified in about 30% of patients, and a general risk factor in 70%.
- An abdominal sonogram with Doppler is the imaging study of choice in diagnosing PVT.

Section 1: Background
Definition of disease
- Partial or complete occlusion of the portal vein by a thrombus. Thrombosis of the portal vein is due to a combination of factors, both local and systemic. It may present with a catastrophic ischemia of the bowel or occur in the absence of symptoms in the chronic state with the formation of collateral circulation over time.

Disease classification
- PVT can be classified as acute (thrombus formation without evidence of portal hypertension or collateral circulation) or chronic, also known as portal cavernoma with the formation of a network of collateral circulation.

Incidence/prevalence
- Increasingly recognized as imaging modalities to detect PVT are improving.
- The lifetime risk of developing PVT in the general population is reported to be 1%.

Etiology
- One of the causes of PVT is tumor thrombus. The more common tumors associated with PVT include hepatocellular carcinoma, neuroendocrine tumors, pancreatic cancer and unknown primary.
- Cirrhosis with extended duration of hepatopetal flow may lead to PVT.

Mount Sinai Expert Guides: Hepatology, First Edition. Edited by Jawad Ahmad, Scott L. Friedman, and Henryk Dancygier.
© 2014 John Wiley & Sons, Ltd. Published 2014 by John Wiley & Sons, Ltd.
Companion website: www.mountsinaiexpertguides.com

- In both the acute and chronic form of PVT (excluding tumors), the cause of PVT is multifactorial with both local and systemic factors contributing to the thrombus formation.

Pathology/pathogenesis
- PVT from tumor is due to a direct extension of the tumor cells into the portal vein. In patients with cirrhosis, thrombus formation is related to increased portal pressure leading to decreased portal blood flow and possibly a decrease in inherent anticoagulants (protein C, protein S, antithrombin III) from decreased hepatic functioning in the setting of cirrhosis.
- In patients without cirrhosis, the most common cause is a systemic hypercoagulable condition in the presence of a prothrombotic disorder. Local factors contributing to the thrombus formation include intra-abdominal infections and inflammatory conditions.

Predictive/risk factors

Risk factor	Incidence
Well compensated cirrhosis	0.6–16%
Decompensated cirrhosis	35%
Non-cirrhotic	5–10%

Section 2: Prevention

> **CLINICAL PEARLS**
> - In patients with PVT secondary to cirrhosis, anticoagulation is generally not recommended.
> - In patients without cirrhosis, long-term anticoagulation is recommended as the most likely cause of thrombus formation in an underlying hypercoagulable condition.

Screening
- Any patient with a previous history of venous thrombus formation should be screened for a prothrombotic condition and anticoagulation should be initiated if the risks of bleeding are low.

Section 3: Diagnosis (Algorithm 28.1)

> **CLINICAL PEARLS**
> - History should include symptoms of portal hypertension: abdominal distention, GI bleeding, change in mental status, or in the cases of acute PVT, acute onset of abdominal pain. History should also include any previous episodes of venous thrombus formation. Previous known history of liver disease leading to cirrhosis should also be ascertained.
> - Signs of portal hypertension include presence of ascites, varices, encephalopathy and splenomegaly in patients with cirrhosis. In the cases of acute PVT, an acute abdomen with tenderness on examination may be present and liver function is usually preserved.
> - Laboratory examinations should include a comprehensive metabolic panel to assess for hepatic functioning (albumin, PT INR, bilirubin), CBC with platelets to reveal elevated white blood cell count possibly indicating an infection as local factors leading to thrombus formation, and evidence of polycythemia or thrombocytosis.
> - Color Doppler ultrasonography is the imaging modality of choice. Contrast enhanced CT scan and MRI of the abdomen may also be used for the diagnosis of thrombus in the portal vein.

Differential diagnosis

Differential diagnosis	Features
BCS	Doppler sonography can distinguish location of thrombus

Typical presentation
- The presentation may differ slightly depending upon the acuteness of the thrombosis.
- In acute PVT (symptoms develop within 60 days of presentation), signs and symptoms of portal hypertension/collateral circulation may be absent. Typically, the patient presents with acute abdominal pain and fever. If the thrombus extends to the mesenteric veins, mesenteric ischemia may ensue leading to life-threatening complications of infarction and sepsis.
- In chronic PVT, the presentation is usually that of complications of portal hypertension including variceal bleeding, ascites and encephalopathy.

Clinical diagnosis
History
- The history should focus in attempting to determine the time course of PVT, whether acute or chronic, and potential local abdominal factors that may be contributing to thrombus development.
- The distinguishing symptoms of acute thrombosis include abdominal pain and fever.
- Chronic PVT usually presents with symptoms related to cirrhosis such as previous known history of liver disease and subsequent complications of portal hypertension. Additionally, as non-cirrhotic PVT is mostly related to a hypercoagulable condition, a history of previous episodes of other venous thrombus complications should be taken as well as a family history of pro-thrombotic conditions.
- Local contributing factors include a recent history of abdominal surgery or infections such as appendicitis, diverticulitis, pancreatitis or cholecystitis.

Physical examination
- The presence of fever and abdominal tenderness should alert the physician to the possibility of an acute thrombus and investigations should be initiated to confirm the diagnosis, with the need for immediate intervention to avoid further complications, including mesenteric ischemia. In the cirrhotic patient, signs are related to the chronicity of the liver disease. These signs include a shrunken liver, muscle wasting, spider angiomata, ascites, encephalopathy and the presence of varices. With advanced cirrhosis, splenomegaly is usually present. Chronic gastrointestinal bleeding from portal gastropathy may lead to signs of chronic anemia including pale conjunctivae.

Laboratory diagnosis
List of diagnostic tests
- CBC with platelets: thrombocytosis and polycythemia vera may provide initial clues to an underlying hypercoagulable condition. In patients with cirrhosis and portal hypertension, thrombocytopenia alone or pancytopenia may be present secondary to splenomegaly. In patients with abdominal infections leading to local factors contributing to thrombus formation in the absence of cirrhosis, the WBC count may be elevated.

- Comprehensive metabolic panel: in the rare case of hepatic ischemia from acute massive thrombus formation in the portal vein, the AST/ALT may be dramatically elevated from hepatic ischemia. In the cirrhotic patient, the elevations in AST/ALT are modest and signs of hepatic dysfunction including low albumin and elevated bilirubin may be present instead.
- Liver biopsy is rarely needed to confirm cirrhosis as this is usually evident from history and examination.
- Biopsy of the portal vein thrombus to confirm a tumor thrombus from a thrombus secondary to cirrhosis and not tumor, may be rarely needed. However, this distinction is critical in the prognosis and further management of the patient and should be done if there is uncertainty.
- Hypercoagulable investigation is indicated in the patients with non-cirrhotic PVT.

List of imaging techniques
- Color Doppler sonography has a 98% negative predictive value.
- Contrast-enhanced CT scan or MRI is also useful for diagnosis especially if tumor is suspected. Also, when an acute thrombosis is suspected, CT scan or MRI may be useful in the diagnosis of an inflammatory or infectious condition in the abdomen such as pancreatitis, appendicitis or perforated viscus.

Algorithm 28.1 Diagnosis of portal vein thrombosis

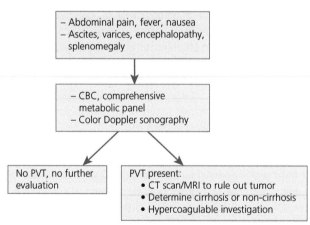

Potential pitfalls/common errors made regarding diagnosis of disease
- Presentation of PVT may mimic outflow obstruction (BCS).
- Must consider local factors contributing to thrombus formation (infections such as appendicitis, pancreatitis, cholecystitis) and treat accordingly.
- In chronic PVT and the formation of enlarged collaterals (portal cavernoma) on the surface of the common bile duct, may rarely lead to external compression and obstruction of the bile duct (portal cholangiopathy) leading to jaundice and cholangitis.

Section 4: Treatment (Algorithm 28.2)
Treatment rationale
- The treatment of tumor thrombus in the portal vein is the treatment of the underlying malignancy.
- In the acute thrombosis without cirrhosis, goals of treatment include thrombolysis to prevent the progression into the mesenteric veins and infarction as well as prevention of chronic PVT which can subsequently lead to complications of portal hypertension. In patients without cirrhosis, an underlying hypercoagulable condition must be investigated and the need for long-term anti-coagulation therapy determined.
- In patients with portal vein thrombus in the setting of cirrhosis, anti-coagulation is not recommended.

When to hospitalize
- Patients with acute portal vein thrombosis in the absence of cirrhosis.
- These patients require prompt diagnosis and intervention for anti-coagulation and interventional therapy including TIPS.
- Exploratory laparotomy for those patients suspected to have mesenteric ischemia and intestinal infarction.

Table of treatment

Treatment	Comment
Conservative treatment	Patients with PVT secondary to cirrhosis do not require any further intervention (i.e. anticoagulation)
Medical	Chronic PVT with portal hypertension and varices, prophylaxis with non-selective beta blocker is recommended: nadolol Acute PVT: consider systemic or *in situ* thrombolysis (streptokinase or tissue plasminogen activator)
Surgical	Acute PVT: consideration for surgical thrombectomy in those patients who are undergoing exploratory laparotomy for intestinal infarction
Radiological	Acute PVT: consideration for TIPS for those patients high risk for bleeding from medical thrombolysis therapy
Other	Liver transplantation for decompensated cirrhosis

Prevention/management of complications
- In-situ or systemic thrombolysis with streptokinase or tissue plasminogen activator may lead to increased morbidity from bleeding complications and result in only partial resolution of the clot. The decision to initiate this therapy must balance overall risks and benefits.

CLINICAL PEARLS
- Investigations into a potential hypercoagulable condition and long-term use of anti-coagulation is essential in preventing progression of disease and need for liver transplantation in the future. Investigations should include for both genetic (Factor V Leiden, prothrombin gene mutation, protein C, protein S, and antithrombin III) and acquired (oral contraceptive use, myeloproliferative disorder, antiphospholipid syndrome, paroxysmal nocturnal hemoglobinuria) causes.
- In select patients with acute PVT, TIPS should be a consideration for management to prevent further propagation of thrombus.

Algorithm 28.2 Management/treatment of portal vein thrombosis

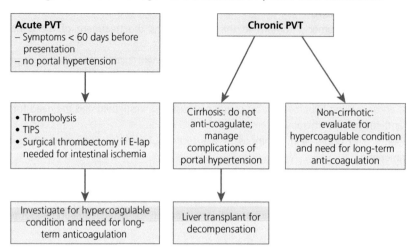

Section 5: Special Populations
Pregnancy
- During pregnancy, anti-coagulation with warfarin is contraindicated and other therapies need to be considered.

Children
- Umbilical cannulation, omphalitis, and abdominal infections may lead to extrahepatic portal vein obstruction in children manifesting as complications of portal hypertension with preserved hepatic functioning.
- Management of variceal bleeding include band ligation and surgical shunting with mesenteric-to-left portal vein bypass.

Section 6: Prognosis

- The current outcome of acute and chronic PVT in the absence of cirrhosis is good with appropriate investigations into underlying hypercoagulable conditions and appropriate management with anticoagulation.
- Overall, anticoagulation has a favorable benefit–risk ratio.
- In patients with decompensated cirrhosis, liver transplantation remains an option with excellent long-term survival.

Section 7: Reading List

Condat B, Pessione F, Hillaire S, Denninger M, et al. Current outcome of portal vein thrombosis in adults: risk and benefit of anticoagulation. Gastroenterology 2001;120:490–7

DeLeve L, Valla D, Garcia-Tsao G. Vascular disorders of the liver. Hepatology 2009;49:1729–64

Plessier A, Darwish-Murad S, Hernandez-Guerrs M, et al. Acute portal thrombosis unrelated to cirrhosis: a prospective multicenter follow-up study. Hepatology 2010; 51: 210–18

Sogaard K, Astrup L, Vilstrup H, Gronbaek H Portal vein thrombosis; risk factors, clinical presentation and treatment. BMC Gastroenterology 2007;7:34

Valla DC, Condat B. Portal vein thrombosis in adults: pathophysiology, pathogenesis and management. J Hepatol 2000;32:865–71

Section 8: Guidelines

Guideline title	Guideline source	Date
AASLD Practice Guidelines: Vascular disorders of the liver	American Association for the Study of Liver Diseases (AASLD) http://www.aasld.org/practiceguidelines/Documents/Bookmarked%20Practice%20Guidelines/VascularDisordersLiver.pdf	2009

Section 9: Evidence

Not applicable for this topic.

Section 10: Images

Not applicable for this topic.

Additional material for this chapter can be found online at:
www.mountsinaiexpertguides.com
This includes a case study and multiple choice questions

CHAPTER 29

Non-Cirrhotic Portal Hypertension

M. Isabel Fiel[1] and Thomas D. Schiano[2]
[1]Department of Pathology, Icahn School of Medicine at Mount Sinai, New York, NY, USA
[2]Division of Liver Diseases, Icahn School of Medicine at Mount Sinai, New York, NY, USA

OVERALL BOTTOM LINE
- Cirrhosis is the most common cause of portal hypertension.
- Causes of NCPH include hepatovenous or portomesenteric thrombosis, alcoholic hepatitis and sinusoidal obstruction syndrome.
- Atypical patterns of intrahepatic fibrosis associated with NCPH include schistosomiasis, sarcoidosis, congenital hepatic fibrosis and cystic fibrosis.
- Increasingly recognized causes of NCPH are OPV and NRH.
- Typically, hepatic synthetic function is normal and liver chemistry tests are only mildly deranged in the setting of NCPH.

Section 1: Background
Definition of disease
- NCPH is the clinical manifestation of portal hypertension, i.e. ascites, variceal bleeding, occurring in the absence of cirrhosis.

Disease classification
- NCPH may be related to vascular thrombosis and their associated causes pylephlebitis, arteriovenous fistula, alcoholic hepatitis and sinusoidal obstruction syndrome (veno-occlusive disease).
- In addition, NCPH may be due to atypical patterns of hepatic fibrosis as seen in schistosomiasis, sarcoidosis, congenital hepatic fibrosis and cystic fibrosis.

Incidence/prevalence
- The true incidence of NCPH is unknown but NRH and OPV are increasingly being recognized on liver biopsy.
- A recent FDA Advisory was issued regarding the use of certain HAART medications, specifically didanosine and the development of NCPH.
- PVT may occur in conjunction with a hypercoagulable state and spontaneously in a small percentage of patients with long-standing cirrhosis.

Mount Sinai Expert Guides: Hepatology, First Edition. Edited by Jawad Ahmad, Scott L. Friedman, and Henryk Dancygier.
© 2014 John Wiley & Sons, Ltd. Published 2014 by John Wiley & Sons, Ltd.
Companion website: www.mountsinaiexpertguides.com

Etiology
- Dependent upon the cause of NCPH.
- Portal and mesenteric vein thrombosis as well as hepatic venous outflow obstruction or sinusoidal obstruction syndrome are most commonly related to hypercoagulable states, such as JAK2 V617F mutation.
- NRH may be secondary to medications, collagen vascular disease or myeloproliferative disorders while OPV is currently considered idiopathic.

Pathology/pathogenesis
- Portal hypertension in the absence of cirrhosis results from either vascular thrombosis or architectural distortion of the liver.
- NRH arises as a consequence of an altered intrahepatic blood flow whereas in OPV the main histopathological finding is either diminished or, in severe cases, obliterated portal vein branches.

Predictive/risk factors

Common Causes of Non-Cirrhotic Portal Hypertension

NRH
OPV
Idiopathic portal hypertension
Incomplete septal cirrhosis
Sinusoidal obstruction syndrome
Alcoholic hepatitis
BCS
Schistosomiasis
Sarcoidosis
PBC/PSC
Congenital hepatic fibrosis
Hepatic arterio-portal fistula/splanchnic arteriovenous fistula
Extrahepatic portal vein obstruction
Hereditary hemorrhagic telangiectasia (Osler–Weber–Rendu)
Splenic vein thrombosis
Massive splenomegaly
Right-sided heart failure/constrictive pericarditis
Pylephlebitis

Section 2: Prevention

- No interventions have been demonstrated to prevent the disease aside from the anticoagulation in patients having hypercoagulable or myeloproliferative disorders.

Screening
- Appropriate radiologic studies are performed in patients manifesting clinically with portal hypertension.
- Liver biopsy should be performed in the absence of vascular thrombosis to rule out an intrinsic liver disease.

Primary prevention
- Anticoagulation when appropriate.
- Antibiotic treatment of pylephlebitis.
- Medical treatment of schistosomiasis and sarcoidosis.

Section 3: Diagnosis (Algorithm 29.1)

- Diagnosis based on needle liver biopsy is difficult; it is imperative for the clinician to alert the pathologist as to the presence of portal hypertension in the patient. Because some patients have overlapping features of these conditions, these entities should be considered as morphologic variants within the wide spectrum of NCPH, related to intrahepatic impediment to blood flow.

Differential diagnosis

Differential diagnosis	Features
Cirrhosis	Typical histology, known etiology of intrinsic liver disease in the setting portal hypertension
Chronic liver disease	Significant fibrosis despite the absence of established cirrhosis, e.g. sarcoidosis
Vascular thrombosis	Typical radiographic findings in the presence or absence of intrinsic liver disease

Typical presentation
- Patients present with clinical evidence of portal hypertension usually manifested by varices with or without bleeding or ascites. Hepatic synthetic function is typically well-preserved or normal and there may be only minimal if any abnormal liver tests.
- Patients may also present with thrombocytopenia in the absence of clinical portal hypertension with hematologic investigations identifying hypersplenism as its etiology.

Clinical diagnosis
History
- Ask if the patient has a history of other thrombotic events, malignancy or family history of hypercoagulability or liver disease. Careful inquiry regarding past and present medication use is necessary.
- Ascertaining whether any systemic disease is present such as cystic fibrosis is important. Arterio-portal fistulas can occur after liver interventions. Patients may have developed PVT as children due to omphalitis from catheter replacement. It is important to exclude all forms of liver disease that may lead to cirrhosis.
- OPV has been associated with vinyl chloride and arsenic poisoning and, more recently, along with NRH, has been implicated in the development of NCPH in HIV patients receiving didanosine.
- Congenital hepatic fibrosis can be seen in conjunction with Caroli syndrome (Figure 29.1). Pylephlebitis is an ascending infection of the portal venous system that can lead to PVT and

liver abscess. There is typically bacteremia arising from a right-sided abdominal process, e.g., diverticulitis, appendicitis, Crohn's disease-related abscess.

Physical examination
- Findings of portal hypertension such as ascites, splenomegaly or caput medusae may be seen. Patients with sinusoidal obstruction syndrome or hepatic venous outflow obstruction may have ascites and peripheral edema. Alcoholic hepatitis may manifest with jaundice and cutaneous stigmata of chronic liver disease.
- NCPH due to systemic disease may exhibit physical findings of those illnesses such as chronic lung disease in cystic fibrosis, or skin and eye disease in patients with sarcoidosis.

Laboratory diagnosis
List of diagnostic tests
- Liver biopsy findings: NRH is defined as diffuse nodularity of the liver parenchyma composed of small nodules consisting of two-cell thick hepatocyte plates surrounded by condensed reticulin fibers and accompanied by little or no fibrosis with the portal tracts located in the center of the nodule ("reverse lobulation") (Figure 29.2). On hematoxylin and eosin staining, the architectural changes may not be apparent and therefore a reticulin stain is often necessary to establish the diagnosis. NRH arises as a consequence of the alteration of intrahepatic blood flow. The table – Diseases associated with the development of NRH – outlines the different diseases frequently associated with NRH.
- OPV is also known as idiopathic portal hypertension or non-cirrhotic portal fibrosis and is also seen in the spectrum of ISC. ISC is characterized by slender fibrous septa that outline incomplete macronodules and by occlusive venous changes. In OPV, the primary hepatic lesions are found in the portal tracts which show varying degrees of fibrosis and sclerosis of portal vein branches; marked dilatation of sinusoids may also be present (Figure 29.3). Portal vein changes range from marked wall thickening to total obliteration of the lumen known as phlebosclerosis within a densely fibrotic portal tract. Occasional septa originate from portal areas and often end blindly within the parenchyma.
- Bone marrow biopsy to exclude blood dyscrasia.
- Hypercoagulability testing.

Diseases associated with the development of NRH
PBC
HIV
Celiac disease
Congenital abnormalities of the portal vein
Post-liver transplantation
Rheumatologic disorders • SLE • Scleroderma • Rheumatoid arthritis • Polyarteritis nodosa • Anti-phospholipid antibody syndrome

(Continued)

Myeloproliferative disorders

Hodgkin and non-Hodgkin lymphoma

Chronic lymphocytic leukemia

Medications
- Azathioprine
- 6-thioguanine
- Didanosine
- Chemotherapeutic agents

Chronic diseases (TB, chronic osteomyelitis)

List of imaging techniques
- Abdominal US to establish patency of hepatic veins, inferior vena cava and a porto-mesenteric access.
- US, MRI or CT scan will identify mass lesions in the liver or spleen, as well as identify the presence of lymphadenopathy.
- Arterio-porto fistulas may be seen with angiography.

Algorithm 29.1 Diagnosis of non-cirrhotic portal hypertension

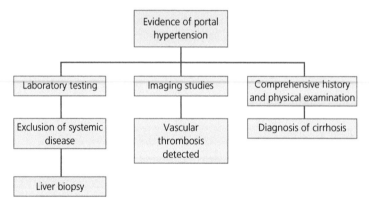

Potential pitfalls
- Increasingly recognized causes of NCPH are NRH and OPV.
- Both entities typically cause clinical portal hypertension in the absence of hepatic synthetic compromise and liver chemistry tests may be normal or only mildly deranged. Radiological and gross appearance of the liver may be normal or show only slight nodularity.
- The diagnosis may be missed if the information regarding portal hypertension is not provided.
- Needle liver biopsy may be difficult to read in small samples (NRH).
- Primary hematologic disorders may at times be difficult to diagnose and appropriate hematologic referral is essential.
- NRH and OPV can be idiopathic disorders.

Section 4: Treatment (Algorithm 29.2)
Treatment rationale
- Therapy of underlying portal hypertensive symptoms is of primary importance. Medical, endoscopic or radiologic intervention for variceal bleeding, i.e. TIPS and medical, dietary or radiologic management of ascites is the primary treatment. Timely diagnosis of the underlying cause should then be undertaken. For example, immunosuppressive treatment for sarcoidosis, antibiotics for pylephlebitis, anti-coagulation for hypercoagulable states and removal of the offending medication that could be causing NRH, e.g. azathioprine.

When to hospitalize
- Patients should be hospitalized for treatment of variceal bleeding or in an effort to establish a diagnosis.

Table of treatment

Treatment	Comment
Conservative	Observe if clinical portal hypertension not present
Medical	Medical control of portal hypertension via beta-blockade, discontinuation of all medications potentially causing NRH or OPV, anti-coagulation if hypercoagulability exists, treatment of myeloproliferative disorders, immunosuppressive therapy of sarcoidosis, antibiotics for infection if necessary
Surgical	Porto-systemic shunting
Radiological	TIPS, embolization of fistulas or varices

Prevention/management of complications
- Adequate treatment of underlying disease to prevent further thrombosis or worsening of portal hypertension.
- Discontinuation of medications or avoidance of toxins that might be contributing to NRH or OPV.
- Screen adequately for cardiopulmonary disease in patients with HHT.
- Rarely, patients with NRH and OPV have synthetic compromise and liver failure and require liver transplantation. In most cases the primary diagnosis had gone unrecognized.

Algorithm 29.2 Treatment of non-cirrhotic portal hypertension

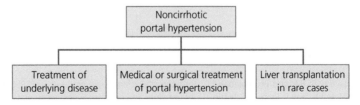

CLINICAL PEARLS

- OPV has been associated with vinyl chloride and arsenic poisoning and, more recently, along with NRH, has been implicated in the development of NCPH in HIV+ patients receiving didanosine.
- Patients with NRH or OPV may have other concurrent liver disease that contributes to hepatic synthetic dysfunction.
- OPV, NRH and sarcoidosis alone can result in liver failure and in these cases, the liver volume is small.
- Patients may initially be seen by a hematologist initiating an investigation for thrombocytopenia when liver disease and NCPH are first suspected.
- Cavernous transformation of the portal vein suggests long-standing thrombosis and may be associated with portal hypertensive biliopathy (cholestasis due to bile duct obstruction by the portal cavernoma).
- It is incumbent upon clinicians and pathologists to be aware of the diagnosis of OPV so as not to miss it on a liver biopsy.

Section 5: Special Populations

- Pregnant women may be at risk for the development or worsening of hypercoagulable conditions and the presence of increased plasma volume can exacerbate pre-existing portal hypertension.
- Patients immigrating from endemic areas, i.e. Central America and Puerto Rico, endemic areas for schistosomiasis, should have appropriate serological screening. Liver biopsy may show the classic pathognomonic features.

Section 6: Prognosis

- NCPH may occur early in the setting of sarcoidosis and if adequately treated, patients rarely require transplantation.
- NRH may occur in the setting of PSC and PBC and may contribute to the early portal hypertension seen in these conditions.
- Patients with NCPH due to HHT may have ongoing GI bleeding as well as high-output cardiomyopathy and pulmonary A–V malformation. Liver transplantation is sometimes undertaken to treat the cardiopulmonary disease.
- The portal hypertension due to NRH may persist and worsen despite the removal of the offending medication.
- Arterio-portal fistula may be a cause of worsening hepatic fibrosis that occurs even without other concurrent disease.
- NRH and OPV are causes of liver dysfunction and portal hypertension in patients with myeloproliferative disorders.

Section 7: Reading List

Bioulac-Sage P, Le Bail B, Bernard PH, Balabaud C. Hepatoportal sclerosis. Semin Liver Dis 1995;15:329–39
Fiel MI, Thung SN, Hytiroglou P, Emre S, Schiano TD. Liver failure and need for liver transplantation in patients with advanced hepatoportal sclerosis. Am J Surg Pathol 2007;31:607–14.

Garcia-Pagan JC, Hernandez-Guerra M, Bosch J. Extrahepatic portal vein thrombosis. Semin Liver Dis 2008;28:282–92

Geller SA, Dubinsky MC, Poordad FF, et al. Early hepatic nodular hyperplasia and submicroscopic fibrosis associated with 6-thioguanine therapy in inflammatory bowel disease. Am J Surg Pathol 2004;28: 1204–11

Ibarrola C, Colina F. Clinicopathological features of nine cases of non-cirrhotic portal hypertension: current definitions and criteria are inadequate. Histopathology 2003;42:251–64

Jha P, Poder L, Wang ZJ, Westphalen AC, Yeh BM, Coakley FG. Radiologic mimics of cirrhosis. Am J Roentgenol 2010;194:993–9

Khalid SK, Garcia-Tsao G. Hepatic vascular malformations in hereditary hemorrhagic telangiectasis. Semin Liver Dis 2008;28:247–58

Krasinskas AM, Eghtesad B, Kamath PS, Demetris AJ, Abraham SC. Liver transplantation for severe intrahepatic noncirrhotic portal hypertension. Liver Transpl 2005;11:627,34; discussion 610–1.

Li Y, Chen D, Ross AG, et al. Severe hepatosplenic schistosomiasis: clinicopathologic study of 102 cases undergoing splenectomy. Human Pathology 2011;42:111–9

Maida I, Garcia-Gasco P, Sotgiu G, et al. Antiretroviral-associated portal hypertension: a new clinical condition? Prevalence, predictors and outcome. Antivir Ther 2008;13:103–7

Reshamwala PA, Kleiner DE, Heller T. Nodular regenerative hyperplasia: not all nodules are created equal. Hepatology 2006;44:7–14

Sarin SK, Kumar A. Noncirrhotic portal hypertension. Clin Liver Dis 2006;10:627–51

Schiano TD, Kotler DP, Ferran E, Fiel MI. Hepatoportal sclerosis as a cause of noncirrhotic portal hypertension in patients with HIV. Am J Gastroenterol 2007;102:2536–40

Schiano TD, Uriel A, Dieterich D, Fiel MI. The development of hepatoportal sclerosis and portal hypertension due to didanosine use in HIV. Virchows Arch 2011;458:231–5

Singh MM, Pockros PJ. Hematologic and oncologic diseases of the liver. Clin Liver Dis 2011;15:69–87

Section 8: Guidelines

Not applicable for this topic.

Section 9: Evidence

Not applicable for this topic.

Section 10: Images

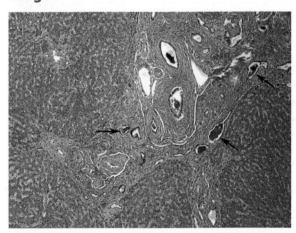

Figure 29.1 Congenital hepatic fibrosis in a patient with Caroli syndrome. Abnormally situated bile ducts (arrows) at the periphery of a densely fibrotic portal tract is characteristic of this entity. H & E. Original magnification ×40.

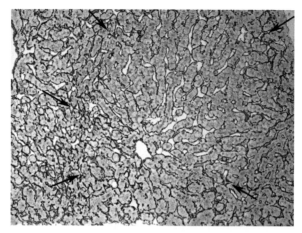

Figure 29.2 NRH in a patient taking azathioprine. Note the nodular appearance of the parenchyma with each nodule surrounded by condensed reticulin fibers (arrows).

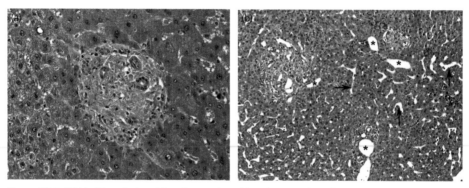

Figure 29.3 OPV incidentally found in a liver explant. (a) A close up view of a fibrotic portal tract with no visible portal vein lumen. H & E. Original magnification ×100. (b) Three portal tracts are portrayed in this photomicrograph. The portal veins are herniated into the surrounding parenchyma (asterisks). Also note that the sinusoids are markedly dilated (arrows). H & E. Original magnification ×40.

Additional material for this chapter can be found online at:
www.mountsinaiexpertguides.com
This includes a case study and multiple choice questions

CHAPTER 30

Liver Lesions

James S. Park

Division of Gastroenterology, NYU School of Medicine, New York, NY, USA

OVERALL BOTTOM LINE

- The medical evaluation of liver lesions is often challenging to clinicians. When a patient is diagnosed with a liver lesion, it is important to consider the clinical situation in which it was discovered.
- Careful history taking and physical examination often give important clues to diagnosis.
- The laboratory evaluation and morphological features on radiological imaging frequently lead to diagnosis without a biopsy.
- Primary hepatic neoplasm should be high on the list of differential diagnoses in patients with chronic liver diseases presenting with new focal liver lesions.

Section 1: Background
Disease classification

- Liver (hepatic) lesions are classified into non-malignant (benign) lesions, primary malignant neoplasms and secondary malignant (metastatic) neoplasms.
- The most common benign hepatic lesions are hepatic hemangioma, hepatic cysts and hepatic adenoma and FNH. Common infectious lesions include pyogenic and amebic liver abscesses and echinococcal cyst.
- Common primary hepatic neoplasms include HCC and cholangiocarcinoma.
- The liver is a common organ for metastatic disease. The secondary or metastatic neoplasm sources include malignancies from colon, breast, lymphoma, thyroid, pancreas, melanoma, lungs and neuroendocrine tumors.

Incidence/prevalence

- The most common benign solid hepatic tumor is hemangioma and its prevalence is 3–10%. Hepatic hemangioma is often found in the right lobe of the liver and in females predominantly.
- Simple hepatic cysts are discovered in 5–10% of asymptomatic adults. These are benign and often are found in the right lobe of the liver. Large cysts are found frequently in women over 50 years of age.
- The second most common of primary solid liver tumor is FNH.
- Prevalence of FNH and hepatic adenoma are 3–8% and less than 1%, respectively. Both are more common in females. FNH is benign; however, the hepatic adenomas is associated with malignant transformation and spontaneous hemorrhage.

Mount Sinai Expert Guides: Hepatology, First Edition. Edited by Jawad Ahmad, Scott L. Friedman, and Henryk Dancygier.

© 2014 John Wiley & Sons, Ltd. Published 2014 by John Wiley & Sons, Ltd.

Companion website: www.mountsinaiexpertguides.com

- The prevalence of HCC and metastatic lesions are less than 1% of the general population. It develops in patients with chronic liver disease, is the fourth leading cause of cancer-related death among males and its incidence is on the rise worldwide.

Economic impact
- The increased use of radiological tests such as CT scan, MRI and ultrasound has increased incidental findings of liver lesions. Many of these are benign and are found incidentally during the investigation of unrelated matters. These lesions frequently cause diagnostic dilemmas and challenges to physicians.
- Liver lesions found incidentally often lead to several blood and radiological tests and occasionally invasive tests such as biopsy which may impact overall economic cost. However, there is no clear data on the precise economic impact of liver lesions found incidentally.

Predictive/risk factors
- There are no clear risk factors for hemangioma, hepatic cyst and FNH.
- The risk of developing hepatic adenoma is associated with estrogen, oral contraceptive pills, anabolic steroid use and glycogen storage disease.
- The risk of developing a hepatic neoplasm such as HCC is associated with exposure to aflatoxins and cirrhosis of the liver from hepatitis C, NASH and chronic hepatitis B infection. The risk of developing HCC in cirrhotic patients is roughly 3–5% yearly.

Section 2: Prevention

> **BOTTOM LINE/CLINICAL PEARLS**
> - There is no preventive measure for benign hepatic hemangioma, cyst and FNH.
> - The primary prevention should be focused on identifying and screening patients at risk of developing a primary hepatic neoplasm such as HCC.
> - Hepatitis A and hepatitis B vaccinations should be offered routinely to those patients with chronic liver diseases who are not immune.

Screening
- For asymptomatic patients without any underlying liver disease, a routine liver lesion screening is not recommended. However, serum liver function should be offered to patients during a routine physical check-up to identify patients at risk of developing chronic liver diseases.
- For patients with liver cirrhosis and/or chronic hepatitis B infection, HCC screening such as ultrasound should be offered every 6 months to detect the cancer at an early stage.

Section 3: Diagnosis

> **BOTTOM LINE/CLINICAL PEARLS**
> - Clinical context is very important in diagnosis of focal liver lesions. For healthy patients with no evidence of chronic liver disease, malignant hepatic neoplasm is less likely.
> - For patients with a focal liver lesion and with evidence of chronic liver diseases such as cirrhosis and/or hepatitis B infection, primary hepatic neoplasm such as HCC should be ruled out with further blood and radiological tests.
> - The diagnosis requires evaluation of clinical situations, performing appropriate blood tests and radiological tests.

Typical presentation

- Most commonly, benign hepatic cyst, hemangioma and FNH are found incidentally. Most commonly the patients have no symptoms from the liver lesions. However, some patients may complain of vague RUQ discomfort when the lesions are complex and large.
- Patients with pyogenic abscess or amebic abscess may have fever, chills and abdominal pain associated with infection.
- Patients with small adenomas are asymptomatic. Those with larger adenomas (>5 cm) infrequently present with acute abdominal pain due to tumor rupture and intratumor hemorrhage.
- Cirrhotic patients with small HCC often have no specific symptoms. As the HCC grows, the patient tends to experience vague RUQ discomfort from the space-occupying lesion. As the tumor becomes more advanced, the patients may present with new hepatic decompensation such as variceal bleed, jaundice, ascites and hepatic encephalopathy.

Clinical diagnosis

History (please see Algorithms 30.1 and 30.2)

- Clinical context is very important in diagnosis of focal liver lesions. For healthy patients with no symptoms and no evidence of chronic liver disease, malignant hepatic neoplasm is less likely.
- In young patients with no predisposing medical problem or symptoms, the most common etiology of a hepatic lesion is hepatic cyst, followed by hemangioma. Hepatic cyst is hypo- or anechoic where as hemangioma tends to have peripheral rim contrast enhancement on the delay phase of a CT scan or MRI.
- In healthy young females with hypervascular lesions there should be concern about FNH or hepatic adenoma. Differentiating FNH from hepatic adenoma is important since the latter is not considered to be benign. The hepatic adenoma is associated with complications such as rupture, hemorrhage and malignant transformation.
- FNH is usually found as a slowly enhancing lesion with a characteristic central vascular scar on dynamic contrast imaging. It is benign and biopsy is often not helpful in making diagnosis. Unlike hepatic adenomas, there is no strong correlation between use of oral contraceptive pills to development of FNH. Liver biopsy should be avoided in hepatic adenomas due to increased risk of complications such as bleeding and tumor rupture.
- The liver is a highly vascular organ and therefore it is the most common place for metastasis in the body. In those with history of or suspected extrahepatic malignancies, investigations for metastatic liver disease should be pursued.
- In patients with chronic liver diseases such as hepatitis B and cirrhosis, the most common primary liver tumor is HCC. HCC can usually be diagnosed radiographically in patients with cirrhosis or hepatitis B infection. It has a characteristic radiographic feature of arterial enhancement of tumor followed by washout of contrast during the venous or delay phase of a CT scan or MRI. AFP is often helpful but not always elevated in HCC.
- Histological confirmation of HCC is not usually needed if the lesion meets the radiological criteria for HCC in patients with chronic liver disease. However, histological confirmation by core biopsy should be obtained when the diagnosis is not clear between HCC and cholangiocarcinoma.
- Focal liver lesions found on US smaller than 1 cm should be followed up with US at intervals of 3 months up to 1 year. If there has been no growth over a period of up to 1–2 years, one can revert to routine 6-month surveillance for patients with chronic liver diseases or stop following the lesions in healthy asymptomatic patients.

- Lesions larger than 1 cm in diameter should be studied with triple phase CT scan or MRI. If the appearance is typical for HCC in patients with chronic liver diseases, no further diagnostic evaluation is required. If the radiological characteristics are not typical for HCC, the second contrast imaging test such as MRI should be performed (if CT scan was done). If the focal liver lesions are found to be atypical on both MRI and CT scan, one should pursue a core biopsy of the suspected lesion.

Physical examination

- The physical examination would be most likely normal in healthy young patients presenting with incidental finding of benign hepatic cyst, hemangioma and FNH.
- The patient with liver cirrhosis may have various stigmata of chronic liver diseases such as jaundice, icteric sclera, spider nevi in the upper body, palmar erythema, muscle wasting from protein energy malnutrition, ascites, peripheral edema, splenomegaly and asterixis from hepatic encephalopathy.
- The abdominal examination sometimes reveals a palpable large HCC and audible hepatic bruit.

Laboratory diagnosis
List of diagnostic tests

- Elevated serum AFP may also be seen in patients with chronic liver disease without HCC such as acute or chronic viral hepatitis, e.g. hepatitis C. A rise in serum AFP from the baseline level in a patient with cirrhosis should raise a concern for new HCC. However, HCC is often diagnosed at a lower AFP level in screened patients which indicating a low sensitivity of the test.
- Carbohydrate antigen 19-9 (CA19-9) may be elevated in patients with cholangiocarcinoma or certain types of HCC.

List of imaging techniques

- US examination can be done easily at low cost. There is, however, greater inter-observer variability in reading affecting overall sensitivity. The test can be less accurate in patients with more advanced cirrhosis stage with ascites.
- Contrast imaging modalities such as CT scan and MRI are useful for detecting and differentiating the focal hepatic lesions. If the typical vascular pattern of HCC (arterial enhancement with venous phase contrast "washout") is seen in cirrhotic patients, it is considered to be diagnostic for HCC regardless of AFP level and no liver biopsy is needed.

Potential pitfalls/common errors made regarding diagnosis of disease

- Benign liver lesions found incidentally in healthy patients may lead to multiple investigations with minimal yield.
- HCC is relatively frequent in cirrhosis and the diagnosis can be missed as the majority of patients do not develop symptoms until HCC progresses to advanced stage.

Section 4: Treatment
Treatment rationale

- If the liver lesion is benign, no further treatment would be indicated.
- Differentiating FNH from hepatic adenomas is important because the latter has a potential for malignant transformation and also has risk of tumor rupture and bleed. Therefore, hepatic adenomas should be surgically removed whenever possible.

Algorithm 30.1 Diagnostic approach to patient with liver mass

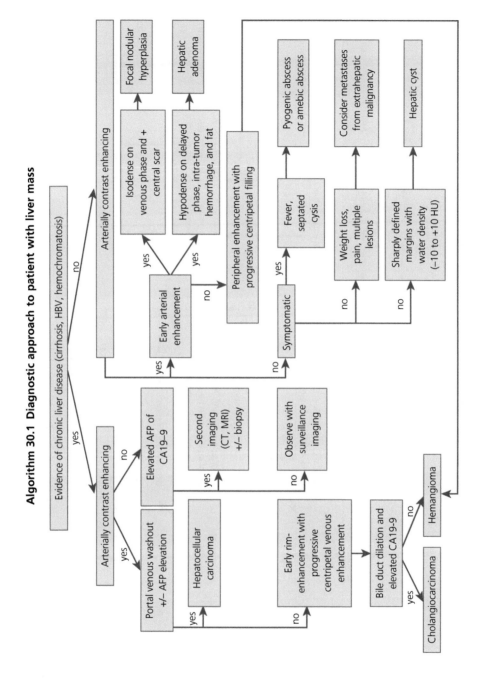

Algorithm 30.2 Benign and malignant liver tumors

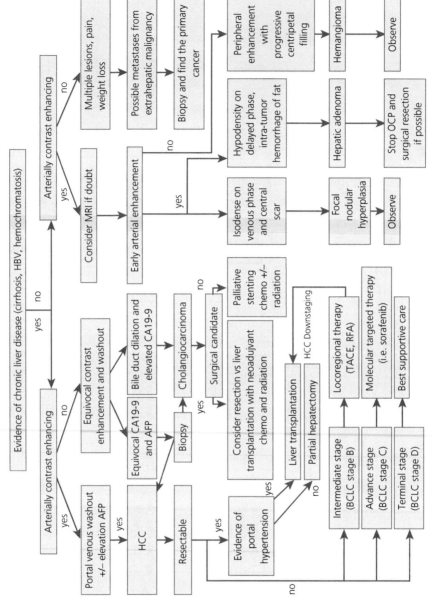

- If the liver lesion is a HCC, the treatment is based on type of malignancy, extent of spread, functional status of the patient and overall liver function.
- If HCC is small and solitary in patients without portal hypertension, curative surgical resection should be sought after.
- In patients with an intermediate stage (T2) of HCC or cirrhotic HCC patients with portal hypertension, liver transplantation would offer the best chance for cure.
- Local regional therapy such as chemoembolization or radiofrequency ablation can be used as a bridge to liver transplantation in selected HCC patients.

CLINICAL PEARLS
- If the liver lesion is found to be benign, no further treatment would be needed.
- FNH can be watched if the patient remains asymptomatic. However, hepatic adenomas should be surgically removed whenever possible.
- If the liver lesion is HCC, the treatment is based on type of malignancy, extent of spread, functional status of the patient and overall liver function.
- In appropriate patients, surgical resection and liver transplantation can be offered with curative intent.

Section 5: Special Populations

Not applicable for this topic.

Section 6: Prognosis
Follow-up tests and monitoring
- For benign liver lesions, no further monitoring is required unless the patient develops new symptoms such as abdominal pain and abnormal LFTs.
- All cirrhotic patients should receive HCC surveillance (liver imaging +/– AFP) every 6 months.
- For cirrhotic patients with liver lesions which have not been growing over a period of up to 1–2 years, one can revert to routine 6-month surveillance.

Section 7: Reading List

Assy N, Nasser G, Djibre A, et al. Characteristics of common solid liver lesions and recommendations for diagnostic workup. World J Gastroenterol 2009;15:3217–27

Blachar A, Federle M, Sosna J. Liver lesions with hepatic capsular retraction. Semin Ultrasound CT MR 2009;30:426–35

Bruix J, Sherman M. Management of hepatocellular carcinoma. Hepatology 2005;42:1208–36

Malhi H, Gores GJ. Cholangiocarcinoma: modern advances in understanding a deadly old disease. J Hepatol 2006;45:856–67

Mortele KJ, Ros P. Benign liver neoplasms. Clin Liver Dis 2002;6:119–45

Section 8: Guidelines
International guidelines

Guideline title	Guideline source	Date
ESPEN Guideline	http://www.aasld.org/practiceguidelines/Documents/ Bookmarked%20Practice%20Guidelines/HCCUpdate2010.pdf	2010

Section 9: Evidence

Not applicable for this topic.

Section 10: Images

Not applicable for this topic.

Additional material for this chapter can be found online at:
www.mountsinaiexpertguides.com
This includes a case study and multiple choice questions

CHAPTER 31

Cystic Lesions of the Liver

Abdulelah Alhawsawi[1], Juan P. Rocca[2] and Marcelo E. Facciuto[1]
[1]Recanati/Miller Transplantation Institute, Mount Sinai Hospital, New York, NY, USA
[2]Department of Surgery, Icahn School of Medicine at Mount Sinai, New York, NY, USA

OVERALL BOTTOM LINE
- Cystic lesions of the liver represent a heterogeneous group of disorders, most of them with an indolent and benign course.
- Cystic lesions of the liver are frequent and usually an incidental finding.
- Widespread use of modern imaging has dramatically increased reports of the prevalence of simple cysts with rates as high as 18% on CT scan.
- In some circumstances a surgical intervention is indicated by symptoms or to treat specific potential complications and morbidity related to the etiology of the cyst. Thus, efforts to characterize these lesions and arrive at a specific diagnosis should be made.

Section 1: Background
Definition of disease
- Liver cysts are congenital or acquired fluid-filled spaces within the liver parenchyma that are lined by epithelium (true cysts) or that do not possess an epithelial lining (pseudocysts).

Disease classification
- Primary hepatic and biliary cysts:
  - Simple cysts.
  - PCLD.
  - Cystadenoma/cystadenocarcinoma.
  - Bile duct cysts (Caroli disease).
- Secondary hepatic and biliary cysts:
  - Pyogenic liver abscess.
  - Parasitic liver cysts (hydatid cysts, amebic liver abscess).
  - Post-trauma.

Incidence/prevalence
- Simple cysts: the female to male ratio is 4:1, and the prevalence is approximately 3%.
- PCLD: the exact prevalence in the general population is unknown but it tends to be greater in women and increases with advancing age, severity of renal cystic disease and renal dysfunction.

Mount Sinai Expert Guides: Hepatology, First Edition. Edited by Jawad Ahmad, Scott L. Friedman, and Henryk Dancygier.
© 2014 John Wiley & Sons, Ltd. Published 2014 by John Wiley & Sons, Ltd.
Companion website: www.mountsinaiexpertguides.com

- Cystadenoma/cystadenocarcinoma: these are rare tumours (5% of the reported hepatic cystic lesions). Most occur in women older than 40 years of age.
- Bile duct cysts (Caroli disease): more than 200 cases of Caroli disease have been reported in the literature. Caroli disease is a rare congenital disorder, defined by bile ductular ectasia without other hepatic abnormalities. Caroli syndrome is more frequent than the pure form of Caroli disease where there is associated hepatic fibrosis. The incidence of cholangiocarcinoma in Caroli disease is 10–20%.
- Pyogenic liver abscess: the incidence is 25 per 100 000 pediatric admissions in the USA.
- Parasitic liver cysts (amebic liver abscess): worldwide, approximately 40–50 million people are infected annually, with the majority of infections occurring in developing countries. The prevalence of infection is higher than 5–10% in endemic areas like South Africa and Bangladesh.
- Parasitic liver cysts (hydatid cysts): the incidence of hydatid disease in the USA is very low, with approximately 200 cases presenting per year while in rural areas of developing countries it is largely endemic.
- Post-trauma: rare.

Etiology
- Simple cysts: simple cysts are believed to be the result of excluded hyperplastic bile duct rests.
- PCLD: AD-PCLD is an autosomal dominant disease that is associated with PKD. Affected individuals are found to have mutations of PKD1 (40–75%), and approximately 25% have mutations of the PKD2 gene.
- Cystadenoma/cystadenocarcinoma: unknown.
- Bile duct cysts (Caroli disease): development of these biliary cystic dilations is believed to result from the arrest of or a derangement in the normal embryologic remodeling of the large intrahepatic ducts.
- Pyogenic liver abscess: hematogenous (portal, arterial), biliary or direct inoculation of bacterial infection from trauma.
- Parasitic liver cysts (amebic liver abscess): *Entamoeba histolytica*
- Parasitic liver cysts (hydatid cysts): *Echinococcus granulosus* (cystic echinococcosis) or *E. multilocularis* (alveolar echinococcosis), *E. vogelii* and *E. oligarthros* (extremely rare).
- Post-trauma: trauma.

Section 2: Prevention

Not applicable for this topic.

Section 3: Diagnosis
Simple cyst
- Clinical: most of them are asymptomatic and found incidentally on imaging. Rarely, they may cause pain due to pressure, enlarging size, or bleeding into the cyst. Other causes for abdominal pain should be ruled out first before attributing the symptoms to simple cysts.
- Laboratory: no changes on LFTs.
- Histology: single layer of cuboidal or columnar epithelium (resembling biliary epithelium).
- Imaging: found incidentally – see Figure 31.1.
- On US a simple cyst is an anechoic unilocular lesion, with sharp, smooth borders and posterior acoustic enhancement.

- On CT well-demarcated water attenuation lesion (water density −10 to +10 HU).
- On MRI: simple cysts look hyperintense (bright) on T2-weighted images.

Cystadenoma
- Clinical: abdominal pain, swelling, nausea, and anorexia.
- Laboratory: no changes in LFTs unless the biliary tree is involved, then it can present with cholestasis (elevated direct bilirubin and AP).
- Carbohydrate antigen 19-9 (CA 19-9) levels in the fluid may be increased. Pre-operative fluid sampling is not recommended because of the risk of disseminating malignancy in case of cystadenocarcinoma.
- Histology: large multilocular mucin-filled cyst, with papillary projections resembling ovarian stroma. The lining epithelium is cuboidal or columnar. The cyst wall must be carefully assessed at surgical resection to rule out malignant transformation (cystadenocarcinoma).
- Imaging:
  - US: single, large, anechoic cysts. Some internal echoes showing septation secondary to papillary projections.
  - CT: large cyst, with mural nodules, septations and calcifications.
  - MRI: highly hyperintense on T2-weighted images. Can offer better resolution than CT to show septations and nodules (see Figure 31.2).

PCLD
- Clinical: abdominal pain, distention, postprandial fullness. Complications include: intracystic bleeding, extrinsic compression of the biliary tract and/or infection.
- There is an association with cerebral artery aneurysm.
- Laboratory: no changes unless the biliary tree is obstructed, then it can present with cholestasis (elevated direct bilirubin and AP).
- Histology: single layer of cuboidal or columnar epithelium.
- Imaging:
  - US and CT: multiple fluid-filled round or oval cysts, with distinct margins in the liver and/or kidneys (see Figure 31.3).
  - MRI: hyperintense on T2-weighted images and hypointense on T1-weighted images, except when they are complicated by hemorrhage.

Caroli disease
- Clinical: recurrent cholangitis which is the main cause of morbidity and mortality in these patients.
- Laboratory: leukocytosis and cholestasis during cholangitis.
- Histology: single layer of cuboidal or columnar epithelium.
- Imaging: multiple hepatic cysts on CT and US. Communicating with the biliary tree (can be the only distinction from PCLD).
- MRI: dilated segmental intrahepatic biliary ducts can be seen on MRI. MRCP reveals similar findings as ERCP but has the advantage of being non-invasive (see Figure 31.4).

Hydatid cyst
- Clinical: small – asymptomatic; large – abdominal pain, jaundice (communication with biliary tree).
- Laboratory: serology (ELISA) is 90% sensitive. Can present with cholestatic jaundice in cholangitis.

- Histology: three layers – inner germinal layer, middle laminated layer and an outer fibrous layer (host reaction).
- Imaging:
  - US and CT: shows a large multilayered cyst with partial or full calcification (see Figure 31.5). Daughter cysts can be seen.
  - MRI: is more sensitive than CT scan in showing the different layers of the cyst wall and daughter cysts.

Pyogenic (bacterial) liver abscess
- Clinical: typically fever with RUQ pain and non-specific abdominal symptoms such as nausea, vomiting, malaise and weight loss. Can also present with hepatomegaly and jaundice.
- Laboratory: evidence of infection with elevated white cell count, elevated liver enzymes (particularly AP) and bilirubin. Blood cultures are positive in up to half of all cases. Gram stain and culture of aspirate obtained by CT- or US-guided drainage.
- Imaging:
  - US and CT: show a fluid collection with surrounding edema and occasionally loculation or stranding. A pleural effusion or right lower lung lobe infiltrate can sometimes be seen.

Amebic liver abscess
- Clinical: typically fever with RUQ pain and non-specific abdominal symptoms such as nausea, vomiting, malaise and weight loss. Can also present with hepatomegaly but jaundice is less common than with pyogenic abscess. A history of recent travel (within the last 4–5 months) to endemic areas is usual but occasionally can be much more remote. A diarrheal illness can sometimes accompany the presentation but can also precede the abdominal symptoms.
- Laboratory: evidence of infection with elevated white cell count, elevated liver enzymes (particularly AP). Serology or antigen testing for *Entamoeba histolytica* in blood or stool. Aspiration for diagnosis is usually not required.
- Imaging:
  - Amebic abscess is typically found in the right lobe.
  - US: shows a well-defined hypoechoic mass.
  - CT: typically low density with some peripheral enhancement.
  - MRI: low signal lesion on T1- and high signal on T2-weighted images.
  - Chest X-ray can show a right-sided pleural effusion and/or elevated right hemidiaphragm.

Section 4: Treatment
Simple cyst
- Management:
  - Asymptomatic: best managed with observation.
  - Symptomatic: percutaneous aspiration alone is associated with high recurrence rate and is not recommended Aspiration followed by sclerotherapy is a reasonable option and can provide symptomatic relief in up to 80% of patients. Laparoscopic cyst fenestration is the current treatment of choice with a better long-term relief for up to 90% of patients.

Cystadenoma
- Management: complete surgical resection of the cyst is the only option to prevent recurrence, which usually can be accomplished with cyst enucleation if the location and size permits. If

the diagnosis of cystadenocarcinoma is made, then a formal liver resection with free margins must be performed.

Polycystic liver disease
- Management (challenging – must be patient – tailored):
  - Asymptomatic: observation.
  - Symptomatic: percutaneous aspiration followed by sclerotherapy; cyst fenestration (open or laparoscopic); liver resection; liver transplantation.

Caroli disease
- Management: antibiotics for cholangitis; anatomic liver resections for segmental Caroli disease; liver transplantation for severe and persistent cases.

Hydatid cyst
- Management:
  - Chemotherapy: albendazole (10–15 mg/kg PO divided three times a day for 3–6 months) and mebendazole (40–50 mg/kg PO divided three times a day for 3–6 months) – used as adjuncts to other treatment modalities. Recommended prior to any procedure for 1–3 months to decrease cyst viability.
  - Percutaneous aspiration (under albendazole or mebendazole coverage), injection and re-aspiration: image-guided aspiration for confirmation; followed by injection of a proto-scolicidal agent and then re-aspiration to collapse the treated cavity. Only applicable to uncomplicated cysts surrounded by liver parenchyma.
  - Marsupialization: has the goal of evacuating contents of the cyst and preventing spillage to other areas.
  - Formal and complete cyst resection is more aggressive but the most effective therapy and has the advantage of lower recurrence rate. It should be reserved for experienced centers.

Amebic liver abscess
- Management: the principles of management include parenteral antibiotics (even large abscesses heal with antibiotics), abscess drainage and treatment of the underlying condition.
  - The treatment of uncomplicated cases is metronidazole 500–750 mg PO three times a day for 7–10 days or tinidazole 2 g PO once a day for 5 days. Typically after the initial treatment, therapy is required to clear luminal cysts using diiodohydroxyquin (650 mg PO three times a day for 3 weeks) or paromomycin (25–30 mg/kg PO divided three times a day for 7 days).
  - Patients with imminent rupture of cyst, or failure of symptom resolution, should be considered for percutaneous drainage under metronidazole coverage.

Table of treatment

Cyst type	Conservative treatment	Medical	Surgical	Radiological
Simple	Asymptomatic: observation	N/A	Cyst fenestration (open or laparoscopic)	Percutaneous aspiration followed by sclerotherapy

(Continued)

Cyst type	Conservative treatment	Medical	Surgical	Radiological
Cystadenoma/ cystadenocarcinoma	N/A	N/A	Cystadenoma: complete surgical resection of the cyst Cystadenocarcinoma: formal liver resection with free margins	N/A
PCLD	Asymptomatic: observation	N/A	Percutaneous aspiration followed by sclerotherapy Cyst fenestration (open or laparoscopic) Liver resection Liver transplantation	Percutaneous aspiration followed by sclerotherapy
Caroli disease	Asymptomatic: observation	Antibiotics for cholangitis	Liver resection Liver transplantation for severe cases	N/A
Hydatid cyst	N/A	Albendazole and mebendazole	Cyst marsupialization or resection	Percutaneous aspiration, injection and re-aspiration
Amebic liver abscess	N/A	Metronidazole	N/A	Percutaneous drainage
Pyogenic liver abscess	N/A	Antibiotics	Surgical drainage	Percutaneous drainage

Section 5: Special Populations

Not applicable for this topic.

Section 6: Prognosis

Not applicable for this topic.

Section 7: Reading List

Blessmann J, Ali IK, Nu PA, et al. Longitudinal study of intestinal Entamoeba histolytica infections in asymptomatic adult carriers. J Clin Microbiol 2003;41:4745–50

Boyle MJ, Doyle GD, McNulty JG. Monolobar Caroli's disease. Am J Gastroenterol 1989;84:1437–44

Carrim ZI, Murchison JT. The prevalence of simple renal and hepatic cysts detected by spiral computed tomography. Clin Radiol 2003;58:626–9

Charlesworth P, Ade-Ajayi N, Davenport M. Natural history and long-term followup of antenatally detected liver cysts. J Pediatr Surg 2007;42:494–9

Dixon E, Sutherland FR, Mitchell P, McKinnon G, Nayak V. Cystadenomas of the liver: a spectrum of disease. Can J Surg 2001;44:371–6

Juran BD, Lazaridis KN. Genetics of hepatobiliary diseases. Clin Gastroenterol Hepatol 2006;4:548–57

Nasseri Moghaddam S, Abrishami A, Malekzadeh R. Percutaneous needle aspiration, injection, and reaspiration with or without benzimidazole coverage for uncomplicated hepatic hydatid cysts. Cochrane Database Syst Rev 2006;2:CD003623.

Pineiro-Carrero VM, Andres JM. Morbidity and mortality in children with pyogenic liver Abscess. Am J Dis Child 1989;143:1424–7

Reid-Lombardo KM, Khan S, Sclabas, G. Hepatic cysts and liver abscess. Surg Clin N Am 2010;90:679–97

Sherlock S, Dooley J. Diseases of the Liver and Biliary System. 11th edition. Oxford: Blackwell Science, 2002: 583

Siren J, Karkkainen P, Luukkonen P, et al. A case report of biliary cystadenoma and cystadenocarcinoma. Hepatogastroenterology 1998;45:83–9

Yagci G, Ustunsoz B, Kaymakcioglu N, et al. Results of surgical, laparoscopic, and percutaneous treatment for hydatid disease of the liver: 10 years experience with 355 patients. World J Surg 2005;29:1670–9

Zhang W, McManus DP. Concepts of immunology and diagnosis of hydatid disease. Clin Microbiol Rev 2003;16:18–36

Zinner MJ, Ashley SW. Maingot's Abdominal Operations, 11th edition. New York: McGraw Hill, 2007

Section 8: Guidelines

Not applicable for this topic.

Section 9: Evidence

See Section 7: Reading List.

Section 10: Images

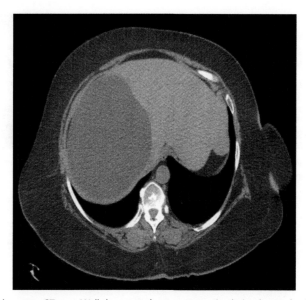

Figure 31.1 Simple cyst on CT scan. Well-demarcated water attenuation lesion (water density −10 to +10 HU)

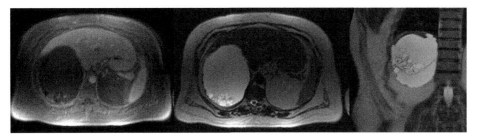

Figure 31.2 Cystadenoma on MRI scan. Arterial-enhancing solid components on posterior wall, nodules and septations

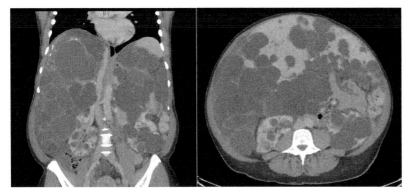

Figure 31.3 Coronal and axial CT scan showing extensive PCLD and PKD

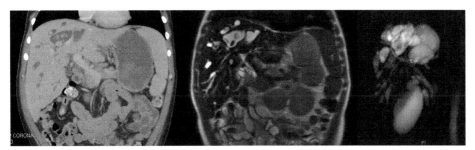

Figure 31.4 CT, MRI/MRCP of a patient with Caroli disease (MRCP showing the communication of the cysts with the biliary system)

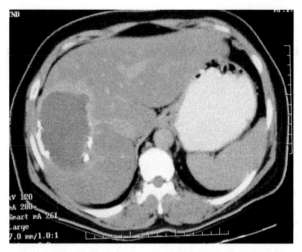

Figure 31.5 CT scan showing a hydatid cyst in the right lobe of liver, complex thick wall with calcifications

Additional material for this chapter can be found online at:
www.mountsinaiexpertguides.com
This includes a case study and multiple choice questions

CHAPTER 32

Surgery in Patients with Liver Disease

Jawad Ahmad

Division of Liver Diseases, Icahn School of Medicine at Mount Sinai, New York, NY, USA

OVERALL BOTTOM LINE
- Patients with underlying acute and chronic liver disease are at risk of morbidity and mortality after surgery.
- The magnitude of the risk is related to the severity of liver disease, the type of surgery and the urgency of the surgery.
- The severity of liver disease as measured by the MELD score and the CTP score can be used to risk stratify patients with liver disease undergoing surgery.
- Even in patients with well-preserved liver synthetic function, the presence of significant portal hypertension can lead to adverse outcomes after surgery, particularly if it involves hepatic resection.
- Acute liver failure and acute AH are generally contraindications for any type of surgery.

Section 1: Background
Definition of disease
- Underlying acute and chronic liver disease has a predictable effect on morbidity and mortality after surgery.
- Quantifying this effect is important prior to surgery to ensure an informed decision is made whether to proceed or not.

Disease classification
- Two scoring systems, the CTP and the MELD have been adapted and evaluated to help clinicians determine perioperative morbidity and mortality in patients with liver disease undergoing surgical procedures.
- The type of surgery and anesthesia also influences the outcome with emergency surgery carrying a particularly high mortality.

Incidence/prevalence
- Based on studies in the 1980s it is estimated that up to 10% of patients with advanced liver disease require a surgical procedure in the final 2 years of life.
- The number of hospital discharges for cirrhosis-related illnesses is close to 400000 annually in the USA and a large number of patients with liver disease will require surgical intervention.

Mount Sinai Expert Guides: Hepatology, First Edition. Edited by Jawad Ahmad, Scott L. Friedman, and Henryk Dancygier.
© 2014 John Wiley & Sons, Ltd. Published 2014 by John Wiley & Sons, Ltd.
Companion website: www.mountsinaiexpertguides.com

Etiology
- The risks of surgery in liver disease vary according to the severity of liver disease, type of surgery and the urgency of the procedure.
- Although all causes of cirrhosis can lead to higher morbidity and mortality after surgery, AH has an extremely high mortality after surgery.
- Fulminant liver failure and acute hepatitis with jaundice also appear to have prohibitive risk for surgery.

Pathology/pathogenesis
- The pathogenesis of worsening liver function after surgery is unclear but several mechanisms have been postulated.
- The fact that the risk of surgery is dependent on the severity of liver disease and to a lesser extent on the type of surgery suggests that changes induced by anesthesia and medications used during surgery play a major role, perhaps affecting hepatic blood flow.
- Advanced liver disease is typically associated with systemic and splanchnic vasodilation that leads to activation of the sympathetic nervous system in an attempt to maintain arterial perfusion.
- The normal cardiac inotropic and chronotropic response to stress may be decreased in cirrhotic patients and the combination of a hyperdynamic circulation without compensatory mechanisms can lead to hepatic hypoperfusion during surgery. This can be exacerbated by the type of surgery (particularly laparotomy or cardiac surgery), hemorrhage, vasoactive medications and even patient positioning.
- Underlying liver disease can significantly impair the metabolism of anesthetics and certain medications used during surgery such as benzodiazepines and narcotics and can lead to prolonged depression of the CNS precipitating HE.
- Anesthesia can lead to changes in blood flow to the liver that can occur with general or regional anesthesia, meaning the risk of decompensation after surgery is not necessarily reduced even if local or spinal anesthesia is employed.

Predictive/risk factors for decompensation after surgery in cirrhotic patients
- Child's C.
- MELD score >15.
- Acute liver failure.
- Jaundice (serum bilirubin >11 mg/dL).
- Emergent surgery.
- Cardiac surgery.
- Abdominal surgery.

Section 2: Prevention

BOTTOM LINE
- No intervention has been shown to prevent the development of hepatic decompensation after surgery in patients with significant liver disease.

Screening

- In patients already known to have liver disease or cirrhosis no screening is required but risk stratification is important.
- However, since liver disease can often be asymptomatic it is important to take a thorough history and physical examination in all patients due to undergo surgery.
- The history will provide any risk factors for viral or alcoholic liver disease.
- A full review of medications is important since drug induced liver disease is common.
- Physical examination should concentrate on looking for stigmata of chronic liver disease.
- There is limited utility in looking for underlying liver disease with blood tests unless there is a clinical suspicion.
- An older study demonstrated only 11 of 7620 patients undergoing elective surgery had abnormal liver tests.
- In addition, liver tests can be normal in well-compensated cirrhotics.

Section 3: Diagnosis (Algorithm 32.1)

> **BOTTOM LINE/CLINICAL PEARLS**
> - The history and physical examination remain key in detecting liver disease in patients undergoing surgery.
> - In patients with known liver disease, jaundice, prior gastrointestinal bleeding, ascites and encephalopathy in the history may demonstrate evidence of decompensated liver disease.
> - In such patients, the physical examination should look for stigmata of chronic liver disease and portal hypertension.
> - Laboratory investigations should include a chemistry panel with emphasis on serum bilirubin, albumin, prothrombin time, creatinine and a CBC.
> - Abdominal imaging may be required to look for evidence of cirrhosis or portal hypertension.

Typical presentation

- Gastroenterologists or hepatologists are commonly asked to provide a risk assessment before surgery on patients with known liver disease.
- In this situation it is important to determine the severity of liver disease based on the CPT and MELD scores, the type of surgery and anesthesia and the urgency of the surgery.
- Other than deferring surgery in some patients who may have a reversible liver illness, there are no real interventions that can decrease the risk of surgery.
- The primary role of the consultant is to provide an opinion as to the perioperative risk which can then lead to a discussion as to whether to proceed depending on the risk–benefit ratio.

Clinical diagnosis

History

- Patients without a prior history of liver disease should be questioned regarding risk factors such as prior remote blood transfusions, tattoos, illicit drug use, alcohol intake, sexual history, personal history of jaundice, or a family history of liver disease.
- The medication history should include prescription medications but it is important to ask about over-the-counter analgesics and complementary or alternative medications, particularly herbal supplements.

Algorithm 32.1 Diagnostic algorithm for pre-operative assessment in patients with suspected liver disease

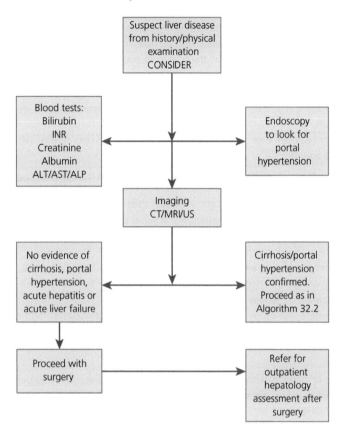

- The review of systems should discuss any excessive fatigue, pruritus and easy bruisability which may be indicators of underlying liver dysfunction.
- In patients with known liver disease the history should concentrate on complaints that might suggest decompensated disease such as:
  - Hematemesis, melena or symptoms compatible with gastrointestinal bleeding.
  - Abdominal distension and ankle edema.
  - Forgetfulness or confusion.

Physical examination
- The physical examination should look for stigmata of chronic liver disease such as the presence of jaundice, palmar erythema, spider nevi, parotid gland enlargement, Dupuytren's contracture, splenomegaly, ascites, dilated abdominal veins, lower extremity edema, gynecomastia, testicular atrophy and temporal wasting or loss of muscle mass.

Useful clinical decision rules and calculators

- In patients with cirrhosis, grading the severity of the liver disease is important in determining the perioperative risk.
- The CTP score and the MELD score have been evaluated and are useful predictive models to determine the risk of surgery in patients with cirrhosis.
- Several studies have demonstrated that the CTP score correlates with outcome after abdominal surgery with mortality rates of:
  - Child's A 10%
  - Child's B 30%
  - Child's C 80%
- The MELD score has been even more extensively investigated. It uses serum bilirubin, creatinine and INR in the equation:

$$\text{MELD score} = (9.6 \times \log_e[\text{creatinine}]) + (3.8 \times \log_e[\text{bilirubin}]) + (11.2 \times \log_e[\text{INR}]) + 6.4$$

(value of creatinine, bilirubin or INR cannot be less than 1.0 for the equation. Creatinine and bilirubin in mg/dL and values >40 are assigned a value of 40).

- In general a MELD score of <10 is considered low risk, MELD score 10–15 intermediate risk and MELD score >15 is high risk.
- The largest study looked at almost 800 patients undergoing major digestive, orthopedic or cardiac surgery and determined that for each point increase in the MELD score above 8, there was a 14% increase in 30 day and 90 day mortality.
- The type of surgery also influences outcome. Emergency surgery carries high mortality in cirrhotic patients but cardiac surgery involving cardiopulmonary bypass and abdominal surgery including colectomy, cholecystectomy, gastric surgery and liver resection appear to have the greatest risk.
- Several groups of patients without cirrhosis also have prohibitive risk for surgery and hence it should be avoided unless the situation is life threatening:
  - Acute liver failure.
  - Acute AH.
  - Serum bilirubin >11 mg/dL.

Disease severity classification

- The CTP and MELD scores are accurate methods to determine the severity of liver disease in patients undergoing surgery.

Laboratory diagnosis

List of diagnostic tests

- In patients without known liver disease and no concern for cirrhosis or portal hypertension on history and physical examination, routine laboratory tests to screen for liver disease are not necessary.
- If patients have had laboratory tests already drawn as part of the pre-surgery investigations and liver test abnormalities are detected it is reasonable to defer elective surgery until a more thorough investigation can be performed to determine the nature, chronicity and severity of any underlying liver disease.
- For patients who are asymptomatic with mild elevations in aminotransferases and normal total bilirubin concentration, cancellation of surgery should not usually be required.

- However, elevations in aminotransferase levels greater than three times the upper limits of normal or abnormalities in synthetic function such as bilirubin and prothrombin time require further investigation.
- This should include viral hepatitis serology for hepatitis B and C, specific tests for metabolic liver disease such as iron studies for hemochromatosis, ceruloplasmin level for Wilson disease, alpha-1 antitrypsin level and phenotyping, and serum markers for autoimmune liver disease.
- In patients with known liver disease presenting for surgery it is important to determine their CPT and MELD score with serum bilirubin, albumin, creatinine and prothrombin time and an assessment of the degree of portal hypertension such as platelet count.

List of imaging techniques
- In patients without known liver disease undergoing surgery, no imaging study is necessary unless the history and physical examination suggests evidence of cirrhosis or portal hypertension. Patients undergoing abdominal surgery will most likely have already had imaging.
- If significant liver disease is suspected, an abdominal imaging study such as ultrasound or CT or MRI scan would not be unreasonable.
- If abdominal surgery is planned, particularly if it involves liver resection, an upper GI endoscopy to look for portal hypertension can be performed.

Potential pitfalls/common errors made regarding diagnosis of disease
- Patients with cirrhosis can have normal liver synthetic function yet still have significant portal hypertension that can influence outcome after surgery, particularly intra-abdominal or hepatic surgery.
- Failure to detect cirrhosis can lead to decompensated liver disease several months after routine surgery – a not uncommon finding in patients presenting for liver transplant evaluation.

Section 4: Treatment (Algorithm 32.2)
Treatment rationale
- In patients who are about to undergo elective surgery, a thorough history and physical examination is sufficient to look for underlying liver disease and if negative no further investigation is required.
- In patients with known liver disease it is important to determine the CPT and MELD score and the degree of portal hypertension.
- The decision to proceed with the surgery will depend on the severity of liver disease, the urgency and type of surgery and the type of anesthesia.
- Well-compensated cirrhotic patients with a MELD score <10 and minimal or no portal hypertension or patients without cirrhosis and mild elevation of liver enzymes should be able to proceed.
- In Child's B patients or MELD score 10–15, there needs to be a discussion with the surgery team and patient regarding the risk–benefit ratio of proceeding.
- In Child's C patients or MELD score >15, elective or non-life threatening condition surgery should not proceed. In a life-threatening situation or in other selected situations, surgery can proceed after ensuring all interested parties are aware of the risks.
- Acute liver failure and acute AH are typically contraindications to any type of surgery.

Algorithm 32.2 Pre-operative assessment in patients with known liver disease

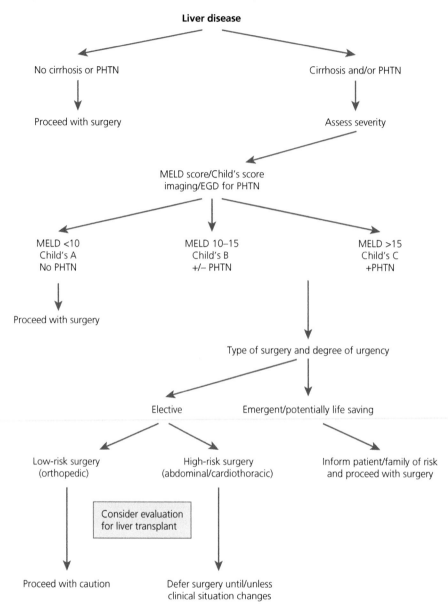

Table of treatment

Treatment	Comment
Medical	No medical treatment has been proven effective in reducing the risk of surgery in cirrhotic patients
	However, if surgery is planned it is reasonable to optimize the patient medically by correcting coagulopathy, minimizing ascites, correcting electrolyte abnormalities and avoiding precipitants of hepatic encephalopathy and hepatorenal syndrome
Surgical treatment in cirrhotic patients: Abdominal surgery	Child's A patients have 10% mortality Child's B patients have 30% mortality Child's C patients have 80% mortality
Cardiac surgery	Child's A patients have 0–11% mortality Child's B patients have 18–50% mortality Child's C patients have 67–100% mortality
Abdominal/cardiac/orthopedic surgery	MELD <8 associated with 5.7% mortality MELD >20 associated with >50% mortality
Radiological: TIPS	Several case series have tried using TIPS to decrease portal hypertension prior to abdominal surgery with mixed results so cannot be recommended

Prevention/management of complications
- The only way to prevent liver-related morbidity and mortality in patients after surgery is to avoid the surgery.
- There are no real pharmacological methods to optimize patient outcome in this situation other than waiting for acute liver disease to improve or occasionally waiting until after liver transplantation (such as with umbilical hernia surgery), or very rarely performing surgery at the same time as liver transplantation (such as transplant and Whipple procedure, transplant and cardiac surgery and combined liver and kidney transplant).

CLINICAL PEARLS
- Child's class A or MELD score <10 are at low risk for death after elective surgery.
- Child's B or MELD 10–15 are at moderate risk, and surgery should be considered depending on the indication and urgency.
- Child's C or MELD >15 are at high risk, and surgery should be avoided or deferred until the clinical situation changes.

Section 5: Special Populations
Others
- Patients with acute AH have a very high mortality risk after surgery and hence elective surgery is contraindicated.

Section 6: Prognosis

> **BOTTOM LINE**
> - The prognosis after surgery in patients with liver disease can be predicted reasonably accurately based on their pre-operative CPT or MELD score and the type and urgency of surgery.
> - Decompensation of liver disease can occur in the immediate post-operative period but can also occur up to several months later.
> - It is important to discuss the risk of surgery with the patient and family prior to the surgery so that an informed decision can be made to proceed with or defer the procedure.

Follow-up tests and monitoring
- After any type of surgery in patients with liver disease, regular follow up for several months should include assessment clinically to look for evidence of decompensation with ascites, encephalopathy, hepatorenal syndrome and portal hypertensive bleeding.
- Regular laboratory studies should be undertaken including liver synthetic function and renal function.
- In patients with worsening liver function and no contraindication, early evaluation for liver transplant should be offered.

Section 7: Reading List

Farnsworth N, Fagan SP, Berger DH, et al. Child-Turcotte-Pugh versus MELD score as a predictor of outcome after elective and emergent surgery in cirrhotic patients. Am J Surg 2004;188:580–3

Garrison RN, Cryer HM, Howard DA, Polk HC Jr. Clarification of risk factors for abdominal operations in patients with hepatic cirrhosis. Ann Surg 1984;199:648–55

Malik SM, Ahmad J. Preoperative risk assessment for patients with liver disease. Med Clin North Am 2009;93:917–29

Schemel W. Unexpected hepatic dysfunction found by multiple laboratory screening. Anesth Analg 1976;55:810–12

Suman A, Barnes DS, Zein NN, et al. Predicting outcome after cardiac surgery in patients with cirrhosis: a comparison of Child-Pugh and MELD scores. Clin Gastroenterol Hepatol 2004;2:719–23

Teh SH, Nagorney DM, Stevens SR, et al. Risk factors for mortality after surgery in patients with cirrhosis. Gastroenterology 2007;132:1609–11

Suggested website
A model to calculate the post-operative mortality risk in patients with cirrhosis can be found at http://www.mayoclinic.org/meld/mayomodel9.html

Section 8: Guidelines

Not applicable for this topic.

Section 9: Evidence

Type of evidence	Title, date	Comment
Case series	Abdominal operations in patients with cirrhosis: still a major surgical challenge. Surgery 1997;122:730	Demonstrated very high (50%) mortality after emergent abdominal surgery in cirrhotic patients
Case series	Surgical resection of hepatocellular carcinoma in cirrhotic patients: prognostic value of pre-operative portal pressure. Gastroenterology 1996;111:1018	Demonstrated that portal hypertension is an important factor in predicting decompensation after hepatic resection
Case series	Risk factors for mortality after surgery in patients with cirrhosis. Gastroenterology 2007;132:1261	Demonstrated that the MELD score was an accurate predictor of post-operative mortality in cirrhotic patients, irrespective of the type of surgery

Section 10: Images

Not applicable for this topic.

Additional material for this chapter can be found online at:
www.mountsinaiexpertguides.com
This includes a case study and multiple choice questions

CHAPTER 33

Nutrition in Liver Diseases

James S. Park

Division of Gastroenterology, NYU School of Medicine, New York, NY, USA

OVERALL BOTTOM LINE
- The risk of malnutrition is shown to correlate with severity of disease in cirrhotic patients. PEM is frequently found in decompensated cirrhotic patients at the time of liver transplantation.
- Malnutrition is linked to an increased risk of complications and death in cirrhotic patients awaiting liver transplantation. Poor nutritional status affects the transplant surgical outcome and post-transplant survival.
- Early recognition and treatment of malnutrition are important in the management of cirrhotic patients, especially those who are listed for transplantation.

Section 1: Background
Definition of disease
- Malnutrition is the condition where the human body does not get or process the right amount of the vitamins, minerals and other nutrients necessary to maintain health of tissues and organ function.

Disease classification
- Malnutrition can be classified into macronutrient and micronutrient deficiencies. The macronutrients include protein, lipid and carbohydrate which are cellular building blocks. The micronutrients include mineral (trace elements), electrolytes and vitamins which are key factors for many metabolic regulatory processes.
- The most common form of macronutrient deficiency in ESLD is protein–energy malnutrition (PEM which is also called protein–calorie malnutrition) characterized by wasting of muscle mass and loss of fat stores.

Incidence/prevalence
- Prevalence for malnutrition is varied; however, virtually all cirrhotic patients at the time of liver transplantation have a form of malnutrition.

Mount Sinai Expert Guides: Hepatology, First Edition. Edited by Jawad Ahmad, Scott L. Friedman, and Henryk Dancygier.
© 2014 John Wiley & Sons, Ltd. Published 2014 by John Wiley & Sons, Ltd.
Companion website: www.mountsinaiexpertguides.com

- Most studies suggest that malnutrition is routinely under-diagnosed and under-treated in cirrhotic patients.

Economic impact
- There is no clear data on the economic impact of malnutrition. However, it has been shown that cirrhotic patients with PEM have an increased risk of infection, encephalopathy, prolonged hospitalization and death before and after liver transplantation.

Etiology
- The etiology of malnutrition in cirrhosis is complex and multifactorial.
- Protein, carbohydrate, and lipid metabolism are all affected by liver disease.
- Poor nutritional intake, impaired absorptive function, altered metabolism and iatrogenic effect from medical treatment are all thought to contribute to malnutrition in cirrhosis.

Pathology/pathogenesis
- Poor dietary intake is common in cirrhotic patients with ascites. This is often due to anorexia and early satiety associated with large ascites affecting gastric emptying and motility.
- Patients often complain of loss of appetite due to strict sodium restriction imposed by clinicians for treatment of ascites. A low sodium diet makes food unpleasant to taste.
- Cholestasis from cirrhosis or cholestatic liver disease leads to a decreased amount of bile flow which is necessary for digestion and absorption of fat and fat-soluble such as vitamins A, D, E and K.
- The use of laxatives such as lactulose and non-absorbable antibiotics for treatment of encephalopathy further increase the risk of malabsorption of protein, fat and micronutrients such as calcium and zinc. These patients frequently have occult steatorrhea which is a clinical sign of fat digestion and malabsorption.
- Gastrointestinal mucosal edema from portal hypertension and low gastric acid output state from portal gastropathy or from use of PPIs further make intestinal absorption of various nutrients such as iron, calcium and protein difficult.
- The liver is a key organ responsible for metabolism of macronutrients such as protein, carbohydrate and lipid. Metabolism and processing of these macronutrients are affected by hepatic dysfunction caused by cirrhosis.
- There is impaired storage of glycogen in the liver which affects glycogenolysis and gluconeogenesis in the fasting state. This leads to accelerated starvation with early recruitment of alternative fuel sources such as protein first, followed by fat second. This leads to a catabolic state with negative nitrogen balance. This is a central reason why cirrhotic patients develop PEM with loss of muscle and fat mass.
- Liver cirrhosis is a hyperinsulinemic state due to impaired clearance of insulin and peripheral insulin resistance. Peripheral insulin resistance with abnormal glucose is seen early in the course of cirrhosis. As the severity of hepatic dysfunction worsens, patients often develop nocturnal hypoglycemia due to impaired hepatic gluconeogenesis in the fasting state.

Predictive/risk factors
- The severity of hepatic dysfunction in cirrhosis correlates with the degree of malnutrition.
- Other risk factors for malnutrition include alcoholic liver disease and cholestatic liver diseases such as PBC, PSC and biliary atresia.

Section 2: Prevention

> **BOTTOM LINE/CLINICAL PEARLS**
> * It is important to identify and screen patients at risk of developing malnutrition.
> * Clinicians should assume that inadequate dietary intake and PEM are present in almost all cirrhotic patients.
> * Nutritional assessment, screening, counseling and treatment should be offered to all cirrhotic patients routinely.
> * Balanced diet, exercise and nutritional supplements can prevent and treat malnutrition.

Screening
* A thorough nutritional assessment should be performed routinely in patients with cirrhosis and cholestatic liver disease. These patients should be routinely screened for fat soluble vitamins (A, D, E, K) and for anemia (iron, folate and vitamin B12).
* Patients with hepatic encephalopathy, chronic renal insufficiency and lactulose-induced diarrhea should be screened for zinc deficiency.
* Serum nutritional markers become less reliable as the severity of hepatic dysfunction and cirrhosis worsens.

Primary prevention
* Nutritional screening for malnutrition and dietary education should be offered to all patients with chronic liver disease.

Secondary prevention
* Periodic assessment should be undertaken to evaluate overall nutritional status.

Section 3: Diagnosis

> **BOTTOM LINE/CLINICAL PEARLS**
> * The approach to patients with chronic liver disease includes a thorough history including nutritional assessment, physical examination and appropriate laboratory studies.
> * Body weight can be misleading in patients with ascites and peripheral edema.
> * Protein catabolism is a hallmark of advanced cirrhosis. Assessment of plasma proteins such as albumin and pre-albumin are less reliable in cirrhosis due to impaired visceral protein synthesis in the liver.
> * Several studies have shown that anthropometric measurements to assess muscle and fat mass and hand grip strength assessments are well correlated to other sophisticated tests such as bioelectrical impedance and dual X-ray absorptiometry.

Typical presentation
* The typical presentation of malnutrition can be elicited from nutritional history and physical findings. Occasionally the patient may have symptoms related to specific micronutrient deficiency. However, the majority of patients often do not have specific symptoms.

Clinical diagnosis

History

- Nutritional assessment can be difficult in cirrhotic patients as conventional nutritional assessment tools become less reliable as hepatic function worsens.
- Fluid excess such as ascites and edema causes overestimation of BMI and actual body weight.
- Hepatic dysfunction impairs protein synthesis such as coagulation factors, albumin and pre-albumin. Therefore, these laboratory tests become less reliable in cirrhotic patients.
- SGA is a technique that combines multiple parts to assess nutritional status. These parts are weight change during the past 6 months, change in dietary intake via dietary recall, gastrointestinal symptoms (emesis, diarrhea and steatorrhea), functional capacity, metabolic demands, signs of muscle wasting and the presence of pre-sacral or pedal edema. SGA has a high interobserver reproducibility rate of 80%.
- Qualitative stool fat should be performed intermittently in patients with cholestatic and alcoholic cirrhosis.
- The assessment of muscle function measuring hand-grip strength and respiratory muscle strength has also been used in nutritional evaluation. Serial hand-grip strength is a good predictor of complications in patients with advanced liver cirrhosis.
- The assessment of muscle function measuring hand-grip strength and respiratory muscle strength has also been used in nutritional evaluation.
- Several studies have shown that anthropometric measurements to assess muscle and fat mass and hand grip strength assessments are well correlated to other sophisticated tests such as bioelectrical impedance and dual x-ray absorptiometry.

Physical examination

- During physical examination, signs of hepatic decompensation, such as encephalopathy, jaundice, ascites, edema, rash and bruising should be noted.
- Height and weight should be recorded with special attention to ascites and edema which can affect the actual body weight.
- It is important to look for signs and symptoms of specific micronutrient deficiencies such as acrodermatitis and change in taste from zinc deficiency, osteoporosis from vitamin D deficiency, glossitis and angular stomatitis from vitamin B deficiency and pale oral mucosa from iron deficiency.
- The table "Nutritional problems in liver diseases" summarizes the potential findings seen in different nutritional deficiencies.

Nutritional problems in liver diseases		
Mineral deficiency	• Iron	• Microcytic hypochromic anemia
	• Selenium	• Cardiomyopathy
	• Zinc	• Alopecia, rash, diarrhea, poor wound healing, encephalopathy
	• Chromium	• Glucose intolerance, encephalopathy, peripheral neuropathy
	• Iodine	• Hypothyroidism, goiter

(Continued)

Vitamin deficiency	• A (Retinol)	• Night blindness, dysgeusia (taste change)
	• B1 (Thiamine)	• Beriberi, cardiac problems, Wernicke's encephalopathy
	• B2 (Riboflavin)	• Cheilosis, angular stomatitis
	• B3 (Niacin)	• Pellagra (dermatitis, dementia, diarrhea)
	• B5 (Pantothenic acid)	• Paresthesias, weakness
	• B6 (Pyridoxine)	• Seborrheic dermatitis, glossitis
	• B7 (Biotin)	• Seborrheic dermatitis, alopecia, encephalopathy
	• B9 (Folic acid)	• Megaloblastic anemia, glossitis
	• B12 (Cobalamin)	• Megaloblastic anemia, ataxia, decreased vibratory or position sense
	• C (Ascorbic acid)	• Scurvy, gingival bleeding, depression
	• D (Ergocalciferol)	• Rickets, osteomalacia, neuropathy
	• E (α-tocopherol)	• Hemolysis, retinopathy, neuropathy
	• K (Phylloquinone)	• Easy bruising and bleeding
Macronutrient deficiency	Protein (PEM)	• Temporal wasting, thenar atrophy, triceps skinfold thickness <3 mm, alopecia, weakness
	Essential fatty acids (alpha-linolenic acid and linoleic acid)	• Dermatitis
	Carbohydrates	• Nocturnal hypoglycemia

Useful clinical decision rules and calculators
- The total BMI = weight in kg/height in m^2. Normal range is from 18 to 25.
- IBW – estimated IBW in (kg):
  - Males: IBW = 50 kg + 2.3 kg for each inch over 5 feet.
  - Females: IBW = 45.5 kg + 2.3 kg for each inch over 5 feet.
- ABW – estimated ABW (kg):
  - If the actual body weight is greater than 30% of the calculated IBW, calculate the ABW:
    ABW = IBW + 0.4(actual weight – IBW)

Laboratory diagnosis
List of diagnostic tests
- Conventional laboratory tests for malnutrition such as albumin, pre-albumin, prothrombin time, and triglycerides are useful in early chronic liver diseases. However, these tests become unreliable with more severe hepatic dysfunction.

Potential pitfalls/common errors made regarding diagnosis of disease
- Malnutrition is often under-diagnosed and under-treated.

Section 4: Treatment
Treatment rationale
- In patients with compensated cirrhosis, the European Society for Clinical Nutrition and Metabolism recommend that patients consume 25–35 kcal/kg ABW per day of total energy source and 1.0–1.2 g/kg ABW per day of protein to maintain a positive nitrogen balance.

- Patients with decompensated cirrhosis with clinical features of muscle wasting are in a higher degree of catabolic state. They should have 35–40 kcal/kg ABW per day and 1.2–1.5 g/kg ABW per day of protein intake to keep a positive nitrogen balance.
- Patients with alcoholic liver disease and cholestatic liver disease are at higher risk of micronutritional deficiencies such as vitamins and trace elements. They should be routinely screened with appropriate blood tests and treated accordingly.
- Parenteral and enteral nutrition has been used in patients with advanced liver disease to improve their nutritional status, especially before surgery. Enteral nutrition is preferable to parenteral nutrition due to the higher risks of infection and liver dysfunction (parenteral nutrition associated cholestasis) linked to parenteral nutrition.
- Protein restriction is not recommended for treatment of encephalopathy. The vast majority of patients with advanced cirrhosis and alcoholic liver disease can tolerate a large quantity of protein in the diet. In cases of refractory encephalopathy, no more than 2–3 days of protein reduction should be used.
- Fasting should be avoided unless it is absolutely necessary. Even a short period of fasting puts the cirrhotic patient in an accelerated starvation and protein catabolism state which is an important source of endogenous ammonia production and hepatic encephalopathy.
- The use of branch-chain amino acids in patients with refractory hepatic encephalopathy is controversial but may have a distinct role.
- Salt restriction makes foods less desirable. Therefore, the degree of salt restriction should be balanced with amount of caloric intake and food palatability.
- Patients with decompensated liver cirrhosis and/or alcoholic cirrhosis should have their calorie intake spread throughout the day with five to seven small meals in the forms of complex carbohydrate, lipid and protein.
- Lipids are a good source of energy in cirrhotic patients and should supply 20–40% of caloric need.
- Late night snacks with complex carbohydrates is an important way to combat protein catabolism and nocturnal hypoglycemia.
- In hospitalized decompensated liver patients, enteral feeding is safe even in patients with non-bleeding esophageal varices. A short course of enteral feeding improves liver function, encephalopathy and survival.

Section 5: Special Populations

Not applicable for this topic.

Section 6: Prognosis

BOTTOM LINE/CLINICAL PEARLS
- Malnutrition is associated with significant mortality in patients with cirrhosis.
- Untreated malnutrition affects mortality and morbidity in patients waiting for liver transplantation.

Follow-up tests and monitoring
- SGA.
- Body weight change.

- Anthropometric measurement such as mid-arm muscle circumference to measure muscle mass and triceps skin fold thickness to assess fat mass.
- Hand-grip strength test.
- Appropriate blood tests for micronutrient deficiency.

Section 7: Reading List

Cabre E, Gassull M. Nutritional aspects of liver disease and transplantation. Curr Opin Clin Nutr Metabol Care 2001;4:581–9

Figueiredo FA, Dickson ER, Pasha TM, et al. Utility of standard nutritional parameters in detecting body cell mass depletion in patients with end-stage liver disease. Liver Transpl 2000;6:575–81

Lautz, HU, Selberg, O, Korber, J et al. Protein-calorie malnutrition in liver cirrhosis. Clin Investig 1992;70:478

Matos C, Porayko MK, Francisco-Ziller N, et al. Nutrition and chronic liver disease. J Clin Gastroenterol 2002;35:391–7

Nompleggi DJ, Bonkovsky HL. Nutritional supplementation in chronic liver disease: an analytical review. Hepatology 1994;19:518–33

Plank LD, Gane EJ, Peng S, et al. Nocturnal nutritional supplementation improves total body protein status of patients with liver cirrhosis: a randomized 12-month trial. Hepatology 2008;48:557–66

Section 8: Guidelines

International society guidelines

Guideline title	Guideline source	Date
ESPEN practice guidelines	The European Society for Clinical Metabolism and Nutrition (ESPEN) http://espen.info/documents/0909/Hepatology.pdf http://espen.info/documents/ENSurgery.pdf	2009 2006

Section 9: Evidence

Type of evidence	Title, date	Comment
Randomized control study	Nocturnal nutritional supplementation improves total body protein status of patients with liver cirrhosis: a randomized 12-month trial. Hepatology 2008;48:557–66	First large randomized control study to demonstrate benefit of nocturnal nutrition supplement to improve the nutritional status

Section 10: Images

Not applicable for this topic.

Additional material for this chapter can be found online at:
www.mountsinaiexpertguides.com
This includes a case study and multiple choice questions

PART 2

PEDIATRICS

CHAPTER 34

Diagnosis and Management of Acute Liver Failure: A Pediatric Perspective

Tamir Miloh

Department of Gastroenterology and Hepatology, Phoenix Children's Hospital, Phoenix, AZ, USA

OVERALL BOTTOM LINE
- Diagnosis of ALF in children is more complex than in adults, as encephalopathy may be subtle, appear late and may even remain unrecognized.
- History is usually taken from the family in younger children and should focus on age of presentation (neonate, toddler, adolescent), family history and consanguinity, perinatal course, newborn screen results, growth and development, feeding (breast milk, fructose), episodes of fasting, school performance, available drugs and over-the-counter medications.
- The most common etiology for ALF in children in the Western world remains indeterminate (non-A-E hepatitis) and is a diagnosis of exclusion.
- Children with ALF should be referred to a pediatric liver transplant center. Children with encephalopathy or an INR >4 (without encephalopathy) should be admitted to an ICU for continuous monitoring.
- In neonatal liver failure, IV acyclovir should be started at the earliest opportunity, while awaiting definitive diagnosis. Specific therapies are available for HSV, acetaminophen overdose, several metabolic diseases, neonatal hemochromatosis, hemophagocytic syndrome, Wilson disease and AIH.
- Liver transplantation remains the definitive treatment with utility of reduced (split) and living donor grafts to increase the donor pool.

Section 1: Background
Definition
- The definition of ALF in children is more complex than in adults – encephalopathy may be subtle, appear late and may even remain unrecognized.
- A practical definition of ALF suggested by the PALF study group is "coagulopathy with INR of ≥1.5 with encephalopathy or INR ≥2 without encephalopathy due to a liver cause, not correctable by intravenous vitamin K," with biochemical evidence of acute liver injury and no evidence of chronic liver disease.

Mount Sinai Expert Guides: Hepatology, First Edition. Edited by Jawad Ahmad, Scott L. Friedman, and Henryk Dancygier.
© 2014 John Wiley & Sons, Ltd. Published 2014 by John Wiley & Sons, Ltd.
Companion website: www.mountsinaiexpertguides.com

Disease classification

- The 1993 classification defines hyperacute, acute and subacute liver failure as coagulopathy and encephalopathy developing within 1 week, 8–28 days and 4–12 weeks within onset of jaundice.

Incidence and prevalence

- A USA population-based surveillance for ALF conducted in 2007 showed an annual incidence of 5.5 per million among all ages.
- The exact frequency of ALF in children is unknown.

Etiologies of ALF in children

- The etiology for ALF in children differs from adults and varies by age and geography (in the developing world, hepatitis A and other infections are more common).
- The most common etiology for ALF in children in the Western world remains indeterminate (non-A-E hepatitis) and is a diagnosis of exclusion.
- In children 0–3 years: indeterminate 54%, metabolic 15% (tyrosinemia, galactosemia, hereditary fructose intolerance), viral 8% (HSV, echovirus, adenovirus, HBV), ischemia 4% (congenital heart disease, cardiac surgery, myocarditis, severe asphyxia), autoimmune 4%, acetaminophen 3% and other 12% (neonatal hemochromatosis, sepsis, medications [valproate, isoniazid], hemophagocytic syndrome).
- HBV is less common in children as a cause for ALF. Infants born to mothers who have active hepatitis and are HBeAg negative are at risk for ALF presenting around 3 weeks to 3 months of age.
- In children 3–18 years: indeterminate 47%, acetaminophen 18%, autoimmune 8% (mostly LKM positive, type 2), metabolic 7% (Wilson disease), drugs 6%, viral 4%, ischemia 4% (Budd–Chiari syndrome), and other 6% (including malignancy and hyperthermia).

Pathology/pathogenesis

- The mechanisms that underlie the poor regenerative response in ALF are not well defined. Massive destruction of hepatocytes may represent a direct cytotoxic effect (virus), accumulation of potentially hepatotoxic metabolites (drugs, inborn errors of metabolism) or oxidative damage (Wilson disease or neonatal hemochromatosis).
- Patchy or confluent, massive necrosis of hepatocytes is commonly found on liver biopsy or explant. Centrilobular necrosis is found in acetaminophen intoxication or circulatory shock and microvesicular fatty change of hepatocytes in inborn errors of metabolism and valproate hepatotoxicity. Hepatocyte death may occur predominantly by apoptosis rather than by necrosis in some metabolic disorders. Liver biopsy is rarely helpful in ALF and is usually contraindicated because of the presence of coagulopathy.
- Children who develop ALF may have an underlying altered immune response that increases the risk of ALF and infections.

Predictive/risk factors

- The prognosis is dependent on the etiology.
- Poor prognostic factors:
  - INR >4: 73% of children with an INR <4 surviving without OLT compared with 16.6% with an INR >4.
  - Grade 3–4 encephalopathy.
  - Factor V concentration <25%.
  - Metabolic acidosis with arterial pH <7.3 after the second day of acetaminophen overdose in adequately hydrated patients is associated with 90% transplant free mortality.

- Hepatorenal syndrome.
- Jaundice for more than 7 days prior to the onset of encephalopathy.
- ALF in Wilson disease, non-acetaminophen drug-induced ALF, indeterminate (non-A-E) hepatitis and AIH with encephalopathy.
- A prognostic score is available predicting the outcome of decompensated Wilson disease, incorporating bilirubin, INR, AST, WBC, and albumin at presentation.

Section 2: Prevention

Not applicable for this topic.

Section 3: Diagnosis

> **BOTTOM LINE**
> - History is usually taken from the family in younger children and should focus on age of presentation (neonate, toddler, adolescent), family history and consanguinity, perinatal course, newborn screen results, growth and development, feeding (breast milk (lactose), fructose), episodes of fasting, school performance, available drugs and over-the-counter medications.
> - Physical examination is similar to adults. However, encephalopathy may be subtle and special attention given to dysmorphic features (genetic disease) and growth and development.
> - Laboratory tests should include blood glucose (particularly in infants), electrolytes, INR and daily CBC with surveillance blood and urine cultures. For testing for etiology see Algorithm 34.1.
> - Liver biopsy is rarely helpful and usually contraindicated due to coagulopathy.

Differential diagnosis
- Other causes of coagulopathy in the presence of liver disease should be considered.

Differential diagnosis	Features
Vitamin K deficiency	History of cholestasis or biliary obstruction Factors II, VII, IX, X low Factor V (not vitamin K dependent) and factor VIII (extrahepatic production) are normal
Sepsis	Fever, other signs and symptoms of infection (cardiovascular, etc.) Elevated fibrinogen split products Low fibrinogen and platelets All factors (II, V, VII, VIII, IX, X) low as consumption coagulopathy
Chronic liver disease	Onset of jaundice >8 weeks Other signs and symptoms of chronic liver disease and portal hypertension: ascites, splenomegaly, growth failure, caput medusae, clubbing

Typical presentation
- The child with fulminant hepatic failure usually has been previously healthy. Progressive jaundice, anorexia, vomiting and abdominal pain are commonly observed. Hepatic encephalopathy

Algorithm 34.1 Diagnosis of acute liver failure in children

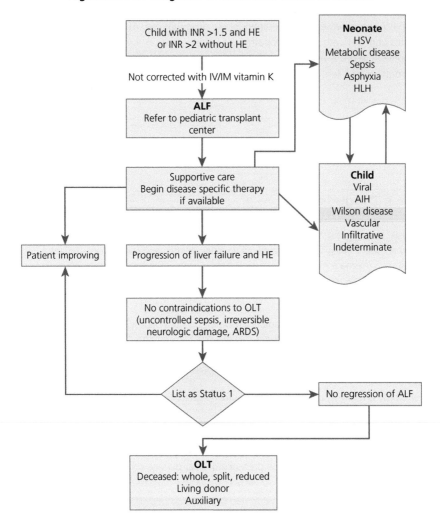

may be initially characterized by irritability, poor feeding, and a change in sleep rhythm in infants and disturbances of consciousness or motor functioning in older children.
- Progression can occur over the course of a few days or weeks.
- Bleeding from the GI tract and easy bruising, as a result of severe coagulopathy.

Clinical diagnosis
History
- History is usually taken from the family in younger children and should focus on age of presentation (neonate, toddler, adolescent), family history (liver disease, miscarriages or neonatal deaths) and consanguinity, antenatal and perinatal course, newborn screen results, growth and development, feeding (breast milk, lactose, fructose), episodes of fasting, sick contacts, constitutional symptoms, fever, fatigue, abdominal pain, progression of jaundice, vomiting and diarrhea, rashes, other comorbidities (autoimmune disease), school performance and medications.

- For acetaminophen: careful review of dose and frequency should be taken, including other remedies that may contain acetaminophen (i.e. cough medicine).
- Over-the-counter medications should be investigated.

Physical examination
- Physical examination is similar to adults. However, encephalopathy may be subtle (see table "Hepatic encephalopathy stages in children").

Hepatic encephalopathy stages in children

Stage	Clinical presentation	Reflexes	Neurological examination
1	Irritability, poor feeding, change in sleep rhythm, child not acting like self to parents	Normal or hyper-reflexive	Tremor, apraxia, impaired handwriting. Difficult to test adequately in infants
2	Drowsy, inappropriate behavior, decreased inhibitions	Normal or hyper-reflexive	Dysarthria, ataxia Difficult to test adequately in infants
3	Somnolence, stupor, combativeness, obeys simple commands	Hyper-reflexive, positive Babinski	Rigidity
4	Comatose, arouses with painful stimuli (4a) or no response (4b)	Absent	Decerebrate or decorticate

- Special attention given to jaundice, dysmorphic features (genetic disease), growth and development, fetor hepaticus, fever, respiratory rate (increased in hyperammonemia), decrease in liver size, splenic size, presence of ascites, excoriation marks, xanthomas, eye findings (cataracts, KF rings, pupil response and papillary edema) and gastrointestinal, subcutaneous and mucosal bleeding.

Laboratory diagnosis
List of diagnostic tests
- CBC:
  - WBC: elevated in infection, low in viral infection, certain metabolic disease).
  - Anemia: GI bleeding, non-autoimmune hemolytic anemia in Wilson disease.
  - Reticulocytes.
  - Direct Coombs test.
  - Platelet count: thrombocytopenia in chronic liver disease, DIC.
  - Pancytopenia: non-A-E hepatitis.
  - Bone marrow aspiration/biopsy (HLH, hematologic malignancy).
- Coagulation studies:
  - Prothrombin time or INR.
  - Factors II, VII, IX, X (vitamin K dependent).
  - Factor V (synthesized in liver not vitamin K dependent, short half-life, predictor of liver regeneration if >25%.
  - Factor 8: not synthesized by the liver.
  - Fibrinogen, fibrinogen split products (DIC).
- Blood for grouping and crossmatching.

- Chemistry:
  - Glucose (particularly in infants), electrolytes, calcium, phosphorus, magnesium, uric acid, cholesterol/triglyceride, amylase.
  - Liver enzymes (ALT, AST, GGT, ALP) often declining in the setting of worse synthetic hepatic function as necrosis progresses.
  - Total and direct bilirubin.
  - Albumin.
  - Acetaminophen levels.
  - Ammonia.
  - Serum amino acids (inborn errors of metabolism).
  - Alpha-1 antitrypsin phenotype.
  - Plasma acylcarnitines (fatty oxidation defects).
  - Blood gas analysis.
  - Increased lactate/pyruvate (mitochondrial disease).
  - Galactose-1-phosphate uridyl transferase (galactosemia).
  - Serum copper and ceruloplasmin (Wilson disease).
  - Serum quantitative IgG, ASMA, ANA, LKM (AIH).
  - Serum AFP (tyrosinemia).
  - Results of newborn screening.
  - High ferritin (>1000 μg/L), low total iron binding capacity (neonatal hemochromatosis).
  - High ferritin and triglycerides, hypofibrinogenemia, low or absent NK-cell activity, high soluble IL-2 receptor (HLH).
- Serology:
  - Hepatitis A: anti-HAV IgM antibody.
  - Hepatitis B: HBsAg, HBcAb(IgM), HBV DNA.
  - Hepatitis C: anti-Hep C antibody, Hep C PCR.
  - Hepatitis D: anti-Hep D antibody.
  - Hepatitis E: anti-HE antibody (IgM).
  - Cytomegalovirus (serology, PCR or culture).
  - Epstein–Barr virus (serology or PCR).
  - HIV.
  - Herpes simplex virus (neonates) IgM, direct fluorescent antibody, PCR and culture.
  - If indicated: measles/varicella/adenovirus/echovirus/toxoplasmosis/leptospirosis/listeriosis.
- Cultures:
  - Bacterial cultures: blood, urine, stool, throat swab, sputum, skin lesion if present, ascitic fluid if present.
  - Viral culture of urine and skin lesion if present.
  - Surveillance – daily culture.
- Urine:
  - Toxicology.
  - Chemical analysis, osmolality, and electrolytes.
  - Positive urine non-glucose reducing substances (galactosemia).
  - Amino/organic acids.
  - Succinyl acetone (tyrosinemia).
  - 24 hour urinary copper pre and post penicillamine (two doses of 500 mg 12 h apart) for Wilson disease.
- Biopsy:
  - Liver biopsy rarely required and usually contraindicated due to coagulopathy. May rule out AIH.

- Salivary gland biopsy: iron deposition in neonatal hemochromatosis.
- Muscle or skin biopsy: mitochondrial and other inborn errors of metabolism.

List of imaging techniques
- Abdominal US Doppler, CT angiography or MRI may show necrotic liver and vasculature (Budd–Chiari syndrome). Important to know anatomy prior to listing for liver transplantation. MRI of abdomen (extrahepatic iron deposition in neonatal hemochromatosis).
- Brain CT for cerebral bleeding and edema.
- Brain MRI (metabolic disease).

Potential pitfalls/common errors in diagnosis
- Failure to recognize or late recognition of hepatic encephalopathy.
- Coagulopathy responsive to vitamin K (vitamin K deficiency).
- Reassurance by decline in transaminases (may be a sign of progressive hepatic necrosis).
- No history of acetaminophen ingestion (acetaminophen may be found in many over-the-counter cough remedies).
- Failure to recognize HSV in neonates: acyclovir should be started empirically until HSV ruled out.
- Failure to diagnose metabolic crisis and hypoglycemia in infants: patients should be started on IV dextrose.
- Infants may be positive for CMV IgG (placental transmission) and be asymptomatic carriers (positive urine culture) for CMV.
- Children with ALF and sepsis often do not show the classic signs of fever and leukocytosis.
- Important to diagnose a multisystem disease (i.e. metabolic disease) which may exclude candidacy for liver transplantation.

Section 4: Treatment
Treatment rationale
- There is no proven therapy that is known to reverse hepatocyte injury or to promote regeneration of hepatocytes.
- The treatment of fulminant hepatic failure involves primarily supportive care.
- ALF is a life-threatening condition and warrants immediate referral to a pediatric liver transplant center. Progression may be rapid and unexpected.
- Children with encephalopathy or an INR >4 (without encephalopathy) should be admitted to an ICU for continuous monitoring.
- A quiet environment is necessary to avoid increase in intracranial pressure.
- In neonatal liver failure, intravenous acyclovir should be started at the earliest, while awaiting definitive diagnosis.
- Prophylactic broad-spectrum antibiotics and antifungals should be started.
- Specific therapies are available for HSV (acyclovir), acetaminophen (N-acetylcysteine), metabolic disease, HLH and neonatal hemochromatosis, Wilson disease (plasmapheresis, plasma exchange or albumin dialysis while awaiting for OLT) and autoimmune hepatitis (steroids).
- Patients should be managed in the pediatric ICU with frequent monitoring. Vital signs, urine output, neurologic observations, blood glucose (particularly in infants), electrolytes, INR, and daily CBC with surveillance blood and urine cultures should be obtained.
- Hypoglycemia should be avoided by use of intravenous glucose infusion or by ensuring adequate enteral intake.

- Total fluid intake is restricted to two-thirds maintenance if there is no evidence of dehydration.
- Protein intake should not be restricted.
- Acid suppression should be given to prevent GI bleeding.
- IV/SC or IM vitamin K should be given in an attempt to correct coagulopathy – at least 3 doses.
- Correct INR with fresh frozen plasma, cryoprecipitate, or Factor VIIa prior to procedures or active bleeding.
- The role of N-acetylcysteine in non-acetaminophen ALF is under investigation and currently controversial.
- Elective intubation and mechanical ventilation should be instituted when grade 3 encephalopathy develops or when patients in grade 1 or 2 encephalopathy require sedation.
- Sedation should be avoided due to the possibility of encephalopathy aggravation.
- Corticosteroid replacement should be considered in patients with abnormal short Synacthen test and hypotension unresponsive to conventional therapy.
- Cerebral perfusion pressure (mean arterial blood pressure – intracranial pressure) should be maintained at more than 50 mmHg and signs of elevated intracranial pressure should be monitored frequently (neurochecks, hypertension, bradycardia, pupils).
- Treatment of hepatic encephalopathy is similar to adults: lactulose (to achieve two to three soft stools per day with a pH below 6), oral antibiotics, mannitol if serum osmolarity <320 mOsm/L, sodium thiopental, mild cerebral hypothermia (32–35°C), hypernatremia (serum sodium >145 mmol/L), sodium benzoate and maintenance of PCO_2 <25 (temporary).
- Some studies advocate the advantage and safety of invasive intracranial pressure monitoring after correction of coagulopathy in improving morbidity and mortality.
- Renal dysfunction commonly occurs from dehydration, from acute tubular necrosis from the initial toxic insult and from hepatorenal syndrome. Hemodiafiltration and hemodialysis should be considered when the urine output is <1 mL/kg/hour.
- Plasmapheresis is used in some clinical settings of ALF (refractory coagulopathy, encephalopathy). However, it is not evidence based.
- Treatment of hepatic encephalopathy, cerebral edema, coagulopathy, infection, renal and metabolic derangements were discussed in Chapter 26.

Liver transplantation
- Children with ALF are listed as status 1A by UNOS if they had no pre-existing liver disease, life expectancy without OLT <7 days, onset of encephalopathy within 8 weeks of first symptoms of liver disease and one of the following three: ventilator dependent or requiring dialysis/CVVH/CVVHD or INR >2. Acute decompensated Wilson disease can be listed as status 1 A.
- Multisystem disorders must be excluded before considering liver transplantation. Absolute contraindications for OLT: fixed and dilated pupils, uncontrolled sepsis, and severe respiratory failure (ARDS). Relative contraindications: progressive or severe neurologic disease, treated infection and accelerating inotropic requirements.
- In children reduced (split) and living donor grafts may increase the donor pool. Auxiliary liver transplant (partial graft leaving recipient liver *in situ*) has been utilized in children with ALF. Once the native liver recovers, immunosuppression is weaned and eventually stopped, resulting in gradual donor liver atrophy.
- Hepatocyte transplantation and liver-assisted devices remain experimental.

Treatment for pediatric unique causes of ALF

Disease	Clinical presentation	Diagnostic approach	Treatment
Galactosemia	Vomiting and hypoglycemia after lactose (breast milk) ALF E. coli sepsis Cataracts	Results of newborn screening Positive urine non-glucose reducing substances Low activity of galactose-1-phosphate uridyl transferase in red blood cells	Exclusion of lactose: usually leads to a quick recovery Some progress to ALF
Hereditary fructosemia	Vomiting, hypoglycemia and tremor after exposure to fructose (fruit) ALF Renal dysfunction	Low fructose-1-phosphate aldolase B activity in liver tissue Liver biopsy with electron microscopy Genetic analysis	Exclusion of fructose
Tyrosinemia	ALF Severe coagulopathy Cirrhosis Early HCC Neurologic crisis Renal dysfunction	Results of newborn screening High serum tyrosine and methionine levels High serum AFP Succinylacetone detection in urine	Exclusion of tyrosine NTBC 2(2-nitro-4-trifluoromethyl benzoyl)-1,3-cyclohexenedione OLT
Mitochondrial respiratory chain disease	Brain, muscle, heart and liver are most affected Hypoglycemia, vomiting, coagulopathy, acidosis, myopathy, hypotonia, seizure	Increased lactate/pyruvate Biopsy (muscle, liver, and skin fibroblast culture) with molecular genetic studies Brain MRI Ophthalmologic examination Echocardiography	Respiratory chain cofactors (coezymeQ10) Antioxidants Carnitine Avoid certain drugs (valproate)
Fatty chain oxidation defect (MCAD-medium chain acyl-CoA dehydrogenase)	Recurrent liver failure with hypoglycemia, precipitated by minor illness Cardiomyopathy	Results of newborn screening Lack of serum and urine ketones Carnitine/acylcarnitine Free fatty acids Urine organic acids	Avoid fasting High carbohydrate Avoid fat when ill Carnitine (?)
Inborn errors of bile acid metabolism	Jaundice without pruritus	Serum low GGT and bile acids Urinalysis for bile acids	UDCA or cholic acid

Neonatal hemochromatosis
- ALF in the neonate – coagulopathy in the presence of near normal transaminases.
- History of previous fetal loss and neonatal ALF.
- Diagnosis: high ferritin (>1000 µg/L), low total iron binding capacity. Demonstration of extra-hepatic iron – buccal or salivary gland biopsy with iron stain, MRI (typical pattern of iron deposition in the pancreas).
- Treatment: IVIG, exchange transfusion, antioxidants (deferoxamine, vitamin E, N-acetylcysteine, selenium and prostaglandin-E) have not been validated, antenatal maternal IVIG if previous pregnancy/child was affected, OLT.

Hemophagocytic lymphohistiocytosis
- Familial (primary) HLH and secondary (post-infectious, immunodeficiency or autoimmunity) HLH.
- Presenting symptoms: fever, hepatosplenomegaly, neurologic symptoms, rash, lymphadenopathy.
- Laboratory: cytopenia in at least two cell lines, high ferritin and triglycerides, hypofibrinogenemia, low or absent NK-cell activity, high soluble IL-2 receptor and tissue demonstration of hemophagocytosis.
- Treatment: steroids, immunoglobulins, cyclosporine, chemotherapy, bone marrow transplant.

CLINICAL PEARLS
- Children with ALF should be referred promptly to a tertiary pediatric liver transplant center and monitored carefully in a pediatric ICU (vitals, CBC, chemistry, INR and surveillance cultures).
- In neonates acyclovir should be started empirically until HSV can be excluded and lactose-free formula should be given until galactosemia screening is negative.
- Vitamin K should be administered in an attempt to correct coagulopathy induced by vitamin K deficiency.
- Other treatable causes (HSV, acetaminophen, metabolic, neonatal hemochromatosis, hemophagocytic syndrome, AIH, ischemic) should be investigated.
- Children are listed as status 1 in UNOS for liver transplantation and reduced (split), auxiliary and living donor grafts may be utilized.

Section 5: Special Populations
Neonates
- HSV infection, inborn errors of metabolism, neonatal hemochromatosis and familial hemophagocytic syndrome are more common etiologies for ALF among neonates than in older children. Therefore, empiric therapy with acyclovir and lactose-free formula should be initiated promptly, until HSV infection and galactosemia can be ruled out.
- HSV ALF usually presents towards the end of the first week of life. It may manifest with fever, lethargy, poor feeding, seizures and abdominal distension. Vesicular rash is not always present. The majority of women have no history of genital herpes before delivery.

- A metabolic screening should be obtained (newborn screening, serum PH, ammonia, serum aminoacids, urine organic acids and succinyl acetone). Neonatal hemochromatosis should be suspected in the setting of jaundice, coagulopathy with only moderately elevated transaminases (two to three times above normal) and high ferritin. Confirmation is via buccal salivary gland biopsy or evidence of extrahepatic iron on MRI.

Section 6: Prognosis

- The prognosis is dependent on the etiology.
- The worse prognosis for neonatal ALF is HSV infection (14% 200 day survival), HLH (42% survival), hemochromatosis (52%), metabolic (71%) and others (91%).
- Poor prognostic factors: INR >4, Grade 3–4 encephalopathy, Factor V concentration <25%, hepatorenal syndrome, jaundice for more than 7 days prior to the onset of encephalopathy, ALF in Wilson disease, non-acetaminophen drug induced ALF, indeterminate (non A-E) hepatitis and AIH with encephalopathy.
- Outcomes after OLT for ALF have been improving and are comparable with other indications.

Section 7: Reading List

Cochran JB, Losek JD. Acute liver failure in children. Pediatr Emerg Care 2007;23:129–35

Dhawan A. Etiology and prognosis of acute liver failure in children. Liver Transpl 2008;14(Suppl 2): S80–4

Hansen K, Horslen S. Metabolic liver disease in children. Liver Transpl 2008;14:713–33

Kortsalioudaki C, Taylor RM, Cheeseman P, Bansal S, Mieli-Vergani G, Dhawan A. Safety and efficacy of N-acetylcysteine in children with non-acetaminophen-induced acute liver failure. Liver Transpl 2008;14: 25–30

Lee WM, Squires RH Jr, Nyberg SL, Doo E, Hoofnagle JH. Acute liver failure: summary of a workshop. Hepatology 2008;47:1401–15

Miloh T, Kerkar N, Parkar S, et al. Improved outcomes in pediatric liver transplantation for acute liver failure. Pediatr Transplant 2010:14;863–9

Shanmugam NP, Bansal S, Greenough A, Verma A, Dhawan A. Neonatal liver failure: aetiologies and management – state of the art. Eur J Pediatr 2011;170:573–81

Squires RH Jr, Shneider BL, Bucuvalas J, et al. Acute liver failure in children: the first 348 patients in the pediatric acute liver failure study group. J Pediatr 2006;148: 652–8

Squires RH Jr. Acute liver failure in children. Semin Liver Dis 2008;28:153–66

Section 8: Guidelines

Not applicable for this topic.

Section 9: Evidence

Not applicable for this topic.

Section 10: Images

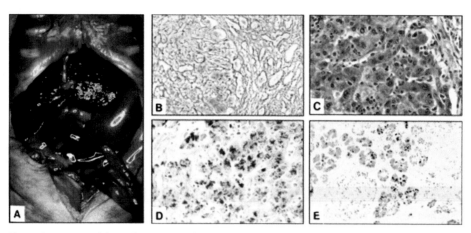

Figure 34.1 Neonatal hemochromatosis. (A) Macroscopic appearances of abdominal contents at necropsy showing enlarged liver with multiple dark surface nodules; generalized edema and ascites were also present. (B, C) Microscopic features of disrupted liver architecture showing nodule formation and pigmented and hypertrophic hepatocytes with cirrhosis (B, silver reticulin stain. ×100; C, H & E. ×400). (D) Liver section stained to show massive deposition of iron in hepatocytes (Perls' stain. ×400). (E) Deposition of iron in pancreatic tissue; note heavy staining of glandular acini of exocrine pancreas and also isolated punctate staining with islet cells (lower left of section) (Perls' stain. ×100). Source: Kelly et al. Classification and genetic features of neonatal haemochromatosis: a study of 27 affected pedigrees and molecular analysis of genes implicated in iron metabolism. J Med Genet 2001;38:599–610. Reproduced with permission of the BMJ Publishing Group.

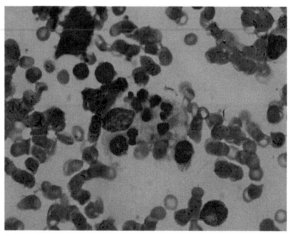

Figure 34.2 Hemophagocytic syndrome. Bone marrow aspirate containing phagocytic histiocytes with ingested platelets and red cell precursors.

Additional material for this chapter can be found online at:
www.mountsinaiexpertguides.com
This includes a case study and multiple choice questions

CHAPTER 35

Liver Function Tests in Childhood

Nanda Kerkar

Children's Hospital of Los Angeles, University of Southern California, Los Angeles, CA, USA

OVERALL BOTTOM LINE
- The term LFTs is often misused to refer to serum chemistry tests.
- Liver disease is evaluated by tests that detect liver injury, impaired bile flow or cholestasis, synthetic capacity, excretory function and metabolic function.
- Interpretation of abnormalities of the specific tests in the context of pediatric liver disease is described.
- Screening tests that need to be performed when abnormal aminotransferases are noted are described.
- An algorithm suggesting an approach when a child presents with abnormal aminotransferases is presented.

Section 1: Tests that Evaluate Liver Injury (Algorithm 35.1)

- Serum aminotransferases include ALT and AST.
- LDH is a cytoplasmic enzyme present in many tissues including liver and therefore has limited specificity.
- ALT (formerly SGPT) is primarily localized to liver and in the cytosol.
- AST (formerly SGOT) is present in liver (mitochondria and cytosol), heart, skeletal muscle, kidney and brain.
- The aminotransferases lack some sensitivity as values may be normal despite presence of inflammation on liver biopsy and also lack specificity as they may be elevated in non-hepatic conditions like myopathy and hypothyroidism.
- The ULN for ALT varies widely and many use a value around 50 IU/L. More recently, a study using National Health and Nutrition Examination Survey data showed that the 95th percentile levels for ALT in healthy weight, metabolically normal, liver disease-free, pediatric participants were 25.8 IU/L (boys) and 22.1 IU/L (girls), much lower than is used in clinical practice.
- The most common cause of elevated aminotransferases in pediatric practice is NAFLD; BMI >85th percentile overweight, BMI >95th percentile obese.

Mount Sinai Expert Guides: Hepatology, First Edition. Edited by Jawad Ahmad, Scott L. Friedman, and Henryk Dancygier.
© 2014 John Wiley & Sons, Ltd. Published 2014 by John Wiley & Sons, Ltd.
Companion website: www.mountsinaiexpertguides.com

Algorithm 35.1 Diagnosis of abnormal transaminases in children

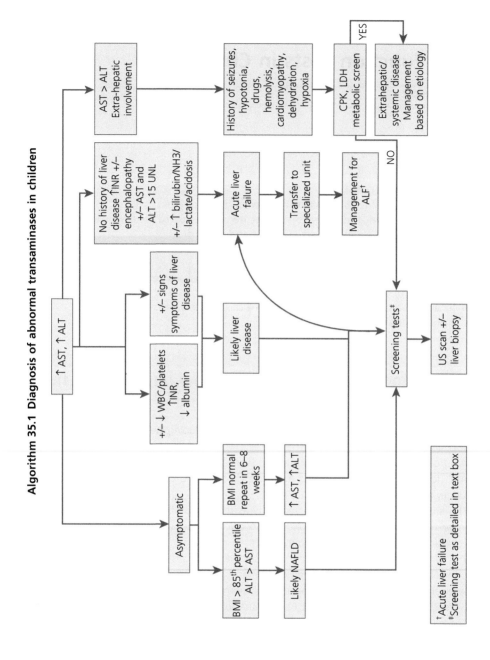

Elevated ALT and AST commonly seen in children
- NAFLD.
- Chronic liver disease:
  - Viral hepatitis.
  - Autoimmune hepatitis.
  - Wilson disease.
  - Cholestatic liver disease.
  - Cryptogenic cirrhosis.

AST and ALT >15 times normal
- Acetaminophen/toxin induced.
- Hypoxia/hypoperfusion – "shock liver".
- Acute viral hepatitis.

AST > ALT
- Hemolysis.
- Acute rhabdomyolysis – viral illness/vigorous physical activity.
- Myopathy.
- Myocardial disease.
- Macro AST.

ALT > AST
- NAFLD.
- Celiac disease.

Screening laboratory tests for abnormal aminotransferases
- CBC, INR.
- BUN, creatinine, electrolytes, albumin, GGT, total and direct bilirubin.
- Toxicology screen, glucose, ammonia (when ALT, AST >10 times normal).
- Viral hepatitis: hepatitis A IgG and IgM, hepatitis B surface antigen and antibody, hepatitis C antibody.
- Autoimmune hepatitis screen: immunoglobulin G, antinuclear antibody, smooth muscle antibody, liver kidney microsomal (LKM) antibody.
- Wilson disease screen: ceruloplasmin, 24 hour urinary copper.
- Alpha-1 antitrypsin deficiency: alpha-1 phenotype.
- Creatinine phosphokinase, aldolase, LDH (AST > ALT, concern for extra-hepatic cause of elevated aminotransferases).

Section 2: Tests that Evaluate Impaired Bile Flow or Cholestasis

- ALP.
- GGT.
- 5'nucleotidase.

Serum GGT
- Serum GGT varies by age: normal value up to 400 IU/L in neonates and reducing to 50 IU/L by a year of age.

- GGT is elevated typically in biliary obstruction.
- Cholestasis with low/normal GGT is characteristically seen in progressive familial intrahepatic cholestasis (PFIC 1 and 2) and inborn errors of bile acid synthesis.

Increased GGT
- Biliary atresia.
- Choledochal cyst.
- Biliary stones/stricture.
- Inspissated bile syndrome.
- Sclerosing cholangitis.
- Alagille syndrome.
- Alpha-1 antitrypsin deficiency.
- Anticonvulsants like phenobarbitone, phenytoin.

ALP

- The most likely source of ALP are liver and bone.
- Normal growing children and adolescents have elevation of ALP of bone origin.
- Increased ALP associated with elevated GGT or 5'nucleotidase is considered of hepatic origin.
- Increased ALP in the absence of liver disease may be:
  - Secondary to chronic renal failure.
  - Familial inheritance, blood type B or O.
  - Pregnancy.
  - Transient hyperphosphatemia of infancy.
- Decreased ALP is seen in:
  - Zinc deficiency (zinc is a co-factor for ALP).
  - Wilson disease.

PFIC
- Is a rare but important familial cause of cholestasis in the newborn.
- Is divided into three types based on mutations in genes encoding transport proteins responsible for the production of bile.
- Mothers of children with PFIC, who are heterozygous for the mutation especially ABCB4 have intrahepatic cholestasis of pregnancy, pruritus during pregnancy, post-natal resolution.

PFIC1 (Byler disease)
- Mutation in ATP8B1, a P-type ATPase that is an aminophospholipid flippase that is responsible for maintaining canalicular lipid asymmetry.
- Presents by 1 year of age with low GGT cholestasis, elevated transaminases, pruritus, hepatosplenomegaly, malabsorption, failure to thrive and rickets.
- Given the protein is present in other epithelia – there is also extrahepatic involvement with diarrhea, deafness, pancreatitis, renal tubular acidosis and/or lung disease.
- Histology reveals a bland hepatocellular, canalicular cholestasis with coarse granular bile on electron microscopy.
- Biliary diversion may help the pruritus. Liver transplantation is not the preferred option in view of extra-hepatic involvement.

PFIC2
- Mutation in ABCB11 which codes for bile salt export pump that is responsible for bile acid transport across the canalicular membrane.
- Similar to PFIC1 there is low GGT cholestasis in infancy, with transaminases elevated >5 ULN, but there is no extra-hepatic involvement.
- Rapid progress to cirrhosis and possibility of development of HCC and cholangiocarcinoma in the first year of life.
- Histology shows giant-cell hepatitis and lobular cholestasis with finely granular/filamentous bile in dilated bile canaliculi on electron microscopy.
- Monitoring of AFP and regular US scans important.
- Biliary diversion and liver transplantation are required in many.

PFIC3
- Mutation in ABCB4, which codes for MDR3 (multidrug resistance protein 3), causing malfunction of a transporter required for biliary phosphatidylcholine secretion → reduced biliary phospholipid → renders the biliary epithelium susceptible to damage by the biliary bile acids.
- Age of onset is variable but usually after infancy and GGT is high.
- Histology shows bile ductular proliferation and mixed inflammatory infiltrates. Periductal sclerosis affecting the interlobular bile ducts and biliary cirrhosis eventually occurs.
- Oral ursodeoxycholic acid is useful.
- Liver transplantation is required once cirrhosis develops.

Benign recurrent intrahepatic cholestasis (BRIC)
- Milder form of low GGT cholestasis.
- BRIC1 and BRIC2 are thought to be secondary to missense mutations of ATP8B1 and ABCB11 respectively.
- Intermittent episodes of cholestasis and severe pruritus.
- Chronic liver damage does not occur.

Section 3: Tests that Evaluate Synthetic Capacity of the Liver

- Serum albumin.
- PT.
- PTT.
- Clotting factors including factor V, VII.
- Lipid (cholesterol, triglyceride, lipoprotein).

Albumin
- Albumin is synthesized only in the liver.
- Albumin has a long half-life (T1/2) of 20 days
- Reduced serum albumin:
  - Chronic liver disease.
  - Chronic disease and malnutrition.
  - After a large GI bleed.
  - Secondary to loss of protein:
    - in any protein losing enteropathy.
    - nephrotic syndrome.

Clotting factors

- Factors V, VII, IX, X, XI, prothrombin and fibrinogen are synthesized in the liver.
- Factors II, VII, IX and X are vitamin K dependent.
- Factor V is vitamin K independent.
- Factor VII has the shortest T1/2 at 3–5 hours
- INR or PT:
  - Evaluates the extrinsic pathway of coagulation.
  - Is an excellent test for liver function, especially in ALF.
  - If the INR remains prolonged despite parenteral vitamin K, it reflects poor synthetic function, in the absence of sepsis causing disseminated intravascular coagulation, and congenital deficiencies of clotting factors or drugs.
- Factor VIII is normal in liver disease but abnormal in DIC and is useful in distinguishing between the two conditions when INR is prolonged.

Section 4: Tests that Evaluate Excretory Function of the Liver

- Clearance of endogenous substances like bilirubin, bile acids and exogenously administered dyes like indocyanine green.
- Bilirubin:
  - Is produced from the breakdown of heme and is unconjugated.
  - Is converted by glucuronyl transferase to a water soluble glucuronide form (conjugated bilirubin) excreted in bile.
  - Has a half-life of 4 hours.
  - In urine is a sensitive indicator of conjugated hyperbilirubinemia.
  - A small portion of the conjugated fraction is covalently bound to albumin – δbilirubin – long t1/2 of 17–20 days.
- Jaundice:
  - Is the yellow discoloration of sclerae, skin and other tissues caused by accumulation of bilirubin.
  - Is an important sign of disease or functional disorder of the hepatic, biliary or hematological systems.
  - Appears in children and adults when serum bilirubin >2 mg/dL.
  - Appears in neonates when serum bilirubin >5 mg/dL.
- Unconjugated hyperbilirubinemia:
  - Is characterized clinically by jaundice without bile in urine.
  - When less than 15% of the total bilirubin is conjugated.
  - Can pass through the blood–brain barrier if the serum concentration of unconjugated bilirubin exceeds the capacity of serum proteins, particularly albumin to bind bilirubin.
- Kernicterus:
  - Is a disorder in which unconjugated bilirubin is deposited in parts of the brain causing death or permanent neurologic damage, typically nerve deafness, choreoathetosis, cerebral palsy and mental retardation.
  - Risk is increased when serum bilirubin >20 mg/dL and at lower levels if there is associated acidosis, asphyxia, prematurity and hypoalbuminemia.
  - Phototherapy and exchange transfusion is performed to reduce unconjugated bilirubin and avoid kernicterus.
- Neonatal hyperbilirubinemia (predominantly unconjugated):

- Prematurity.
- Sepsis.
- Hemolytic disorders:
  - blood group incompatibility – ABO, RH.
  - defects of red cell membranes – spherocytosis.
  - red cell enzyme deficiencies – glucose 6-phosphate dehydrogenase, pyruvate kinase.
- Increased red cell mass:
  - placental transfusion, twin to twin transfusion.
  - infant of diabetic mother.
  - late clamping of cord.
  - excessive bruising, cephalhematoma.
- Hypoxia.
- Hypothyroidism, galactosemia, fructosemia, tyrosinemia.
- Meconium retention, high intestinal obstruction.
- Intrauterine infection.
- Uridine phosphate glucuronyl transferase deficiency:
  - Crigler-Najjar types 1 and 2.
  - Gilbert's.
- Conjugated bilirubin vs direct bilirubin:
  - Direct bilirubin:
    - so called as it reacts "directly" with diazo reagent without accelerant.
    - conjugated bilirubin + δbilirubin.
    - if total bilirubin is very high, some unconjugated bilirubin also reacts "directly" causing overestimation of the "direct" fraction.
  - Conjugated bilirubin measured by BuBc slide method – direct spectrophotometry is more accurate as it is not influenced by unconjugated bilirubin even when levels of total bilirubin are high.
- Conjugated hyperbilirubinemia or cholestasis: conjugated fraction of bilirubin exceeds 15% of the total:
  - In infancy, the differential diagnosis of cholestasis in association with abnormal transaminases includes biliary atresia, choledochal cyst, Alagille syndrome, TORCH, alpha-1 antitrypsin deficiency, progressive familial intrahepatic cholestasis, metabolic and other causes (please see Chapter 36).
  - As the infant improves, bilirubin is often the last parameter to normalize.
- Bile acids:
  - Are synthesized from cholesterol exclusively in the hepatocytes.
  - Are elevated in cholestasis and are usually associated with high GGT.
  - Are elevated with low GGT in progressive familial intrahepatic cholestasis types 1 and 2 (see text box).
  - Primary bile acids are low in defects of bile acid synthesis:
    - low GGT cholestasis.
    - screening urine by fast ion bombardment mass spectrometry aids diagnosis.
    - prognosis good with early bile acid replacement therapy in majority.

Section 5: Tests that Evaluate Metabolic Function

- Ammonia, lactate, pyruvate and specific profiles based on inherited deficiencies of enzymes.

- Ammonia:
  - ➤ is produced in the large intestine by the action of bacterial urease on dietary protein and aminoacids.
  - ➤ is converted into urea via the urea cycle and then to glutamine.
  - ➤ is also produced in a small amount by the kidney and this renal production may increase in the presence of drugs like valproate.
- Almost 80% of portal ammonia is removed by the liver in a single pass. In chronic liver disease, disturbed urea cycle function and porto-systemic shunts cause ammonia to by-pass the liver and may cause encephalopathy.
- Ammonia is elevated in:
  - ➤ liver failure.
  - ➤ metabolic disorders – urea cycle defects, tyrosinemia.
  - ➤ portosystemic shunts.
  - ➤ GI bleeding.
  - ➤ sepsis.
  - ➤ large protein load.
- Lactate:
  - ➤ is derived from pyruvic acid by LDH.
  - ➤ is elevated when liver function is impaired and in inborn errors of metabolism.
  - ➤ is an excellent marker of graft function in the immediate post-transplant period and in ALF setting.

Section 6: Other Laboratory Tests

- Serum globulins:
  - Alpha fraction: alpha-1 antitrypsin, ceruloplasmin and haptoglobin which are also acute phase reactants.
  - Beta fraction: transferrin, β-lipoprotein.
  - Gamma fraction: immunoglobulin (Ig) – IgG, IgA and IgM.
- Plasma and urine aminoacids.
- Autoantibodies – markers of autoimmune hepatitis:
  - Antinuclear antibody.
  - Smooth muscle antibody.
  - Liver kidney microsomal antibody.
- AFP:
  - Is produced by the fetal liver.
  - Is considered with albumin to be amongst the earliest liver specific markers in development.
  - Levels may be as high as 100000ng/mL in the neonatal period and reduce to <10ng/mL by a year of life.
  - Level may remain elevated in:
    - ➤ metabolic conditions like tyrosinemia.
    - ➤ ataxia telangiectasia.
    - ➤ tumors like hepatoblastoma and hepatocellular carcinoma.
    - ➤ pregnancy.
  - It may used as a marker of liver regeneration in ALF or after partial liver resection.
- CBC:
  - Hemoglobin, WCC and platelet count are not included in liver function tests.

- Decreased platelet count and WCC in the absence of hematological disease is suggestive of hypersplenism secondary to portal hypertension.

Section 7: Reading List

Green RM, Flamm S. AGA technical review on the evaluation of liver chemistry tests. Gastroenterology 2002;123:1367–84

Mowat A. Liver Disorders in Childhood, 3rd edition. London: Butterworth-Heinemann, 1994.

Ng VL. Laboratory assessment of liver function and injury in children. In Suchy F, Sokol R, Balistreri W (eds), Liver Disease in Children, 3rd edition. Cambridge: Cambridge University Press, 2007

Schwimmer J, Dunn W, Norman G, et al. SAFETY study: alanine aminotransferase cutoff values are set too high for reliable detection of pediatric chronic liver disease. Gastroenterology 2010;138:1357–64

Suggested website
Childhood Liver disease Research and Education Network (ChiLDREN): http://www.childrennetwork.org/

Section 8: Guidelines

Not applicable for this topic.

Section 9: Evidence

Not applicable for this topic.

Section 10: Images

Not applicable for this topic.

Additional material for this chapter can be found online at:
www.mountsinaiexpertguides.com
This includes a case study and multiple choice questions

CHAPTER 36

Approach to Jaundice in Infancy

Jaime Chu
Division of Hepatology, Icahn School of Medicine at Mount Sinai, New York, NY, USA

OVERALL BOTTOM LINE
- Neonatal cholestasis is a condition characterized by the elevation of conjugated bilirubin.
- Infants with cholestasis often depend on the general practitioner for proper diagnosis and appropriate initial investigations, namely a fractionated serum bilirubin with early referral to a pediatric hepatologist.
- The NASPGHAN Cholestasis Guideline Committee has developed a systematic approach to the evaluation of the cholestatic infant.
- Early diagnosis of the etiology of the cholestasis is essential for effective treatment, most importantly in cases of EHBA, metabolic, or infectious liver diseases, and for management of complications of chronic liver disease.

Section 1: Background
Definition of disease
- Cholestasis is not a disease but is a symptom of underlying disease. It is characterized by abnormal bile formation or flow.
- In cholestatic disorders, there is an elevation of conjugated bilirubin with a direct bilirubin >1 mg/dL or >20% of total bilirubin if total bilirubin is >5 mg/dL.

Incidence/prevalence
- Jaundice may be seen in up to 15% of all newborns.
- However, neonatal cholestasis occurs in approximately one in every 2500 infants and must be distinguished from entities causing an unconjugated hyperbilirubinemia, such as physiologic jaundice or breast milk jaundice.

Etiology
- The differential diagnosis of neonatal cholestasis is broad.
- The most common causes are:
  - EHBA: 40%.
  - Idiopathic neonatal hepatitis: 10–15%.
  - Alpha-1 antitrypsin deficiency: 10%.
  - Inborn errors of metabolism: 20%.
  - Congenital infections: 5%.

Mount Sinai Expert Guides: Hepatology, First Edition. Edited by Jawad Ahmad, Scott L. Friedman, and Henryk Dancygier.
© 2014 John Wiley & Sons, Ltd. Published 2014 by John Wiley & Sons, Ltd.
Companion website: www.mountsinaiexpertguides.com

Pathology/pathogenesis

- The major determinant of bile flow is the enterohepatic circulation of bile acids. Cholestasis results from impaired bile formation by the hepatocyte (with alteration of key hepatobiliary transporter expression) or from obstruction of bile flow through the intra- or extrahepatic biliary tree with resulting decreased bile flow.
- The neonatal liver is more susceptible to developing cholestasis from a variety of disease processes compared with an older child or adult as there is a smaller bile acid pool and immaturity of hepatic bile acid uptake and excretion systems, leading to reduced enterohepatic circulation of bile acid.

Section 2: Prevention

> **BOTTOM LINE**
> - No interventions have been demonstrated to prevent the development of neonatal cholestasis.

Screening

- Currently, there is no screening test to predict which infants will develop cholestasis. Conjugated bilirubin measured in plasma of neonates between 6 and 10 days of life was found to be a sensitive and specific marker of neonatal liver disease. However, development of methods to detect conjugated bilirubin in dried blood spots would be needed for large-scale neonatal screening. In the case of EHBA where timely intervention improves outcomes, Taiwan has implemented a universal screening program for biliary atresia by providing parents with a stool color card on discharge after birth and parents return the stool card at 1 month of age. This screening program has led to earlier detection of EHBA and improved surgical outcomes.

Section 3: Diagnosis (Algorithm 36.1)

> **BOTTOM LINE**
> - Parents or the primary care physician are the first to recognize signs of cholestasis – jaundice, dark urine or pale colored stools.
> - The presentation of a jaundiced infant can reflect either unconjugated or conjugated hyperbilirubinemia – thus formal laboratory testing must be done to test for cholestasis.
> - The AAP and NASPGHAN recommend measurement of total and direct serum bilirubin for any infant who is jaundiced at 2 weeks of age. However, breast-fed infants with no history of dark urine or pale stools and normal physical examination who can be reliably monitored may wait until 3 weeks of age to have testing done if jaundice persists at that time.

Differential diagnosis

- First and foremost, it is paramount to distinguish between conjugated and unconjugated hyperbilirubinemia.
- Second, the practitioner must differentiate between physiologic jaundice and pathologic hyperbilirubinemia. The age of the infant and the duration of the abnormal bilirubin level may

Algorithm 36.1 Diagnostic approach to neonatal cholestasis

Source: Adapted from Moyer V et al 2004. Reproduced with permission of Wolters Kluwer Health.

aid in differentiating the disorders. Pathologic hyperbilirubinemia often occurs during the first 24 hours of life and may be associated with anemia or hepatosplenomegaly, may demonstrate a rapid rise (>5 mg/dL per day), may be prolonged (>7–10 days in a full-term infant), or may present with elevated conjugated bilirubin level (>1 mg/dL or >20% of TSB).

Differential diagnosis	Features
Physiologic jaundice	Transient elevation of bilirubin values during the second or third day of life
Breastfeeding jaundice	Within the first 7 days of life; occurs when breast-fed newborn does not receive adequate breast milk intake due to delayed or insufficient milk production or poor feeding by the newborn. Signs/symptoms of dehydration and weight loss with fewer bowel movements (decreased bilirubin excretion from the body)
Breast milk jaundice	Breast-fed newborn; TSB >5 mg/dL but with mildly increased levels that do not require intervention. Typically begins after the first 3–5 days of life, peaks within 2 weeks after birth, and normalized over 3–12 weeks
Other causes of unconjugated hyperbilirubinemia	Hemolysis, hypothyroidism, rare inherited disorders of bilirubin excretion or conjugation

Typical presentation
- The presentation of a patient with neonatal cholestasis is specific to the etiology of the cholestasis.
- Infants with EHBA (most common etiology) will typically be full-term with normal birth history. Weight gain and activity are normal for the first several weeks at which point parents may notice the development of jaundice or scleral icterus. Often infants are not scheduled to see the pediatrician until the 2-month well-child visit, so it is incumbent on the caregivers to bring the jaundice to the attention of medical care.
- On physical examination, EHBA patients are likely well-appearing with jaundice, scleral icterus, and acholic stools.

Clinical diagnosis
History
- A good history can be useful in the differential diagnosis of neonatal cholestasis. Historical questioning should include familial diseases, consanguinity, maternal infection/prenatal findings, and birth history. In addition, questions of feeding, weight gain, neonatal infection or fever, and urine and stool color are also important.

Physical examination
- On physical examination, assessment for general health and nutrition status, along with inspection for dysmorphic facies, murmurs, rashes and neurologic status can be helpful. Abdominal examination should include inspection for distention, ascites, and liver and spleen size and consistency, as well as direct visualization of urine and stool color.

Laboratory diagnosis

List of diagnostic tests
- Total and direct bilirubin:
  - A fractionated bilirubin is the most important test in the evaluation of a jaundiced infant.
  - In neonatal cholestasis, direct bilirubin >1 mg/dL or >20% of total bilirubin if total bilirubin is greater than 5 mg/dL.
  - Any elevation of direct bilirubin should be considered abnormal and prompt further investigation and consultation with a pediatric hepatologist is recommended.
- Albumin, INR:
  - Markers of hepatic synthetic function.
- AST, ALT:
  - Evaluate the extent of hepatocellular injury.
- GGT, AP:
  - May indicate obstructive causes of cholestasis.
  - A very low GGT level may be useful to exclude obstruction and may suggest a genetic or metabolic cause of intracellular cholestasis.
  - The degree of elevation of GGT is not useful in discriminating the etiology of the cholestasis.
- Given the broad span of etiologies for neonatal cholestasis, including non-hepatic conditions, evaluation should also include alpha-1 antitrypsin phenotype, glucose, bacterial cultures, viral serologies, and review of the newborn screen for diseases causing neonatal cholestasis, especially hypothyroidism and galactosemia. Further testing, including specialized blood and urine tests for inborn errors of metabolism or storage disorders, should be tailored to the individual patient.
- Percutaneous liver biopsy:
  - Remains the most important diagnostic test in the evaluation and is recommended in cases of undiagnosed neonatal cholestasis.
  - Can be safely and expediently performed in infants and should be interpreted by an experienced pediatric liver pathologist.
  - The NASPGHAN Cholestasis Guideline Committee recommends performing a percutaneous liver biopsy before a surgical procedure to diagnose biliary atresia.
  - It is important to note that some cholestatic diseases are dynamic over time and if the biopsy is performed before 6 weeks of age and the results are equivocal (e.g. EHBA may resemble idiopathic neonatal hepatitis), the disease may still be in its early stages and the biopsy may have to be repeated.

List of imaging techniques
- Abdominal US:
  - A useful initial imaging modality to evaluate liver structure, size and composition. Also detects extrahepatic anomalies such as choledochal cysts, gall bladder anatomy, obstructing gallstones, or sludge.
  - Best performed at a referral center by experienced personnel due to operator-dependency.
- Hepatobiliary scintigraphy scans:
  - Uses technetium-labeled imino-diacetic derivatives to view the biliary tract.
  - Injected radioactive material is normally excreted into the intestine. Non-visualization of radioactivity within the intestine 24 hours after injection is considered to be abnormal, indicating biliary obstruction or hepatocellular dysfunction.

- Can be 100% sensitive for infants with EHBA but specificity for EHBA can be as low as 33% (non-excretion may also occur in infants with non-EHBA intrahepatic cholestasis, such as paucity of intrahepatic bile ducts or various forms of neonatal hepatitis).
  - From NASPGHAN Cholestasis Guidelines: hepatobiliary scintigraphy generally adds little to the routine evaluation of the cholestatic infant but may be of value if other means for excluding biliary obstruction are not available.
- ERCP:
  - Not routinely recommended in the evaluation of neonatal cholestasis.
  - However, may be useful and utilized at tertiary centers experienced with ERCP in the neonate and in very select cases where the diagnosis is still uncertain after liver biopsy.
- MRCP:
  - An exciting modality to aid in diagnosis in cases of neonatal cholestasis.
  - Non-invasive with high sensitivity and specificity in evaluating the pancreatobiliary tree in children.

Potential pitfalls/common errors made regarding diagnosis of disease

- Total serum bilirubin level alone is not sufficient to screen neonates with jaundice. It is extremely important to differentiate between indirect hyperbilirubinemia and direct hyperbilirubinemia, which is always pathologic and requires urgent investigation.
- Do not presume the 2-month-old breast-fed infant has breast-milk jaundice. Diagnosis of neonatal cholestasis must be done promptly, as patients with early diagnosis of biliary atresia (<60 days of life) have a better prognosis following portoenterostomy. A missed diagnosis of biliary atresia leads to progressive liver disease and the need for liver transplantation.
- Although patients with biliary atresia classically have acholic stools, the presence of pigmented stools does not rule out biliary atresia.

Section 4: Treatment
Treatment rationale
- First line treatment should focus on the primary disease responsible for the cholestasis.
- Treatment of neonatal cholestasis is primarily focused on maintaining growth and development in the setting of cholestasis. The consequences of cholestasis are predominantly related to the reduced secretion of bile acids into the intestines, which leads to decreased absorption of long-chain fats and fat-soluble vitamins.

When to hospitalize
- The decision to hospitalize the infant with cholestasis depends on the age, suspected etiology (especially EHBA or biliary obstruction requiring early surgical intervention) and clinical appearance.
- Ill-appearing patients with jaundice and fever require admission and evaluation for a possible underlying infectious disorder. Additionally, jaundice in an otherwise asymptomatic newborn can be an early indication of sepsis or UTI and requires evaluation and initiation of antibiotics when warranted.
- Transfer to a tertiary care facility should be considered in cases of neonatal cholestasis, especially in any patient with evidence of liver failure or who is at risk for the development of liver failure.

Table of treatment

Treatment	Comment
Medical treatment	
Increased energy requirements	Patients should receive 125% of the recommended daily allowance based on ideal body weight Weight for height can be misleading, especially in those with ascites; anthropometric measurements can offer a better estimation of nutritional status
Decreased absorption of long-chain fatty acids	Infant formula high in medium-chain triglycerides; may be further concentrated up to 30 kilocalories per ounce to improve caloric intake and minimize fluid volume
Decreased absorption of fat-soluble vitamins	Supplementation of vitamins A, D, E, and K (ADEK) or, for better absorption, the combination of TPGS-vitamin E, multivitamin, and vitamin K may be used. Vitamin levels should be followed periodically
Pruritus	Ursodeoxycholic acid, rifampin, cholestyramine, diphenhydramine, hydroxyzine – each can be used with varying efficacy and side effects
Surgical interventions	Dependent on etiology of cholestasis

CLINICAL PEARLS
- Treatment is based on underlying etiology of cholestasis.
- Early recognition of neonatal cholestasis and diagnosis of underlying etiology is essential to ensure timely intervention, especially with regards to metabolic, infectious and obstructive diseases.
- Even when etiology of cholestasis is under investigation, the infant will still benefit from supportive management to prevent complications related to chronic cholestasis.

Section 5: Special Populations

Not applicable for this topic.

Section 6: Prognosis

BOTTOM LINE
- The prognosis of an infant with cholestasis is specific to the underlying etiology.
- Some conditions are easily managed with an excellent prognosis, while others are chronic and require lifelong medical care.
- In both situations, it is important to remember that many of the causes of neonatal cholestasis require expeditious diagnosis and treatment, which can impact the prognosis and further progression of liver disease.

Section 7: Reading List

Hartley JL, Davenport M, Kelly DA. Biliary atresia. Lancet 2009;374:1704–13

Lien TH, Chang MH, Wu JF, et al. Taiwan Infant Stool Color Card Study Group. Effects of the infant stool color card screening program on 5-year outcome of biliary atresia in Taiwan. Hepatology 2011;53:202–8

Mack CL, Sokol RJ. Unraveling the pathogenesis and etiology of biliary atresia. Pediatr Res 2005; 57:R87–R94

Mieli-Vergani G, Howard ER, Portman B, Mowat AP. Late referral for biliary atresia – missed opportunities for effective surgery. Lancet 1989;1:421–3

Moyer V, Freese DK, Whitington PF, et al. Guideline for the evaluation of cholestatic jaundice in infants: recommendations of the North American Society for Pediatric Gastroenterology, Hepatology and Nutrition. J Pediatr Gastroenterol Nutr 2004;39:115-28

Powell JE, Keffler S, Kelly DA, Green A. Population screening for neonatal liver disease: potential for a community-based programme. J Med Screen 2003;10:112–16

Sokol RJ, Shepherd RW, Superina R, Bezerra JA, Robuck P, Hoofnagle JH. Screening and outcomes in biliary atresia: summary of a National Institutes of Health workshop. Hepatology 2007;46:566–81

Suchy FJ. Approach to the infant with cholestasis. In: Suchy FJ, Sokol RJ, Balistreri WF (eds), Liver Disease in Children, 3rd edition. New York: Cambridge University Press, 2007:179–89

Trauner M, Meier PJ, Boyer JL. Molecular pathogenesis of cholestasis. N Eng J Med 1998;339:1217–27

Suggested website
http://www.childrennetwork.org/

Section 8: Guidelines
National society guidelines

Guideline title	Guideline source	Date	Summary
Guideline for the evaluation of cholestatic jaundice in infants: recommendations of the North American Society for Pediatric Gastroenterology, Hepatology and Nutrition	North American Society for Pediatric Gastroenterology, Hepatology and Nutrition (NASPGHAN) http://www.naspghan.org/user-assets/Documents/pdf/PositionPapers/CholestaticJaundice InInfants.pdf	2004	Also endorsed by the American Academy of Pediatrics

Section 9: Evidence

See NASPGHAN Guidelines.

Section 10: Images

Not applicable for this topic.

Additional material for this chapter can be found online at:
www.mountsinaiexpertguides.com
This includes a case study and multiple choice questions

CHAPTER 37

Management of End-Stage Liver Disease in Children

Ronen Arnon

Department of Pediatrics, Icahn School of Medicine at Mount Sinai, New York, NY, USA

OVERALL BOTTOM LINE
- ESLD, is an irreversible condition that leads to imminent complete failure of the liver.
- Most chronic liver diseases of childhood result in cirrhosis characterized by widespread hepatic fibrosis and regenerative nodules. Diagnosis of cirrhosis is based on clinical, laboratory, imaging and histologic findings.
- PHT, acute variceal bleeding and hypersplenism, ascites, spontaneous bacterial peritonitis, encephalopathy, coagulopathy and malnutrition, are complications of decompensated cirrhosis.
- Bleeding esophageal varices are managed endoscopically (banding/sclerotherapy), medically (non-selective beta blockers, octreotide) or surgically (portosystemic shunts, TIPS or liver transplantation).
- Fluid and salt restriction with/without diuretics are effective in managing ascites.
- Spontaneous bacterial peritonitis should be diagnosed promptly by paracentesis and treated with antibiotics.
- Hepatic encephalopathy can be subtle in infants and managed with antibiotics, lactulose and low protein diet.
- Coagulopathy is managed with vitamin K and blood products prior to procedures.
- Malnutrition requires high caloric formulas containing medium-chain triglycerides and fat-soluble vitamin supplements.
- Patients with cirrhosis should be screened for HCC (periodic abdominal US and serum AFP level) and for hepatopulmonary syndrome (upright hypoxemia). Children with decompensated cirrhosis should be evaluated for liver transplantation.

Section 1: Background
Definition of disease
- ESLD is an irreversible condition that leads to imminent complete failure of the liver. The etiology of ESLD in children varies with age of presentation.
- In infants biliary atresia, parenteral nutrition-induced cholestasis, Alagille syndrome and metabolic syndromes are the main causes for ESLD. In older children and adolescents autoimmune hepatitis, cryptogenic cirrhosis, PSC or Wilson disease are the leading etiologies for ESLD.
- The main causes of chronic liver disease in children are presented in the table – Causes of liver disease in children that result in cirrhosis.

Mount Sinai Expert Guides: Hepatology, First Edition. Edited by Jawad Ahmad, Scott L. Friedman, and Henryk Dancygier.
© 2014 John Wiley & Sons, Ltd. Published 2014 by John Wiley & Sons, Ltd.
Companion website: www.mountsinaiexpertguides.com

- ESLD can be with compensated and decompensated liver disease. In compensated liver disease, there may be no symptoms and the indication of liver disease may be incidental findings of liver/spleen or elevation of liver enzymes or direct bilirubin. Decompensated liver disease is characterized by clinical complications (jaundice, ascites, variceal bleeding) and laboratory findings of synthetic failure such as increased INR and hypoalbuminemia.
- The complications of ESLD in children include:
  - PHT and variceal bleeding.
  - Ascites.
  - Bacterial infection, SBP.
  - Hepatopulmonary syndrome and pulmonary hypertension.
  - Hepatic encephalopathy.
  - Coagulopathy.
  - Malnutrition.
  - Hepatorenal syndrome.
  - Hepatocellular carcinoma.

Causes of liver disease in children that result in cirrhosis

Infectious disease	**Toxic/drugs disorders**
Chronic hepatitis B	Organic solvents
Chronic hepatitis C	Hepatotoxic drugs
Herpes simplex disease	Hypervitaminosis A
Cytomegalovirus	Total parenteral nutrition
Genetic/metabolic disorders	**Vascular lesions**
Alpha-1 antitrypsin deficiency	Budd–Chiari syndrome
Cystic fibrosis	Congenital heart failure
Galactosemia	Veno-occlusive liver disease
Tyrosinemia	**Autoimmune diseases**
Wilson disease	Autoimmune hepatitis
Hemochromatosis	PSC
Glycogen storage disease type 3	**Biliary diseases**
Glycogen storage disease type 4	Biliary atresia
Progressive familial intrahepatic cholestasis type 1	Alagille syndrome
(Byler disease)	Choledochal cyst
Progressive familial intrahepatic cholestasis type 2	Congenital hepatic fibrosis
Progressive familial intrahepatic cholestasis type 3	Intrahepatic cystic biliary dilatation
Zellweger	(Caroli disease)
Congenital disorders of glycosylation	**Idiopathic diseases**
Non-alcoholic steatohepatitis	Neonatal hepatitis
	Cryptogenic

Section 2: Prevention

Not applicable for this topic.

Section 3: Diagnosis

- The diagnostic approach is provided in each of the following complications of chronic liver disease (including physical examination, laboratory parameters and imaging studies when relevant).

- PHT and variceal bleeding.
- Ascites.
- Bacterial infection, SBP.
- Hepatopulmonary syndrome and pulmonary hypertension.
- Hepatic encephalopathy.
- Coagulopathy.
- Malnutrition and nutrition support.
- Hepatorenal syndrome.
- Hepatocellular carcinoma.

> Please note: as many of the complications of chronic liver disease appear in adults as well, an algorithm was provided only for nutrition and nutrition support part, which is unique for children.

Section 4: Treatment

- The treatment (medical/surgical) is provided in each of the different complications of chronic liver disease (see relevant chapters on complications of cirrhosis as listed under Section 3: Diagnosis, and under the individual headings in this chapter). A treatment algorithm was provided to the nutritional part which is unique to children.

Section 5: Special Populations

Not applicable for this topic.

Section 6: Prognosis

- The prognosis is provided in each of the different complications of chronic liver disease (see relevant chapters on complications of cirrhosis as listed under Section 3: Diagnosis, and under the individual headings in this chapter).

PHT and variceal bleeding
- PHT is defined by a portal venous pressure above 5 mmHg and an elevated pressure gradient between the portal vein and the inferior vena cava, which is measured by the HVPG above 10–12 mmHg.
- HPVG is elevated in cirrhosis and its response to pharmacotherapy may predict the recurrence of gastrointestinal bleeding.

Clinical manifestations
- Acute variceal bleeding is the presenting symptom of PHT in up to two-thirds of children.
- No particular peak age of presentation has been demonstrated and GIB was reported as early as 2 months of age.
- Splenomegaly may be first discovered on routine physical examination.
- Cytopenias (thrombocytopenia and/or leucopenia) may present as a result of hypersplenism which may cause petechiae and ecchymoses.

- Abdominal vascular marking may be prominent as a result of subcutaneous portocollateral shunting.
- Rectal varices and hypertensive rectopathy may be found.
- Peristomal varices are a common site of bleeding in children with short gut.

Diagnosis
- PHT should be suspected in any child with significant GIB or unexplained splenomegaly.
- Physical examination should focus on the liver, spleen, cutaneous markings and growth.
- Laboratory studies should examine cytopenias and the liver function.
- US with Doppler is the primary investigation of choice in children. Other imaging studies, such as triple phase CT, magnetic resonance venography and selective angiography may be helpful diagnostically in complex cases.
- The gold standard in the diagnosis of varices is EGD.
- Capsule endoscopy, a minimally invasive procedure that uses special video capsules, has a sensitivity of 63–100% for screening of esophageal varices and may be used in children older than 10 years.
- Gastroesophageal varices are an extension of the esophageal varices and isolated gastric varices occur in the absence of esophageal varices and are less common in children.
- Portal gastropathy was found in 25% of children with PHT.

Natural history
- Cirrhotic patients without varices develop them at a rate of 8% per year.
- GIB may occur in the first year of life. Patients with biliary atresia and bilirubin >4 mg/dL have lower survival after the first variceal bleeding without liver transplantation (LT). Complications of PHT are a leading cause of mortality in untreated biliary atresia.
- Mortality rate from variceal bleeding in children is 0–8% in published studies.
- Continuous bleeding at the time of EGD is a poor prognostic sign.

Therapy
- Approaches to the management of PHT in children are mostly descriptive and anecdotal and mostly adapted from the adult literature.
- The management of varices can be divided into pre-primary (before esophageal varices develop), primary (before GIB develops), secondary (before recurrent GIB) and acute variceal bleed.
- In patients with small varices who have not bled but are at increased risk of bleeding (progressive liver disease, esophageal varices with red wales), non-selective beta blockers (i.e. propranolol) are recommended in adults with scant data on efficacy in children. The dose is titrated to decrease the basal heart rate by 25% with a wide dosing range (0.6–8 mg/kg/day) two to four times a day.
- In patients with medium to large varices at high risk of bleeding, either beta blockers or endoscopic therapy (sclerotherapy or banding) may be recommended.
- The initial management of acute variceal bleeding is patient stabilization. Fluid and blood resuscitation is critical, with optimal hemoglobin in adults between 7 and 9 g/dL to avoid overfilling.
- Fresh frozen plasma, recombinant factor 7 and vitamin K may be of benefit in coagulopathic patients. Platelets should be given if the count is <50 000.
- Intravenous antibiotics are recommended to decrease the risk of severe infectious complications.

- Somatostatin (octreotide) or vasopressin should be considered the first line treatment of variceal bleeding. Octreotide is tolerated by children and was effective in treatment of GIB.
- EGD should be initiated once the diagnosis of acute variceal bleeding is suspected and endoscopic therapy performed.
- Variceal band ligation was found to achieve variceal eradication more quickly, with a lower rebleeding rate and fewer complications compared with sclerotherapy.
- Sclerotherapy, also effective in aborting variceal bleeding, is recommended in patients in whom banding is not technically feasible, especially children younger than 2 years, due to difficulty in passing the device.
- Surgical shunts and TIPS are effective rescue therapies. LT may be effective if a donor is found rapidly.
- Given the high rebleeding rate, secondary prophylaxis is recommended. Combination endoscopic plus beta blockers are warranted.

Ascites

- The accumulation of ascitic fluid is the product of a complex process involving hepatic, renal, systemic, hemodynamic and neurohormonal factors. PHT is key to the development of ascites and portal pressure below 12 mmHg in adults is rarely associated with ascites.
- Fluids and salt restriction to reduce ascites can be effective but may have a negative effect on growth unless balanced by high caloric concentrated formula.
- The diuretic of choice is the aldosterone antagonist, spironolactone (starting dose of 1 mg/kg, to be increased gradually up to 6 mg/kg/day). Furosemide (1–2 mg/kg) can be used to control the hyperkalemia (side-effects of spironolactone) and to promote strong and rapid response.
- Children, and especially infants, are vulnerable to the complications of ascites. Tense ascites may lead to extrahepatic organ dysfunction, including compromise of gastrointestinal, renal and pulmonary function.
- Abdominal paracentesis is indicated in non-responsive tense ascites that leads to severe extrahepatic organ dysfunction.
- A modest amount of ascites, as long as extrahepatic organ function is not compromised, is somewhat desired if the patient is to be considered for LT to allow for room for donor transplant organs and subsequent ease of fascial and skin closure with minimal intra-abdominal compression and compromise of donor organ vascular flow.

SBP

- SBP refers to bacterial peritonitis not associated with intestinal perforation or any "secondary" source. It occurs in children with cirrhosis and ascites and is potentially fatal.
- SBP should be suspected in patient with new-onset ascites, increased abdominal girth in patients with ascites, fever, abdominal pain, worsening encephalopathy or elevation of peripheral WBC.
- The diagnosis is established by abdominal paracentesis which reveals cloudy fluid, a positive ascitic fluid bacterial culture and an elevated ascitic fluid absolute polymorphonuclear count (i.e. 250 cells/mm^3) without an evident intra-abdominal, surgically treatable source of infection.
- Characteristically SBP is caused by a single species, often enteric bacteria such as *Klebsiella* spp, *E. coli*, Enterococcus or by *Streptococcus pneumoniae*.
- Cefotaxime is the antibiotic of choice in most pediatric patients, because it effectively covers the most common organisms.

- According to the recent AASLD guidelines adults who have survived an episode of SBP should receive long-term (secondary) prophylaxis with daily norfloxacin (or trimethoprim/sulfamethoxazole). Given the concern of long-term quinolone use in infants and young children, regarding arthralgia or cartilage toxicity, trimethoprim-sulfamethoxazole may be for used in children.

Hepatopulmonary syndrome and pulmonary hypertension

- Hepatopulmonary syndrome is the association of liver disease, hypoxemia and intrapulmonary vascular dilatations.
- The prevalence of hepatopulmonary syndrome in cirrhotic children is reported as 8–19%.
- Clinically, hepatopulmonary syndrome is evidenced by decreased oxygen saturation in the upright position in subjects with chronic liver disease (orthodeoxia) and platypnea – improved dyspnea while lying down. Patients often manifest signs of pulmonary disease including dyspnea, exercise intolerance and digital clubbing.
- Agitated saline echocardiography and macroaggregated albumin scanning are the best diagnostic measures for hepatopulmonary syndrome.
- Screening for hepatopulmonary syndrome with upright saturation is recommended for children with cirrhosis and/or PHT.
- Portopulmonary hypertension is pulmonary hypertension associated with PHT as a result of medial hypertrophy, concentric intimal proliferation of the small pulmonary arteries.
- Endothelin-1 receptor antagonists, prostacyclin analogues, sildenafil and LT in combination with heart and lung transplant may be effective in some cases of portopulmonary hypertension. Severe pulmonary hypertension >50 mmHg is a contraindication to LT due to high perioperative mortality.

Hepatic encephalopathy

- Hepatic encephalopathy can develop in pediatric patients with either acute liver failure or chronic liver disease. In children, the development of early grades of encephalopathy can be difficult to assess. Many of the symptoms of early grades of hepatic encephalopathy, such as irritability, are relatively non-specific findings for moderate to severely ill infants.
- Children with chronic ESLD with PHT may develop minimal hepatic encephalopathy, leading to subtle impairment of cognitive function, specifically in areas affecting memory and attention span.
- Precipitating factors for hepatic encephalopathy include an oral protein load, GI bleeding, infection and use of sedatives or after surgical shunts for PHT.
- Serum ammonia levels are usually elevated in encephalopathy and correlate with the severity of hepatic encephalopathy.
- Oral antibiotics (rifaximin) and synthetic disaccharides (lactulose) are used to minimize ammonia production in patients with hepatic encephalopathy.

Coagulopathy

- Coagulation disorders associated with liver disease may occur secondary to hepatocellular damage (reduced synthesis of coagulation factors), vitamin K malabsorption, hypersplenism (thrombocytopenia) or multifactorial as seen in DIC.
- These disturbances are important in evaluation of the synthetic function of the liver, in prognostic assessment of the liver disease and in management of variceal bleeding.

- Severe coagulopathy may lead to intracerebral bleeding and DIC. Factor VII is the first coagulation factor that decreases, probably because of its short half-life (4–6 hours).Reductions in synthesis of factors II, V, IX, X, and XI also correlate with the extent of cirrhosis and the loss of liver parenchymal cells. Factor VIII levels remain normal or elevated, even in cirrhotic patients because of either extrahepatic synthesis (e.g. endothelial cells) or reduced clearance of the factor VIII–von Willebrand factor complex in the liver.
- Abnormalities in both platelet number and platelet function are common in chronic liver disease due to:
  - Splenomegaly secondary to PHT and subsequent sequestration of platelets in the spleen (hypersplenism).
  - Reduced hepatic production of the thrombopoietin (thrombopoietic growth factor).
  - Impaired platelet aggregation secondary to variety of intrinsic platelet defects.
- The treatment of coagulopathy of liver disease consists of:
  - Parenteral (usually subcutaneously) vitamin K (1–2 mg in an infant and 5–10 mg in an older child).
  - Blood products like fresh frozen plasma, cryoprecipitate and platelets are reserved for use in the setting of active bleeding or before surgical procedures.
  - Recombinant factor VIIa may improve coagulopathy caused by liver failure.

Malnutrition and nutrition support in infants and children with chronic liver disease

- Liver disease results in complex pathophysiologic disturbances affecting nutrient digestion, absorption, distribution, storage and use.
- Routine nutritional assessment should be performed at every visit of an infant or child with chronic liver diseases and includes clinical history, physical examination and laboratory investigations (see table: Assessment of nutritional status of a child with chronic liver disease).
- The conventional technique of assessment, such as body weight and weight adjusted for height, may not be accurate in children with chronic liver disease because of ascites and organomegaly. Using parameters that are less affected by fluid retention, e.g. height, muscle wasting, triceps skin folds, biochemical tests for albumin/prealbumin, and vitamin and micronutrients deficiency, are more reliable.
- The etiology of failure to gain weight in patients with chronic liver disease is multifactorial although insufficient dietary intake is probably the most important cause and is correctable. Decreased caloric intake is related to decreased desire to feed and early satiety from delayed gastric emptying or gastroesophageal reflux due to the presence of large-volume ascites or hepatosplenomegaly.
- Fat malabsorption occurs in cholestatic disorders with accompanying fat-soluble vitamin and essential fatty acid deficiencies.
- Other vitamin and trace elements such as thiamine, folic acid, vitamin D, vitamin E, magnesium and zinc may also be deficient.
- Severely malnourished infants with ESLD are at increased risk for death while awaiting LT and have poor outcome following LT.
- Failure to gain weight represents one of the components of the Pediatric End-Stage Liver Disease scoring system currently in use for risk-based allocation of liver donor organs to potential pediatric transplant (below 12 years old) recipients in the USA.
- Patients with chronic liver disease require increased caloric intake, usually 120–150% of their estimated daily requirements.

- Formulas containing medium-chain triglycerides are used to maximize fat absorption in the setting of severe cholestasis (see table: Nutrition support for children with chronic liver disease).
- Daily supplements of fat-soluble vitamins (A, D, E, K) must be added (see table: Vitamin supplementation for children with chronic liver disease).
- In children with growth retardation who are unable to take adequate protein and calories, supplementations with high caloric drinks and night-time nasogastric enteral tube feedings should be considered. Continuous nasogastric tube feeding may be necessary for patients experiencing regurgitation or volume intolerance due to ascites or organomegaly.
- Algorithm 37.1 details the approach to assessment and management of malnutrition in children with chronic liver disease.

Algorithm 37.1 Assessment and management of malnutrition in children with chronic liver disease

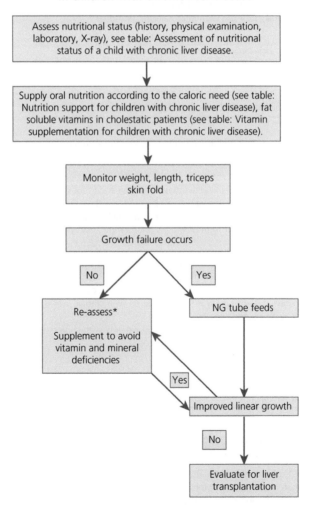

Assessment of nutritional status of a child with chronic liver disease

History
- Breast feed, type of formula, volume of feeds, total caloric intake/24 hours
- Frequency and volume of vomiting, stool, presence of steatorrhea
- Presence of epistaxis, easy bruising (vitamin K deficiency), night blindness (vitamin A deficiency) or bone fractures (vitamin D deficiency)

Physical examination
- Height, weight, head circumference, muscle bulk, subcutaneous tissue
- Rachitic rosaries, craniotabes, delayed closure of fontanelle (vitamin D deficiency)
- Excessive bruising (vitamin K deficiency)
- Depressed lower limb tendon reflexes (vitamin E deficiency)

Laboratory investigations
- CBC, liver enzymes, albumin, prealbumin (low levels in protein malnutrition)
- INR (vitamin K deficiency)
- Serum retinol (vitamin A deficiency)
- Plasma tocopherol and tocopherol/cholesterol ratio (vitamin E deficiency)
- Triene/tetraene ratio (essential fatty acid deficiency)
- Serum 25-OH vitamin D, 1.25 OH vitamin D, calcium, phosphor

Imaging
- Plain X-ray (vitamin D deficiency and its complications)

Nutrition support for children with chronic liver disease.

Caloric need
Based on the infant/child weight and according to validated tables in the literature. Ideal body weight should be used in these calculations (50th percentile weight for the child height).

Formula
MCT-enriched formulae like Progesemil/Alimentum is recommended for cholestatic infants. Concentrating formulae (by adding less water) can be used in order to increase the caloric density. For breast fed infants, human milk fortifier can be added. Adding carbohydrates (usually in the form of glucose polymers) or/and fat in a form of MCT is another practical option.

Nutrients
- Carbohydrates: children with chronic liver disease are at risk for hypoglycemia during intercurrent infections or when fasting. Monitoring glucose levels and IV glucose may be needed in these circumstances. High concentration of carbohydrates may cause osmotic diarrhea.
- Proteins: protein dose of 3–4 g/kg/day is safe in children with chronic liver disease. Lower dose is needed in patients with encephalopathy.
- Fat: nearly half of the total fat should be provided in patients with cholestasis as MCT. LCT are needed to provide essential fatty acids.

Vitamin supplement for children with chronic liver disease

Fat soluble vitamins

Vitamin A: vitamin A dose is 5000–25 000 IU/day, monitor to adjust the dose and to prevent hypervitaminosis A as a high level of vitamin A is hepatotoxic.

Vitamin D: vitamin D dose is 400 IU/day. The main formulations are vitamin D2 that is fat soluble and 25-OH D3 that is more water soluble. Monitor levels of 25-OH and 1,25-OH vitamin D, calcium and phosphor. Monitor clinically and radiologically as needed.

Vitamin E: dose of vitamin E is 15–25 IU/kg/day preferably as TPGS. Monitor plasma tocopherol and/or tocopherol /cholesterol ration to screen for deficiency and monitor treatment response. Spinocerebellar degeneration secondary to vitamin E is not reversible.

Vitamin K: dose of oral vitamin K is 2.5–5 mg/day. Vitamin K status can be monitored by PT or INR and the response to subcutaneously or intramuscular vitamin K (0.3/mg/kg).

Water soluble vitamins and trace elements.

These should be provided to infant and children with chronic liver disease according to the RDA (Recommended Dietary Allowance).

HRS

- HRS is a functional progressive renal failure of unknown cause in patients with acute or chronic liver disease. It is characterized with renal arterial vasoconstriction and marked reduction of renal cortical blood flow. The histologic findings are minimal and the changes of HRS are reversible after LT or recovery from the underlying liver disease.
- The clinical presentation of HRS varies in the severity and rapidity of renal dysfunction:
  - In type 1 HRS there is a drop of more than 50% of creatinine clearance within a 2 week period usually precipitated by acute deterioration of circulatory function, gastrointestinal bleeding, spontaneous bacterial peritonitis or aggressive diuretics. It is associated with very poor patient prognosis.
  - In type 2 HRS there is a mild slow progressive renal dysfunction in patient with refractory ascites. The survival of these patients is shorter than patients with ascites without HRS.
- The differential diagnosis of HRS includes pre-renal failure, which responds to acute volume expansion, and acute tubular necrosis.
- Typically the renal failure of HRS is oliguric, with normal urine sediment. The urine sodium concentration is low (<10 mEq/L), urine osmolarity is above plasma osmolarity and there is brief or no diuresis in response to rapid volume expansion.
- There is no known effective treatment for HRS other than LT. It is important to avoid agents and conditions that precipitate HRS such as nephrotoxic drugs (aminoglycosides), dehydration and gastrointestinal hemorrhage. Supportive treatment including low protein diet and correction of electrolyte abnormality is recommended. Hemodialysis and continuous arteriovenous hemofiltration have been successfully used in children while waiting for LT.
- Terlipressin a vasopressin analogue, has frequently been used in adults with HRS. There was no apparent impact of terlipressin therapy on survival in HRS patients and there are no studies in children as yet.

HCC

- Patients with tyrosinemia type 1 or progressive familial intrahepatic cholestasis type 2 may develop HCC in infancy or early childhood. Patients with chronic hepatitis B, even without cirrhosis, and patients with cirrhosis secondary to hepatitis C or other etiologies may develop HCC.
- The presenting symptoms may be abdominal pain or abdominal mass with an increased AFP, but HCC can be found incidentally at LT.
  - CT and MRI (triple phase) are the best imaging studies for evaluation of liver lesions in patient with cirrhosis. Although there are no established recommendations for screening

children with cirrhosis for HCC, we do recommend yearly abdominal US and serum AFP levels in these patients.

• Treatment of children with HCC is based on the adult experience. The therapies that are known to offer a high rate of complete responses are surgical resection, transplantation and percutaneous ablation.

Section 7: Reading List

Al-Hussaini A, Taylor RM, Samyn M, Bansal S, Heaton N, Rela M, Mieli-Vergani G, Dhawan A. Long-term outcome and management of hepatopulmonary syndrome in children. Pediatr Transplant 2010;14: 276–82

Bass NM, Mullen KD, Sanyal A, et al. Rifaximin treatment in hepatic encephalopathy. N Engl J Med 2010;362:1071–81

Bruix J, Sherman M. Management of hepatocellular carcinoma: an update. American Association for the Study of Liver Diseases. Hepatology 2011;53:1020–2. doi: 10.1002/hep.24199

Cohen MJ, Sahar T, Benenson S, Elinav E, Brezis M, Soares-Weiser K. Antibiotic prophylaxis for spontaneous bacterial peritonitis in cirrhotic patients with ascites, without gastro-intestinal bleeding. Cochrane Database Syst Rev 2009;2:CD004791

Fabrizi F, Dixit V, Messa P, Martin P. Terlipressin for hepatorenal syndrome: a meta-analysis of randomized trials. Int J Artif Organs 2009;32:133–40

Garcia-Tsao G, Sanyal AJ, Grace ND, Carey W. Prevention and management of gastroesophageal varices and variceal hemorrhage in cirrhosis. Hepatology 2007;46:922–38

Leonis MA, Balistreri WF. Evaluation and management of end-stage liver disease in children. Gastroenterology 2008;134:1741–51

Nightingale S, Ng VL. Optimizing nutritional management in children with chronic liver disease. Pediatr Clin North Am 2009; 56:1161–83

Novy MA, Schwarz KB. Nutritional considerations and management of the child with liver disease. Nutrition 1997;13:177–84

Peck-Radosavljevic M. Review article: coagulation disorders in chronic liver disease. Aliment Pharmacol Ther 2007;26(Suppl 1):21–8

Runyon BA. AASLD Practice Guidelines Committee. Management of adult patients with ascites due to cirrhosis: an update. Hepatology 2009; 49:2087–107

Sabri M, Saps M, Peters JM. Pathophysiology and management of pediatric ascites. J Pediatr Gastroenterol Nutr 2001;33:245–9

Sanyal AJ, Bosch J, Blei A, Arroyo V. Portal hypertension and its complications. Gastroenterology 2008;134:1715–28

Section 8: Guidelines

National society guidelines

Guideline title	Guideline source	Date
Prevention and Management of Gastroesophageal Varices and Variceal Hemorrhage in Cirrhosis	American Association for the Study of Liver Diseases (AASLD) http://www.aasld.org/practiceguidelines/Documents/ Bookmarked%20Practice%20Guidelines/Prevention%20 and%20Management%20of%20Gastro%20Varices%20 and%20Hemorrhage.pdf	2007
Management of Adult Patients with Ascites Due to Cirrhosis: An Update	American Association for the Study of Liver Diseases (AASLD) http://www.aasld.org/practiceguidelines/Documents/ ascitesupdate2013.pdf	2013
Management of Hepatocellular Carcinoma: An Update	American Association for the Study of Liver Diseases (AASLD) http://www.aasld.org/practiceguidelines/Documents/ Bookmarked%20Practice%20Guidelines/HCCUpdate2010.pdf	2010

Section 9: Evidence

See AASLD Guidelines.

Section 10: Images

Not applicable for this topic.

Additional material for this chapter can be found online at:
www.mountsinaiexpertguides.com
This includes a case study and multiple choice questions

CHAPTER 38

Liver Transplantation: A Pediatric Perspective

Nanda Kerkar
Children's Hospital of Los Angeles, University of Southern California, Los Angeles, CA, USA

OVERALL BOTTOM LINE
- There are key differences between adult and pediatric LT with respect to indications, evaluation of candidates, timing and priority for transplant, and management.
- Biliary atresia is the most common indication for LT in children in comparison with hepatitis C-related cirrhosis in adults.
- The PELD score is used to prioritize organ allocation in children <12 years, while the MELD score is used for those >12 years, similar to adults.
- Growth and development as well as psychosocial aspects require special attention in children requiring LT.
- Exposure to EBV for the first time after LT poses unique challenges in pediatrics.

Section 1: Background

- LT in children has become the standard of care for children with acute liver failure and ESLD since the early 1980s

---

History
- 1963 – First LT in a child with biliary atresia by Thomas Starzl.
- 1978 – Cyclosporin used as an immunosuppressant.
- 1989 – Tacrolimus introduced (primary immunosuppression in USA today).
- 1991 – First living donor transplantation was performed in a child as there was an organ shortage crisis particularly in small children.
- 2002 – PELD and MELD scores introduced to prioritize patients waiting for LT in the USA.

- The major issue in transplantation today is the organ shortage, causing longer waiting times and increasing waiting list mortality.
- To overcome this, various strategies including live donor transplantation, split LT, extended criteria donors such as elderly donors, hepatitis B core antibody positive donors, and donation after cardiac death have been employed.
- Due to poorer outcome after transplant, we typically avoid using extended criteria donors and donation after cardiac death unless the benefit outweighs the risks in pediatric LT.

Mount Sinai Expert Guides: Hepatology, First Edition. Edited by Jawad Ahmad, Scott L. Friedman, and Henryk Dancygier.
© 2014 John Wiley & Sons, Ltd. Published 2014 by John Wiley & Sons, Ltd.
Companion website: www.mountsinaiexpertguides.com

Incidence/prevalence
- Around 12000 pediatric LTs have been performed in the USA.
- Approximately 600 transplants are performed annually.
- Initial survival rates 40 years ago were in the 30% range, but now 1-year survival rates are as high as 90%.

Economic impact
- LT is one of the most expensive medical and surgical procedures performed in the world today.
- Conservative estimates of the cost of a single uncomplicated LT in the USA are several hundred thousand dollars.
- The direct and indirect costs associated with liver disease and associated treatment exceeds $180 billion annually in the USA.
- It is generally believed that when compared with other accepted medical technologies, LT meets the cost-effectiveness criterion of having an additional benefit worth the added cost.

Indications for LT in children
- Cholestatic liver disease:
  - Extrahepatic biliary atresia.
  - Alagille syndrome.
  - Sclerosing cholangitis.
  - Progressive familial intra-hepatic cholestasis.
  - Idiopathic neonatal hepatitis.
- Fulminant liver failure.
- Metabolic liver disease:
  - Structural damage to the liver: Wilson disease, alpha-1 antitrypsin deficiency, tyrosinemia, cystic fibrosis, glycogen storage disease.
  - No structural damage to the liver: Urea cycle defects, primary hyperoxaluria.
- Autoimmune hepatitis.
- Liver tumors:
  - Infantile hepatic hemangioendothelioma.
  - Hepatoblastoma.
- Miscellaneous:
  - Cryptogenic cirrhosis.
  - Congenital hepatic fibrosis.
  - Drug overdose/toxicity.
  - Viral hepatitis.
  - Retransplantation secondary to complications of first transplant.

Contraindications to LT in pediatrics
- Coma with irreversible brain injury.
- Uncontrolled systemic infection including AIDS.
- Liver tumors with extrahepatic metastasis.
- Terminal progressive systemic disease.
- Inadequate cardiac or pulmonary function.

Timing of LT
- Early referral is key to a successful LT
- In acute liver failure

- INR >2 despite parenteral Vitamin K supplementation.
- INR >1.5 and encephalopathy.
- In biliary atresia:
  - Persistence of cholestasis 6–8 weeks after Kasai portoenterostomy.
  - Failure to thrive, weight and height < third centile.
  - Recurrent cholangitis.
  - Portal hypertension complications – ascites, GI bleeding.
  - Poor synthetic function with prolonged INR, reduced albumin.
- In metabolic disorders:
  - Failure of medical therapy.
  - Repeated metabolic decompensations increase the risk of neurological deficits.

Evaluation for LT
- Initial consultation by pediatric hepatologist:
  - To confirm diagnosis and establish need for LT.
  - To discuss other therapeutic options versus LT.
  - To explain sequence of events involved in LT evaluation, listing, surgery and subsequent course and introduce to LT surgeon and coordinator.
  - To begin to establish relationship with family and answer any concerns before initiating formal evaluation by the rest of the team.
- Evaluation by the transplant surgeon:
  - To assess suitability for LT and assess need for specialized imaging.
  - To discuss type of organ, deceased versus living donor, scoring system and waiting list.
  - To explain technical aspects of surgery including complications.
  - To discuss outcomes after LT and side effects of immunosuppression.
- Evaluation by nutritionist:
  - To assess recipient's nutritional status and caloric intake.
  - To initiate tube feeding in conjunction with the hepatologist if failure to thrive.
- Evaluation by infectious disease specialist:
  - To ensure there are no infection issues that preclude LT.
  - To ensure immunization schedule is expedited especially live vaccines in infants and babies.
- Evaluation by cardiologist:
  - To ensure that the child has stable cardiac status and can undergo transplant surgery.
- Evaluation by social worker:
  - To ensure that the child comes from a stable home and is able to comply with the post-transplant regimen and provide support as required.
- Evaluation by transplant coordinator:
  - To coordinate the child's evaluation for LT.
  - To go over the LT process including scoring, donor types and outcomes and take informed consent for evaluation and listing.
  - To provide education about the transplant process and give appropriate manuals.
  - To organize listing of the patient after evaluation is completed.
  - To provide liaison between physicians, the family and the referring doctor.
- Repeat consult by the hepatologist at the end of evaluation:
  - To reinforce the information given by other members of the team.
  - To ensure that the family understands implications of being listed for LT.
  - To answer any concerns and repeat information as required.
  - To ensure there is an interim plan for management until LT.

Laboratory tests and imaging for LT assessment
- Blood type and screen ×2.
- Serologies:
  - HIV, hepatitis A, B and C.
  - CMV urine shell vial culture <1 year, CMV IgG for children >1 year.
  - EBV IgG and IgM.
  - Varicella IgG, MMR IgG, toxoplasma IgG, RPR, HSV in select cases
- Disease specific:
  - Hepatitis B: HBsAg/Ab, HBeAg/Ab, HBV DNA, anti-HDV, AFP.
  - Autoimmune hepatitis/sclerosing cholangitis: antinuclear antibody, SMA, LKM antibody, quantitative IgG.
  - Alpha-1 antitrypsin phenotype.
  - Wilson disease: ceruloplasmin, 24 hour urine copper.
  - Metabolic: glucose, lactate, ammonia, pyruvate, urinary organic acids including succinyl acetone, serum aminoacids, AFP, acyl carnitine profile, arterial blood gas.
  - Neonatal hemochromatosis: ferritin, iron studies, salivary gland biopsy, MR pancreas.
  - Malignancy: AFP, CA 19-9, carcinoembryonic antigen.
  - Cholestasis: serum bile acids.
- Pro-coagulant screen in selected cases.
- Imaging:
  - Chest X-ray.
  - Liver US scan.
  - ECG/echocardiogram.
  - CT or MR of the abdomen.

Growth and development
- Chronic organ failure leads to retarded growth and delayed puberty.
- In children with ESLD, growth retardation is inversely correlated with age, leading to the notion that liver failure is more critical to the nutrition-dependent growth phase of infancy.
- In genetic disorders like Alagille syndrome or PFIC, there may be intra-uterine growth retardation and there is little catch-up growth after LT.
- Anthropometric measurements should be plotted regularly on growth charts in all children with chronic liver disease.
- Cholestatic infants and babies require formula high in MCTs.
- Supplementation with fat soluble vitamins A, D, E and K in cholestasis.
- Parenteral vitamin K in cholestatic children if INR is prolonged.
- Nasogastric tube feeds if failure to thrive.
- Parenteral nutrition in extreme cases.

Interim care
- Nutritional support.
- Complete immunization, particularly live vaccination (MMR, varicella).
- Ursodeoxycholic acid 10 mg/kg twice a day in cholestasis.
- Rifampin trial (10 mg/kg/day) in those with persistent pruritus.
- Diuretics for control of ascites – typically combination of furosemide (1 mg/kg/dose) and spironolactone (up to 6 mg/kg/day in divided doses).
- Prophylactic antibiotics in selected cases.
- Patient and family education.
- Liaison with referring physician.

Listing for LT
- Children with fulminant liver failure get listed as Status 1A which is the highest priority for transplant.
- Status IB is designed for children who do not have typical abnormalities of liver function as required for PELD/MELD:
  - Metabolic disease.
  - Hepatoblastoma.
  - Chronic liver disease with a calculated MELD/PELD >25 and:
    - on a ventilator.
    - Glasgow coma scale <10, within 48 hours of listing.
    - GI bleeding requiring at least 30 mL/kg of packed red blood cell replacement in the previous 24 hours.
    - renal failure/insufficiency requiring dialysis/continuous venovenous filtration.
- Children with chronic liver disease get listed using PELD/MELD.

PELD
- PELD score was derived from a population of children enrolled in the Studies of Pediatric Split Transplantation as a means of stratifying children awaiting LT based on a continuous objective score that reflects risk for death or moving to an ICU in the ensuing 3 months.
- PELD has been in use since 2002.
- PELD is used to prioritize children for LT <12 years, MELD for >12 years.
- Parameters used are INR, total bilirubin, serum albumin, age <1 year and height less than 2 SD from the mean for age and gender.
- PELD score = 0.436 (age (<1 year)) – 0.687 × Log_e (albumin g/dL) + 0.480 × Log_e (total bilirubin mg/dL) + 1.87 × Log_e (INR) + 0.667 (growth failure (<–2 SD present)).

Types of LT
- Source of organ:
  - Deceased donor.
  - Living donor.
- Type of graft:
  - Whole graft.
  - Reduced graft.
  - Partial graft – right lobe, left lobe, left lateral segment, monosegment.
- Orthotopic LT – graft put in same position after removing native liver, standard in LT today.
- Auxiliary partial orthotopic LT (APOLT) – part of native liver left *in situ*, part of graft liver used:
  - Transplanted graft provides missing enzyme as in Crigler–Najjar syndrome.
  - Transplanted graft provides adequate liver function to act as bridge until native liver recovers as in fulminant liver failure.
- Domino LT – three patients benefit – typically graft of a patient with familial amyloidosis is given to an elderly patient with a lower calculated score, the new liver is split between the adult with amyloidosis and a pediatric patient.
- Combined transplant:
  - Liver and kidney.
  - Liver and small bowel.

Liver
- The liver is divided into eight functional segments each with independent arterial, venous and biliary connections – Couinaud's segments.
- Couinaud's segments:

- Caudate lobe (segment I).
- Left lateral segment (II and III).
- Left lobe (I [usually], II, III and IV).
- Right lobe (V, VI, VII and VIII).
- The liver constitutes 2% of body weight:
  - The left lateral segment is 25%.
  - The left lobe lobe is 40%.
  - The right lobe is 60% of the liver volume.
- As a rule of thumb:
  - Infants get the left lateral segment.
  - Small children <12 years get the left lobe.
  - Children >12 years get the right lobe.
- Graft recipient ratio (expressed as percentage of body weight) 0.8–4 is required.
- Inadequate graft volume can cause 'small for size syndrome':
  - Cholestasis.
  - Coagulopathy.
  - Oliguria.
  - Intractable ascites.

Technical aspects of LT in children

- Piggy-back technique is often used in infants and small children, avoiding the venovenous bypass used in adults.
- Entire retrohepatic vena cava is preserved and the new liver is anastomosed to a cuff from one or more of the main supra-hepatic veins.
- Diameter of the vessels is very small and vascular grafts are used often in arterial and venous anastomoses.
- The biliary anastomosis in infants and small children is often a choledochojejunostomy (to a Roux-en-Y defunctioning intestinal loop) rather than a duct to duct as seen in adults.

Living donor transplantation in children

- Living donor LT was first started in response to a waiting list mortality of >25% in children.
- Advantages:
  - Safety net for family and clinician if sudden deterioration.
  - Increases the organs available to children.
  - Elective operation, improved morbidity and mortality compared with adults.
  - Use of healthy donors and minimal cold ischemia time reduces primary graft non-function.
  - Psychological benefit to the donor.
- Disadvantages:
  - Risk to healthy donor.

EBV and PTLD

- PTLD following LT is a significant cause of morbidity and mortality in children.
- The majority of cases of PTLD in childhood is associated with primary EBV infection.
- PTLD is usually diagnosed in the first 2 years after LT and though the incidence historically has been 6–15%, it has reduced with EBV surveillance and preemptive immunosuppression reduction.
- EBV donor-recipient mismatching and intensified immunosuppression are risk factors for developing PTLD.
- Molecular EBV monitoring routinely after LT and using prophylactic antiviral therapy in the post-transplant period is essential.

- Reducing immunosuppression after detection of EBV by PCR or a rise in EBV is the first step towards preventing PTLD.
- Diagnosis of PTLD is based on histology.
- The WHO classification:
  - Early lesions – reactive plasmacytic hyperplasia or infectious mononucleosis-like.
  - Polymorphic PTLD (polyclonal or monoclonal).
  - Monomorphic PTLD.
- The hepatic infiltration in PTLD is predominantly B-cell in comparison to that seen in rejection where it is T-cell predominant.
- *In situ* hybridization for EBV-encoded nuclear RNA (EBER) confirms that the infiltrating lymphoid cells are EBV positive.
- Reducing or stopping immunosuppression is key in controlling PTLD.
- There is no consensus for the role of anti-virals in treatment of PTLD.
- Rituximab, a humanized anti-CD20 monoclonal antibody has been used successfully to treat PTLD.
- Surgery, radiotherapy and chemotherapy have been used in more advanced stages to control disease.
- Molecular monitoring of EBV post-transplant in pediatric LT recipients and reducing immunosuppression after detection of EBV have led to improved outcomes.

Adherence
- Adherence is defined by the WHO as 'the extent to which a person's behavior – taking medication, following a diet, and/or executing lifestyle changes, corresponds with agreed recommendations from a healthcare provider'.
- LT recipients receive life-long immunosuppressive medications.
- Non-adherence to medications is a leading cause of morbidity in pediatric LT.
- Underlying risk factors for non-adherence include depression, low socio-economic status, post-traumatic stress syndrome and complicated medical status.
- Responsibility of taking the medication is shifted to the child between the ages of 9 and 16 years (average 12 years).
- The most common reason given for non-adherence is forgetfulness.
- Adolescents are most likely to be non-adherent.

Assessment of adherence
- Subjective:
  - Direct questioning of child, parent or health care personnel.
  - Answering questionnaires.
- Objective:
  - Pill counts.
  - Medication refill rates.
  - Electronic monitoring devices (device registers each time medication is taken out of the container).
  - Blood levels of medication especially the degree of fluctuation between individual blood levels.

- Measures used to reinforce adherence:
  - Increase in clinic visits and stressing the importance of adherence.
  - Monitoring of graft function and tacrolimus levels more frequently.
  - Making medication regimen as simple as possible and palatable.

- Text messaging to remind recipients to take their medications.
- Involvement of psychologist.
- Involvement of social worker.

Transition to adult services
- Successful transfer to the adult service may depend on the pediatric recipient being able to independently manage his/her healthcare while in the pediatric setting.
- Lack of personal responsibility for health has been cited as a barrier to successful transition.
- Adherence status should be regularly monitored before, during and after the transition.
- Systematic research is needed to ensure successful transition while efficiently using the resources that are available.

Algorithm 38.1 Approach to LT in children

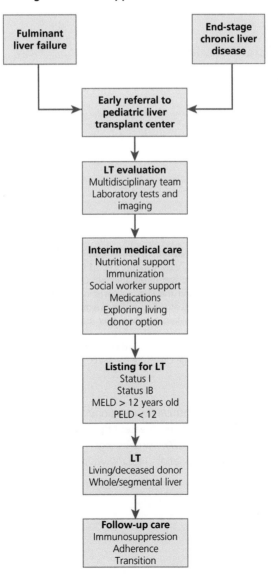

Fulminant liver failure

End-stage chronic liver disease

Early referral to pediatric liver transplant center

LT evaluation
Multidisciplinary team
Laboratory tests and imaging

Interim medical care
Nutritional support
Immunization
Social worker support
Medications
Exploring living donor option

Listing for LT
Status I
Status IB
MELD > 12 years old
PELD < 12

LT
Living/deceased donor
Whole/segmental liver

Follow-up care
Immunosuppression
Adherence
Transition

Section 2: Prevention

Not applicable for this topic.

Section 3: Diagnosis

Not applicable for this topic.

Section 4: Treatment

Not applicable for this topic.

Section 5: Special Populations

Not applicable for this topic.

Section 6: Prognosis

Not applicable for this topic.

Section 7: Reading List

Eghtesad B, Kadry Z, Fung J. Technical considerations in liver transplantation: what a hepatologist needs to know (and every surgeon should practice). Liver Transpl 2005;11; 861–71

Kerkar N, Emre S. Issues unique to pediatric liver transplantation. Clin Liver Dis 2007;11:323–36

McDiarmid SV, Ananda R, Lindblad AS and the Principal Investigators and Institutions of the Studies of Pediatric Liver Transplantation (SPLIT) Research Group. Development of a pediatric end-stage liver disease score to predict poor outcome in children awaiting liver transplantation. Transplantation 2002;74: 173–81

Tiao G, Alonso M, Ryckman F. Liver transplantation in children. In Suchy F, Sokol R and Balistreri W (eds) Liver Disease in Children. New York: Cambridge University Press, 2007

Suggested websites

American Society of Transplantation: http://www.a-s-t.org/

American Association of the Study of Liver Disease: http://www.aasld.org/

United Network of Organ Sharing: http://www.unos.org/

International Pediatric Transplant Association: http://www.iptaonline.org/

Section 8: Guidelines

Not applicable for this topic.

Section 9: Evidence

Not applicable for this topic.

Section 10: Images

Not applicable for this topic.

Additional material for this chapter can be found online at:
www.mountsinaiexpertguides.com
This includes a case study, multiple choice questions and advice for patients

PART 3

TRANSPLANTATION

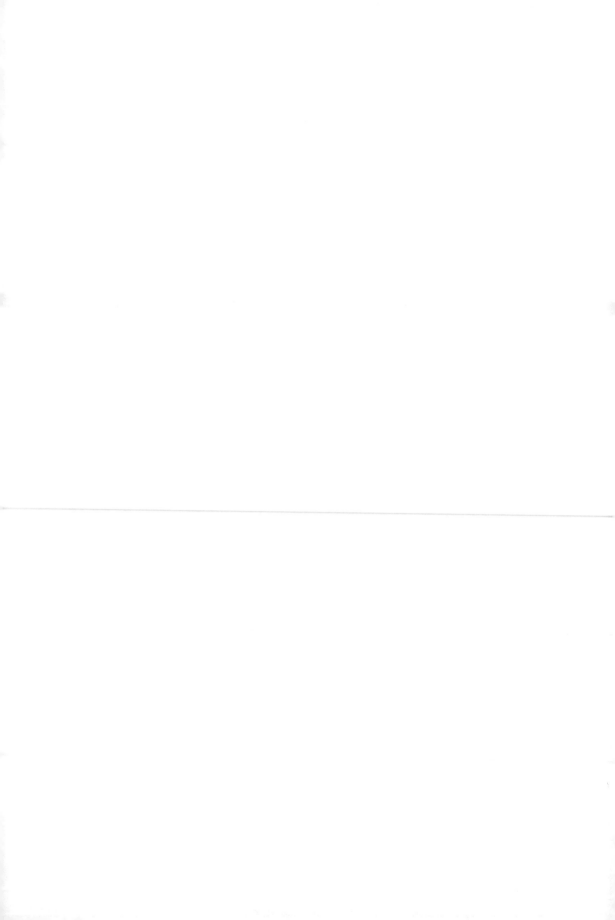

CHAPTER 39

Evaluation of Patients for Liver Transplantation

Lawrence U. Liu

Division of Liver Diseases, Icahn School of Medicine at Mount Sinai, New York, NY, USA

OVERALL BOTTOM LINE
- LT is now accepted as a life-saving treatment modality for patients with ESLD or ALF.
- ESLD causes over 75 000 deaths annually in the USA.
- Currently, over 6000 LTs are performed annually in the USA.
- Not all patients, however, are candidates for this procedure; hence the need for an evaluation process.
- A multidisciplinary system is used to evaluate thoroughly the potential LT candidate, including factors that may affect pre- and post-transplantation survival and quality of life.
- The MELD score is currently utilized to prioritize deceased donor organ allocation for LT.
- There continues to be a significant gap between patients who undergo LT and who die while on the waiting list.

Section 1: Background

- The evaluation of patients for LT initially involves identifying patients that would benefit from this procedure.
- Patients undergo a thorough medical, cardiac, surgical and psychosocial assessment.
- The most common disease processes that lead to LT evaluation are listed under "Common etiologies for an LT evaluation." The majority of patients have ASLD due to cirrhosis from a variety of etiologies. Of those patients that complete the evaluation process and are placed on the waiting list for LT, more than a third have hepatitis C-related liver disease (see table: Patients on the LT waiting list). HCC has become a leading indication as its incidence rises in the USA.
- ALF makes up only 5–10% of all LTs and there are a small number of pediatric and miscellaneous indications.

Common etiologies for an LT evaluation
- Hepatitis C.
- Alcoholic liver disease.
- HCC.
- NASH.
- Hepatitis B.
- ALF.

Mount Sinai Expert Guides: Hepatology, First Edition. Edited by Jawad Ahmad, Scott L. Friedman, and Henryk Dancygier.

- Cholestatic liver diseases: PBC, PSC.
- AIH.
- Cryptogenic cirrhosis.
- Metabolic liver diseases: Wilson disease, alpha-1 antitrypsin deficiency, hereditary hemochromatosis.
- Pediatric liver diseases: biliary atresia, primary hyperoxaluria.

Patients on the LT waiting list: UNOS 2010 Annual Report (representing 2009 results). www.unos.org

Etiology	Percentage
Hepatitis C	30.7
Alcoholic liver disease	22.6
Malignancy	4.2
Hepatitis B	3
ALF	2.8
Others/cryptogenic	36.7

MELD score

- The MELD scoring system was initially developed at the Mayo Clinic for estimating the 3-month survival of patients with ESLD who underwent TIPS placement.
- A modification of the original MELD score was adapted to predict 90-day survival in patients waiting for LT with a very high accuracy and has subsequently been well validated. The MELD score equation uses the serum bilirubin, creatinine and INR to give a continuous variable. Due to the logarithmic scale used the lowest values for each of the three variables is 1.0 and the creatinine is capped at 4 mg/dL (which is also the value used for patients on renal replacement therapy).
- MELD = $0.378 \times \log_e$ (bilirubin mg/dL) + $1.12 \times \log_e$ (INR) + $0.957 \times \log_e$ (creatinine mg/dL) + 0.643; range: 6–40 points.
- The higher the score, the greater the risk of dying and hence a higher priority for LT. Research has shown that both hospitalized and historical patient groups with a MELD score higher than 40 had a 3-month mortality of 100%.
- The MELD score has been used for deceased donor liver allocation for adult patients in the USA since 2002. A different system (the PELD score) is used for pediatric patients and is detailed in Chapter 38.
- The MELD score accurately predicts waiting list mortality but importantly a higher MELD score does not significantly worsen post-transplantation survival (unless the MELD score is very high). Since some patients would benefit from LT but do not necessarily have ESLD, or have other complications of liver disease that are not considered in the MELD score, a MELD exception can be used. The most common reason for a MELD exception is HCC. A seminal study from Milan by Mazzaferro et al. in 1996 observed that a 4-year survival rate of 65% in LT recipients was noted if certain factors (the Milan criteria) were met.

Milan criteria

- One lesion, between 2 and 5 cm in diameter.
- Up to three lesions, each ≤3 cm in diameter.
- No vascular invasion.

- No metastatic disease.
- Patients with HCC within the Milan criteria are eligible for a MELD exception of 22 points, regardless of their actual MELD score. This MELD exception score is increased by 10% every 3 months and hence it is important to identify HCC in LT candidates as this increases their chance of receiving a LT.
- Several other HCC criteria exist which have tried to increase the number of patients eligible for a MELD exception. The UCSF criteria expands the limits set by the Milan criteria. Although some reports demonstrate similar post-transplantation survival, these criteria are currently not established as the standard by UNOS:
- UCSF criteria:
  - One lesion, up to 6.5 cm in diameter.
  - Up to three lesions, each not exceeding 4.5 cm in diameter.
  - Total tumor diameter not exceeding 8 cm.
  - No evidence of vascular invasion and metastatic disease.

Section 2: Prevention

Not applicable for this topic.

Section 3: Diagnosis
Indications for an LT evaluation

- Patients with ESLD with a MELD score ≥15.
- Patients with complications of cirrhosis: ascites, encephalopathy, synthetic dysfunction or variceal bleeding. Prior to 2002, allocation of deceased donor organs was determined largely by the Child–Pugh score. Originally used to assess the risk of mortality in cirrhotic patients undergoing surgery, this score was subsequently used to determine their need to undergo LT.
  - The Child–Pugh score utilizes five variables: total bilirubin, albumin, prothrombin time, degree of ascites and hepatic encephalopathy.
  - Each variable is assigned 1, 2 or 3 points depending on severity, making a maximum score of 15 points.

	1 point	2 points	3 points
Total bilirubin	<2 mg/dL	2–3 mg/dL	>3 mg/dL
Albumin	>3.4 mg/dL	2.8–3.4 mg/dL	<2.8 mg/dL
Prothrombin time (INR)	<1.6	1.6–2.2	>2.2
Ascites	None	Moderate	Severe
Hepatic encephalopathy	None	Mild/moderate	Severe

  - Categories (Child Class A, B, C) are assigned according to the score range:
    - Child Class A: 5–6 points
    - Child Class B: 7–9 points
    - Child Class C: 10–15 points
  - A patient needed to be at least Child Class B for LT candidacy consideration (prior to the current use of the MELD score for organ allocation).

- Patients with ALF are also candidates for LT (see Chapter 26). These patients do not have chronic liver disease but develop hepatic encephalopathy within 8 weeks and/or jaundice within 2 weeks of onset of liver injury. Since mortality in ALF is high and these patients have a very short time frame to be evaluated and listed for transplantation before they may become too sick to undergo LT, they are listed for transplantation using a special 'status 1' designation that gives them a higher priority than patients with a high MELD score.
- Patients with hepatopulmonary syndrome or portopulmonary hypertension also receive a MELD exception if they meet certain criteria (see Chapters 23 and 24).
- Metabolic conditions: these are uncommon indications for LT and typically require a MELD exception. They include familial amyloidotic polyneuropathy, primary hyperoxaluria, Wilson disease, alpha-1 antitrypsin deficiency, urea cycle enzyme deficiencies, glycogen storage disease, tyrosinemia, and intractable acute intermittent porphyria.
- Miscellaneous: several other conditions are indications for LT such as polycystic liver disease, metastatic neuroendocrine tumors and erythropoietic protoporphyria

Contraindications to LT candidacy

Absolute	Relative
Active extrahepatic malignancy	* Depending on the expertise/experience
Advanced HCC (exceeding the Milan/UCSF) criteria	of the center's transplantation team:
AIDS	
Uncontrolled sepsis	Advanced age
Severe cardiopulmonary conditions	Cholangiocarcinoma
Active alcohol and/or substance abuse	Portal vein thrombosis
Poor social support network	Extensive previous abdominal surgery
Inability to comply with post-transplantation	HIV infection
treatment	
Severe physical debilitation	
Technical and/or anatomical barriers	
Extensive portal and mesenteric vein thrombosis	
Irreversible brain injury	

Section 4: Treatment
Treatment rationale
- The potential LT candidate is initially assessed by primary members of the transplantation team (e.g. hepatologist, coordinator, nutritionist, social worker, cardiologist) and may require further specialty consultations when warranted by their clinical condition. A multidisciplinary approach is the key to the evaluation process.
- The patient undergoes basic laboratory tests, abdominal imaging studies and cancer surveillance. Further tests are performed when the need arises.
- Upon completion and evaluation of the various consultations and test results, the patient's transplantation candidacy is discussed at a meeting with the other transplantation team members. The patient will then either be accepted or declined as a candidate, or may need to be re-assessed if further tests/consultations are needed.

Evaluation: multidisciplinary approach
- Hepatologist.
- Surgeon.
- Social worker.

- Transplantation coordinator.
- Nutritionist.
- Financial coordinator.
- Cardiologist.
- When indicated: psychiatrist/psychologist, nephrologist, pulmonologist, ethicist, dentist/oral surgeon, anesthesiologist

Tests
Biochemical
- CBC.
- Basic and liver chemistries.
- Prothrombin time/INR.
- Blood type and screen.
- Alpha fetoprotein.
- Urinalysis.
- Serologies: hepatitis A,B and C, cytomegalovirus, RPR, HIV.
- When indicated: autoimmune markers, antimitochondrial antibody, ceruloplasmin, alpha-1 antitrypsin antibody, iron studies, hereditary hemochromatosis, mutation analysis, hepatitis B or C viral load, immunoglobulins.
- Urine toxicology screen and serum ethanol.

Cancer surveillance
- Colonoscopy.
- Males: PSA.
- Females: Mammogram, Pap smear.

Miscellaneous
- Upper endoscopy.
- Cardiac tests: ECG, echocardiogram, stress test (exercise/pharmacologic), cardiac catheterization (when indicated).
- Abdominal imaging: CT scan or MRI; evaluation for metastatic disease (if the patient has HCC).
- Bone densitometry.

Organ allocation system
- When the patient is determined to be a candidate for LT the patient's current MELD score is calculated and used to prioritize their position on the transplantation list. Their score is updated periodically – with the frequency determined by the score range, with sicker patients being evaluated more frequently.

MELD score	Frequency of re-certification
≥25	Every 7 days
19–24	Every month
11–18	Every 3 months
≤10	Every 12 months

- UNOS Regions: the USA is divided into 11 regions for organ allocation. The duration of waiting time, the MELD score when patients undergo transplantation, and importantly, the patient mortality while waiting on the transplantation list, can differ among these regions due largely to the number of patients on the waiting list and the availability of donor organs. Patients being evaluated at transplantation centers are given the option to be listed simultaneously at other regions' centers to expand their options.

- Patients may have associated conditions that allow them priority points (i.e. a higher assigned MELD score than their actual one). As detailed above these include HCC, HPS, recurrent cholangitis and metabolic disorders.
- In these patients the MELD score is re-certified every 3 months; if the patients continue to meet the eligibility criteria, their assigned score increases (generally a new score that reflects 10% increased mortality while on the waiting list) each time. For example, patients with HCC that meet the Milan criteria are assigned an initial score of 22 points (even if their actual MELD score does not reach this number); if they continue to meet the criteria after 3 months, the score is increased to 25 points.

Types of liver grafts
- Patients who are listed for LT typically will receive an organ from a deceased donor. Occasionally a whole liver can be split into two with a smaller left (lateral) lobe being used for a child and the rest for an adult. In recent years the types of donor organ that are accepted for use have increased to try and increase the number of LTs and reduce the number or people dying on the waiting list. These organs are termed 'extended criteria-donor' or 'marginal' donor (although there is no consensus definition) and are discussed in more detail in the surgical transplantation chapters.
- If patients have a relative that is willing to donate part of their liver as a live donor this can be explored (see Chapter 40).

Section 5: Special Populations
Pregnancy
- Pregnant patients are generally not involved in situations that require LT as most pregnancy-related liver disease resolve post-partum.
- A notable exception may be ALF which should be handled on a case by case basis due to the absence of a current guideline.
- In rare instances, immediate post-partum patients may be at risk for developing hepatic rupture and require urgent LT evaluation.

Children
See Chapter 38.

Elderly
- Patients of advanced age have inherent increased risks of peri-operative complications. A maximum age of 75 years appears to be accepted by most transplantation centers.
- LT eligibility for elderly patients should also focus on the estimated life expectancy and quality of life from this surgery.

Others
- Various reports demonstrate worse outcomes in certain populations such that care needs to be taken in these patients:
  - Obesity – outcome improved if BMI <35.

- HIV – patients need to have undetectable RNA and a CD4 count above 100 for at least 16 weeks before transplantation.
- Diabetes – patients should have absence of end-organ damage. Patients with kidney failure may require the addition of renal transplantation.
- LT can be performed together with other organs (e.g. kidney, pancreas, heart, lung, small bowel, multivisceral) and are best done at centers with adequate expertise in this field.

Section 6: Prognosis

CLINICAL PEARLS
- Since the advent of LT, patient survival rates have generally improved. The current 1-year survival rate ranges between 85 and 90%, with 5-year rates exceeding 65%.
- The etiology of liver disease affects survival after LT, with the best results seen in cholestatic liver disease and the worst in hepatitis C.
- Recurrence of the original disease is relatively common and can lead to organ failure in certain cases, particularly hepatitis C (which explains the worse survival). Other examples include hepatitis B infection, alcoholic liver disease, NAFLD, AIH, PBC, and PSC, but these seldom lead to graft loss.

Natural history of untreated disease
- There continues to be a discrepancy between patients who undergo LT and those who are removed from the waiting list. According to the 2010 UNOS Annual Report: 15 625 patients were on the waiting list at the end of 2009; 5748 patients underwent LTs that year, and 2396 patients died on the waiting list.

Prognosis for treated patients
Outcome after transplantation
- The current 1-year survival rate ranges between 85 and 90%, with 5-year rates exceeding 65%.

Follow-up tests and monitoring
- Patients waiting on the LT list undergo periodic updates with new MELD scores according to a defined schedule (see Section 4: Treatment).
- Those with priority points from HCC undergo imaging studies every 3 months to monitor the malignancy and determine if further treatment is required or if the cancer exceeds transplantation eligibility. Patients with priority points for other reasons (e.g. HPS, recurrent cholangitis) also require re-certification of their priority points every 3 months.

Section 7: Reading List

Kamath PS, Wiesner RH, Malinchoc M, et al. A model to predict survival in patients with end-stage liver disease. Hepatology 2001;33:464–70

Mandell MS, Lindenfeld J, Tsou MY, Zimmerman M. Cardiac evaluation of liver transplant candidates. World J Gastroenterol 2008;14:3445–51

Mazzaferro V, Regalia E, Doci R, et al. Liver transplantation for the treatment of small hepatocellular carcinomas in patients with cirrhosis. N Engl J Med 1996;334:693–9

Merion RM. Current status and future of liver transplantation. Semin Liver Dis 2010;30:411–21

O'Leary JG, Lepe R, Davis GL. Indications for liver transplantation. Gastroenterology 2008;134:1764–76

Russo MW. Current concepts in the evaluation of patients for liver transplantation. Expert Rev Gastroenterol Hepatol 2007;1:307–20

Sharma P, Rakela J. Management of pre-transplant patients – Part 1. Liver Transpl 2005;11:124–33

Yao FY, Ferrell L, Bass NM, et al. Liver transplantation for hepatocellular carcinoma: expansion of the tumor size limits does not adversely impact survival. Hepatology 2001;33:1394–403

Suggested website

www.UNOS.org

Section 8: Guidelines

Guideline title	Guideline source	Date
Evaluation of the Patient for Liver Transplantation	AASL http://www.aasld.org/practiceguidelines/Documents/ Bookmarked%20Practice%20Guidelines/Liver%20Transplant.pdf	2008

Section 9: Evidence

Not applicable for this topic.

Section 10: Images

Not applicable for this topic.

Additional material for this chapter can be found online at:
www.mountsinaiexpertguides.com
This includes a case study and multiple choice questions

CHAPTER 40

Live Donor Transplantation Evaluation

Lawrence U. Liu

Division of Liver Diseases, Icahn School of Medicine at Mount Sinai, New York, NY, USA

OVERALL BOTTOM LINE

- LDLT is a viable alternative to the liver graft supply shortage when both donor and recipient are carefully chosen and when the surgery and donor evaluation are performed at a transplantation center with expertise in this procedure.
- In the USA, LDLT makes up less than 5% of the total number of LTs performed annually.
- The potential donor must have an established emotional relationship with the recipient, and be free of any coercion to undergo this type of surgery.
- Donor mortality, although rare, remains a reality. The estimated donor mortality rate ranges from 0.2 to 2%. The most common post-operative donor complications are biliary-related and infections.
- There appears to be no long-term effects in patients who have undergone liver donation surgery. Long-term data continue to be collected on donor outcomes.

Section 1: Background
Overview

Over 6000 LDLT have been performed worldwide. Milestones include the first successful LDLT (adult-to-pediatric) in 1989 and the first successful adult-to-adult LDLT in 1997. LDLT significantly increase the donor pool. For adult recipients, the patient and graft survival rates after LDLT are comparable, or better than, DDLT.

Advantages of a LDLT (over a DDLT)

- Surgery is performed electively – no waiting time, optimal time is chosen for the transplantation (i.e. before the recipient becomes too sick).
- Liver graft is in excellent condition (pre-selected organ quality, decreased ischemia time).
- The possibility of saving the recipient from waiting-list mortality.

Basic principles of live liver donation (Vancouver Forum Criteria)

- Live liver donation to be performed only if the donor risk is justified by expectation of an acceptable recipient outcome.
- Patient and graft survival of a LDLT should approximate the expected outcome for a recipient (with the same disease etiology) undergoing a DDLT.

Mount Sinai Expert Guides: Hepatology, First Edition. Edited by Jawad Ahmad, Scott L. Friedman, and Henryk Dancygier.
© 2014 John Wiley & Sons, Ltd. Published 2014 by John Wiley & Sons, Ltd.
Companion website: www.mountsinaiexpertguides.com

- Indications for LDLT should be the same as those established for DDLT.
- LDLT should offer an overall advantage to the recipient when compared with waiting for the availability of a DDLT.
- Any outcome that penalizes living donors for the act of donation is not acceptable.

Benefits to the donor

- Psychologic – the concept of altruism; the traditional end-points of medical and surgical therapy do not apply to living donors.

Section 2: Prevention

Not applicable for this topic.

Section 3: Diagnosis
Donor selection criteria

- Age between 18 and 55 years.
- Presence of donor–recipient genetic and/or emotional relationship.
- ABO compatibility.
- Absence of medical contraindications or prior major abdominal surgery.
- BMI not greater than 28–30 kg/m^2.
- Free from coercion to donate.

Types of donation

Left lateral lobe	25% (segments II and III)
Left lobe	40% (segments I–IV)
Right lobe	60% (segments V–VIII)

- The selection of recipient eligibility for LDLT should be similar for those being evaluated to receive grafts from deceased donors.
- HCCs should still be within the Milan criteria.
- An elevated MELD score (e.g. above 25) and/or increased portal hypertension may preclude eligibility for LDLT since the effects of advanced liver dysfunction may not be relieved by a partial graft immediately post-transplantation. However, this decision is not universal and will be determined by each transplantation center performing LDLT.
- In the USA, it is currently not the standard practice to perform LDLT for patients with ALF due to the low benefit:risk ratio.
- To avoid selection bias and to protect donor welfare, separate teams (medical and surgical) are maintained for evaluation of both potential recipient and donor.
- In donors with relative contraindications for donation that can be decreased/reversed (e.g. fatty liver disease, current smoking and alcohol use), and if the potential recipient has the time to wait, individualized management strategies (e.g. weight loss, cessation of smoking and alcohol use) can be formulated. The donor can then be re-assessed periodically to determine the suitability for donation.

- Before making a decision to donate, the donor should be aware of the potential recipient's chance of survival post-transplantation. For example, HCC and viral hepatitis may recur after the transplantation.

Section 4: Treatment (Algorithm 40.1)
Donor evaluation
- The main priority for the donor team is to ensure donor safety.
- Blood tests: CBC, basic and liver chemistries, prothrombin time/INR, blood type and screen, viral serologies, HIV, iron studies, urinalysis, urine toxicology screen, serum ethanol, pregnancy test (if indicated).
- Evaluations: hepatologist, transplantation coordinator, social worker, psychiatrist, ethicist, cardiologist, surgeon.
- Imaging studies: volumetric imaging, delineation of vascular and biliary anatomy. The donor must have >30% residual liver volume post-hepatectomy and the graft-to-recipient weight ratio (in g/kg) must be at least 0.8–1.0. This ratio corresponds to 40–50% of the standard recipient liver volume and generally fulfills the metabolic requirements of adequate liver function in the recipient post-transplantation. SFSS is a condition that occurs when the recipient has a small graft, resulting in delayed graft function (e.g. hyperbilirubinemia, coagulopathy, ascites, hepatic encephalopathy) or a lack of it. The risk of developing SFSS is seen when the graft-to-recipient weight ratio is less than 1.0. An "all-in-one" multidetector CT scan has the advantage over MRI in assessing the biliary anatomy accurately. Fatty liver detection in imaging studies has improved and may obviate the need for assessment through a liver biopsy.
- Liver biopsy: if indicated (e.g. to assess for etiology of abnormal liver chemistries, steatosis, familial liver disease).
- Informed consent: to understand the risks of liver donation and the possible benefits/outcomes of the recipient.
- Medical out – "time-out" period after evaluation completion and date of surgery; the donor may opt out of donation at any time and be offered a "medical out" as a reason for withdrawing. Up to 40% of living donors are eventually excluded from liver donation. Withdrawal from the evaluation process and recipient death (while donor evaluation is ongoing) are the most common reasons.

Prevention/management of complications
Post-operative complications
- Biliary pathology and infections are the most common.
- Variations in biliary anatomy can be as high as 44% and may contribute to post-operative complications such as bile leak, biloma and stricture formation.
- In a study of 405 donors by the A2ALL (Adult-to-Adult Living Donor Liver Transplantation) Cohort Study, 9% had biliary complications beyond post-operative day 7, and 12% had bacterial/viral/fungal infections.
- Clavien classifies donor operative morbidity according to the severity of events; recommended by the Vancouver Forum.
- This classification was originally created to assess cholecystectomy outcomes and was subsequently adopted to look at other post-operative results including living liver donors.
- Clavien's classification stratifies complications into Grades 1–4, ranging from minor (Grade 1) to severe (re-transplantation and/or death) (Grade 4). Ghobrial's A2ALL study found 37% of donors to have complications: 27% had Grade 1, 26% Grade 2, 2% Grade 3 and 0.8% Grade 4.

Outcomes

Donor mortality rates	
~0.5%	Right lobe donor
~0.1%	Left lobe donor
0.2-2%	Overall

Algorithm 40.1 Management/treatment of potential donors

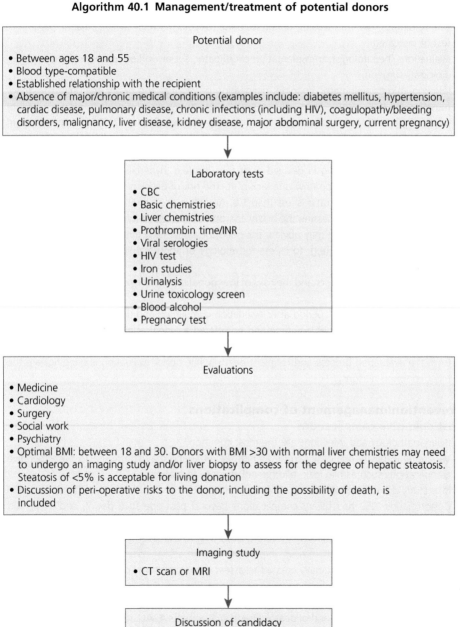

> **CLINICAL PEARLS**
> - Ultimately only 15% of donor-recipient pairs eventually undergo LDLT.
> - Anatomical, medical and psychosocial contraindications are the main reasons for excluding potential donors.
> - LDLT should only be a consideration in patients who would benefit from liver transplantation, and not as a potential solution for stable patients with a low MELD score and therefore low priority for DDLT, or patients with advanced HCC (beyond Milan or UCSF criteria).
> - The risk to the donor is only justified if there is significant potential benefit to the recipient after liver transplantation.

Section 5: Special Populations

Not applicable for this topic.

Section 6: Prognosis

> **CLINICAL PEARLS**
> - The most common complications post-donation are biliary-related (9%) and infections (12%).
> - Estimated donor mortality rate ranges from 0.2 to 2%.
> - Most post-operative complications are similar to patients who have undergone abdominal surgery for other reasons (e.g. hernia formation, incisional neuropathy, intra-abdominal adhesions).

Follow-up tests and monitoring
- There is a projected 3-month recovery time for most donors from the time they undergo surgery until they resume their pre-operative level of activity. Some donors have been able to recover within 6–8 weeks.
- Long-term data continue to be collected on the donor outcomes. They are either seen in the office or contacted by phone annually. Currently, there have been no long-term effects from liver donation that are different from those who have undergone abdominal surgery.

Section 7: Reading List

Araújo CCV, Balbi E, Pacheco-Moreira LF, et al. Evaluation of living donor liver transplantation: causes for exclusion. Transplant Proc 2010;42:424–5

Barr ML, Belghiti J, Villamil FG, et al. A report of the Vancouver Forum on the care of the live organ donor: lung, liver, pancreas, and intestine data and medical guidelines. Transplantation 2006;81:1373–85

Berg CL, Gillespie BW, Merion RM, et al.; A2ALL Study Group. Improvement in survival associated with adult-to-adult living donor liver transplantation. Gastroenterology 2007;133:1806–13

Bramstedt KA. Living liver donor mortality: where do we stand? Am J Gastroenterol 2006;101:755–9

Campos BD, Botha JF. Strategies to optimize donor safety with smaller grafts for adult-to-adult living donor liver transplantation. Curr Opin Organ Transplant 2012;17:230–4

Clavien PA, Camargo Jr CA, Croxford R, Langer B, Levy GA, Grieg PD. Definition and classification of negative outcomes in solid organ transplantation. Application in liver transplantation. Ann Surg 1994;220: 109–20

Clavien PA, Sanabria JR, Strasberg JM. Proposed classification of complications of surgery with examples of utility in cholecystectomy. Surgery 1992;111L518–26

Dindo D, Demartines N, Calvien PA. Classification of surgical complications: a new proposal with evaluation in a cohort of 6336 patients and results of a survey. Ann Surg 2004;220:109–20

Fisher RA, Kulik LM, Freise CE, et al.; A2ALL Study Group. Hepatocellular carcinoma recurrence and death following living and deceased donor liver transplantation. Am J Transplant 2007;7:1601–8

Freise CE, Gillespie BW, Koffron AJ, et al.; A2ALL Study Group. Recipient morbidity after living and deceased donor liver transplantation: findings from the A2ALL Retrospective Cohort Study. Am J Transplant 2008;8:2569–79

Ghobrial RM, Freise CE, Trotter JF, et al.; the A2ALL Study Group. Donor morbidity after living donation for liver transplantation. Gastroenterology 2008;135:468–76

Ghobrial RM, Saab S, Lassman C. Donor and recipient outcomes in right lobe adult living donor liver transplantation. Liver Transpl 2002;8:901–9

Nadalin S, Malagò M, Radtke A, et al. Current trends in live liver donation. Transpl Int 2007;20:312–30

Olthoff KM, Abecassis MM, Emond JC; A2ALL Study Group. Outcomes of adult living donor liver transplantation: comparison of the Adult-to-adult Living Donor Liver Transplantation Cohort Study and the national experience. Liver Transpl 2011;17:789–97

Olthoff KM, Merion RM, Ghobrial RM, et al.; A2ALL Study Group. Outcomes of 385 adult-to-adult living donor liver transplant recipients: a report from the A2ALL Consortium. Ann Surg 2005;242:314–23

Shaked A, Ghobrial RM, Merion RM, et al.; A2ALL Study Group. Incidence and severity of acute cellular rejection in recipients undergoing adult living donor or deceased donor liver transplantation. Am J Transplant 2009;9:301–8

Terrault NA, Shiffman ML, Lok AS, et al.; A2ALL Study Group. Outcomes in hepatitis C virus-infected recipients of living donor vs deceased donor liver transplantation. Liver Transpl 2007;13:122–9

Trotter JF, Wachs M, Everson GT, Kam I. Adult-to-adult transplantation of the right hepatic lobe from a living donor. N Eng J Med 2002;346:1074–82

Trotter JF, Wachs M, Trouillot T, et al. Evaluation of 100 patients for living donor liver transplantation. Liver Transplant 2000;6:290–5

Varotti G, Gondolesi GE, Goldman J, et al. Anatomic variations in right liver living donors. J Am Coll Surg 2004;198:577–82

Section 8: Guidelines

Not applicable for this topic.

Section 9: Evidence

Not applicable for this topic.

Section 10: Images

Not applicable for this topic.

Additional material for this chapter can be found online at:
www.mountsinaiexpertguides.com
This includes a case study and multiple choice questions

CHAPTER 41

Surgical Evaluation for Liver Transplantation

Hiroshi Sogawa
Thomas E. Starzl Transplantation Institute, University of Pittsburgh Medical Center, Pittsburgh, PA, USA

OVERALL BOTTOM LINE
- There are four key components of the surgical evaluation of patients for LT based on necessity, suitability, strategy and informed consent:
  1. Necessity: does this patient need LT?
  2. Suitability: is this patient a good candidate for LT?
  3. Strategy: how do we get a liver for this patient or are there other alternative options?
  4. Informed consent (choice): a detailed discussion of the risks and benefits of the procedure.

Section 1: Background

- Evaluation of patients for LT is a multidisciplinary process that involves medical, surgical, cardiac, infectious disease and psychosocial assessment.
- Surgical evaluation is an essential part of the process and it is the first bond between a patient and a surgeon.
- Four key components should be addressed in the surgical evaluation:
  1. Necessity.
  2. Suitability.
  3. Strategy.
  4. Informed consent (choice).
- The overall surgical risk must be considered and evaluated by a surgeon and an anesthesiologist in high risk cases.
- It is essential to physically see the patient as an "eye ball" test is frequently more useful than information reported from your colleagues or laboratory results when assessing the patient's surgical risk.
- Anatomical evaluation and a surgical plan need to be made well in advance of surgery.

Mount Sinai Expert Guides: Hepatology, First Edition. Edited by Jawad Ahmad, Scott L. Friedman, and Henryk Dancygier.
© 2014 John Wiley & Sons, Ltd. Published 2014 by John Wiley & Sons, Ltd.
Companion website: www.mountsinaiexpertguides.com

Section 2: Prevention

Not applicable for this topic.

Section 3: Diagnosis (Algorithm 41.1)
Necessity
Key questions
- Does the patient need liver transplantation?
- Does this patient have significant complications due to irreversible liver disease?
- Is this patient too early for transplantation? Well-compensated liver cirrhosis?
- If the MELD score is <15, what is the indication for the transplantation? Is this due to HCC? Is this patient sicker than the calculated MELD score (e.g. a patient with recurrent ascites who requires large volume paracentesis every week?).
- Does the patient have an alternative treatment such as TIPS?
- Does the patient have an alternative treatment such as liver resection for HCC?
- Does the patient need one organ, or more organs such as liver/kidney or multi-visceral transplantation?

Typical presentation
- The patient is a 55-year-old obese (BMI 35) male with history of HCV liver cirrhosis /HCC who came here to be seen by a surgeon for LT evaluation. Screening US showed a 2 cm mass in segment VIII. CT scan showed that the mass had arterial enhancement and portal phase wash out. Platelet count was 55. His natural MELD score was 7. No ascites or encephalopathy was noted. He was treatment-naïve for hepatitis C. Should he have a LT or liver resection?
- The patient is a 27-year-old otherwise healthy female who took one bottle of Tylenol and NSAIDs to commit suicide. N-acetylcysteine was administered within 24 hours after taking these drugs. She is encephalopathic. Total bilirubin is 15 mg/dL, lactate is 3 mmol/L, phosphorous is 2 mg/dL and creatinine is 2 mg/dL. She is on levophed 4 µg/minute. Could this patient recover without liver transplantation? What are risk factors for fulminant liver failure?

Useful clinical decision rules and calculators
- MELD score 15–17 is the cut-off for liver transplantation risk/benefit: the benefit of LT will overweigh its risk when a patient's MELD score exceeds 15–17.
- If a patient with lower MELD (<15) needs LT, the patient should have strong indications such as HCC, refractory ascites or very poor quality of life.

Disease severity classification
- Child-Turcot-Pugh (CTP) score.
- MELD/PELD score.

Potential pitfalls/common errors made regarding diagnosis of disease
- Hepatoportal sclerosis and other causes of non-cirrhotic portal hypertension can sometimes mimic liver cirrhosis. If the patient has hepatoportal sclerosis with portal vein thrombosis, the treatment of choice may be the shunt surgery rather than LT.
- Liver resection might be the better or equivalent option, if feasible (single tumor without significant portal hypertension) for the patients with HCC in regions of the country where a very high MELD score is required for DDLT.

Algorithm 41.1 Key questions for surgical evaluation

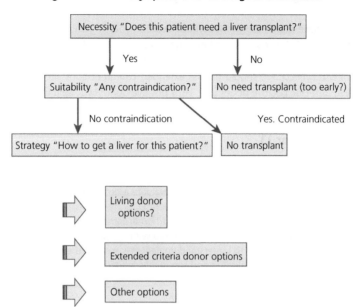

Suitability: Does the patient have a contraindication for liver transplantation?

Contraindications to transplantation
- Hemodynamic instability.
- Cardiopulmonary dysfunction which prevents the patient from undergoing major vascular surgery such as liver transplantation.
- Active systemic infection.
- Invasive cancer.
- Social or psychiatric contraindications (lack of social support).

High-risk patients
- Re-transplantation (particularly for HCV infection).
- Patients with multiple co-morbidities.
- Recent infection.
- Portal vein thrombosis.
- Previous hepatectomy.
- Multi-drug resistance bacterial colonization.

- How much can you stretch the limit surgically? If portal vein thrombosis extends to the superior mesenteric vein completely, should you try caval hemi-transposition, renal vein-portal bypass, or multi-visceral transplantation?
- If the patient has end-stage renal disease (more than 3 months), should we do combined liver/ kidney transplantation?

Strategy: How to get a liver for the patient

Key questions
- Does the patient have high enough MELD/PELD score in your region for transplantation?
- If the patient's MELD/PELD score is not high enough in your UNOS region, you should think about LDLT or multiple listing in low MELD/PELD regions.
- Regardless of MELD/PELD, we should discuss extended criteria options such as older donors' liver, fatty liver, anti-HBc positive donor liver, HCV positive donor liver, split liver, donation after cardiac death (DCD) liver.

Informed consent for LT

> **CLINICAL PEARLS**
> - Surgical evaluation is not only an opportunity to evaluate a potential candidate but also for a surgeon to inform the patient of all the facts about LT.
> - You should spend enough time with a patient and his/her family at the surgical evaluation as it is the start of a long and important relationship with the patient.
> - You should not expect a patient to understand immediately what you explain. Transplantation matters are complicated and sometimes intimidating for a patient. This is the start of education process.

What should you tell a patient?
- Process of evaluation and listing.
- Donor selection and options including extended donor criteria.
- Transplantation surgical procedure.
- Peri-operative mortality and possible complications.
- The risk of primary graft non-function.
- Hepatic artery thrombosis, portal vein thrombosis, bile leak/stricture.
- Other surgical complications (intra-abdominal abscess, bowel injury).
- Current national transplantation outcome data and your transplantation center's outcomes.
- Need for life-long immunosuppression and its possible complications.
- Importance of compliance and post-transplantation care.
- Risk of disease transmission or cancer transmission from a donor.
- Patients have a right to decline organs and multiple listing.

Section 4: Treatment

Management/treatment algorithm
- Low MELD patients but need liver transplantation: need a strategy!
  - Donor options and its strategy:
    - Extended Criteria Donors (ECD):
      - older donor liver.
      - fatty liver.
      - anti-HBc positive donor.
      - HCV positive donor.
      - split liver.
      - donation after cardiac death liver.
    - Living donor liver.
    - Multiple listing.

- Concept of the Donor Risk Index (DRI) (see Feng et al. in Reading List)
  - ➤ numerical value derived from multiple variables including: older donor, cause of death, ethnicity, height, cold ischemia time, split, donation after cardiac death, that is a measure of donor liver quality.

CLINICAL PEARLS
- Tailor the donor/treatment option for each individual patient.
- Older donor livers can be transplanted to non-HCV patients
- Avoid using donors older than 65 years of age in HCV patients.

Section 5: Special Populations
Pregnancy
- LT is contraindicated in the pregnant woman and pregnancy prevention for patients with decompensated cirrhosis is advised.
- However, a post-LT patient can safely conceive and deliver. This needs to be in conjunction with high-risk pregnancy specialist. Pregnancy is best avoided within the first year after transplantation.

Children
- The issue is how to get an organ. Split LT or LDLT should be strongly considered for a small child.

Elderly
- There is no recipient age limit for LT. However careful consideration of the risks and benefits is imperative in potential recipients over the age of 70.

Others
- HIV patients: under NIH protocol, several centers have successfully transplanted this patient population with reasonable outcome. However, immunosuppression management is somewhat difficult and unconventional due to drug interaction with anti-retroviral medications.
- Portal vein thrombosis: prepare jump graft from the same or different donors. In this case excellent local donor liver is preferable rather than marginal imported liver because of potential longer warm ischemia time.

Section 6: Prognosis

Not applicable for this topic.

Section 7: Reading List

Ahmed A, Keeffe EB. Current indications and contraindications for liver transplantation. Clin Liver Dis 2007;11:227–47
Busuttil RW, Klintmalm GB (eds) Transplantation of the Liver, 2nd edition. Philadelphia: Elsevier Saunders, 2005

Feng S, Goodrich NP, Bragg-Gresham JL, et al. Characteristics associated with liver graft failure: the concept of a donor risk index. Am J Transplant 2006;6:783–90

Murray KF, Carithers RL Jr; AASLD.AASLD practice guidelines: evaluation of the patient for liver transplantation. Hepatology 2005;41:1407-32

Section 8: Guidelines
National society guidelines

Guideline title	Guideline source	Date
AASLD Practice Guidelines: Evaluation of the Patient for Liver Transplantation	American Association for the Study of Liver Disease (AASLD) http://www.aasld.org/practiceguidelines/Documents/Bookmarked%20Practice%20Guidelines/Liver%20Transplant.pdf	2005

Section 9: Evidence

Not applicable for this topic.

Section 10: Images

Not applicable for this topic.

Additional material for this chapter can be found online at:
www.mountsinaiexpertguides.com
This includes a case study and multiple choice questions

CHAPTER 42

Post-Operative Care of The Liver Transplantation Patient

Alan G. Contreras Saldivar
Recanati/Miller Transplantation Institute, Mount Sinai Hospital, New York, NY, USA

OVERALL BOTTOM LINE
- Success in liver transplantation depends on coordination of care among a multidisciplinary team.
- Initial assessment should start with careful review of the entire patient history including details of the donor and the surgery.
- LFTs early after transplantation are unreliable in determining allograft function and clinical parameters must be used to guide therapy.
- Continual assessment and support of organ function and a high suspicion of potential complications are the goal during the immediate post-operative period.
- The etiology of graft dysfunction early after transplantation is multiple and includes ischemia reperfusion injury, primary non-function, technical complications, rejection and infections.
- Immunosuppression starts in the operating room. Triple therapy including steroids, calcineurin inhibitors and mycophenolate mofetil are the most commonly used.
- Prophylaxis against perioperative infections has to be based on previous known infections and should include prophylaxis against *Pneumocystis carinii* and cytomegalovirus.

Section 1: Background

- Before the advent of LT, liver failure was nearly universally fatal but currently the patient survival after LT is 85% at 1 year and more than 75% at 5 years.
- Satisfactory quality of life has been described up to 30 years after LT.

Incidence/prevalence
- By the end of 2006, there were almost 40 000 people known to be alive with functioning LTs in the USA and over 6000 LTs are performed annually.
- Improved long-term survival is possible due to a better understanding of the pathophysiology related to ESLD, improvement in surgical techniques and post-operative care and novel therapeutic approaches.
- Immediately after completion of the transplantation operation most patients are transferred to an ICU where optimal post-operative care can only be provided by a dedicated multidisciplinary team.

Mount Sinai Expert Guides: Hepatology, First Edition. Edited by Jawad Ahmad, Scott L. Friedman, and Henryk Dancygier.
© 2014 John Wiley & Sons, Ltd. Published 2014 by John Wiley & Sons, Ltd.
Companion website: www.mountsinaiexpertguides.com

Pathology/pathogenesis

- Patients with ESLD usually have a marked reduction in systemic vascular resistance, mean arterial pressure and increase in cardiac output. This hyperdynamic stage may last several weeks following LT.
- Moreover, myocardial contractility can be impaired due to a decreased number of adrenergic receptors in these patients. The progressive vasodilatation seen in cirrhosis leads to the activation of endogenous vasoconstrictors, sodium and water retention, and increasing renal vasoconstriction.
- Patients with cirrhosis usually demonstrate increased total body sodium, and dilutional hyponatremia. Other electrolyte abnormalities are common including hypomagnesemia and hypocalcemia.
- Renal perfusion may initially be maintained due to vasodilators such as prostaglandins and nitric oxide. However, the natural progression of liver disease overcomes these protective mechanisms, leading to progressive renal hypoperfusion, a gradual decline in the glomerular filtration rate, and, in some patients, hepatorenal syndrome. Up to 25% of LT candidates have impaired renal function. Continued loss of ascites during the operation and surgical bleeding increases intravascular hypovolemia and the risk of acute kidney injury.
- The respiratory system can also been compromised. Mild hypoxemia is common among cirrhotic patients, and can result from the compression of lung parenchyma by ascites or pleural fluid. Severe hypoxemia is less common and, in the absence of associated cardiopulmonary disease, strongly suggests hepatopulmonary syndrome – estimated to be present in 4–47% of patients with chronic liver disease. Hepatic hydrothorax and portopulmonary hypertension are other pulmonary complications that may develop in patients with cirrhosis. During the transplantation surgery, severe lung edema with hypoxemia may occur following reperfusion, or as a consequence of massive release of cytokines due to pre-existing antibodies against blood components causing transfusion-related acute lung injury.
- Coagulopathy in ESLD patients results from inadequate clotting factor synthesis, fibrinolysis and thrombocytopenia. Platelet dysfunction is also common in patients with coexisting renal insufficiency.
- Most ESLD patients present with hypoalbuminemia and many patients are severely malnourished before transplantation and will require significant nutritional support.

Section 2: Prevention

Not applicable for this topic.

Section 3: Diagnosis
Initial evaluation and general considerations
History

- The immediate perioperative care starts by obtaining a good history of events prior to and during the transplantation surgery.
- General characteristics of the patient at the moment of the transplantation, etiology of liver disease, history of previous surgeries and co-morbidities, history of complications from the liver disease including hepatopulmonary syndrome, portopulmonary syndrome, hydrothorax, GI bleeding due to portal hypertension, ascites, previous spontaneous bacterial peritonitis or other infections including the microorganisms involved and sensitivities, renal function and the prior need of renal replacement therapy, are all valuable information.

- Some donor and surgical characteristics impact on the risks of several complications after surgery. Hence general information from the donor including age, co-morbidities, type of donor (live, brain dead or donor after cardiac death), type of graft (whole liver or segment of the liver), ischemia time, serologies, and technical aspects of the surgery including anatomical variations, surgical technique, the need for venovenous bypass or hemodialysis/hemofiltration and perioperative anesthetic care including hemodynamic stability, post-reperfusion syndrome, the need for vasopressors and the total amount of fluids and blood products should be noted.

Physical examination and initial tests

- On arrival in the ICU an initial assessment of the vital signs and complete physical examination must be performed. A chest radiograph is taken to confirm placement of lines and the endotracheal tube position. The nasogastric tube and Foley catheter output must be recorded and if intra-abdominal drains were left, the quantity and the characteristics of the drainage must be determined, whether it is clear, bloody or bilious stained. Patients may arrive hypothermic from the operation room to the ICU and attempts must be done to normalize the body temperature and keep it above 37 °C. Immediate laboratory tests should be ordered including arterial blood gas, CBC, serum electrolytes, glucose, blood urea nitrogen, creatinine, LFTs and serum lactic acid.

Cardiovascular system

- Most patients have a Swan-Ganz catheter and cardiac output and systemic vascular resistance can be calculated. The high cardiac output and low vascular resistance that characterize patients with ESLD can persist for several weeks following transplantation. Hemodynamic stabilization is clinically assessed by adequate organ and tissue perfusion. The intravascular hypovolemic state of these patients requires aggressive volume resuscitation with IV fluids. However, some patients may require vasoconstrictive therapy such as noradrenaline and vasopressin.

Respiratory system

- Pulmonary management consists of standard ventilator support. Some patients with good general condition and functional capacity with uncomplicated surgery can be awakened and extubated in the operating room. However, most of the patients are in a chronic debilitated state and they are typically extubated in the ICU after it has been determined that hemodynamic stability has been achieved and they fulfill the criteria for extubation. In our institution, this occurs most commonly within the first 24 hours after the operation. Patients with intracranial hypertension in the setting of ALF require particular attention to ventilation to prevent abrupt shifts in pressure and the arterial tension of carbon dioxide. Good pain control, chest physiotherapy and incentive spirometry following extubation are mandatory to avoid pulmonary complications.

Renal system

- Prior to transplantation 25% of patients have renal dysfunction and this is an independent predictor of post-transplantation morbidity and mortality. After LT, more than 50% of recipients will show impaired renal dysfunction. Oliguria may be the earliest warning sign. The etiology includes hepatorenal syndrome, perioperative hypotension, acute tubular necrosis, graft dysfunction and drug-induced injury. Those with hepatorenal syndrome are most likely to required renal replacement therapy. The initiation of renal replacement therapy remains a clinical decision where fluid overload, electrolyte disturbances and metabolic acidosis are the most common triggers. Continues venovenous hemodialysis is preferable soon after transplantation because it offers superior cardiovascular stability. If necessary, conventional hemodialysis can be used later. Nephrotoxicity is a known side effect of CNIs used to prevent rejection. Reducing the dose or delaying introduction of CNIs are useful strategies in long-term renal protection in those with a high probability of renal dysfunction.

Electrolytes
- Electrolyte abnormalities are common after transplantation. Hyponatremia is often seen in patients with fluid retention. Rapid correction can result in central pontine myelinolysis and could lead to permanent brain injury. Fluids high in sodium are generally avoided. However, they may be needed in cases of severe hyponatremia. Post-transplantation, fluids should be administered based on the serum sodium level. If the sodium concentration is <125 mEq/L, normal saline (0.9%) should be the fluid of choice. If serum sodium is >135 mg/mEq/L, half normal saline (0.45%) can be used. Plasmalyte solution resembles the electrolyte content of plasma and is often used for resuscitation and maintenance after transplantation. Hypomagnesemia is common in cirrhotic patients and may be exacerbated in the immediate postoperative period by blood loss or medications such as tacrolimus, cyclosporine or loop diuretics and should be corrected. A recovering graft has a high requirement for phosphate and magnesium and these should be replaced adequately. Citrate toxicity from transfusion of blood or blood products may cause a profound reduction in calcium levels. Ionized serum calcium levels should be monitored as total calcium levels depend on the albumin concentration.

Coagulopathy
- Platelet dysfunction due to renal insufficiency can be managed with desmopressin. Replacement of blood products is necessary in the presence of active bleeding or any planned intervention. Otherwise, maintenance of an INR between 1.5 and 2, a platelet count >50 × 10⁹/L and a fibrinogen level >100 mg/dL is acceptable.

Gastrointestinal system
- Many patients are severely malnourished before transplantation and early enteral nutrition is an achievable goal for most patients.

Assessment of graft function
Clinical
- The assessment of liver function starts after reperfusion. The appearance of the liver, early bile production, hemodynamic stability and correction of coagulopathy ('oozing' from all cut surfaces) are all good signs that can be assessed intraoperatively. A smooth ICU course after LT is dependent on satisfactory graft function which can be assessed by clinical parameters including awakening from the anesthetized state, stable respiratory effort, hemodynamic stability and good urine output.

Laboratory
- The absolute transaminase elevation is not as useful a parameter as the trend after transplantation. However, elevation >2500 IU/L is suggestive of significant parenchymal injury and AST >5000 IU/L may indicate primary non-function. Both, AST and ALT peak during the first 2 days and slowly level off. Normalization of the prothrombin time is a good parameter of the synthetic recovery of the liver allograft. Resolution of metabolic acidosis and clearance of serum lactate are good indicators of the liver's ability to metabolize acids, as well as perfusion of systemic tissue.

Radiology
• An US Doppler is performed on post-operative day 1 to assess the patency of the vascular anastomosis and when necessary thereafter.

Assessment of potential complications
Post-operative bleeding
• The most common cause of post-operative hypotension is intra-abdominal bleeding which may be heralded by tachycardia, decrease in CVP and urine output, prolongation of the pro-thrombin time, persistently low platelet count, decrease in hematocrit or a fall in the mixed venous oxygen saturation. The increase in bloody output from the drains can be obvious but significant bleeding can occur without any change in the drains if they are obstructed. If there is hemodynamic instability due to intra-abdominal bleeding, immediate return of the patient to the operative room is required. If the patient is hemodynamically stable, attempts must be made to improve coagulopathy and body temperature. Normothermia is essential in maintaining the integrity of the coagulation system. In more than half of the patients, a major source of bleeding is not found and the blood loss can often be attributed to initial coagulopathy and fibrinolysis.

Graft dysfunction
• LFT abnormalities and coagulopathy can persist for several days after transplantation. Continuous elevation of transaminases suggests significant hepatic necrosis. Elevation of AP and bilirubin is suggestive of cholestasis. However, these two patterns of liver function can occur simultaneously. The etiological reasons for graft dysfunction early after transplantation are multiple and include ischemia, reperfusion injury, primary non-function, technical complications, rejection and infections.

Causes of early hepatic dysfunction following LT

Cause	Features

Primary non-function	• 5% of LTs
	• Severe liver dysfunction: hepatic coma, coagulopathy, jaundice, hypoglycemia, renal dysfunction, hemodynamic instability
	• Treatment: urgent re-transplantation as a medical urgency (status 1A) if:
	  • Within 7 days of transplantation: AST ≥3000 and one or both of the following:
	    ➤ INR ≥2.5 or
	    ➤ acidosis, defined as having an arterial pH ≤7.3 or venous pH of 7.25 and or lactate ≥4 mmol/L

Hepatic artery thrombosis	• 3–9% of LTs. Higher risk in pediatrics or when complex arterial reconstruction was done during the transplantation • Occurs early following transplantation and may present with elevation of liver enzymes or as an incidental finding on Doppler. Further investigation with angiography or immediate surgical exploration is required • Associated with biliary complications, bilomas, liver abscess and graft loss • Treatment: revascularization. Urgent re-transplantation as a medical urgency (status 1A) if the same criteria as primary non-function • Hepatic artery thrombosis in a transplanted liver within 14 days of implantation not meeting the above criteria can be listed as a MELD of 40

(Continued)

Cause	Features
Hepatic artery stenosis	• Consequence of anastomosis narrowing or kinking. If left unattended increases the risk of thrombosis • Mild elevation of bilirubin and transaminases may occur • Doppler study showing increase flow velocity (>200 cm/second) • Angiography confirms the diagnoses and angioplasty (and stent placement) can be done at the same time or repaired by surgery
Portal vein thrombosis	• Uncommon • Can occur in the setting of portal vein stenosis or previous portal vein thrombosis in the recipient • Severe elevation of LFTs is common. May present with ascites and GI bleeding secondary to portal hypertension • Surgical revision and thrombectomy should be attempted to save the graft. Re-transplantation may be necessary
Hepatic vein thrombosis	• Most common on piggyback operations but can occur following the standard technique • Venous outflow obstruction causes a Budd–Chiari-like syndrome and significant elevation in transaminases results from acute congestion. Ascites and evidence of portal hypertension are common • Doppler US is helpful and is followed by venography where a percutaneous angioplasty with stent placement could be therapeutic
Caval stenosis	• Constriction at the anastomotic suture line of the upper cava • Clinically the patient has congestion below the anastomosis that may include outflow obstruction with liver congestion with elevation of transaminases and signs of portal hypertension, ascites, renal dysfunction and low extremity edema • Doppler shows increase in velocity at the site of the anastomosis • If suspected, an angiogram should be performed and a pressure gradient measurement of >10 mmHg or greater is confirmatory. Percutaneous angioplasty with stent placement can be therapeutic but if it fails, surgical intervention may be needed
Biliary leak	• Clinically evident if biliary output is seen from the drains but may present with localized or generalized peritonitis • Total bilirubin can be tested on the drains if the serum bilirubin level is elevated and the diagnosis is uncertain • Anastomotic biliary leaks can occur as a result of technical problems but hepatic artery thrombosis and ischemic damage has to be ruled out • Early anastomotic leaks are best treated with reoperation and surgical revision. Biliary leaks from the cut surface of partial livers can be treated conservatively if the leak is contained and adequately drained • ERCP with sphincterotomy and/or stent placement is a useful therapeutic option for a localized leak
Biliary stenosis	• Slower increase in bilirubin but a higher increase in AP and GGT • Biliary stenosis can occur as a result of technical problems but hepatic artery thrombosis and ischemic damage has to be excluded • Biliary strictures can be treated with ERCP and stent placement or percutaneous techniques. Strictures that fail to respond may need to be revised surgically and conversion to Roux-en-Y choledochojejunostomy may be necessary
Rejection	• Rejection may occur within the first weeks following transplantation. Patients that have not reached appropriate levels of immunosuppression are at increased risk • LFT abnormalities may be cholestatic, hepatocellular or both • Clinical signs are non-specific and unreliable • Diagnosis is made by liver biopsy (portal infiltrates, lymphocyte-mediated bile duct injury and endothelialitis)

Cause	Features
Infection	• Bacterial and fungal systemic infections may result in abnormal LFTs, usually in a cholestatic pattern. Patients usually have signs of systemic inflammatory response • A complete investigation to find the source should be performed. Body cultures should be sent and empirical antimicrobial therapy started taking into consideration previous cultures and sensitivities • Liver abscess secondary to cholangitis occurs typically as a result of hepatic artery thrombosis. CT scan of the abdomen can be diagnostic and percutaneous drainage can be attempted at the same time by interventional radiology • Viral infections occur more common 1–6 months following transplantation. CMV, HSV, VZV, EBV and adenovirus are among the most common and they all may present with hepatitis. PCR, viral cultures and immunohistochemistry are useful diagnostic tools

Section 4: Treatment
Immunosuppression and prophylaxis

• Triple therapy is generally given in most centers in the immediate post-operative period and consists typically of steroids, CNI (tacrolimus or cyclosporine) and antiproliferative agents (mycophenolate mofetil). In patients with kidney failure, delaying the introduction of CNI is a good strategy to avoid further kidney injury. As an alternative, if serum creatinine is >2 mg/dL or the patient is on renal replacement therapy, tacrolimus is started at a low dose on POD 4 and basiliximab (anti IL-2 receptor monoclonal antibody) 20 mg IV is given on POD 0 and POD 3. Appropriate surgical antibiotic prophylaxis should be given, and in addition, prophylaxis against *P. carinii* and CMV should be started. Hepatitis B prophylaxis is started for those patients with hepatitis B or any recipient that received a hepatitis B core positive donor. Most patients should also receive peptic ulcer disease prophylaxis especially when receiving high dose steroids as well as calcium supplements.

Induction immunosuppression guidelines*

Drug	Dose	
Methylprednisolone	Intraoperatively POD 1 POD 2 POD 3 POD 4	500 mg IV × 1 dose 80 mg IV every 12 hours × 2 doses 60 mg IV every 12 hours × 2 doses 40 mg IV every 12 hours × 2 doses 20 mg IV every 12 hours × 2 doses
Prednisone	POD 5-8 POD 9-12 POD 13-	20 mg PO daily 15 mg PO daily 10 mg PO daily – for 3 months from the date of transplantation. Then 5 mg PO daily for 3 months and discontinue.
	Note: patients with AIH will remain on maintenance steroids at the discretion of the hepatologist	
Tacrolimus (FK-506, Prograf) or cyclosporine	0.25 mg/kg PO twice a day starting in SICU on POD 0 Adjust regimen to maintain trough level of 8–12 ng/mL 6-8 mg/kg PO twice a day starting on SICU on POD 0 Adjust regimen to maintain through level of 300–400 ng/mL	
Mycophenolate mofetil (MMF, CellCept)	1000 mg PO twice a day until tacrolimus trough levels reach goal, then MMF can be decreased to 500 mg PO twice a day at the discretion of the hepatologist or transplantation surgeon. Start on POD 0 Adjust appropriately for leucopenia. Hold if WBC <2000	

* Guidelines for immunosuppression post-LT in patients with serum creatinine <2.0 mg/dL

Prophylaxis guidelines

Strategy	Drug	Dose
Surgical antibiotic prophylaxis	• No significant history of infection: ampicillin–sulbactam	3 g IV pre-operatively and then every 6 hours × 24 hours*
	• Alternative for patients allergic to penicillin: • Aztreonam and • Vancomycin	1 g IV pre-operatively and then every 8 hours × 24 hours*
	• Patients with significant history of infections: regimen should be individualized	1 g IV pre-operatively and then every 12 hours × 24 hours*
Antifungal prophylaxis	• All patients: clotrimazole troche	Troche PO three/four times a day for 1 month
	• High risk patients (re-transplants, fulminant liver failure, renal failure, complicated LT surgery, reoperations): fluconazole	10 mg IV/PO daily until transfer from SICU (or for 7 days whichever is longer)
P. carinii prophylaxis (+)	• Trimethoprim/sulfamethoxazole	400 mg/60 mg PO daily for 3 months
	• Alternative for patients who are allergic or intolerant: • Atovaquone or	1500 mg PO daily or 750 mg twice a day for 3 months
	• Pentamidine	4 mg/kg IV/IM every month for 3 months
CMV prophylaxis (+)	• For all CMV IgG + recipients (D-/R+ AND D+/R+): valgancyclovir	450 mg PO daily for 90 days*
	• CMV IgG+ donor/CMV IgG- recipient (D+/R-): valgancyclovir	900 mg PO daily for 90 days*
	CMV IgG-donor/CMV IgG-recipient (D-/R-): valacyclovir	500 mg PO daily for 30 days
Hepatitis B prophylaxis	• All recipients with hepatitis B: HBIg	10 000 U (6 vials) starting during the LT (anhepatic phase), POD 0, POD 1. 4 vials: POD 2 to discharge, then monthly Anti-HBs quantitative must be checked POD 2, 5 and 8. If titer <500 mIU/mL, dose should be repeated
	• Continue with nucleoside analog • Recipient hepatitis B negative with a hepatitis B core positive donor: entecavir	0.5 mg daily*
Others	• Calcium carbonate	1250 mg PO twice daily while taking prednisone
	• Aspirin	81 mg PO daily
	• Famotidine	20 mg PO twice daily*

* Adjust to renal function

• (+)Prophylaxis should be extended in patients profoundly immunosuppressed (antithymo-globulin initial treatment, rejection treatment, etc.).
• After the initial care in the SICU, once the patients are extubated and hemodynamically stable, they are transferred to the transplantation ward. Diet should be advanced as tolerated and early ambulation should be encouraged. In some instances, early physical therapy and social

work assessment is necessary because some patients will require transfer to an acute rehabilitation facility. Drains are usually removed 2–3 days after the surgery regardless of the volume of ascites. Staples are usually removed 2–3 weeks after the operation during an office visit. Teaching lessons for the appropriate use of medications, lifestyle precautions and diet are provided to the patients and family members and the patients are discharged and followed with office visits and blood tests initially twice a week.

Section 5: Special Populations

Not applicable for this topic.

Section 6: Prognosis

Not applicable for this topic.

Section 7: Reading List

Gelb B, Feng S. Management of the liver transplant patient. Expert Rev Gastroenterol Hepatol 2009;3:631–47
Huprikar S. Update in infectious diseases in liver transplant recipients. Clin Liver Dis 2007;11:337–54
Koffron A, Stein JA. Liver transplantation, pretransplant evaluation, surgery, and posttransplant complications. Med Clin North Am 2008;92:861–88
Lee SO, Razonable RR. Current concepts on cytomegalovirus infection after liver transplantation. World J Hepatol 2010;2:325–36
Pillai AA, Levitsky J. Overview of immunosuppression in liver transplantation. World J Gastroenterol 2009;15:4225–33
Razonable, RR, Findlay JY, O'Riordan A, et al. Critical care issues in patients after liver transplantation. Liver Transpl;17:511–27
http://optn.transplant.hrsa.gov/policiesAndBylaws/policies.asp

Section 8: Guidelines

Not applicable for this topic.

Section 9: Evidence

Not applicable for this topic.

Section 10: Images

Not applicable for this topic.

Additional material for this chapter can be found online at:
www.mountsinaiexpertguides.com
This includes a case study and multiple choice questions

CHAPTER 43

Diagnostic Approach to Abnormal Liver Tests Following Liver Transplantation

Charissa Y. Chang
Division of Liver Diseases, Icahn School of Medicine at Mount Sinai, New York, NY, USA

OVERALL BOTTOM LINE
- Routine monitoring of liver tests throughout the early and late post-transplantation period is essential in screening for allograft dysfunction.
- Many causes of graft dysfunction including rejection and hepatic artery thrombosis do not cause symptoms.
- Liver test elevations are usually the first indication of a problem, and early diagnosis and intervention can be crucial in preventing graft loss.
- This chapter summarizes the diagnostic approach to abnormal liver tests following transplantation.
- Specific management for each diagnosis is addressed in separate chapters.

Section 1: Background
Definition of disease
- The differential diagnosis of abnormal LFTs following transplantation differs depending on the time period following transplantation.

Disease classification

Time course of graft dysfunction following LT	
0–3 days:	Primary graft non-function
	Hepatic artery thrombosis
	Hyperacute rejection (rare)
3–4 days:	Acute cellular rejection
	Hepatic artery thrombosis
	Bile leak, cholangitis
	Portal vein thrombosis
	Drug hepatotoxicity

Mount Sinai Expert Guides: Hepatology, First Edition. Edited by Jawad Ahmad, Scott L. Friedman, and Henryk Dancygier.
© 2014 John Wiley & Sons, Ltd. Published 2014 by John Wiley & Sons, Ltd.
Companion website: www.mountsinaiexpertguides.com

14 days–3 months:	Rejection (acute)
	Recurrent HCV
	Biliary complications
	Drug hepatotoxicity
	Delayed hepatic artery thrombosis (less common after first month)
3–12 months:	Rejection (acute or chronic)
	Recurrent hepatitis C (including fibrosing cholestatic hepatitis)
	Infection: CMV, EBV, adenovirus
	Outflow obstruction
	Hepatic artery stenosis
>12 months:	Rejection (acute or chronic)
	Recurrent HCV
	Reactivation of HBV (cAb + graft)
	Biliary stricture (anastomotic or ischemic)
	Hepatic artery stenosis
	De novo autoimmune hepatitis
	Plasma cell hepatitis
	Drug hepatotoxicity
	Steatohepatitis

Etiology

- Causes of abnormal liver tests after transplantation can be related to allograft integrity (primary graft non-function, delayed graft function), vascular problems (hepatic artery thrombosis, outflow obstruction), biliary problems (bile leak, biliary strictures), infections, immune reactions (allo and autoimmune) and recurrent disease.
- Most biliary complications occur within the first 3–6 months following transplantation.

  Infections are most likely to occur within the first year, particularly following withdrawal of prophylaxis.

  Acute and chronic rejection is diagnosed by liver biopsy. The threshold to perform a liver biopsy is low in the transplantation recipient due to benefits of early intervention in improving long-term graft survival when rejection is treated in a timely manner. The risk for acute rejection is highest during the first year after transplantation, but can occur at any time. Untreated acute rejection leads to bile duct loss and chronic rejection, which can manifest as cholestatic liver test elevation with or without pruritus.
- Many diseases (hepatitis C, PSC, AIH, PBC, NASH and HCC) can recur following transplantation.
- Recurrent HCV can cause liver test elevations as early as within the first 2 weeks following transplantation, although clinically significant disease usually takes at least several weeks to manifest. An uncommon form of recurrent viral hepatitis called fibrosing cholestatic hepatitis can occur within the first year in patients transplanted for HCV. This is associated with jaundice, accelerated graft dysfunction and poor patient survival. Biopsy findings in the patient with recurrent HCV can overlap with rejection, making the diagnosis challenging. While recurrent HCV remains a significant clinical problem, recurrent HBV is now rare with the advent of HBIg and effective antiviral agents.

Pathology/pathogenesis

- The time frame of liver enzyme abnormalities after transplantation can be helpful in determining the cause.

Early post-transplantation period (first 6 months)

- Aminotransferases, bilirubin and INR should improve daily following LT. AST is generally the first hepatic enzyme to normalize. A peak AST >5000 IU/L following transplantation is associated with lower rates of patient and graft survival.

  Hepatic artery thrombosis and primary graft non-function are causes of persistently abnormal tests in the first 24–72 hours following transplantation. Hepatic artery thrombosis is diagnosed using Doppler US of the hepatic artery. If Doppler evaluation is equivocal, angiography may be needed to diagnose suspected hepatic artery thrombosis.

- Primary graft non-function is a clinical diagnosis based on failure of adequate bile production, hemodynamic instability, encephalopathy, and lactic acidosis in combination with abnormal liver tests (AST >3000) and coagulopathy (INR >2.5). This can occur in the setting of hepatic artery thrombosis or due to donor-related problems such as small size or prolonged ischemia time.

  Hyperacute rejection, caused by preformed antibodies and complement-mediated destruction of endothelial cells followed by graft thrombosis, presents within minutes to hours following transplantation and is rarely seen. Risk factors include transplantation of an ABO incompatible graft.

- Most cases of acute cellular rejection occur between 7 and 28 days following transplantation. Symptoms are absent early in the course and the only indication may be elevation of liver tests, hence the need for frequent monitoring of laboratory tests during the first month after transplantation. Diagnosis is made by liver biopsy demonstrating a triad of endothelialitis, bile duct injury and mixed inflammatory infiltrate (see Chapter 44).

- Other considerations if liver biopsy does not demonstrate evidence of rejection include:
  - Delayed graft function, particularly if the allograft comes from an extended criteria donor (donation after cardiac death, prolonged ischemia time, older age, steatosis >30%).
  - Sepsis.
  - Drug toxicity.
  - Technical complications including bile leak.

- Delayed hepatic artery thrombosis or hepatic artery stenosis can lead to biliary strictures, cholangitis, and hepatic abscesses. More sensitive imaging including MRCP, MRA or CT angiography may aid in diagnosis if a bile duct or hepatic artery problem is suspected despite a normal US.

Late post-transplantation period (beyond 6 months)

- Similar principles apply in the approach to causes of allograft dysfunction beyond the first 6 months, specifically imaging to assess for biliary complications and hepatic artery flow and maintaining a low threshold to perform liver biopsy to assess for rejection.

- Recurrent disease, particularly HCV, becomes more of a consideration in the differential as time progresses following LT. There is significant overlap between pathologic findings seen with rejection and recurrent HCV which can pose a diagnostic challenge. Elevated HCV RNA levels (beyond several million IU/mL) may support a diagnosis of HCV whereas recent subtherapeutic immunosuppression levels may favor rejection.

- NASH, whether recurrent or *de novo*, is another cause of abnormal liver tests in the transplantation recipient and is exacerbated by diabetes, hypertension and dyslipidemia associated with side effects of immunosuppression.

- Chronic rejection occurs following bouts of acute rejection and is characterized by bile duct loss. Patients may report pruritus or have jaundice and allograft failure during later stages;

however often the patient may have asymptomatic AP elevation as the only manifestation. A rare variant of rejection-termed plasma cell hepatitis can occur in patients with recurrent HCV following interferon therapy and should be considered in any LT recipient being treated with interferon who develops rising liver tests.

- Biopsy is important in the diagnosis of rejection and assessing for recurrent disease; however, findings must be correlated with a thorough history including underlying liver disease leading to transplantation, operative complications, donor quality, compliance with immunosuppression, risk factors for infectious causes of hepatitis, and medications associated with liver test abnormalities. This emphasizes the importance of open communication within a multidisciplinary team that includes a pathologist, transplantation surgeon and hepatologist.
- Older donor age, prolonged ischemia time, early hepatic artery complications and living donor transplantations can lead to late causes of biliary complications.
- Donor/recipient CMV mismatch (donor seropositive, recipient seronegative) should raise the suspicion for CMV as a cause of elevated tests following withdrawal of antiviral prophylaxis.
- Recidivism with alcohol use is ideally minimized with stringent selection criteria prior to transplantation. However, it should also be considered in the differential of liver test elevations.
- A particular cause of drug-induced toxicity following transplantation worth mentioning is nodular regenerative hyperplasia which is associated with azathioprine.

Section 2: Prevention

- Although there are many causes of abnormal LFTs after transplantation, in general most of them are not preventable.

Section 3: Diagnosis

- Patterns of liver test elevation are variable and are not reliable in distinguishing between different causes.
- Liver biopsy is essential in making the diagnosis of rejection or recurrent disease.
- Imaging can aid in diagnosing hepatic artery thrombosis or biliary strictures.
- Please see the Differential diagnosis table and Algorithms 43.1 and 43.2.

Differential diagnosis

Differential diagnosis	Features
Primary graft non-function	Failure of adequate bile production, hemodynamic instability, encephalopathy, lactic acidosis, markedly abnormal liver tests (AST >3000) and coagulopathy (INR >2.5). Concurrent hepatic artery thrombosis. History of donor-related problems such as small size or prolonged ischemia time

(Continued)

Differential diagnosis	Features
Acute rejection	History of low immunosuppression levels (i.e. non-compliance, drug interactions or GI losses leading to low levels) Liver biopsy demonstrating triad of endothelialitis, mixed inflammatory infiltrate, bile duct injury
Chronic rejection	History of low immunosuppression levels Recent or prior history of acute rejection Liver biopsy demonstrating bile duct loss Pruritus on history, cholestatic liver test elevation
Hepatic artery thrombosis	Decreased hepatic artery flow on imaging (Doppler US, CT angiography, MRA)
Biliary stricture	Cholestatic liver test elevation History of impaired hepatic arterial flow (hepatic artery thrombosis or stenosis) Dilated bile ducts on US or MRCP
Recurrent disease	Liver biopsy demonstrating features of original disease (HCV, PSC, PBC, NASH) MRCP showing recurrent PSC
Drug-induced liver injury	Recent new medications or herbal products

Typical presentation
- Typically abnormal LFTs after LT are picked up on routine laboratory tests. Occasionally, depending on the cause, the patient can present with fever, abdominal pain or jaundice.

Clinical diagnosis
History
- The history should include a detailed review of the operative note record for organ and surgical characteristics, the cause of liver disease and the immunosuppression protocol.
- The abnormal tests will usually be picked up incidentally and the patient will be asymptomatic but it is important to ask about systemic symptoms such as pain, fever, change in urine or stool color and any medication changes.

Physical examination
- The physical examination will usually be unrevealing.

Laboratory diagnosis
- Please see Section 1: "Pathology/pathogenesis" and Algorithms 43.1 and 43.2.

Potential pitfalls/common errors made regarding diagnosis of disease
- There should be a low threshold to perform a liver biopsy, particularly when trying to differentiate between rejection and recurrent hepatitis C.

Section 4: Treatment
Treatment rationale
- The treatment for the different causes of abnormal LFTs after transplantation will depend on the etiology.

Algorithm 43.1 Approach to investigation of elevated liver tests within first 6 months following transplantation

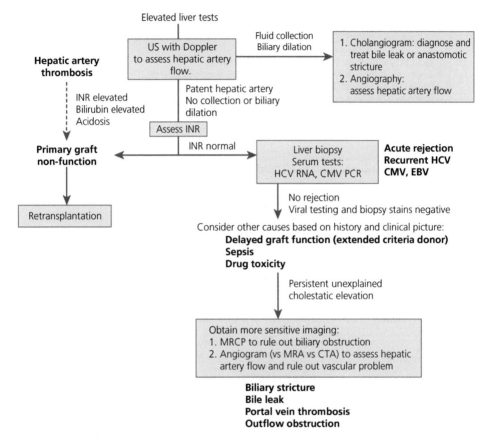

- See Algorithm 43.1 and 43.2 and individual chapters dealing with rejection, recurrent disease and other complications after transplantation.

Section 5: Special Populations
Children
- Please see Chapter 38.

Section 6: Prognosis

BOTTOM LINE
- Prognosis will depend on the cause (please see individual chapters).
- Primary non-function and early hepatic artery thrombosis require re-transplantation.
- Acute rejection is typically easily treated, chronic rejection much less so.
- Biliary complications can be treated endoscopically or percutaneously with some success.
- Recurrent disease can be difficult to treat, particularly hepatitis C, but often occurs several years after transplantation and patients can do reasonably well.

**Algorithm 43.2 Approach to investigation of elevated liver tests
after 6 months following transplantation**

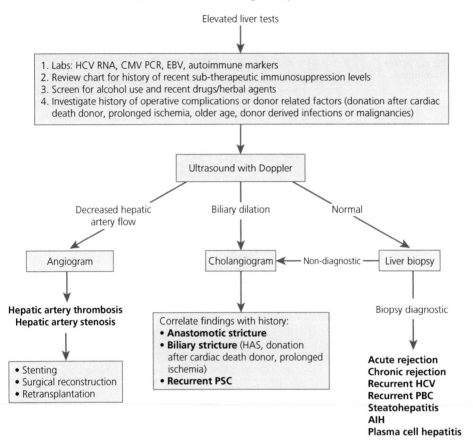

Section 7: Reading List

Banff Working Group. Liver biopsy interpretation for causes of late liver allograft dysfunction. Hepatology 2006;44:489–501

Briceno J, Ciria R. Early graft dysfunction after liver transplantation. Transplantation Proceedings 2010;42:631–3

Everson G, Kam I. Immediate postoperative care. In Maddrey W, Schiff E, Sorrell M (eds) Transplantation of the Liver, 3rd edition. Philadelphia: Lippincott Williams and Wilkin, 2001:131–62

Fiel M, Agarwal K, Stanca C, et al. Posttransplant plasma cell hepatitis (de novo autoimmune hepatitis) is a variant of rejection and may lead to a negative outcome in patients with hepatitis c virus. Liver Transplantation 2008;14:861–71

Wiesner R, Menon K. Late hepatic allograft dysfunction. Liver Transpl 2001;7:S60–73

Section 8: Guidelines

Not applicable for this topic.

Section 9: Evidence

Not applicable for this topic.

Section 10: Images

Not applicable for this topic.

Additional material for this chapter can be found online at:
www.mountsinaiexpertguides.com
This includes a case study and multiple choice questions

CHAPTER 44

Acute Rejection

Costica Aloman
University of Illinois, Chicago, IL, USA

OVERALL BOTTOM LINE
- From a clinical perspective it is very important to distinguish between "histological" and "clinically relevant" AR.
- The majority of AR episodes occur in the first 6 weeks after LT.
- The diagnosis of AR needs confirmation on liver biopsy.
- The differential diagnosis includes conditions that cause elevation of liver injury tests, jaundice and even fever in the first 3 months after LT.
- The severity of rejection dictates the treatment strategy, particularly in the presence of HCV infection.

Section 1: Background
Definition of disease
- Allograft rejection can be defined as an immunological reaction to the presence of foreign tissue or organ, which has the potential to result in graft dysfunction and failure.
- AR is defined as an inflammation of the allograft, elicited by genetic disparity between the donor and recipient, primarily affecting interlobular bile ducts and vascular endothelium, including portal veins, hepatic venules and occasionally the hepatic artery and its branches.

Disease classification
- Several methods for classifying acute rejection exist:
  - Based on the timing of onset after LT:
    - early AR in the first 3–6 months after LT.
    - late AR after 3–6 months from LT.
  - Based on the presence of abnormal liver chemistry tests:
    - histological (only histological signs of AR).
    - clinically relevant AR (abnormal liver chemistry tests with histological proved AR).
  - Based on the histological severity of AR (Banff classification).
  - Based on steroid treatment response:
    - steroid-responsive.
    - steroid-resistant.

Mount Sinai Expert Guides: Hepatology, First Edition. Edited by Jawad Ahmad, Scott L. Friedman, and Henryk Dancygier.
© 2014 John Wiley & Sons, Ltd. Published 2014 by John Wiley & Sons, Ltd.
Companion website: www.mountsinaiexpertguides.com

Incidence/prevalence
- The cumulative incidence of AR was reported to be as high as 65% by 1 year post-transplantation in the earlier studies after the introduction of CNI.
- The incidence at 3 months has decreased to less than 10% after introduction of interleukin-2 receptor alpha (IL-2Rα) blockers.
- The majority of AR episodes occur in the first 6 weeks post-transplantation.

Etiology
- Acute rejection is the end result of the acute immune response directed against the presence of alloantigens in the transplanted liver, which has the potential to result in endothelial and bile duct damage that may progress to chronic rejection and allograft failure.

Pathology/pathogenesis
- Allograft injury is the result of complex interaction between:
  - Hepatic antigen-presenting cells (donor/recipient).
  - Recipient helper, effector and regulatory T cells.
  - Immune-induced activation of TNF-α superfamily receptors on target cells (mainly cholangiocytes and endothelial cells) that results in bile duct inflammation, endothelial damage and presence of mixed inflammatory infiltrate in the portal areas.
- Direct presentation of alloantigens by donor dendritic cells from the transplanted liver is thought to be the main mechanism responsible for AR.

Predictive/risk factors for early AR

Risk factor	Relative risk
Recipient age (>60 years)	0.81 (0.73–0.90, CI 95%)
Creatinine >2 mg/dL without dialysis	0.48 (0.29–0.80, CI 95%)
Pre-operative AST <40 IU/L vs >200	0.52 (0.30–0.90, CI 95%)
Pre-operative AST 40–199 IU/L vs >200	0.66 (0.48–0.90, CI 95%)
Presence of edema immediately pre-transplantation	0.71 (0.56–0.91, CI 95%)
Cold ischemic time ≥15 hours	1.61 (CI 1.19–2.20, CI 95%)
Donor age ≥30 years	1.27 (1.0002–1.61, CI 95%)

Section 2: Prevention

- Improved immunosuppressive strategies and the use of IL-2Rα blockers decreases the risk of AR

Screening
- There are no screening strategies for AR although periodic liver injury tests and measurement of immunosuppressive medication levels are performed in order to detect abnormalities at an early stage and avoid low levels of immunosuppression.

Primary prevention
- Maintain corticosteroid treatment during the first 3–6 months after LT.
- For corticosteroid-free regimens use IL-2Rα or alemtuzumab for induction.

- Close monitoring of tacrolimus, cyclosporine or sirolimus levels as dictated by the timing from transplantation.
  - Monitor and adjusting the dose of tacrolimus/cyclosporine in correlation with newly introduced medications that may affect pharmacokinetics of immunosuppressive medications.

Secondary prevention

- Maintain higher level of maintenance immunosuppression after an episode of AR.
- If patient only on tacrolimus maintenance consider adding mycophenolate mofetil.

Section 3: Diagnosis (Algorithm 44.1)

- The diagnosis is suggested by elevated liver enzymes, followed by the appearance of jaundice and sometimes fever in LT recipients.
- MRI/MRCP, CT scan or US of the liver are required in order to rule out other conditions that can cause abnormal liver injury tests in the first 3–6 months after LT such as vascular insufficiency, biliary complications and recurrent disease (particularly in the case of hepatitis C).
- The diagnosis of AR needs to be confirmed by core liver biopsy.
- At least two of the following three features are required for a histopathological diagnosis of AR:
  1. Mixed but predominantly mononuclear portal inflammation, containing blastic (activated) lymphocytes, neutrophils and frequently eosinophils;
  2. Bile duct inflammation/damage;
  3. Subendothelial inflammation of portal veins, terminal hepatic venules or hepatic arteries (Figure 44.1).

Differential diagnosis

Differential diagnosis	Features
Obstructive cholangiopathy	History of difficult surgical biliary tract reconstruction; presentation with clinical findings suggestive of cholangitis: fever, RUQ pain; imaging studies with intrahepatic biliary ductal dilatation
Hepatic artery thrombosis/stenosis	History of difficult surgical hepatic artery reconstruction; imaging studies with absence of blood flow in the hepatic artery
Recurrent disease	History of HCV, PSC, PBC, AIH: • High levels of HCV-RNA suggestive of recurrent cholestatic form of HCV which is confirmed by biopsy • Recurrent PBC/AIH is confirmed by biopsy Recurrence of AIH with a cholestasis variant confirmed by biopsy
Sepsis	Presence of high fever with chills and positive blood cultures
Opportunistic infections	Positive CMV PCR or EBV PCR or anti-HSV1 IgM

Typical presentation
- The diagnosis of AR is suspected in patients with non-compliance with immunosuppressive medication or low levels of CNI in the first 3–6 months after LT, who develop progressive increases in AST, ALT, AP and jaundice.

Clinical diagnosis
History
- The key features the clinician should enquire about when taking the patient's history are:
  - Compliance with immunosuppressive medications and documentation of tacrolimus, cyclosporine or sirolimus levels.
  - The cause of liver disease pre-transplantation.
  - Recently introduced medications.
- It is very important to obtain and review the surgical report of the LT.

Physical examination
- During physical examination special attention should be paid to the following findings that help in assessing the severity of AR or help in the differential diagnosis:
  - Fever.
  - Jaundice.

Useful clinical decision rules and calculators
- Compliant jaundiced patient with severe AR, therapeutic levels of tacrolimus and no HCV infection consider thymoglobulin rather than corticosteroids.

Disease severity classification
- The specific histological features of AR represented by mixed inflammatory infiltrate, bile duct inflammation/damage, and subendothelial inflammation are scored on a 0 to 3 scale (mild, moderate, severe), added together to arrive at a final RAI using Banff schema.
- The RAI scores between 0 and 9:
  - 0–2 no rejection.
  - 3 borderline.
  - 4–5 mild rejection.
  - 6–7 moderate rejection.
  - 8–9 severe rejection.
- The RAI grading system has proven to be reproducible and has prognostic significance.

Laboratory diagnosis
List of diagnostic tests
- Elevated AST, ALT, AP and GGT.
- In severe cases also increased total bilirubin and INR.
- Liver biopsy is diagnostic.

List of imaging techniques
- MR or CT angiography to rule out hepatic artery stenosis/thrombosis.
- MRCP to rule out biliary obstruction.

Algorithm 44.1 Diagnosis of AR

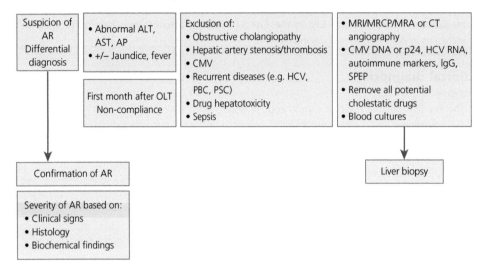

Potential pitfalls/common errors made regarding diagnosis of disease

- Undiagnosed obstructive cholangiopathy or hepatic artery stenosis/thrombosis.
- Ongoing infection/sepsis.
- Undiagnosed infiltrative process as amyloidosis, neoplasm, fungal infection.

Section 4: Treatment (Algorithm 44.2)
Treatment rationale

- Treatment for AR is targeting down-regulation of immune response against allograft antigens. Corticosteroids have represented the first line treatment in AR after LT for the last three decades. Other possible additional/alternative treatments are thymoglobulin, mycophenolate mofetil, anti- IL-2Rα blockers, OKT3 and deoxyspergualin.
- Two major factors are involved in making the decision of the specific immunosuppressive treatment strategy in face of confirmed AR:
  - Severity of rejection. Subclinical/mild AR versus severe histological AR with jaundice. Histological diagnosis of AR does not necessarily imply requirement for treatment. Careful monitoring of the graft function and adjustment of the CNI levels is advisable in this category of patients.
  - Presence of HCV infection. Over the last two decades studies have suggested that the use of high dose steroids has a negative impact on graft function and HCV recurrence so avoiding high doses of steroids and OKT3 if possible in this category of patients is recommended.

When to hospitalize

- Patient with proved AR that required IV steroids or thymoglobulin.
- Proved AR with jaundice and/or increased INR.

Algorithm 44.2 Treatment of AR

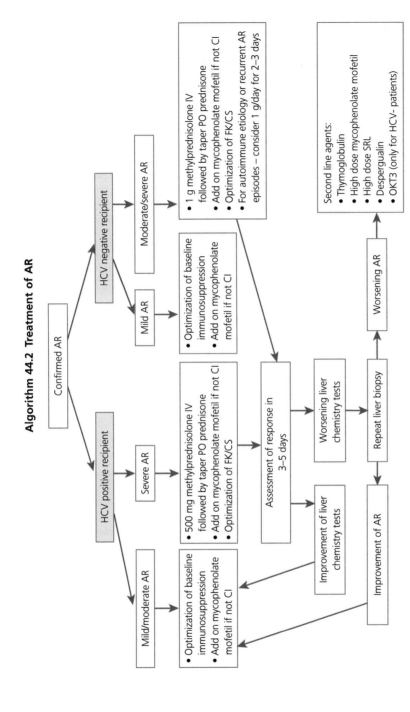

CI, contra-indication; CS, cyclosporine; FK, tacrolimus; SRL, sirolimus.

Table of treatment

Treatment	Comment
Conservative treatment	In cases of mild rejection with normal liver chemistry tests Optimization of maintenance immunosuppression
Medical : 1. Methylprednisolone: 500 mg–1 g for 1–3 days 2. Thymoglobulin: 1.5 mg/kg/day for 5–7 days 3. Addition of sirolimus: target level of 12–20 ng/mL 4. Addition of mycophenolate mofetil: target dose of 3 g every 8 hours if tolerated 5. Tacrolimus: if patient in cyclosporine regimen 6. Anti-IL-2Rα antibodies 7. OKT3 8. Deoxyspergualin 3: 5 mg/kg/day, 4–14 days	Indicated in cases of at least moderate/severe AR Require prophylaxis against opportunistic infection (anti CMV, candida, herpes viruses, *P. carinii*) Require central line for thymoglobulin administration Close glucose monitoring and tight control of post-transplantation diabetes mellitus

Prevention/management of complications
- Prevention of opportunistic infection after administration of high dose steroids and thymoglobulin.
- Prevention of phlebitis after thymoglobulin administration by using a central line.
- Close monitoring of glucose and control of glycemia with insulin regimen.
- Prevention of GI bleeding with PPI.

CLINICAL PEARLS
- Decision to treat AR is based on the histological severity but also on clinical presentation of AR
- Presence of HCV infection – advise careful assessment of risk/benefits of using high dose steroids.
- Re-evaluate diagnosis of AR if no response to high-dose steroids before escalating immunosuppression.
- After the use of high-dose steroids/thymoglobulin for AR it is critical to start opportunistic infection prophylaxis.

Section 5: Special Populations

Not applicable for this topic.

Section 6: Prognosis

- The pathological diagnosis of AR, especially in the widespread era of protocol biopsies, does not automatically signal that modification of immunosuppressive treatment is indicated, particularly if AR is low grade.

- Transient findings of AR after LT without significant clinical changes or impact on graft function have been observed.
- An episode of AR does not appear to have a negative impact on patient and graft survival in HCV negative patients.
- An episode of AR in HCV positive patients increases the replication of HCV, impairs graft function, and decreases graft and patient survival.

Prognosis for treated patients

- Almost 80% of AR respond after a course of high dose of corticosteroids.
- Biochemical and histological improvement is noted in the first 3–5 days after high dose corticosteroids.

Section 7: Reading List

Demetris A, Batts KP, Dhillon AP, et al. Banff Schema for grading liver allograft rejection: an international consensus document. Hepatology 1997;25:658–63

Eksteen B, Neuberger JM. Mechanisms of disease: the evolving understanding of liver allograft rejection. Nat Clin Pract Gastroenterol Hepatol 2008; 5:209–19

Rosen HR. Transplant immunology: what the clinicians need to know for immunotherapy. Gastroenterology 2008;134:1789–801

Sanchez-Fueyo A, Strom TB. Immunologic basis of graft rejection and tolerance following transplantation of liver or other solid organs. Gastroenterology 2011;140:51–64

Terminology for hepatic allograft rejection. International Working Party. Hepatology 1995; 22:648–54

Volpin R, Angeli P, Galiato A, et al. Comparison between two high-dose methyprednisolone schedules in the treatment of acute cellular rejection in liver transplant recipients: a controlled clinical trial. Liver Transpl 2002;8:527–34

Weisner RH, Demeteris AJ, Belle SH, et al. Acute hepatic allograft rejection: incidence, risk factors and impact outcome. Hepatology 1998;28:638–45

Section 8: Guidelines

Not applicable for this topic.

Section 9: Evidence

Type of evidence	Title, date	Comment
RCT	Comparison between two high-dose methylprednisolone schedules in the treatment of acute cellular rejection in liver transplant; 2002	One dose of 1 g methylprednisolone followed by taper is more effective and safer than three doses of methylprednisolone for three consecutive days
Prospective observational study	Acute hepatic allograft rejection: incidence, risk factors and impact on outcome; 1998	Only a small minority of patients on Prograf
International Consensus Document	Banff schema for grading liver allograft rejection: 1997	Established the common nomenclature and a set of histopathological criteria for the grading of acute liver allograft rejection

Section 10: Images

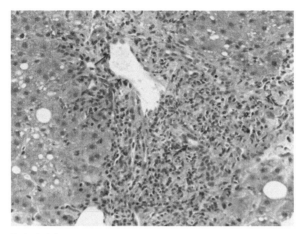

Figure 44.1 AR: pathological features.

Additional material for this chapter can be found online at:
www.mountsinaiexpertguides.com
This includes a case study, multiple choice questions, advice for
patients and ICD codes

CHAPTER 45

Chronic Rejection

Costica Aloman
University of Illinois, Chicago, IL, USA

OVERALL BOTTOM LINE
- The most frequent CR is preceded by one or more episodes of AR that are often resistant to corticosteroid therapy and require anti-lymphocyte or other rescue therapy.
- The early phases of CR are potentially reversible, so it is critical to develop a multidisciplinary management plan with active involvement of an expert liver pathologist.
- There are limited therapeutic options for established CR and none of the options have been compared in a RCT.
- The main challenge in the management of CR is to establish the need for increasing the immunosuppressive regimen versus the option of re-transplantation.
- Signs of allograft failure suggest the need of re-transplantation.

Section 1: Background
Definition of disease
- Allograft rejection can be defined as an immunological reaction to the presence of foreign tissue or organ, which has the potential to result in graft dysfunction and failure.
- Chronic allograft rejection is defined as an immunologic injury to the allograft, which usually evolves from severe or persistent AR and results in potential irreversible damage to the bile duct, arteries and veins that evolves into graft failure.

Disease classification
- The classification of CR is based on the histological findings of early versus late findings of CR.
- This classification provides information regarding the likelihood of reversal and does not absolutely define a point of no return.

Incidence/prevalence
- Historically, CR accounted for up to 20% of all cases of liver allograft failure but this has decreased significantly over the last 20 years due to improvement in immunosuppressive medications and monitoring.
- Currently, CR has an incidence of less than 3–4% of all causes of liver allograft failure.

Mount Sinai Expert Guides: Hepatology, First Edition. Edited by Jawad Ahmad, Scott L. Friedman, and Henryk Dancygier.

Etiology

- CR is the end result of the persistent immune response directed against the presence of alloantigens in the transplanted liver, which has the potential to result in graft dysfunction and failure.

Pathology/pathogenesis

- Graft injury is the result of a complex interaction between:
  - Hepatic antigen presenting cells (donor/recipient).
  - Recipient helper, effector and regulatory T cells.
  - Immune-induced activation of TNF-α superfamily receptors on target cells (mainly cholangiocytes and endothelial cells) that results in ductopenia and obstructive arteriopathy.
- Indirect presentation of donor alloantigens from the transplanted liver by recipient antigen presenting cells which is thought to be the main mechanism responsible for late allograft rejection.
- Direct presentation of alloantigens by donor dendritic cells from the transplanted liver possibly involved in the CR that develops soon after liver transplantation in the setting of multiple episodes of AR and/or in steroid resistant AR.

Predictive/risk factors

Risk factor	Odds ratio
Any episode of AR	3.6
More than one episode of acute rejection	7.86
Moderate or severe acute rejection	4.77
Donor age more than 40	2.14
LT for PBC	10.6
LT for AIH	6.7
Male donor to female recipient	5.83 (in cyclosporine-based regimen)
Recipient age less than 30 years old	3.8
CMV IgG positive donor into negative recipient	3.5
Treatment with IFN for HCV	Unknown
CMV infection	Unknown

Section 2: Prevention

- Improvement of immunosuppressive strategies has decreased the risk of CR from 20% to <4% of all causes of liver allograft failure.
- Continuous patient education regarding the importance of compliance with immunosuppressive medication and monitoring.

Screening

- There are no screening strategies for CR although periodic liver chemistry tests and measurement of immunosuppressive medication levels is performed in order to detect early AR and avoid low levels of immunosuppression.

Primary prevention

- Close monitoring of tacrolimus, cyclosporine or sirolimus as dictated by the timing from transplantation.

- Monitor and adjust the dose of tacrolimus/cyclosporine in correlation with newly introduced medications that may interfere with immunosuppressive medication pharmacokinetics.
- Maintain a higher level of tacrolimus or add mycophenolate mofetil after episodes of AR.
- Start tacrolimus if patient develops AR while on a cyclosporine immunosuppression regimen.

Section 3: Diagnosis (Algorithm 45.1)

- Clinical symptoms are non-specific and present only in the late stages. The onset of jaundice indicates usually severe allograft dysfunction.
- Standard liver injury abnormalities in a patient with CR show a progressive cholestatic pattern that can eventually lead to jaundice.
- MRI/MRCP, CT scan or US of the liver are required in order to rule out other conditions that can cause cholestasis.
- To establish the diagnosis of CR a core liver biopsy is necessary.
- Minimal pathological criteria for CR include:
  - Bile duct atrophy/pyknosis affecting the majority of the bile ducts, with or without bile duct loss.
  - Foam cell obliterative arteriopathy.
  - Bile duct loss greater than 50% of the portal tracts (Figure 45.1).

Differential diagnosis

Differential diagnosis	Features
Obstructive cholangiopathy	History of difficult surgical biliary tract reconstruction; presentation with clinical findings suggestive of cholangitis: fever, RUQ pain; imaging studies with intrahepatic biliary duct dilatation
Hepatic artery stenosis/ thrombosis	History of surgically difficult hepatic artery reconstruction; imaging studies with absence of blood flow in the hepatic artery
Drug-induced liver injury	History of recent introduction medications with potential to induce cholestasis
Recurrent disease	History of HCV, PSC, PBC, AIH: • High levels HCV-RNA suggestive of recurrent cholestatic form of HCV is confirmed by biopsy • Recurrent PSC confirmed by imaging appearance of biliary tree on MRCP • Recurrent PBC is confirmed by biopsy • Recurrence of AIH with a cholestasis variant confirmed by biopsy
De novo AIH	History of recent IFN treatment; new presence of SMA, ANA and high IgG; confirmed by biopsy
Infiltrative process (sarcoidosis, amyloidosis, infiltrative neoplasm)	History of sarcoidosis, paraproteinemia and neoplasm; imaging, biochemistry and critical in differential diagnosis

Typical presentation
- The diagnosis of CR is suspected in a patient with non-compliance with immunosuppressive medications or a history of AR, who develops progressive cholestasis and an increase in the canalicular enzymes (ALP, GGT).

Clinical diagnosis

History
- The key features the clinician should enquire about when taking the patient's history are:
  - The cause of pre-transplantation liver disease.
  - Compliance with immunosuppressive medications.
  - Any change in medications.
  - Past medical history of sarcoid, paraproteinemia and malignancy.
- It is very important to review the surgical operative report of the liver transplantation.

Physical examination
- During the physical examination special attention should be paid to the following findings that help in assessing the severity of graft dysfunction:
  - Jaundice.
  - Edema.
  - Ascites.
  - Encephalopathy.

Disease severity classification
- The early phases of CR are potentially reversible, so in order to effectively manage patients with CR active consultation with an expert liver pathologist to identify features of early or late CR is critical. The features should be described as per Banff schema, established for liver allografts.
- The early CR findings are:
  - Small bile ducts:
    - ➤ degenerative changes involved in the majority of the bile ducts.
    - ➤ bile duct loss less than 50%.
  - Terminal hepatic venules and zone 3 hepatocytes:
    - ➤ intimal inflammation.
    - ➤ mild perivenular fibrosis.
    - ➤ lytic zone 3 necrosis/inflammation.
  - Portal hepatic arterioles:
    - ➤ loss less than 25% of portal tracts.
  - Large perihilar hepatic arteries (usually not present on needle biopsies):
    - ➤ intimal inflammation.
    - ➤ focal foam cell deposition without lumen obliteration.
  - Large perihilar bile ducts (usually not present on needle biopsies):
    - ➤ ductal inflammation.
    - ➤ focal foam cell deposition without lumen obliteration.
  - Other: spotty necrosis of hepatocytes, "transition" hepatitis.
- The late CR findings are:
  - Small bile duct:
    - ➤ loss of more than 50% bile ducts.
    - ➤ degenerative changes in the remaining bile ducts.
  - Terminal hepatic venules and zone 3 hepatocytes:
    - ➤ focal obliteration of hepatic venules.
    - ➤ bridging fibrosis.
  - Portal hepatic arterioles:
    - ➤ loss of more than 25% of portal tracts.

- Large perihilar hepatic arteries (usually not present on needle biopsies):
  - ➤ luminal obliteration by sub-intimal foam cells.
- Large perihilar bile ducts (usually not present on needle biopsies):
  - ➤ fibrointimal proliferation.
- Other: severe hepatocyte cholestasis.

Laboratory diagnosis
List of diagnostic tests
- Elevated ALP and GGT.
- Increased total bilirubin and INR if significant graft dysfunction.
- Liver biopsy is diagnostic.

List of imaging techniques
- MR or CT angiography to rule out hepatic artery stenosis/thrombosis.
- MRCP to rule out biliary obstruction.
- MRI or CT scan with contrast when infiltrative neoplasm/sarcoidosis is in the differential diagnosis.

Algorithm 45.1 Diagnosis of CR

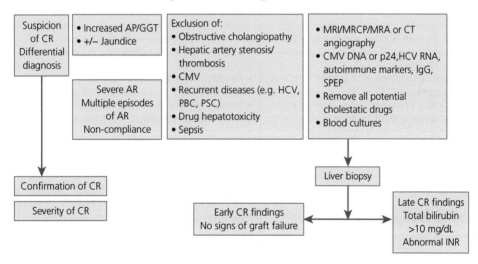

Potential pitfalls/common errors made regarding diagnosis of disease
- Undiagnosed obstructive cholangiopathy or hepatic artery stenosis/thrombosis.
- Ongoing infection/sepsis.
- Undiagnosed infiltrative processes such as amyloidosis, neoplasm, fungal infection.

Section 4: Treatment (Algorithm 45.2)
Treatment rationale
- The main decision regarding CR treatment is choosing between the option of optimizing the immunosuppression regimen with the purpose to save the graft, or evaluation for re-transplantation. Liver biopsy does not define an absolute point of no return so this major

decision needs to be considered in the context of other clinical and biochemical findings, especially the evidence of allograft failure.

- If the patient has evidence of early pathological findings of CR, with a moderate increase in total bilirubin (≤10 mg/dL) and normal hepatic synthetic function, usually in a setting of a recent episode of AR, the most appropriate management will be optimization of immunosuppression by one of the methods indicated in the Table of treatment.
- If the patient has clear pathological evidence of late stage CR, with a significant increase in total bilirubin (>10 mg/dL) and abnormal hepatic synthetic function usually diagnosed in the context of multiple episodes of AR or late CR, a rapid evaluation for re-transplantation is appropriate.

When to hospitalize

- Patients with evidence of complications related to allograft failure including hepatic encephalopathy, hepatorenal syndrome and suspected infection.

Table of treatment

Treatment	Comment
Medical: optimization of immunosuppression: 1. Start tacrolimus if patient in cyclosporine-based regimen 2. Increase tacrolimus dose (goal of 10 ng/mL) 3. Addition of mycophenolate mofetil to tacrolimus (goal of 1 g twice a day) 4. Addition of sirolimus to tacrolimus (goal of 8–10 ng/mL)	Patient with pathological findings of CR and moderate increase in total bilirubin (less than 6–10 mg/dL): • Tacrolimus dose optimization considered first line treatment • Renal insufficiency is the main limiting factor for tacrolimus optimization • If patient develops renal failure during tacrolimus optimization consider adding mycophenolate mofetil or sirolimus • Frequent monitoring of tacrolimus, sirolimus levels and renal function/CBC/triglyceride required, particularly with combination therapy
Surgical: re-transplantation	Clear evidence of late stage CR, with significantly increased total bilirubin (usually more than 10 mg/dL) and abnormal hepatic synthetic function

Prevention/management of complications

- Tacrolimus-induced renal failure:
  - Close monitoring of renal function while increasing the dose of tacrolimus.
  - If acute kidney injury develops , readjust tacrolimus dose and IV fluids.
- Tacrolimus-related neurotoxicity:
  - Decrease tacrolimus dose.
- Mycophenolate mofetil-related leucopenia:
  - Close monitor of CBC.
- Sirolimus-related hypertriglyceridemia:
  - Close monitor of triglyceride levels.

Algorithm 45.2 Treatment of CR

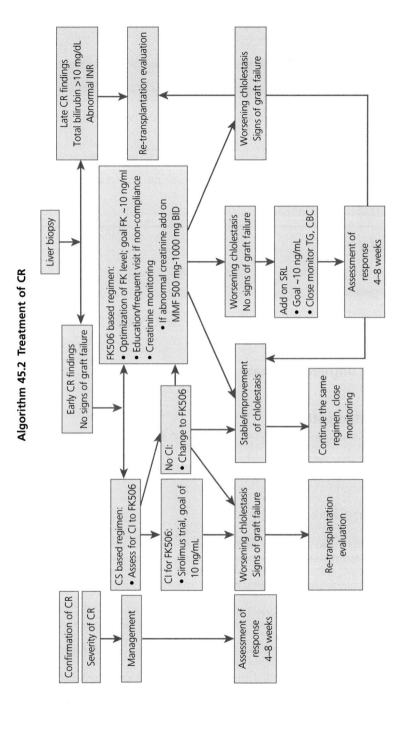

CI, contra-indication; CS, cyclosporine; FK(506), tacrolimus; SRL, sirolimus; TG, triglyceride.

CLINICAL PEARLS
- The presence of liver allograft failure or significant hyperbilirubinemia/increased INR determine the need for re-transplantation.
- Close discussion with an expert liver pathologist for late/early signs of CR is critical for management.
- Early CR needs frequent monitoring of tacrolimus/sirolimus levels and possible side effects from diuretics.
- Development of significant graft dysfunction in spite of augmentation of immunosuppression requires evaluation for re-transplantation.

Section 5: Special Populations

Not applicable for this topic.

Section 6: Prognosis

- Loss of bile ducts greater than 50%, severe /bridging perivenular fibrosis and small arterial foam clusters predicts a greater incidence of graft failure.

Natural history of untreated disease
- Progression to graft failure.

Prognosis for treated patients
- Early conversion of cyclosporine-based regimen (total bilirubin <6 mg/dL) results in 80% graft salvage.
- Addition of sirolimus to tacrolimus regimen results in almost 50% histological response.

Section 7: Reading List

Candinas D, Gunson BK, Nightingale P, et al. Sex mismatch as a risk factor for chronic rejection of liver allograft. Lancet 1995; 346:1117–21

Demetris A, Adams D, Bellamy C, et al. Update of the International Banff Schema for Liver Allograft Rejection: working recommendations for the histopathologic staging and reporting of chronic rejection. An International Panel. Hepatology 2000; 31:792–9

Desai M, Neuberger J. Chronic allograft dysfunction. Transpl Proc 2009;41:773–6

Eksteen B, Neuberger JM. Mechanisms of disease: the evolving understanding of liver allograft rejection. Nat Clin Pract Gastroenterol Hepatol 2008;5:209–19

Evans P, Soin A, Wreghitt T, et al. An association between cytomegalovirus infection and chronic rejection after liver transplantation. Transplantation 2000;69:30–5

Fernandez I, Ulloa E, Colina F, et al. Incidence, risk factors, and outcome of chronic rejection during antiviral therapy for posttransplant recurrent hepatitis C. Liver Transpl 2009;15:948–55

Jain A, Demetris A, Kashyap R, et al. Does Tacrolimus offer virtual freedom from chronic rejection after primary liver transplantation? Risk and prognostic factors in 1,048 liver transplantations with a mean follow-up of 6 years. Liver Transpl 2001;7:623–30

Liver Biopsy Interpretation for Causes of Late Liver Allograft Dysfunction. Banff Working Group. Hepatology 2006; 44:489–501

Randomised trial comparing tacrolimus (FK506) and cyclosporine in prevention of liver allograft rejection. Lancet 1994;344:423–8

Stanca CM, Fiel MI, Kontorinis N, Agarwal K, Emre S, Schiano TD. Chronic ductopenic rejection in patients with recurrent hepatitis C virus treated with pegylated interferon alfa-2a and ribavirin. Transplantation 2007;84:180–6

Terminology for hepatic allograft rejection. International Working Party. Hepatology 1995; 22:648–54

Section 8: Guidelines

Not applicable for this topic.

Section 9: Evidence

Type of evidence	Title, date	Comment
RCT	Randomized trial comparing tacrolimus (FK506) and cylosporin in prevention of liver allograft rejection; 1994	In this trial tacrolimus had advantages over cyclosporin in respect to lower rejection rates
Retrospective observational	Sex mismatch as a risk factor for chronic rejection of liver allograft; 1995	In this retrospective study risk factors for chronic rejection were assessed. The main maintenance therapy was cyclosporine and azathioprine
Retrospective observational	Risk and prognostic factors in 1048 liver transplantations with FK506 maintenance regimen; 2001	Established in a large cohort of patients the long-term incidence of CR, risk factors, prognostic factors, and outcome after OLT with FK506 maintenance regimen

Section 10: Images

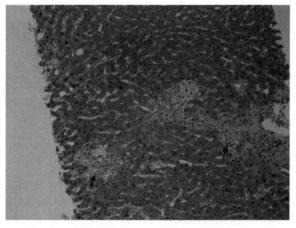

Figure 45.1 Pathological features of CR.

Additional material for this chapter can be found online at:
www.mountsinaiexpertguides.com
This includes a case study, multiple choice questions, advice for
patients and ICD codes

CHAPTER 46

Primary Non-Function

Eric G. Davis[1] and Sander S. Florman[2]
[1]University of Louisville School of Medicine, Louisville, KY, USA
[2]Recanati/Miller Transplantation Institute, Mount Sinai Hospital, New York, NY, USA

OVERALL BOTTOM LINE
- Despite landmark advances in surgical techniques and immunosuppression, PNF following LT remains a major cause of early graft and patient loss.
- Though not fully elucidated, the etiology of PNF lies at the intersection of multiple donor and recipient factors and is characterized by immediate coagulopathy, encephalopathy, acidosis, and poor bile production in the absence of a verifiable technical complication such as vascular thrombosis of the graft.
- Though a uniform definition does not exist, graft function insufficient to sustain life leading to death or re-transplantation in the first week post-operatively characterizes the syndrome.
- Despite modifications in organ allocation that allow for emergent re-transplantation in the event of PNF, early patient loss continues to occur because of persistent organ shortage.

Section 1: Background
Definition of disease
- Graft function insufficient to sustain life leading to death or re-transplantation in the first week post-operatively.
- The diagnosis is made within 24–72 hours of transplantation and is based on a combination of clinical and laboratory abnormalities, with confirmation of absence of secondary causes of graft failure such as vascular thrombosis and compression.

Incidence/prevalence
- Clear delineation of the frequency of PNF is difficult to ascertain as definitions vary from center to center, and in cases in which re-transplantation for graft failure occurs, the ultimate outcome of that graft is unknown.
- An incidence of 5% seems to be an accurate approximation, and PNF accounts for roughly one-third of early re-transplantations.

Etiology
- Though not fully elucidated, the etiology of PNF lies at the intersection of multiple donor and recipient factors.

Mount Sinai Expert Guides: Hepatology, First Edition. Edited by Jawad Ahmad, Scott L. Friedman, and Henryk Dancygier.

Pathology/pathogenesis (Figure 46.1)

- PNF has been associated with prolonged warm and cold ischemia times as well as donor characteristics such as graft steatosis, donor age and hypernatremia.
- Experimental models of PNF exist specifically for graft steatosis and the effects of reperfusion, but not all cases of PNF involve steatotic grafts.
- The inciting event seems to be ischemia–reperfusion injury alone or in the setting of pre-existing donor processes that leads to cell swelling and disturbance of the hepatic sinusoidal microvasculature.
- Synthetic dysfunction, lactic acid conversion, drug and toxin clearance and bile production are all variably affected.
- Graft necrosis is the ultimate histological outcome in cases of true PNF. Cell swelling and purported disturbance of hepatic sinusoidal microvasculature were demonstrated in an elaborate histopathological study, while ultrastructural changes via electron microscopy have been demonstrated on pre-perfusion biopsies in grafts that ultimately failed.

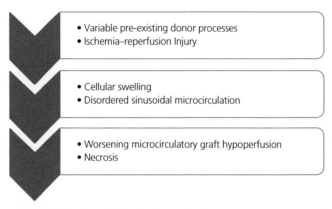

Figure 46.1 Factors involved in the pathology/pathogenesis of PNF

Predictive/risk factors (Figure 46.2)

- Despite multiple identified risk factors, PNF is not completely predictable and involves the interplay of multiple donor, procurement and recipient events.
- Described very early in the age of LT, donor liver steatosis represents one of the most identifiable risk factors for PNF. Frozen-section examination of donor liver biopsies has become standard when suspicion for fatty infiltration exists. Further studies identified macrosteatosis specifically as the dominant risk factor for PNF with the use of fatty livers. Microsteatosis, even severe, is reversible and does not preclude organ usage or predict PNF.
- Unlike kidney transplantation, it is generally well-accepted that the liver does not undergo functional senescence with aging. However, increased donor age seems to be a risk factor for PNF in many observational studies. The severe shortage of donor organs, however, does not preclude the use of older grafts.
- Severe donor hypernatremia, though traditionally associated with worse graft outcomes specifically in terms of PNF following transplantation, has recently been brought into question as a risk factor for PNF. Perhaps more important than absolute hypernatremia is wide fluctuations in sodium concentration in the donors.

- Procurement factors important in minimizing the risk of PNF include shortening the cold ischemic time as much as feasible, especially for marginal organs and when transplanting very ill recipients. The obligatory warm ischemia incurred in donation after cardiac death donors almost certainly contributes to the higher risk of PNF in this donor population.
- Recipient factors are perhaps the least modifiable contributors to PNF. Very ill recipients with high MELD scores, renal failure, and vasopressor requirements represent hostile environments to newly-transplanted grafts. A special scenario unique to living-donor liver transplantation that emulates PNF is small-for-size syndrome in which a partial graft fails to function well in the initial time period following implantation. Native hyperdynamic portal flow to a reduced-size graft leading to portal hyperperfusion is thought to be a major contributor to this phenomenon. Small-for-size syndrome forms the basis for the common practice of denying living-donor liver transplantation to adult patients with advanced disease and severe portal hypertension.

Donor factors	• Steatosis > 30% • Age > 65 • Hemodynamic instability, significant use of vasopressors • Prolonged hospitalization • Hypernatremia, though recent evidence casts this in doubt
Procurement factors	• Prolonged cold ischemic time • Donation after cardiac death
Recipient factors	• Long duration and high severity of illness • Hemodynamic instability • Very ill recipients undergoing living-donor liver transplantation • Contribution of small-for-size syndrome • Repeat transplantation

Figure 46.2 Predictive factors for PNF

Section 2: Prevention

> **BOTTOM LINE/CLINICAL PEARLS**
> - No interventions have been demonstrated to prevent the development of the disease.

Primary prevention
- Avoidance of organs with known risk factors for PNF (macrosteatosis, older donor, longer ischemia time, donation after cardiac death) can reduce the incidence of PNF but is not always feasible due to the current organ shortage.

Section 3: Diagnosis (Algorithm 46.1)

> **BOTTOM LINE/CLINICAL PEARLS**
> - Although a uniform definition does not exist, PNF is defined as graft function insufficient to sustain life leading to death or re-transplantation in the first week post-operatively.
> - It is important to document in the history the characteristics of the transplanted organ.
> - The findings on examination may reflect poor graft function including encephalopathy, coagulopathy and abdominal distension.
> - Laboratory studies will demonstrate coagulopathy, acidosis and poor bile production, and imaging should confirm the absence of a verifiable technical complication such as vascular thrombosis of the graft.

Typical presentation
- The typical presentation of PNF occurs within the first 24–72 hours after transplantation and is characterized by immediate coagulopathy, encephalopathy, acidosis and poor bile production without evidence of a verifiable technical complication such as vascular thrombosis of the graft or compression.

Clinical diagnosis
History
- The patient will not usually be able to provide a history but it is important to review the donor organ characteristics and the operative note for factors associated with PNF.

Physical examination
- The physical examination may be helpful in demonstrating poor hepatic function such as encephalopathy and ascites, and there may be oozing from the wound or line site due to coagulopathy.

Laboratory diagnosis
List of diagnostic tests
- Laboratory studies for PNF will demonstrate poor hepatic function such as elevated pro-thrombin time, bilirubin and other LFTs, poor renal function and features of acidosis. Liver biopsy is not required to make a diagnosis.

List of imaging techniques
- Imaging studies are not diagnostic in PNF but are necessary to rule out other causes of elevated liver enzymes and poor graft function such as hepatic artery thrombosis. A Doppler US is the imaging study of choice.

Section 4: Treatment (Algorithm 46.2)
Treatment rationale
- No treatment has been shown to reverse true PNF. Re-transplantation is the only effective treatment.
- The management algorithm for PNF, unfortunately, is very limited as no modality has been proven efficacious in salvaging a true PNF.

Algorithm 46.1 Diagnostic criteria for PNF

Clinical features	• Shock/hypotension • Obtundation/failure to awaken from anesthesia • Coagulopathy
Laboratory features	• Prolonged PT • Elevated transaminases (frequently > 1000 U/L) • Acidosis • Elevated LDH, cholestatic enzymes • Hypoglycemia
Imaging features	• Primary purpose of imaging to exclude secondary cause of graft dysfunction • Ultrasonography demonstrating adequate portal and arterial inflow and hepatic venous outflow • Absence of large fluid collections creating abdominal compartment syndrome • Absence of profound right heart failure via echocardiography

- Prevention is the mainstay of therapy, beginning with proper donor selection. Minimizing use of steatotic grafts from older donors and avoiding the use of livers from donors in abject hemodynamic collapse and biochemical evidence of shock liver is likely to minimize, but will not abrogate all cases of PNF. Marginal grafts, however, are commonly used as a desperation maneuver in regions where donor scarcity leads to unacceptable waiting list mortality.
- The use of prostaglandin analogues in early anecdotal reports seemed efficacious for enhancing graft survival in PNF, but a subsequent randomized trial demonstrated no survival benefit, though length-of-stay was reduced in the treatment arm.
- Very rarely the failing allograft induces such a severe systemic response that transplantation hepatectomy and temporary portocaval shunting until a replacement graft is found has been performed.
- Re-transplantation remains the only effective therapy once the diagnosis of PNF has been established. The implementation of UNOS exception criteria for Status 1A listing for patients suffering from PNF obviously has improved patient survival, and likely has had the secondary effect of expanding the potential donor pool. With the safety net of priority re-listing for PNF in place, strict avoidance of older livers and steatotic grafts for transplantation has now been replaced with tempered enthusiasm for these grafts as potential life-saving organs in the face of widespread donor shortage.

CLINICAL PEARLS
- Since true PNF is fatal without re-transplantation, prevention is the mainstay of therapy.
- Avoidance of marginal allografts is not always an option, particularly in regions of the country with high waiting list mortality.

Section 5: Special Populations

Not applicable for this topic.

Algorithm 46.2 Management of PNF

Prevention	• Donor selection • Cold ischemic time minimization
Re-transplantation	• Frequently not a clear decision as graft recovery often possible • In many regions, Status 1 listing does not guarantee organ availability in time for patient salvage • Transplantation hepatectomy and porto-caval shunt
Prostaglandin	• Early anecdotal reports of improvement in graft function • Randomized controlled trial failed to demonstrate improvement in survival

Section 6: Prognosis

BOTTOM LINE/CLINICAL PEARLS
• True PNF is fatal without re-transplantation.

Natural history of untreated disease
• Poor without re-transplantation.

Section 7: Reading List

D'Alessandro AM, Kalayoglu M, Sollinger HW, et al. The predictive value of donor liver biopsies for the development of primary nonfunction after orthotopic liver transplantation. Transplantation 1991;51: 157–63

Emond JC, Renz JF, Ferrell LD, et al. Functional analysis of grafts from living donors. implications for the treatment of older recipients. Ann Surg 1996;224:544–52; discussion 552–4

Fishbein TM, Fiel MI, Emre S, et al. Use of livers with microvesicular fat safely expands the donor pool. Transplantation 1997;64:248–51

Henley KS, Lucey MR, Normolle DP, et al. A double-blind, randomized, placebo-controlled trial of prostaglandin E1 in liver transplantation. Hepatology 1995;21:366–72

Lawal A, Florman S, Fiel MI, Gordon R, Bromberg J, Schiano TD. Identification of ultrastructural changes in liver allografts of patients experiencing primary nonfunction. Transplant Proc 2005;37:4339–42

Mangus RS, Fridell JA, Vianna RM, et al. Severe hypernatremia in deceased liver donors does not impact early transplant outcome. Transplantation 2010;90:438–43

Vertemati M, Sabatella G, Minola E, Gambacorta M, Goffredi M, Vizzotto L. Morphometric analysis of primary graft non-function in liver transplantation. Histopathology 2005;46:451–9

Section 8: Guidelines

Not applicable for this topic.

Section 9: Evidence

Not applicable for this topic.

Section 10: Images

Not applicable for this topic.

Additional material for this chapter can be found online at:
www.mountsinaiexpertguides.com
This includes a case study and multiple choice questions

CHAPTER 47

Ischemia Reperfusion Injury after Liver Transplantation

Matthew Y. Suh and Juan P. Rocca

Recanati/Miller Transplantation Institute, Mount Sinai Hospital, New York, NY, USA

OVERALL BOTTOM LINE
- LT, by necessity, subjects the liver allograft to ischemia followed by reperfusion.
- The pattern and severity of IRI that ensues may be clinically irrelevant in the majority of the cases; however, IRI may cause a spectrum of liver dysfunction resulting in DGF or PNF.
- The clinical consequences of IRI may range from prolonged length of stay, post-operative complications, re-transplantation, and ultimately recipient death.
- Recent research has elucidated many molecular pathways involved in hepatic IRI; however, only a few experimental interventional modalities currently exist.

Section 1: Background
Definition of disease
- IRI is a pathologic state characterized by:
  - Ischemic phase injury resulting in significant reduction of microcirculatory blood flow on reperfusion, perpetuating ischemic injury.
  - Inflammatory response, activated during the ischemic phase (initiated by Kupffer cells), which is amplified during the reperfusion phase.
  - Hepatocyte injury and death occurring via inflammatory response (neutrophil activation, complement activation, T cell-mediated apoptosis), as well as directly via ROS resulting in perturbation of ionic homeostasis, depletion of ATP, mitochondrial permeability and transition.
  - Distant organ dysfunction (cardiovascular, lung, kidney) may occur as a direct consequence of hepatic IRI.
- Therefore, IRI is the pathologic state behind DGF and PNF, regardless of cause.
- However, the terminology of IRI is often used to describe the clinical state of DGF where no obvious etiology (i.e. vascular thrombosis) can be identified – therefore, it is a diagnosis of exclusion!

Disease classification
- Normal graft function after LT is characterized by:
  - Intraoperative restoration of hemostasis.
  - Stabilization of hemodynamics.

Mount Sinai Expert Guides: Hepatology, First Edition. Edited by Jawad Ahmad, Scott L. Friedman, and Henryk Dancygier.
Companion website: www.mountsinaiexpertguides.com

- Rapid resolution of encephalopathy.
- Normalization of INR within 24 hours.
- Decrease in AST and ALT within 24–48 hours (AST before ALT, AST t½ ~18 hours, ALT t½ ~48 hours).
- Delayed decrease in bilirubin within 48–72 hours.
- DGF is a clinical state characterized by:
  - Delayed restoration of hemostasis.
  - Delayed stabilization of hemodynamics – may require transient inotropic support.
  - Delayed resolution of encephalopathy.
  - Delayed normalization of INR.
  - Increase in AST and ALT during the first 24–48 hours, followed by decrease.
- PNF = post-operative fulminant hepatic failure:
  - Complete lack of hemostasis, requiring blood product support.
  - Hemodynamic instability, requiring inotropic support.
  - Unresolving encephalopathy.
  - Multisystem organ failure ensues.
  - Continual rise in LFT, bilirubin and lactic acidosis.
  - Massive graft necrosis.

Incidence/prevalence
- Although IRI is a relatively frequent clinical phenomenon in LT, little is known about the incidence of DGF, probably because it is not reported. The incidence of PNF is about 5%.

Etiology
- LT, by necessity, subjects the liver graft to ischemia followed by reperfusion. The transplant liver graft undergoes three phases of ischemia:
  - Warm ischemia – donor ischemic events (codes, "down time") and in donation after cardiac death, from extubation to aortic cross-clamp.
  - Cold ischemia – during cold preservation, from cross-clamp until off ice.
  - Warm ischemia – during vascular anastomoses, from off ice until reperfusion.
- During cold ischemia, sinusoidal endothelial cells are vulnerable, while hepatocytes are relatively protected. During warm ischemia, all cell types are vulnerable; thus, cold ischemia is better tolerated than warm ischemia.

Pathology/pathogenesis
Perfusion abnormality during reperfusion worsens ischemic injury
- Lack of oxygen results in failure of ATPase, leading to intracellular swelling.
- Increase in vasoconstrictors (endothelin and thromboxane A2) and decrease in vasodilators (nitric oxide).
- Results in sinusoidal narrowing.
- During reperfusion, platelet and neutrophil adhesion and sinusoidal narrowing result in reduction of microcirculatory blood flow leading to some areas without reperfusion ("no-reflow").

Inflammatory activation leads to hepatocyte injury
- Kupffer cells initiate inflammatory cascade during the ischemic phase – releasing pro-inflammatory cytokines (TNF-α and IL-1β) – recruiting CD4+ lymphocytes during reperfusion, which in turn recruit neutrophils via IL-17.

- Natural killer cells and platelets are recruited; sinusoidal endothelial cells and hepatocytes are activated.
- Complement pathways are activated leading to membrane attack complex formation.
- Toll-like receptor 4 are activated on Kupffer cells and dendritic cells by danger-associated molecular patterns, resulting in further release of pro-inflammatory cytokines (TNF-α and IL-1β via MyD88 dependent pathway) and IP-10 (leukocyte chemoattractant via MyD88 independent pathway).

ROS cause direct hepatocyte injury

- Kupffer cells release ROS.
- ROS cause oxidative damage to hepatocyte membrane lipids, enzyme complexes of the respiratory chain and DNA.
- ROS injury causes further release of ROS from nearby hepatocyte mitochondria (known as ROS-induced ROS release), self-propagating mitochondrial damage.
- Ionic homeostasis of hepatocyte Ca^{2+}, Na^+ and H^+ is perturbed.
- Mitochondrial Ca^{2+} overload and ATP depletion result in increased permeability of inner mitochondrial membrane via mitochondrial permeability transition.
- When the majority of mitochondria undergo mitochondrial permeability transition, hepatocyte necrosis ensues.

Predictive/risk factors

Donor factors

- Older donors >60 years. May be explained by decreased expression of protective factors (i.e. Nrf2) in older donors.
- Graft macrovesicular steatosis >30%.
- Other underlying liver disease.
- Donation after cardiac death.

Operative factors

- Poor flushing during procurement.
- Mottled reperfusion: may be intraoperative evidence of "no-reflow."
- Increased cold ischemia time.
- Increased warm ischemia time. Higher risk than cold ischemia.

Recipient factors

- Underlying sepsis.

Section 2: Prevention

> **BOTTOM LINE/CLINICAL PEARLS**
> - No intervention has been shown definitely to prevent ischemia reperfusion injury in LT.
> - Surgical ischemic preconditioning (brief periods of ischemia and reperfusion before prolonged ischemia) has shown conflicting outcomes in clinical trials and is considered experimental.
>
> *(Continued)*

- Pharmacologic preconditioning and treatment during transplantation may be the future. Small clinical trials using nitric oxide during LT and sevofluorane during liver resections have shown promising outcomes.
- Administration of immunosuppressive medications (thymoglobulin to recipient and methylprednisolone to donor) have shown some beneficial effects in small clinical trials. Further trials are necessary to confirm these findings.
- N-acetylcysteine had been in use previously, based on the findings of an initial clinical trial. Since then, several other clinical trials have reported conflicting data. Thus, there is no definitive data that N-acetylcysteine has a demonstrable benefit in preventing IRI.
- Two double-blinded randomized clinical trials using prostaglandin E1 (PGE1, alprostadil) have shown no demonstrable benefit in preventing DGF or PNF. While there was a statistically non-significant decrease in LFTs, there were statistically significant decreases in ICU stay and decreases in renal support. Subsequent studies have shown no benefit in post-transplantation renal function.
- Two amino acids (glycine and taurine) have shown beneficial effect, acting on Kupffer cells in experimental models. Currently, there is a European randomized controlled clinical trial to test the efficacy of glycine in the post-transplantation period.

Section 3: Diagnosis (Algorithm 47.1)

BOTTOM LINE/CLINICAL PEARLS
- The clinical diagnosis of IRI is a diagnosis of exclusion!
- Look out for bleeding, coagulopathy, hemodynamic instability, ARDS, MI, acute renal failure, encephalopathy.
- Laboratory studies show increasing LFTs/INR/lactate, decreasing fibrinogen/platelets and metabolic acidosis which stabilizes.
- Abdominal Doppler US is mandatory as vascular thrombosis must be ruled out.
- Assess for underlying sepsis in the recipient (typically pre-transplantation SBP, cholangitis, pneumonia, etc.).
- When evidence of remote IRI or end organ damage is found, the usual etiology of these states must be ruled out (i.e. pre-existing coronary artery disease, aspiration pneumonia, nephrotoxic medications).
- DGF and PNF are a continuum of IRI. The decision to re-list for transplantation (i.e. PNF) must be made within 12–24 hours!

Differential diagnosis

Differential diagnosis	Features
Post-operative bleeding	Hemodynamic instability, drop in hematocrit, oliguria, blood in drains
Vascular thrombosis	No differences!
	Duplex US or angiogram or CT dual phase
PNF	Progressive worsening clinical examination and laboratory tests without improvement
Sepsis	Assess for recent pre-transplantation infections
MI (often with pre-existing coronary artery disease)	EKG changes and/or hemodynamic instability with improvement in coagulopathy, LFTs
Aspiration pneumonia	ARDS and/or sepsis with improvement in coagulopathy, LFTs
Acute kidney injury	Oliguria/anuria with improvement in coagulopathy, LFTs

Typical presentation
- LT is performed with a mildly fatty graft, from an older donor or with a donation after cardiac death graft. Post-operatively, the recipient requires a moderate amount of vasopressor and ventilatory support but stabilizes and does not worsen. The patient's wounds may ooze from operative and line sites. The clinical examination gradually improves, as do the laboratory test abnormalities.

Clinical diagnosis
History
- Recipient factors are not well understood in IRI. Thus, the recipient's history is mostly irrelevant. However, an understanding of how sick the recipient was pre-transplantation (such as hepatorenal syndrome, hepatopulmonary syndrome, infections) will help understand the trends in changes of physical examination and laboratory tests.
- Donor history of prolonged down time, older age, morbid obesity.
- Operative report of problems during preservation, prolonged cold ischemia time or warm ischemia time.

Physical examination
- Look out for evidence of hepatic insufficiency/hepatic failure.
- Encephalopathy/asterixis (if extubated and mental state examination can be done).
- Hemodynamic instability, cardiac ischemia to MI.
- Ventilatory difficulty, increasing oxygen requirement to ARDS.
- Oliguria to acute renal failure.
- Blood loss and coagulopathy.

Useful clinical decision rules and calculators
- If the clinical examination and laboratory tests were improving initially then worsen – suspect vascular thrombosis and all other possible etiologies, except IRI.
- If the clinical examination does not stabilize within the first 24 hours but worsens, strongly consider PNF and relisting for transplantation.
- In the modern era of immunosuppression, immediate post-operative rejection is exceptionally rare, especially in LT, and therefore is not listed among the differential diagnoses.

Laboratory diagnosis
List of diagnostic tests
- LFTs showing increasing AST/ALT/LDH.
- PT/PTT showing increasing PT/PTT/INR.
- CBC and fibrinogen showing decreasing fibrinogen/platelets/hematocrit.
- Arterial blood gas showing metabolic acidosis (increasing lactic acidosis).
- Creatinine kinase MB(CKMB)/troponin (with EKG) if hemodynamically unstable.

List of imaging techniques
- Duplex US of liver.
- Angiogram or dual phase CT scan if Duplex equivocal, or surgical re-exploration.

Potential pitfalls/common errors made regarding diagnosis of disease
- Start the diagnostic investigations early and work quickly.
- If you are not the transplantation surgeon, alert the surgeon ASAP.

Algorithm 47.1 Diagnosis of IRI

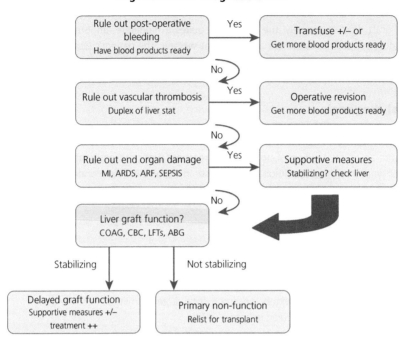

Section 4: Treatment
Treatment rationale
- Supportive therapy is the mainstay of treatment.
- While some clinicians have used N-acetylcysteine in attempts to treat IRI, all clinical trials involving N-acetylcysteine have been in efforts to prevent IRI, not to treat it, even those trials reported conflicting outcomes. Thus, there is no data to support the use of N-acetylcysteine in treatment of IRI.
- Randomized clinical trials looking at prostaglandin E1 (alprostadil) have been in an effort to prevent IRI. A few single center studies looking at the use of PGE1 as treatment of IRI did not show conclusive evidence of benefit. Contradictory data exist as to the benefit in post-transplantation renal function.

Managing the hospitalized patient
- Maintain hemodynamic stability!
- Judicious use of vasopressors and volume is necessary. Maintain euvolemia. Volume overload is dangerous for the liver graft, leading to congestion, and may lead to respiratory difficulty, especially in the setting of acute renal failure. Consider appropriate intervention (Swan–Ganz, pulse contour continuous cardiac output) to measure cardiovascular function (CVP, cardiac output, cardiac index, pulmonary artery wedge pressure, systemic vascular resistance, etc).
- Minimize barotrauma if ARDS (keep tidal volume to 4–6 cm^3/kg).
- Renal replacement therapy (usually continuous veno-venous hemodialysis) is strongly encouraged for acid-base disorder management and volume management.
- Frequent monitoring of laboratory parameters.
- In general, maintain INR <3, hematocrit >21%, platelets >20 × 10^3/μL. Discuss transfusion goal with the transplantation surgery team!

Prevention/management of complications

- Maintaining hemodynamic stability is critical to preventing complications. Further ischemia during recovery of IRI may lengthen the duration of and exacerbate the injury to the liver.
- Infectious complications (such as ventilator-associated pneumonia, catheter-related sepsis, urosepsis) are common with immunosuppression. Rarer are donor-derived infections, which are transmitted via the transplanted organ or perfusate.
- Biliary complications may result after prolonged IRI, and are particularly sensitive to hemodynamic instability (as biliary structures derive all their flows from hepatic arterial flow).

CLINICAL PEARLS
- Supportive therapy is the mainstay of treatment.
- Maintain hemodynamic stability – avoid volume overload!
- Renal replacement therapy is strongly encouraged.
- Transfuse to INR <3, hematocrit >21%, platelets >20 × 10^3/μL.

Section 5: Special Populations
Children
- Children receive priority in allocation of liver allografts in the USA. Therefore, graft selection among the best donors available makes IRI less likely. With an increased risk of vascular thrombosis in a pediatric recipient, other etiologies must be ruled out first.

Section 6: Prognosis

BOTTOM LINE/CLINICAL PEARLS
- If supported properly, DGF patients should recover normal hepatic function. Currently, there is no way to predict which patients will recover (DGF) and those that will not (PNF).
- The risk of infectious complications and biliary complications may be increased.

Section 7: Reading List

Abu-Amara M, Yang SY, Tapuria N, Fuller B, Davidson B, Seifalian A. Liver ischemia/reperfusion injury: processes in inflammatory networks – a review. Liver Transpl 2010;16:1016–32

Alchera E, Dal Ponte C, Imarisio C, Albano E, Carini R. Molecular mechanisms of liver preconditioning. World J Gastroenterol 2010;16;6058–67

Bogetti D, Sankary HN, Jarzembowski TM, et al. Thymoglobulin induction protects liver allografts from ischemia/reperfusion injury. Clin Transplant 2005;19:507–11

de Rougemont O, Lehmann K, Clavien PA. Preconditioning, organ preservation, and postconditioning to prevent ischemia-reperfusion injury to the liver. Liver Transpl 2009;15:1172–82

Henley KS, Lucey MR, Normolle DP, et al. A double-blind, randomized, placebo-controlled trial of prostaglandin E1 in liver transplantation. Hepatology 1995;21:366–72

Hoffmann K Buchler MW, Schemmer P. Supplementation of amino acids to prevent reperfusion injury after liver surgery and transplantation – where do we stand today? Clin Nutr 2010;30: 143–7

Klein AS, Cofer JB, Pruett TL, et al. Prostaglandin E1 administration following orthotopic liver transplantation: a randomized prospective multicenter trial. Gastroenterology 1996;111: 710–15

Kotsch K, Ulrich F, Reutzel-Selke A, et al. Methylprednisolone therapy in deceased donors reduces inflammation in the donor liver and improves outcome after liver transplantation: a prospective randomized controlled trial. Ann Surg 2008;248:1042–50

Lang JDJ, Teng X, Chumley P, et al. Inhaled NO accelerates restoration of liver function in adults following orthotopic liver transplantation. J Clin Invest 2007;117:2583–91

Section 8: Guidelines

Not applicable for this topic.

Section 9: Evidence

Not applicable for this topic.

Section 10: Images

Not applicable for this topic.

Additional material for this chapter can be found online at:
www.mountsinaiexpertguides.com
This includes a case study and multiple choice questions

CHAPTER 48

Vascular Complications of Liver Transplantation

Eric G. Davis[1] and Sander S. Florman[2]
[1]University of Louisville School of Medicine, Louisville, KY, USA
[2]Recanati/Miller Transplantation Institute, Mount Sinai Hospital, New York, NY, USA

OVERALL BOTTOM LINE
- A unique feature of the liver is its dual blood supply via the hepatic artery and portal vein.
- LT requires a minimum of three, and very frequently four, vascular anastomoses to establish inflow and outflow to the allograft.
- Bleeding complications of these anastomoses are readily identified in the operating room, leaving anastomotic stenosis and thrombosis as the leading vascular complications encountered post-operatively.
- Surgical and radiologic approaches play complementary roles in the diagnosis and management of these potentially catastrophic complications and early recognition is key to graft and patient survival.
- Vascular complications following LT generally fall into three categories: hepatic venous, portal venous or arterial complications.

HEPATIC VENOUS OCCLUSION

Section 1: Background

- Hepatic venous outflow is established via one of two methods depending, in part, on surgeon preference as well as graft type.
- Partial grafts from split livers or living donors, by definition, generally do not include the inferior vena cava and direct anastomosis of the donor hepatic vein(s) to the recipient vena cava is necessary. This "piggyback" method is generally technically more demanding with smaller anastomoses and likely accounts for the increased incidence of outflow obstruction in these patients.
- Although some centers perform piggyback reconstruction for all allografts, partial and whole, a more common approach is the caval-replacement method in which the donor vena cava is anastomosed directly to the suprahepatic and infrahepatic vena cavae that remain after recipient hepatectomy.

Mount Sinai Expert Guides: Hepatology, First Edition. Edited by Jawad Ahmad, Scott L. Friedman, and Henryk Dancygier.
© 2014 John Wiley & Sons, Ltd. Published 2014 by John Wiley & Sons, Ltd.
Companion website: www.mountsinaiexpertguides.com

Incidence/prevalence
- The incidence of stenosis of the hepatic vein–caval anastomosis varies from 1 to 6%. This can be due to rotation of the liver graft or true stricture of the anastomosis.

Etiology
- Anastomotic technical error.
- Progressive neointimal hyperplasia.
- Allograft positioning error with torsion or compression of anastomosis.
- A side-to-side cavo-cavoplasty reduces the risk of stenosis.
- Hepatic venous outflow obstruction is more common with the piggyback technique.

Predictive/risk factors
- Partial-liver allografts with piggyback anastomotic technique.
- Budd–Chiari or non-cirrhotic extrahepatic portal vein thrombosis as an indication for OLT.
- Hypercoagulable states.

Section 2: Prevention

Not applicable for this topic.

Section 3: Diagnosis (Algorithm 48.1)
Typical presentation
- Hepatic venous thrombosis threatens graft and patient survival due to early parenchymal dysfunction, necrosis and eventual cirrhotic transformation.
- Very early events are usually technical in nature and require re-operation to prevent immediate graft loss.
- With the exception of late, asymptomatic thromboses, all other hepatic venous stenoses and thromboses should undergo invasive imaging by interventional radiology with the intent to perform angioplasty and stenting.
- The technical success rates as measured by minimization of pressure gradients are extremely high, as evidenced by a report of 13 consecutive balloon angioplasties with stent placements. Technical success was achieved in all 13, with clinical success in all but one patient but who subsequently was found to have diffuse, severe hepatic necrosis and underwent re-transplantation.
- Concomitant azotemia and lower extremity edema often indicate at least partial IVC involvement in post-transplantation hepatic venous occlusion. Very frequently these symptoms are due not to inherent IVC stenosis at the anastomotic site, but to compression of the IVC by the distended, enlarged liver. It is for this reason that a period of observation, after balloon angioplasty and stenting of the hepatic venous stenosis to allow time for allograft distention and symptoms of IVC compression to resolve, seems appropriate.

Clinical features
- Hepatomegaly.
- New-onset ascites.

- Abdominal pain.
- Budd–Chiari syndrome.
- Lower extremity edema (with concomitant IVC occlusion or stenosis).
- Renal insufficiency.

Laboratory features
- Elevated transaminases.
- Hypoalbuminemia.
- Prolonged PTT.
- Azotemia (with IVC involvement).

Imaging features
- US always initial diagnostic test to screen for surrogate markers of outflow occlusion:
  - Hepatomegaly.
  - Ascites.
  - Dilated hepatic veins with monophasic flow and loss of cardiac pulsatility.
  - Reversal of normal portal hepatofugal flow, becoming hepatopedal in extreme cases.
- Contrasted CT and MRI:
  - Well-timed studies show excellent detail of hepatic vein/IVC junction.
  - Helps to exclude concomitant portal vein stenosis or occlusion.
- Invasive venography:
  - Imaging offers advantage of direct measurement of pressure gradients across the stenosis from intrahepatic veins to IVC and right atrium.

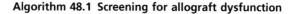

Algorithm 48.1 Screening for allograft dysfunction

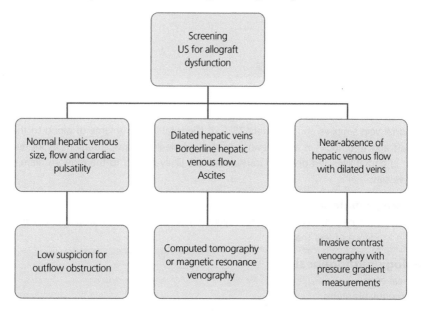

Section 4: Treatment (Algorithm 48.2)

Algorithm 48.2 Management of hepatic venous thrombosis

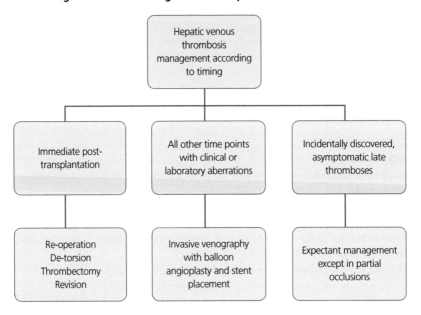

Section 5 Special Populations

Not applicable for this topic.

Section 6 Prognosis

Not applicable for this topic.

PORTAL VEIN THROMBOSIS

Section 1: Background

- The portal vein supplies approximately 75% of the total inflow volume of blood to the liver allograft and thrombosis is a rare event in adult whole-liver transplantation. Its incidence is higher in partial liver and pediatric transplantation, likely related to the reduced diameter of these vessels.

Incidence/prevalence
- Portal vein stricture or thrombosis is a rare event after orthotopic liver transplantation in adults, with an incidence of less than 2%.

Pathology/pathogenesis
- Technical error.
- Hypercoagulable states.
- Inadequate inflow (large pre-existing portosystemic collaterals).

Predictive/risk factors
- Partial liver and pediatric transplantation.
- Pre-existing portal vein thrombus.
- Need for portal venous grafting at time of transplantation.

Section 2: Prevention

Not applicable for this topic.

Section 3: Diagnosis
Typical presentation
- Immediate post-operative portal vein thrombosis usually presents as liver failure with GI bleeding and should be managed with immediate exploration and attempts at thrombectomy and anastomotic revision.
- Portal vein thrombosis discovered at later time periods should undergo invasive transhepatic venography initially with attempts at recanalization via some combination of thrombolytics and balloon angioplasty, except in cases in which long-standing thrombosis has already resulted in cavernous transformation and liver function is normal.
- The same is true for portal vein stenosis without frank thrombosis. Similar to the application of interventional radiologic techniques in outflow occlusions, a series of ten patients with portal vein stenosis managed with percutaneous balloon angioplasty and stenting demonstrated excellent technical results, with resolution of all pressure gradients and continued patency at 10 months.
- An analysis of 84 patients with post-OLT portal vein thrombosis demonstrated a far more deleterious effect on graft and patient survival following portal vein thrombosis than in patients with HAT.

Clinical features
- Gastrointestinal bleeding.
- Encephalopathy.
- Ascites.
- Abdominal pain.

Laboratory features
- Elevated transaminases.
- Thrombocytopenia.

Imaging features
- US:
  - Reduced or absent portal flow.
  - Post-stenotic dilation in near-occlusive stenoses.
- Contrasted CT or MRI:
  - Absence of flow.
  - Arterioportal shunting.

Section 4: Treatment (Algorithm 48.3)

Algorithm 48.3 Management of portal vein thrombosis

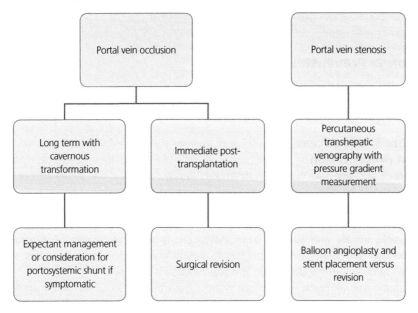

Section 5: Special Populations

Not applicable for this topic.

Section 6: Prognosis

Not applicable for this topic.

HEPATIC ARTERY THROMBOSIS

Section 1: Background

* By far the most common vascular complication of LT, the presence of HAT is routinely sought in the post-operative period in all LT patients via duplex US. Most commonly, the anastomosis is constructed between the donor common hepatic artery and the recipient common hepatic artery, with multiple variations employed for partial allografts and in the pediatric transplantation population.
* Unlike portal and hepatic venous thrombosis, early HAT is frequently clinically quiescent and must be aggressively pursued to maximize graft and patient survival.

Incidence/prevalence
* The incidence of HAT is 3–4% after OLT in adults.

Pathology/pathogenesis
- Technical error.
- Hypercoagulable state.
- Prior intimal damage (transarterial chemoembolization).

Predictive/risk factors
- Pediatric transplantation.
- Complex arterial reconstruction.
- Small-for-size syndrome with excessive, competitive, portal inflow.

Section 2: Prevention

Not applicable for this topic.

Section 3: Diagnosis
Typical presentation
- Most centers employ routine screening for HAT via duplex US after OLT with subsequent studies performed for biliary sepsis or aberrations in transaminases.
- Prevention of HAT via pharmacological means is commonly practiced but likely ineffective. Aspirin usage was studied retrospectively in 529 patients and found to be safe from a bleeding perspective but ineffective in preventing HAT. Many centers utilize post-operative intravenous heparin infusions for patients with known hypercoagulable disorders and in pediatric transplantation, balancing the inherent risk of post-operative hemorrhage.
- Patients with HAT should also be considered for a hypercoagulable evaluation in anticipation of re-transplantation. Hepatic artery stenosis without frank thrombosis discovered via US outside of the immediate post-operative period should be treated much like other vascular complications via angiography. Balloon angioplasty and stenting of these lesions before thrombosis occurs is efficacious, resulting in lower rates of HAT.
- An aggressive approach to HAT including early revascularization and/or re-transplantation in 210 cases in a single-center experience demonstrated no statistically-significant decrease in patient survival. The Mount Sinai experience would suggest that attempts at revascularization for early HAT in asymptomatic patients and reserving primary re-transplantation for symptomatic patients confers the optimum balance of patient survival and resource utilization.
- Late HAT is rarely amenable to surgical intervention. Because the biliary tree is largely dependent upon arterial blood supply, patients with late HAT often present with biliary complications that will not improve with revascularization.

Clinical features
- Frequently no clinical change early after thrombosis.
- Biliary sepsis.

Laboratory features
- Elevated transaminases, subtle or fulminant liver necrosis.
- Prolonged PTT.
- Cholestasis.

Imaging features
- US:
  - Poor or absent arterial waveforms in intrahepatic arteries.
  - Low resistive index (RI): RI = (peak systolic velocity − end diastolic velocity)/peak systolic velocity.
- Contrasted CT and conventional angiography:
  - Absence of intrahepatic arterial contrast.

Section 4: Treatment (Algorithm 48.4)

Algorithm 48.4 Management of hepatic artery thrombosis

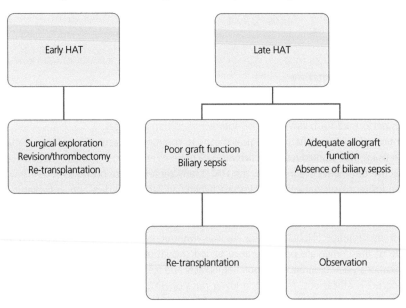

Section 5: Special Populations

Not applicable for this topic.

Section 6: Prognosis

Not applicable for this topic.

Hepatic artery pseudoaneurysms
- An additional complication of the OLT hepatic artery anastomosis with a fortunately infrequent incidence is pseudoaneurysm formation. The vast majority of pseudoaneurysms following OLT are mycotic in nature, with bacteria as well as fungi successfully isolated in the majority of patients.

- Presentation can vary from mild to severe sepsis as well as via massive GI bleeding without overt signs of systemic infection. The majority present within the first 2 months following OLT, and urgent excision and revascularization along with appropriate antimicrobials are the mainstays of therapy. Mortality was 50% in a series of patients who universally underwent aggressive operative therapy, emphasizing the hemorrhagic and septic risks that hepatic artery pseudoaneurysms pose following OLT.
- A role for coil embolization and covered-stent placement by interventional radiology likely exists for bland pseudoaneurysms.

Section 7: Reading List

Duffy JP, Hong JC, Farmer DG, et al. Vascular complications of orthotopic liver transplantation: experience in more than 4200 patients. J Am Coll Surg 2009;208:896–903;discussion 903–5

Leelaudomlipi S, Bramhall SR, Gunson BK, et al. Hepatic-artery aneurysm in adult liver transplantation. Transpl Int 2003;16:257–61

Saad WE, Davies MG, Sahler L, et al. Hepatic artery stenosis in liver transplant recipients: primary treatment with percutaneous transluminal angioplasty. J Vasc Interv Radiol 2005;16:795–805

Sheiner PA, Varma CV, Guarrera JV, et al. Selective revascularization of hepatic artery thromboses after liver transplantation improves patient and graft survival. Transplantation 1997;64:1295–9

Wang SL, Sze DY, Busque S, et al. Treatment of hepatic venous outflow obstruction after piggyback liver transplantation. Radiology 2005;236:352–9

Wang JF, Zhai RY, Wei BJ, et al. Percutaneous intravascular stents for treatment of portal venous stenosis after liver transplantation: midterm results. Transplant Proc 2006;38:1461–2

Wolf DC, Freni MA, Boccagni PM. et al. Low-dose aspirin therapy is associated with few side effects but does not prevent HAT in liver transplant recipients. Liver Transpl Surg 1997;3:598–603

Section 8: Guidelines

Not applicable for this topic.

Section 9: Evidence

Not applicable for this topic.

Section 10: Images

Not applicable for this topic.

Additional material for this chapter can be found online at:
www.mountsinaiexpertguides.com
This includes a case study and multiple choice questions

CHAPTER 49

Biliary Complications after Liver Transplantation

Marie E. Le and Marcelo E. Facciuto

Recanati/Miller Transplantation Institute, Mount Sinai Hospital, New York, NY, USA

OVERALL BOTTOM LINE
- Improvements in organ selection, procurement and preservation have dramatically reduced the incidence of biliary complications after LT.
- Despite standardization of surgical methods in biliary reconstruction, immunosuppression, and post-operative management, biliary complications continue to be a major cause of morbidity and mortality after LT.
- Early and aggressive evaluation of transplant recipients with a suspicion of biliary complication is paramount due to the potential for graft and patient injury.
- Biliary complications include biliary strictures, bile leaks, biliary stones/debris, sphincter of Oddi dysfunction, mucoceles and hemobilia.
- The combination of endoscopic and percutaneous therapy has minimized the need for post-transplant biliary surgery to address complications.

Section 1: Background
Definition of disease
- Two types of biliary reconstruction can typically be performed during a LT: choledocho-choledochostomy (duct-to-duct anastomosis) or choledochojejunostomy (duct-to-bowel anastomosis).
- Instances in which there is pre-existing biliary disease (i.e. PSC), prior biliary surgery, or donor-recipient duct size mismatch, a duct-to-bowel anastomosis is favored.
- Both types of biliary reconstruction can be complicated by strictures, bile leak, obstruction from biliary stones and debris.
- Less common biliary complications include sphincter of Oddi dysfunction, mucoceles and hemobilia.

Disease classification
- Biliary complications can be classified by a post-transplant timeline.
- Early complications consist of those occurring less than 30 days post-transplant and often reflect problems of handling and harvesting the graft, preservation injuries and any unappreciated underlying graft disease.

Mount Sinai Expert Guides: Hepatology, First Edition. Edited by Jawad Ahmad, Scott L. Friedman, and Henryk Dancygier.
© 2014 John Wiley & Sons, Ltd. Published 2014 by John Wiley & Sons, Ltd.
Companion website: www.mountsinaiexpertguides.com

- The most common early biliary complication is a bile leak which is usually attributed to technical failure or vascular insufficiency.
- Late complications consist of those occurring more than 90 days post-transplant.
- Of these complications, biliary strictures are the most prevalent and tend to occur 5–8 months post-transplant.
- The investigation of a patient with suspected biliary complications in the late period requires imaging of the hepatic arterial system and may require a liver biopsy to exclude any rejection or recurrence of disease.

Incidence/prevalence

- Biliary complications after LT are a major source of morbidity with an overall incidence of 5–32%.
- Biliary strictures comprise almost 40% of all biliary complications after LT with an incidence of 5–15% after deceased donor LT but as high as 28–32% after living donor LT.
- Bile leaks are the second most common biliary complication after transplant with an incident of 2–25%.
- Filling defects in the form of biliary stones, debris, and casts comprise 3–12% of biliary complications post-transplant.
- Sphincter of Oddi dysfunction comprises 2–3% of all biliary complications.

Economic impact

- Exact figures are not available but biliary complications have a major impact on the quality of life for a LT recipient – requiring frequent hospital readmissions, repeated imaging and invasive procedures.
- Repeat admissions and imaging, along with occasional re-operation, add to the significant monetary cost of LT and to the emotional toll these patients suffer.

Etiology

- Non-anastomotic stricture:
  - Macroangiopathic – hepatic artery stenosis.
  - Microangiopathic – prolonged cold and warm ischemia times, donation after cardiac death, prolonged use of vasopressors in the donor.
  - Immunogenic (usually presenting later than 1 year post-transplant) – chronic rejection, ABO incompatibility, PSC, AIH.
  - Infection – opportunistic, recurrent hepatitis B or C.
- Anastomotic stricture:
  - Scar formation (fibrosis).
  - Local ischemia.
  - Technical issues.
  - Small caliber of the bile ducts.
  - Mismatch in duct size between donor and recipient.
  - Bile leak in the post-operative period.
- Bile leaks:
  - T-tube biliary reconstruction.
  - Roux-en-Y anastomosis.
  - Reperfusion injury.
  - Hepatic artery thrombosis.
  - Cytomegalovirus infection.

- Inappropriate suture material.
- Tension at the anastomosis.
- Excessive use of electrocauterization for control of bleeding.
- Biliary stones/casts:
  - Sloughed biliary epithelium (due to prolonged cold storage time).
  - Chronic rejection.
  - Infection.
  - Bile stasis.
- Sphincter of Oddi dysfunction:
  - Stenosis – scarring and inflammation, i.e. passage of gallstone through papilla, intraoperative manipulation of the common bile duct.
  - Dyskinesia – secondary to functional disturbance of the sphincter leading to intermittent biliary blockage.
- Use of donation after cardiac death organs, split livers and living donor LTs are efforts to increase the donor pool. However, transplants using these organs are associated with a significant risk of biliary complications due to smaller duct sizes, more complex peripheral anastomosis, and ischemic injury that occurs prior to organ retrieval.

Section 2: Prevention

- In addition to careful donor selection, preservation and retrieval, careful dissection of the hilar area is paramount to guarantee adequate blood supply to the donor duct.
- Likewise, in living donor LTs, preservation of an adequately vascularized right duct is vital.
- As more centers are standardizing biliary reconstruction during LTs, surgeons are favoring duct-to-duct anastomosis when possible.
- A choledocho-choledochostomy allows preservation of the sphincter of Oddi, decreased operative time, less frequent bacterial colonization of the biliary tract and endoscopic access to the biliary tree.
- These factors will lower the frequency of bile leaks and hence biliary strictures.

Screening
- A high index of suspicion should always be maintained for biliary complications in the post-LT patient as the life of the graft and patient are at stake.
- Because of immunosuppression and hepatic denervation, the clinical picture can vary widely.
- The time frame for concern is also broad as bile leaks can occur in the immediate postoperative period and biliary strictures can occur weeks to years after transplant.

Section 3: Diagnosis

- Presentation of biliary complications in the LT patient can vary from asymptomatic with mild elevations in LFTs to a full blown cholangitic picture.
- Patients who do manifest symptoms will often complain of fever, abdominal pain and anorexia.
- The physical examination in a patient with biliary complications can include RUQ pain, jaundice, scleral icterus and pruritus. Sustained output from drain sites is a red flag for biliary problems.

- An elevation in serum aminotransferases, serum AP, serum bilirubin and/or GGT is usually evident.
- Once a biliary complication is suspected, the biliary tree and hepatic vasculature should be evaluated with a Doppler abdominal US. The biliary system can then be further studied with MRCP, ERCP or PTC.

Typical presentation

- The clinical picture for biliary problems in a transplant patient is variable without a typical presentation. Symptomatic patients will present with fever, RUQ pain, jaundice and significant elevations in liver enzymes and bilirubin.

Clinical diagnosis

History

- Abdominal pain (particularly RUQ), change in color of urine (dark) and stools (pale), fevers at home and itching should raise the suspicion for a biliary issue after transplant.

Physical examination

- Fever and tachycardia may be early signs of abdominal sepsis from a bile leak or cholangitis from a biliary obstruction or stricture.
- On abdominal examination, abdominal fullness or substantial, sustained drainage from the incision or drain sites is an obvious sign for concern. Of course, careful determination of jaundice and scleral icterus is helpful.

Laboratory diagnosis

List of diagnostic tests

- Liver function panel – when suspicious of biliary complications, but also routine monitoring during post-operative care (AST, ALT, AP, total bilirubin, GGT).
- Liver biopsy – for late occurring biliary complications to exclude rejection and disease recurrence.

List of imaging techniques

- Doppler US – initial test to evaluate biliary system and hepatic vasculature.
- Hepatic angiogram – when hepatic artery thrombosis or stenosis is suspected.
- MRCP – when suspect biliary obstruction or leak for biliary anatomy.
- ERCP – for biliary anatomy and potential therapeutic intervention in duct-to-duct reconstruction with stenting.
- PTC – for biliary anatomy and potential therapeutic intervention in duct-to-bowel reconstruction and in duct-to-duct reconstruction when ERCP intervention fails.
- HIDA scan – if liver function permits, can be useful as a dynamic study to confirm a biliary leak or stenosis of a biliary–enteric anastomosis.

Potential pitfalls/common errors made regarding diagnosis of disease

- Non-invasive imaging should be the first-line diagnostic test.
- Pulsatile compression of the common bile duct by the hepatic artery can cause a pseudo-obstruction of the bile duct.
- When the cystic duct is parallel to the common bile duct anatomically, the imaging can be mistaken for a dilated common bile duct.

Section 4: Treatment (Algorithm 49.1)
Treatment rationale
- A CT angiogram ideally should be performed to make sure all hepatic vasculature is patent.
- With increasing advancements in endoscopic technique and instrumentation, the primary management of biliary complications has transitioned from predominantly surgical to primarily endoscopic. First line management of biliary strictures and leaks in the LT patient is endoscopic intervention. Identification of a stricture is followed by balloon dilation over a guidewire followed by stent placement, the size depending on the size of the ducts, degree of stricturing and time since transplant. Balloon dilatation alone without stent placement is only successful in approximately 40% of cases. The combination of balloon dilatation and stent placement has a more durable outcome in 75% of patients. When multiple side-by-side stents are placed, the success rate is increased to 80–90%. Patients commit themselves to ongoing ERCP sessions every few months for further dilatation and repeated stent exchange for up to 1–2 years depending on response. Stents must be exchanged to avoid bacterial cholangitis and occlusions from casts and debris.
- Bile leaks are similarly addressed with endoscopic intervention where localization of the leak (cystic duct remnant through inadequate ligation or distal obstruction, T-tube site or tract, surgical anastomosis, cut edge of liver) typically allows treatment with sphincterotomy and stent placement. Any intra-abdominal collections formed by a bile leak should also be drained to prevent secondary infections and late association with adhesions. Multiple biliary anastomoses and peripheral reconstructions limit the efficacy of endoscopic intervention.
- When endoscopy fails, percutaneous modalities are the next option. Percutaneous intervention is considered second line treatment because of its invasive nature and significant morbidity. However, in cases of duct-to-bowel reconstruction, management of biliary complications with PTC is first line and achieves success rates of 50–70%.
- Surgical revision is the next line of intervention when endoscopic and percutaneous transhepatic measures fail. When all else fails, re-transplant is the final option.

When to hospitalize
- Any patient showing signs of intra-abdominal sepsis from a bile leak or cholangitis (secondary to biliary stricture or obstruction) needs to be hospitalized for optimal care and monitoring:
  - Fever.
  - Hypotension.
  - Tachycardia.
- Any patient with intractable pain from biliary complications needs to be admitted for adequate pain control and further investigation.
- Any patient in whom the suspicion for biliary complications is high needs to be referred to a hospital for immediate diagnosis and treatment as graft loss and patient morbidity is high:
  - Jaundice.
  - RUQ pain.
  - Elevated enzymes.

Managing the hospitalized patient
- Standard management should include IV fluids, analgesia and antibiotics.
- The management algorithm will depend on the type of biliary complication as in Section 1: "Etiology." Strictures and leaks should be treated with endoscopic or percutaneous therapy as appropriate and any abdominal collections should be drained.

Prevention/management of complications

* Endoscopic intervention of biliary strictures can be complicated by accumulation of biliary sludge and casts causing rapid stent occlusion which puts the patient at risk of cholangitis. Management consists of stent exchange.
* Percutaneous therapy is associated with hemorrhage and bile leaks both of which can be managed surgically if necessary.

Algorithm 49.1 Management/treatment of biliary leak or stricture

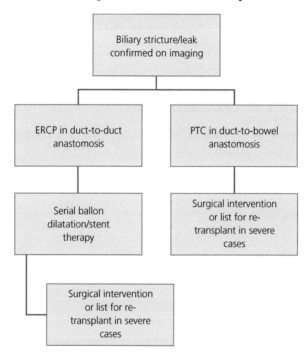

CLINICAL PEARLS
* First – endoscopy; second – percutaneous; third – surgery; last – re-transplant.
* Major drawbacks of endoscopic dilation with stent placement are the need for multiple procedures repeated over extended periods of time and the risk of cholangitis.
* Early bile leaks should be dealt with surgically.

Section 5: Special Populations

Not applicable for this topic.

Section 6: Prognosis

BOTTOM LINE/CLINICAL PEARLS
* Patients can expect lifelong surveillance with pertinent laboratory tests and imaging since biliary strictures, which comprise 40% of all biliary complications, can recur.

Section 7: Reading List

Ayoub WS, Esquivel CO, Martin P, et al. Biliary complications following liver transplantation. Dig Dis Sci 2010;55:1540–6

Buck DG, Zajko AB. Biliary complication after othotopic liver transplantation. Tech Vasc Interventional Rad 2008;11:51–9

Duailibi DF, Ribeiro MA Jr. Biliary complications following deceased and living donor liver transplantation: a review. Transpl Proc 2010;42:517–20

Katz LH, Benjaminov O, Belinki A, et al. Magnetic resonance cholangiopancreatography for the accurate diagnosis of biliary complications after liver transplantation: comparison with endoscopic retrograde cholangiography and percutaneous transhepatic cholangiography- long-term follow-up. Clin Transplant 2010:24:E163–E169

Ostroff, JW. Management of biliary complications in the liver transplant patient. Gastroenterol Hepatol 2010;6:264–72

Porrett PM, Hsu J, Shaked A. Late surgical complications following liver transplantation. Liver Transpl 2009;15(suppl 2): s12–s18

Williams ED, Draganov PV. Endoscopic management of biliary strictures after liver transplantation. World J Gastroenterol 2009;15:3725–33

Yuan Y, Gotoh M. Biliary complications in living liver donors. Surg Today 2010;40:411–7

Section 8: Guidelines

Not applicable for this topic.

Section 9: Evidence

Not applicable for this topic.

Section 10: Images

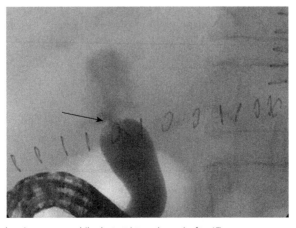

Figure 49.1 ERCP showing common bile duct stricture (arrow) after LT

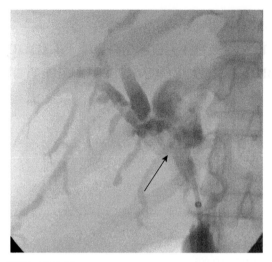

Figure 49.2 Bile duct strictures (arrow)

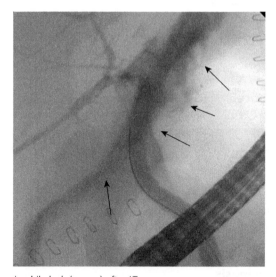

Figure 49.3 ERCP showing bile leak (arrows) after LT

Additional material for this chapter can be found online at:
www.mountsinaiexpertguides.com
This includes a case study and multiple choice questions

Approach to Prophylaxis and Management of Infections after Liver Transplantation

Shirish Huprikar

Division of Infectious Diseases, Department of Medicine, Icahn School of Medicine at Mount Sinai, New York, NY, USA

OVERALL BOTTOM LINE
- The prevention of bacterial, fungal and viral infections after LT is essential to successful outcomes.
- Early recognition of infection is essential for implementing the appropriate treatment strategy and improving outcomes.
- Early consultation with a transplantation infectious diseases specialist is recommended.

Section 1: Background
Disease classification
- Infections in the LT recipient can be classified by community vs hospital acquisition; newly acquired vs reactivation of latent infection; or the type of pathogen (e.g. bacteria, fungi, virus, etc.).

Incidence/prevalence
- Incidence and prevalence of infectious complications can vary depending on type of donor (deceased vs living); type of immunosuppression; local and regional epidemiologic factors; and other donor factors. Bacterial infections are the most frequent infectious complication.

Etiology
- Hospital-acquired.
- Community-acquired.
- Reactivation of latent viral, fungal and mycobacterial pathogens.
- Donor-derived.

Pathology/pathogenesis
- In the first month after transplantation, the pathogenesis of infectious complications is similar to other post-surgical patients and is predominantly healthcare-associated infections. From approximately 1–6 months following transplantation, immunosuppression is most intense and during this period, opportunistic infections in the setting of weak cell-mediated immunity can

Mount Sinai Expert Guides: Hepatology, First Edition. Edited by Jawad Ahmad, Scott L. Friedman, and Henryk Dancygier.
© 2014 John Wiley & Sons, Ltd. Published 2014 by John Wiley & Sons, Ltd.
Companion website: www.mountsinaiexpertguides.com

occur. Following this period, infectious complications are significantly reduced and are similar to community-acquired infections in the general population.

Predictive/risk factors

Type of infection	Risk factors
Bacterial	• Surgical complications • Prolonged intensive care unit stay • Prolonged hospitalization • Treatment of rejection • CMV disease
Fungal	• Fulminant hepatic failure • Re-transplantation • Renal replacement therapy • Treatment of rejection • CMV disease
CMV	• Donor-recipient serostatus mismatch • Rejection

Section 2: Prevention

> **BOTTOM LINE/CLINICAL PEARLS**
> • Prophylaxis strategies to prevent bacterial, fungal and viral infections after LT are considered standard of care.
> • Although studies to support peri-operative antibacterial prophylaxis are lacking, it is widely accepted as standard practice in LT.
> • Clinical studies support strategies to prevent CMV disease in LT recipients.
> • Clinical studies support targeted antifungal prophylaxis in high-risk LT recipients.

Screening
• Blood tests to identify patients at risk for infections are routinely performed in LT candidates:
  • CMV IgG.
  • EBV IgG.
  • Varicella IgG.
  • HIV-1/2 ELISA.
  • Hepatitis A IgG.
  • HBsAg.
  • Antibody to HBsAg (anti-HBs).
  • Anti-HBc.
  • Antibody to hepatitis C.
  • Rapid plasma reagin.
  • *Strongyloides stercoralis* IgG (for patients from endemic regions only).

Primary and secondary prevention

- The following vaccines are recommended for any susceptible LT candidate as early as possible prior to transplantation. It should be noted that vaccine response is poor in patients with advanced liver disease:
  - Influenza (and annually thereafter).
  - Pneumococcal polysaccharide vaccine.
  - Hepatitis A.
  - Hepatitis B.
  - Varicella (should not be administered after transplantation).
  - Tetanus.
  - Polio (inactivated).
- Bacterial prophylaxis is provided to all patients peri-operatively for 24 hours. Ampicillin/ sulbactam is acceptable in most cases. A modified regimen should be considered in the setting of penicillin allergy or colonization with resistant pathogens.
- Viral prophylaxis is provided to all patients for approximately 3 months to prevent CMV and other herpes viruses. Oral valganciclovir is given if the donor or recipient is CMV seropositive. Oral valacyclovir is given if the donor and recipient are seronegative.
- Antifungal prophylaxis is recommended in high-risk situations such as re-transplantation, fulminant hepatic failure and renal failure. Fluconazole is generally used at least until the patient is clinically stable for up to 3 months after transplantation.
- *Pneumocystis jiroveci* pneumonia (PCP) prophylaxis is provided to all patients for at least 3 months after transplantation and should be considered lifelong, particularly in patients with ongoing rejection or graft dysfunction. Trimethoprim-sulfamethoxazole is the preferred agent. Dapsone and atovaquone are alternative agents.
- Testing for latent tuberculosis with tuberculin skin testing or IFN-γ-release assays should be performed in all LT candidates and recipients. Treatment should be considered either early prior to transplantation or once the patient is stable after transplantation.

Section 3: Diagnosis

> **BOTTOM LINE/CLINICAL PEARLS**
> - The diagnosis of infections in LT recipients is guided by three time periods after LT: 0–1 month, 1–6 months, and after 6 months.
> - Most patients will present with fever but sometimes these clinical signs of infection are masked by immunosuppression.
> - In the first period (0–1 months), the majority of infections are typical healthcare-associated infections in a surgical patient.
> - In the second period (1–6 months), opportunistic infections can emerge in the absence of or after discontinuation of prophylaxis.
> - In the third period (>6 months) the majority of infections will be typical community-acquired infections. However, in the setting of rejection and/or graft dysfunction, the risk for healthcare-associated and opportunistic infections can persist.

Clinical diagnosis

0–30 days (Algorithm 50.1)

- The majority of infections will be surgical site infections, pneumonia, catheter-related blood-stream infections, catheter-associated urinary tract infections and *Clostridium difficile* colitis.

Although a detailed physical examination should always be performed, examination of the lungs, abdomen, wound and intravascular catheter sites are particularly essential.

- In the absence of targeted signs or symptoms, the initial evaluation should consist of at least blood cultures and chest X-ray. If there is a high clinical suspicion for pneumonia, a CT scan should be obtained if the chest X-ray is negative. Urinalysis and urine cultures should be obtained in patients with urinary symptoms or patients with an indwelling urinary catheter and unexplained fever and/or leukocytosis. Stool *C. difficile* PCR should be obtained in patients with diarrhea or unexplained abdominal pain.
- If there is no evidence for pneumonia, bacteremia, UTI, or *C. difficile* colitis and signs of infection (e.g. fever and/or leukocytosis) persist, then a CT scan of the chest, abdomen and pelvis should be obtained to identify a deeper surgical site infection or occult pleuro-pulmonary infection.

31–180 days (Algorithm 50.2)
- In addition to any of the infections that are commonly seen during the first month after LT, there should be a heightened suspicion for opportunistic infections during this period.
- CMV disease commonly occurs after prophylaxis has been discontinued particularly in donor positive, recipient negative (D+R-) patients.
- Fungal infections such as *Aspergillus* and *Cryptococcus* may be seen. Other miscellaneous opportunistic infections include *Nocardia* and tuberculosis.

>180 days
- In the absence of rejection or graft dysfunction, the risk for infection dramatically decreases after 6–12 months post-transplantation. Although the recipient remains relatively immunocompromised and theoretically at risk for opportunistic infections, mostly routine community-acquired infections occur in stable LT patients.
- However, most fevers of unknown origin occurring more than one year after LT can be attributed to one of the following infections after routine causes have been excluded: CMV, *Cryptococcus*, tuberculosis, endemic fungi (e.g. histoplasmosis), and EBV-related post-transplantation lymphoproliferative disorder.

Bacterial infections
- Bacterial infections are the most frequent infection following LT and most frequently occur during the first month. The most important and frequently observed infections are surgical site infections, intra-abdominal infections, peritonitis, bloodstream infections, pneumonia, urinary tract infection and *Clostridium difficile* colitis. Diagnosis of bacterial infections is rarely a challenge. Bloodstream infections, urinary tract infections and *Clostridium difficile* colitis are not different from the general patient population and will not be discussed further here.

Surgical site infections
- These include superficial wound infections or deeper infections including intra-abdominal and perihepatic abscesses.
- Diagnosis of superficial wound infections can be made by the presence of tenderness, erythema or purulent discharge from a wound dehiscence.
- Diagnosis of deeper infections is usually triggered by the presence of unexplained fever, leukocytosis, abdominal pain or gastrointestinal symptoms. Radiographic imaging of the abdomen is required to identify hematomas, collections, or abscesses.

- Drainage is required to confirm infection in most situations and microbiologic examination can guide the antimicrobial therapy. Drainage can be performed via interventional radiologic or surgical techniques.

Bilomas

- Bilomas are intrahepatic or perihepatic collections of bile that are a result of complications of the biliary tract (necrosis, stricture and/or leak). In the setting of hepatic artery thrombosis or other known biliary tract complications at the time of LT, clinicians should have a heightened awareness for the presence of bilomas.
- Infection is a frequent complication of bilomas. Fever and abdominal pain are the most common symptoms associated with infected bilomas but approximately one-third of patients may be asymptomatic. Other clues for infected bilomas particularly in the asymptomatic patients are elevations in LFTs or leukocytosis. A contrast-enhanced CT scan is the diagnostic test of choice and bilomas appear as low-attenuation lesions. Although percutaneous drainage of all bilomas should be considered, it is essential in the diagnosis of suspected infected bilomas. Aspirated fluid should be cultured to define the specific bacteria or *Candida* species associated with the infected biloma.

Peritonitis

- Peritonitis after LT is a serious complication associated with significant morbidity and mortality. It is usually associated with surgical site infections, biliary complications, intra-abdominal bleeding, or bowel perforation. Most patients with peritonitis will have fever and significant abdominal pain. Diagnosis is established by positive peritoneal fluid cultures.

Bloodstream infections

- Bloodstream infections are also a serious complication after LT, particularly when associated with any intra-abdominal infection.
- Other common causes of bacteremia include intravascular catheters and pneumonia. The diagnosis is established by positive blood cultures.

Pneumonia

- Pneumonia occurs most frequently in LT recipients who have had a prolonged hospitalization, particularly with mechanical ventilation in the ICU. Diagnosis is established by the presence of new and persistent infiltrate or consolidation on radiographic imaging in combination with clinical signs of pneumonia such as fever, leukocytosis, cough, dyspnea, hypoxia or purulent secretions from the endotracheal tube. The presence of bacteria in respiratory culture alone does not establish the diagnosis of pneumonia.

Urinary tract infections

- Urinary tract infections are most frequently associated with the presence of indwelling urinary catheters. The diagnosis is made in patients with urinary catheters by the presence of unexplained fever and/or leukocytosis in combination with pyuria and >100000 colony forming units of bacteria in culture.
- In the absence of a urinary catheter, fever and/or leukocytosis, the diagnosis of urinary tract infection requires that the patient has urinary symptoms such as dysuria, urinary frequency or

flank pain. A positive urine culture in the absence of clinical signs of infection is defined as asymptomatic bacteriuria and does not require treatment.

Clostridium difficile colitis

- *Clostridium difficile* colitis is usually associated with hospitalization and antibiotic treatment. Patients will usually have watery diarrhea and leukocytosis. Fever and abdominal pain may be present as well.

Viral infections

- Viral infections after LT are typically due to reactivation of herpes viruses such as CMV, HSV, varicella-zoster virus, and EBV. They most frequently occur 3–6 months after transplantation but onset may be delayed by prophylactic strategies or triggered by enhanced immunosuppression to treat rejection.
- CMV infection is diagnosed by detecting viral proteins (pp65 antigenemia) or nucleic acids (DNA PCR) in the blood or other body fluids in the absence of clinical signs or symptoms. CMV disease is established when clinical signs such as fever, leucopenia and thrombocytopenia are present in combination with the detection of CMV DNA in the blood (CMV syndrome) or histologic evidence of CMV in tissues (tissue-invasive CMV disease). Major risk factors for CMV disease include seronegative recipient from seropositive donor; rejection; and intensified immunosuppression.

Fungal infections

- Fungal infections can occur at any time after LT. The most common fungal pathogens in LT recipients are *Candida, Cryptococcus,* and *Aspergillus.*

Candida

- *Candida* infections most frequently occur as healthcare-associated infections in the first month after LT. *Candida* may be involved in all of the previously described bacterial infections with the exception of pneumonia. Diagnosis is established by positive *Candida* cultures from the blood or other sterile sites.

Cryptococcus

- *Cryptococcus* infection most frequently occurs after 3 months and often even later. Most patients will present with subacute meningitis marked by fever and headache. The diagnosis of cryptococcosis is initially established by the detection of cryptococcal antigen in the serum. Meningitis is diagnosed by performing a lumbar puncture and demonstrating positive cryptococcal antigen or culture of cerebrospinal fluid. It is essential that an opening pressure is obtained during the lumbar puncture as further management will be guided by this information.
- Disseminated cryptococcosis is defined by the presence of positive blood cultures or the detection of *Cryptococcus* in two distinct anatomic sites.
- Isolated pulmonary *Cryptococcus* infection can also occur in LT patients. Patients will typically present with cough and fever and radiographic studies will reveal nodules or mass-like lesions. Diagnosis is established by respiratory culture or lung biopsy. Serum cryptococcal antigen can be negative in isolated pulmonary infection.

Aspergillus

- *Aspergillus* infection most frequently occurs after 3 months and often even later. Although previously disseminated infection was a frequent manifestation of aspergillosis, in recent years most cases are pulmonary aspergillosis. Most patients will present with fever and cough and radiographic studies will reveal nodules or mass-like lesions. The diagnosis of proven pulmonary aspergillosis requires the demonstration of the typical hyphal elements in histological examination in combination with positive cultures.
- The diagnosis of probable aspergillosis is made with clinical and radiographic evidence in combination with a positive respiratory culture or serum galactomannan assay.

Algorithm 50.1 Diagnosis of suspected infection in LT recipients (0–30 days)

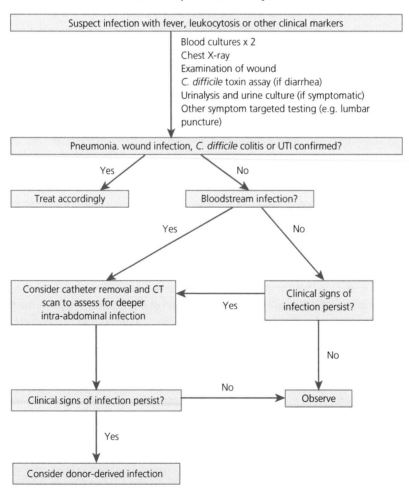

**Algorithm 50.2 Diagnosis of suspected infection
in LT recipients (31–180 days and beyond)**

Suspect infection with fever, leukocytosis or other clinical markers

Acute illness | No | Subacute/chronic illness

Follow Algorithm 50.1
Diagnosis confirmed? → No → Localizing signs or symptoms? → No

Yes

Treat accordingly

Yes

Leukopenia and/or
thrombocytopenia
with fever and
constitutional
symptoms

Fever and
headache

Fever, cough, and
pulmonary
symptoms

Check CMV DNA
PCR and consider
other viral disease

Serum
cryptococcal
antigen + CT scan
of the brain +/–
lumbar puncture
to assess for
cryptococcal
meningitis or other

Serum cryptococcal
antigen +
galactomannan + CT
scan of the chest to
assess for opportunistic
pulmonary infection

If no evidence of
viral infection then
consider TB or
fungal infection

Biopsy of lung
tissue via
bronchoscopy,
surgery, or CT
guidance

Section 4: Treatment
Treatment rationale
Bacterial infections
- A general principle applicable to all bacterial infections is to choose the narrowest antibiotic needed once the bacterial pathogen(s) is known.
- Another important principle is to use the shortest duration of antibiotics needed to clear the infection to avoid toxicity and antibacterial resistance that are associated with prolonged therapies.
- Surgical site infections:
  - Superficial wound infections require debridement of necrotic and devitalized tissue in combination with antibiotic treatment for approximately 5 days.
  - Deeper infections such as intra-abdominal and perihepatic abscesses require drainage and antibiotic treatment for 5–7 days.

- Infected bilomas require drainage often with an indwelling catheter. Surgical or endoscopic intervention to address biliary strictures or leaks may be necessary (see Chapter 49). Antibiotic treatment should be continued until drainage has been fully achieved.
- Peritonitis is treated with antibiotics for 5–7 days after the underlying cause has been treated.
- Bloodstream infections are treated with antibiotics until the source has been eradicated and blood cultures are negative. Catheter-associated bloodstream infections are generally treated with antibiotics until the catheter is removed and the patient is clinically stable with negative blood cultures. *Staphylococcus aureus* bloodstream infections are treated for 14–28 days.
- Pneumonia is treated with antibiotics typically for 5–7 days.
- Urinary tract infections are treated with antibiotics. Cystitis is treated for 3–5 days and pyelonephritis is treated for 7–10 days.
- *Clostridium difficile* colitis is treated with oral metronidazole or oral vancomycin for 10–14 days.

CMV disease after LT

- CMV disease is treated with intravenous ganciclovir (5 mg/kg every 12 hours) until fever has resolved and the patient is able to tolerate oral valganciclovir (900 mg every 12 hours). CMV DNA PCR should be monitored on a weekly basis. The induction phase of therapy is continued until all signs and symptoms of CMV disease have resolved and the serum CMV DNA PCR is not detected.
- Maintenance therapy with a lower dose may be considered in the setting of intensified immunosuppression for rejection but is not mandatory in other settings. Patients should be monitored for clinical relapse. CMV DNA PCR surveillance can be considered to assess for virologic relapse.

Fungal infections

- *Candida* infections are typically treated with 2 weeks of antifungal therapy after the blood cultures have cleared in the setting of candidemia or the source has been treated in other settings.
- *Cryptococcus* is treated based on the site(s) of infection. Disseminated disease or meningitis is treated with a 2-week induction phase of a lipid formulation of amphotericin B in combination with flucytosine. The induction phase may be prolonged if cerebrospinal fluid or blood cultures remain positive. The maintenance phase of fluconazole is generally continued for 6–12 months but may be continued indefinitely in some settings. Isolated pulmonary cryptococcosis can be treated with fluconazole until clinical and radiographic stability have been achieved.
- *Aspergillus* infection is treated with voriconazole until clinical and radiographic stability have been achieved. Lipid formulations of amphotericin B are a reasonable alternative for initial therapy but a switch to voriconazole should be considered as early as possible to avoid the toxicities of amphotericin B.

When to hospitalize

- In general, hospitalization should be considered for all LT recipients with suspected or proven infection unless the diagnosis is clearly established and treatment can safely be given with oral therapy.

Managing the hospitalized patient

- Specific management recommendations depend on the specific infection and clinical status of the patient.

Section 5: Special Populations

Not applicable for this topic.

Section 6: Prognosis

Not applicable for this topic.

Section 7: Reading List

Fishman JA. Infection in solid-organ transplant recipients. N Engl J Med 2007;357:2601–14
Huprikar S. Update in infectious diseases in liver transplant recipients. Clin Liver Dis 2007;11:337–54
http://onlinelibrary.wiley.com/doi/10.1111/ajt.2009.9.issue-s4/issuetoc

Section 8: Guidelines
National society guidelines

Guideline title	Guideline source	Date
AST Infectious Diseases Guidelines, 3rd Edition	American Society of Transplantation (AST) Infectious Diseases Community of Practice http://onlinelibrary.wiley.com/doi/10.1111/ajt.2013.13.issue-s4/issuetoc	March 2013

Section 9: Evidence

Not applicable for this topic.

Section 10: Images

Not applicable for this topic.

> **Additional material for this chapter can be found online at:**
> **www.mountsinaiexpertguides.com**
> **This includes a case study and multiple choice questions**

CHAPTER 51

Malignancy after Liver Transplantation

Lawrence U. Liu

Division of Liver Diseases, Icahn School of Medicine at Mount Sinai, New York, NY, USA

OVERALL BOTTOM LINE

- Due to long-term immunosuppression therapy, the post-LT recipient is at risk for disease conditions (e.g. infection, malignancy) that are generally regulated by the body's immune system.
- Skin cancer is the most common type of *de novo* malignancy after LT.
- Malignancy, either *de novo* type or recurrent HCC, may occur after LT.
- PTLD is a malignancy unique to the transplant recipient.
- Specific screening guidelines have not yet been established for LT recipients; the current ones for immunocompetent persons remain in use. Increased surveillance may be prudent in view of the recipient's immunosuppressed state.
- Treatment can be tailored according to the particular tumor, along with reduction of the immunosuppression regimen to strengthen the individual's immune system.
- Molecular markers may shed more light in the future on risk estimation of HCC recurrence post-transplantation.

Section 1: Background
Definition of disease

- *De novo* malignancy is the second cause of mortality after LT, with cardiovascular disease as the primary reason; cumulative incidence ranges up to 26%.

Incidence/prevalence

- There is a higher incidence of developing malignancy in post-transplant (i.e. immunosuppressed) recipients when compared with the immunocompetent population.
- The cumulative incidence of *de novo* malignancies range up to 26%, with 0.5% for the general non-transplant population.

Mount Sinai Expert Guides: Hepatology, First Edition. Edited by Jawad Ahmad, Scott L. Friedman, and Henryk Dancygier.

© 2014 John Wiley & Sons, Ltd. Published 2014 by John Wiley & Sons, Ltd.

Companion website: www.mountsinaiexpertguides.com

Comparison of the incidence of the common types of malignancy after LT and the incidence in the general population

Cancer type*	Incidence (%) – transplant recipient	Incidence (%) – general population	Mean time to occurrence (in months)
Skin[†]	0.9–3.2	0.02	36.4–50.2
Kaposi's sarcoma	0.14–2.8	500-fold less	
PTLD[‡]	0.9–2.6	0.03	26–32
Colon	0–0.6	0.05	16–50.6
Head and neck	0.1–2	0.01	34.3–61.2
Lung	0–1.2	0.06	42–50
Breast	0.2–0.7	0.1	41–124
Cervix	0–1.5	0.008	1–59
Ovary	0–1.5	0.01	1–59
Kidney/urinary bladder	0–0.4	0.03	20–55.3
Prostate	0.3	0.2	5.8–18.4
Miscellaneous[§]	0.2–0.8		

*Adapted from Chak and Saab.

[†] Equal incidence for both squamous cell and basal cell skin cancer.

[‡] Post-transplantation lymphoproliferative disorder.

[§] Miscellaneous causes include: papillary thyroid cancer, glioblastoma, squamous cell cancer of the conjunctiva, pancreas, small intestine, seminoma, gastric Kaposi's sarcoma, metastasis of primary unknown, angiosarcoma, pituitary, cholangiocarcinoma, stomach, embryonic testicular cancer, hemangioblastoma

Etiology
- The etiology of malignancy after LT is related to long-term immunosuppression use.

Pathology/pathogenesis
- Immunosuppression results in the weakening of the body's natural defenses (e.g. cytotoxic T cells, macrophages, natural killer cells) that generally inhibit oncogenic viral growth and destroy malignant cells *in vitro*.
- Azathioprine use is an independent risk factor for the increased incidence of *de novo* malignancies. By inhibiting purine synthesis, it affects T cell and B cell production.

Predictive/risk factors
- Smoking.
- Alcohol abuse pre-LT.
- Pre-malignant disease (age and gender factors have not been replicated in studies)
  - Barrett's esophagus.
  - Myeloproliferative disorder.
  - Cervical atypia.
  - Colon polyps.
  - Ulcerative colitis.
  - Caroli disease (as a risk factor for cholangiocarcinoma).

Section 2: Prevention

> **BOTTOM LINE/CLINICAL PEARLS**
> - Sirolimus is a mammalian target of rapamycin (mTOR) inhibitor, and in a different drug category from tacrolimus and cyclosporine (calcineurin inhibitors). It has anti-angiogenic properties and has been reported to decrease skin cancer incidence in kidney transplant recipients.
> - mTOR is upregulated in HCC, therefore allowing sirolimus to have a potential effect on HCC recurrence. A recent meta-analysis demonstrated that sirolimus use to reduce HCC recurrence rates post-LT resulted in a lower recurrence rate, longer recurrence-free survival and overall survival, and lower recurrence-related mortality when compared with patients receiving calcineurin inhibitors.

Screening
- There are currently no guidelines on the surveillance schedule for HCC post-LT.
- At Mount Sinai Hospital, the recipients' explants are assessed and classified as either low-risk or high-risk for recurrence, depending on the HCC histology, number of tumors and presence/absence of lymphovascular invasion.

Surveillance imaging protocol for patients who undergo LT for HCC at Mount Sinai Hospital

Imaging schedule*	Low-risk HCC	High-risk HCC
Year 1	At 3 months post-transplantation	Every 3 months
Year 2	At 12 months post-transplantation	Every 6 months
Year 3	End	Every 6 months
Year 4	N/A	Every 12 months
Year 5	N/A	Every 12 months
Year 6	N/A	End

*Imaging studies: chest CT scan (without contrast) and abdomen CT scan or MRI (with intravenous contrast)

- Current guidelines for *de novo* malignancy screening have not yielded consistent benefits in both the liver and kidney transplantation populations to justify the cost-effectiveness of this approach, nonetheless various organizations recommend screening guidelines for the average-risk individual.

Organ/cancer type	Screening guidelines for average-risk individuals	
	Onset	Interval
Breast	Starting age 50	Between 12–24 months
Cervix	Between ages 18 and 20, or when sexual activity begins	Annually
Colon	Fecal occult blood test and flexible sigmoidoscopy starting age of 50	Every 5 years
Skin	Self-examination	Monthly
	Clinician examination	Every 6–12 months
Kidney	No guidelines	N/A
Lung	No guidelines	N/A
Prostate	PSA and DRE starting age of 50	Annually

Primary prevention

- Reduction of immunosuppression drug levels – when applicable – is the key to preserving the balance between graft rejection and decreasing the risk of malignancy.
- Although azathioprine had previously been viewed to increase cancer risk, a recent study among kidney transplant recipients has not shown a difference in cancer incidence rates when comparing its use with cyclosporine.

Secondary prevention

- Sirolimus has shown some promise as an immunosuppressive agent to use for the prevention of skin cancer in kidney transplant recipients and against HCC recurrence.

Section 3: Diagnosis

> **BOTTOM LINE/CLINICAL PEARLS**
> - The key for diagnosing malignancy after LT is to have a high index of suspicion depending on the underlying risk factors.
> - Patients with HCC should be surveyed for recurrence using appropriate imaging.
> - Patients with significant smoking and alcohol history are at risk for most cancers but particularly head and neck cancer.
> - Prior sun exposure and fair skin predispose to skin cancer.
> - Regular cancer screening is imperative in LT recipients, particularly regular dermatology assessment.
> - The tables in Section 2 summarize some screening strategies for *de novo* malignancies and HCC.

Section 4: Treatment

Treatment rationale

- Decreasing immunosuppression regimens has been observed to decrease existing cancers; this strategy is performed in addition to specific cancer treatments recommended to the patient.

Types of malignancy

De novo malignancy

Incidence

- Up to 26% (significantly higher than in the general population).
- Skin cancer – the most common type (squamous cell and basal cell). Incidence: 0.9–3.2%; mean time to occurrence is 36–50 months (see table in Section 1).
- Colon cancer – increased risk in PSC with inflammatory bowel disease. The risk for developing colon cancer in a LT recipient with and without ulcerative colitis was reported as 11% and 0.1%, respectively.
- Head/neck/lung cancer – increased risk in those with smoking and alcohol history.
- The development of PTLD is associated with recipients receiving high immunosuppression regimens and EBV infection.

Risk factors

- Use of tacrolimus and azathioprine.
- Higher immunosuppression regimens can potentially increase the risk of *de novo* malignancy due to their suppression of the body's natural defenses.

- The use of induction therapy (T-cell depleting strategies) has not been found to be associated with an increased risk of *de novo* malignancy development.

Treatment
- Standard treatment of the specific malignancy.
- Changing main immunosuppressive agent to sirolimus.
- Sirolimus has been utilized as an immunosuppressive agent for the prevention of skin cancer in kidney transplant recipients and against HCC recurrence. Its use against other types of cancer remains under investigation.

PTLD
- The second most common cancer in LT recipients; 85% is of B-cell origin.
- The median time for PTLD occurrence after solid organ transplantation ranges from 30 to 72 months.

Incidence
- 0.9–2.8% (although this can be as high as 15% in pediatric recipients).

Mortality rate
- Up to 50%.

Poor prognostic indicators
- High-grade histology, poor performance status, EBV-negativity (incidence rate of 23%), graft involvement.

Risk factors
- EBV infection.
- CMV donor-recipient mismatch.
- Hepatitis C virus.
- Intensive immunosuppression (e.g. muromonab-CD3 [OKT3], antithymocyte globulin).

Signs/symptoms

Typical symptoms and their incidence in PTLD	
Signs/symptoms	**Incidence (%)**
Fever	57
Lymphadenopathy	38
Weight loss	9
Splenomegaly	21

Laboratory tests
- General laboratory profile to include a CBC with differential, hepatic and renal function tests, ESR, LDH, uric acid, serum electrophoresis.
- EBV DNA (by PCR).
- Excisional biopsy – preferred over needle core biopsy and fine needle aspiration.

Evaluation for tumor staging

- CT scan of neck/chest/abdomen/pelvis – extranodal manifestations are found in more than 70% of cases; cranial imaging is also advised due to a 10% risk of CNS involvement.
- Echocardiogram – as a baseline study since one of the treatment strategies – CHOP – may result in cardiac abnormalities.

Treatment

- Reduction of immunosuppression, or withdrawal – if possible, to its minimum level to allow the patient's natural immunity to recover. Acute graft rejection rates, as a result of this management strategy, can reach 30% in adults (and 80% in pediatric patients).
- Targeting of B cells with monoclonal antibodies (e.g. rituximab).
- Chemotherapy (e.g. CHOP).
- Local control (if warranted) – with surgery and radiation.

Recurrent HCC

- Occurs in 10–15% of patients; most occur within the first 18–24 months.
- There are currently no guidelines on the surveillance schedule for HCC post-LT.
- At Mount Sinai, the recipients' explants are assessed and classified as either low risk or high risk for recurrence, depending on the HCC histology, number of tumors and presence/absence of lymphovascular invasion. See table "Surveillance imaging protocol for patients who undergo LT for HCC at Mount Sinai Hospital."

Risk factors

- Moderately to poorly-differentiated histology of the HCC in the explant.
- Certain molecular markers of HCC may predict the risk of recurrence even for tumors that are beyond the Milan criteria.
- Lymphatic and microvascular tumor invasion were noted to significantly decrease both disease-free and over-all survival.
- The etiology of the underlying liver disease requiring transplantation was not found to affect the survival rate from HCC recurrence.

Sites of recurrence

- Lungs, liver, bone, adrenal gland.

Treatment

- There are currently no guidelines regarding treatment of recurrent HCC post-LT. Treatment strategies can include:
  - Surgical resection – strongest independent predictor of long-term survival.
  - Chemoembolization.
  - Systemic chemotherapy, e.g. sorafenib may be offered as adjuvant therapy but varying degrees of drug tolerance remains an issue. Median survival rates also vary, and range from 5 to 25 months.
- Prognosis remains variable and can depend on risk factors and number of lesions; in theory, solitary lesions can be resected and may provide a better prognosis.

Section 5: Special Populations

Not applicable for this topic.

Section 6: Prognosis

> **BOTTOM LINE/CLINICAL PEARLS**
> * Malignancy, either *de novo* type or recurrent HCC, may occur early or years after LT.
> * Specific screening guidelines have not yet been established for LT recipients; the current ones for immunocompetent persons remain in use. Increased surveillance may be prudent in view of the recipient's immunosuppressed state.
> * Treatment can be tailored according to the particular tumor, along with reduction of immunosuppression regimen to strengthen the individual's immune system.
> * PTLD is a malignancy unique to the transplant recipient. Its mortality rate can reach 50%. Acute graft rejection can occur due to the use of immunosuppression reduction as part of its management strategy.
> * Molecular markers may shed more light in the future on risk estimation of HCC recurrence post-transplantation.

Section 7: Reading List

Benlloch S, Berenguer M, Prieto M, Moreno R, San Juan F, Rayón M, Mir J, et al. De novo internal neoplasms after liver transplantation: increased risk and aggressive behavior in recent years? Am J Transplant 2004;4:596–604

Chak E, Saab S. Risk factors and incidence of de novo malignancy in liver transplant recipients: a systematic review. Liver Int 2010;30:1247–58

Chinnakotla S, Davis GL, Vasani S, Kim P, Tomiyama K, Sanchez E, Onaca N, Goldstein R, Levy M, Klintmalm GB. Impact of sirolimus on the recurrence of hepatocellular carcinoma after liver transplantation. Liver Transpl 2009;15:1834–42

Euvrard S, Morelon E, Rostaing L, Goffin E, Brocard A, Tromme I, Broeders N, del Marmol V, Chatelet V, Dompmartin A, Kessler M, Serra AL, Hofbauer GF, Pouteil-Noble C, Campistol JM, Kanitakis J, Roux AS, Decullier E, Dantal J, TUMORAPA Study Group. Sirolimus and secondary skin-cancer prevention in kidney transplantation. NEJM 2012;367:329–39

Fabia R, Levy MF, Testa G, Obiekwe S, Goldstein RM, Husberg BS, Gonwa TA, Klintmalm GB. Colon carcinoma in patients undergoing liver transplantation. Am J Surg 1998;176:265–9

Gallagher MP, Kelly PJ, Jardine M, Perkovic V, Cass A, Craig JC, Eris J, Webster AC. Long-term cancer risk of immunosuppressive regimens after kidney transplantation. J Am Soc Nephrol 2010;21:852–8

Herrero JI. Screening of de novo tumors after liver transplantation. J Gastroenterol Hepatol 2012;27:1011–6

Hosseini-Moghaddam SM, Soleimanirahbar A, Mazzulli T, Rotstein C, Husain S. Post renal transplantation Kaposi's sarcoma: a review of its epidemiology, pathogenesis, diagnosis, clinical aspects, and therapy. Transpl Infect Dis 2012;14:338–45

Jagadeesh D, Woda BA, Draper J, Evens AM. Post transplant lymphoproliferative disorders: risk, classification, and therapeutic recommendations. Curr Treat Options Oncol 2012;13:122–36

Jiménez-Romero C, Manrique A, Marqués E, Calvo J, Sesma AG, Cambra F, Abradelo M, et al. Switching to sirolimus monotherapy for de novo tumors after liver transplantation. A preliminary experience. Hepatogastroenterology 2011;58:115–21

Kornberg A, Küpper B, Tannapfel A, Katenkamp K, Thrum K, Habrecht O, Wilberg J. Long-term survival after recurrent hepatocellular carcinoma in liver transplant patients: clinical patterns and outcome variables. EJSO 2010;36:275–80

Menon KV, Hakeem AR, Heaton ND. Meta-analysis: recurrence and survival following the use of sirolimus in liver transplantation for hepatocellular carcinoma. Aliment Pharmacol Ther 2012 (Epub ahead of print)

Nelson BP, Nalesnik MA, Bahler DW, Locker J, Fung JJ, Swerdlow SH. Epstein-Barr virus-negative posttransplant lymphoproliferative disorders: a distinct entity? Am J Surg Pathol 2000;24:375–85

Opelz G, Dohler B. Lymphomas after solid organ transplantation: a collaborative transplant study report. Am J Transpl 2004;4:222–30

Rodríguez-Perálvarez M, Luong TV, Andreana L, Meyer T, Dhillon AP, Burroughs AK. A systematic review of microvascular invasion in hepatocellular carcinoma: diagnostic and prognostic variability. Ann Surg Oncol 2013;20:325–39

Rubin J, Ayoub N, Kaldas F, Saab S. Management of recurrent hepatocellular carcinoma in liver transplant recipients: a systematic review. Exp Clin Transplant 2012;10:531–43

Schwartz M, Dvorchik I, Roayaie S, Fiel MI, Finkelstein S, Marsh JW, Martignetti JA, Llovet JM. Liver transplantation for hepatocellular carcinoma: extension of indications based on molecular markers. J Hepatol 2008;49:581–8

Sotiropoulos GC, Nowak KW, Fouzas I, Vernadakis S, Kykalos S, Klein CG, Paul A. Sorafenib treatment for recurrent hepatocellular carcinoma after liver transplantation. Transplant Proc 2012;44:2754–6

Staufer K, Fischer L, Seegers B, Vettorazzi E, Nashan B, Sterneck M. High toxicity of sorafenib for recurrent hepatocellular carcinoma after liver transplantation. Transpl Int 2012;25:1158–64

Tessari G, Girolomoni G. Nonmelanoma skin cancer in solid organ transplant recipients: update on epidemiology, risk factors, and management. Dermatol Surg 2012;38:1622–30

Wong G, Chapman JR, Craig JC. Cancer screening in renal transplant recipients: what is the evidence? Clin J Am Soc Nephrol 2008;3:S87–100

Zavaglia C, Airoldi A, Mancuso A, Vangeli M, Viganò R, Cordone G, Gentiluomo M, Belli LS. Adverse effects affect sorafenib efficacy in patients with recurrent hepatocellular carcinoma after liver transplantation: experience at a single center and review of the literature. Eur J Gastroenterol Hepatol 2013;25:180–6

Zimmerman MA, Trotter JF, Wachs M, Bak T, Campsen J, Skibba A, Kam I. Sirolimus-based immunosuppression following liver transplantation for hepatocellular carcinoma. Liver Transpl 2008;14:633–8

Section 8: Guidelines

Guideline title	Guideline source	Date
Long-Term Management of the Successful Adult Liver Transplant	AASLD http://www.aasld.org/practiceguidelines/ Documents/LongTermManagmentofSuccessfulLT.pdf	2012

Section 9: Evidence

Not applicable for this topic.

Section 10: Images

Not applicable for this topic.

Additional material for this chapter can be found online at:
www.mountsinaiexpertguides.com
This includes a case study and multiple choice questions

CHAPTER 52

Hepatitis C Post-Liver Transplantation

Thomas D. Schiano[1] and M. Isabel Fiel[2]
[1]Division of Liver Diseases, Icahn School of Medicine at Mount Sinai, New York, NY, USA
[2]Department of Pathology, Icahn School of Medicine at Mount Sinai, New York, NY, USA

OVERALL BOTTOM LINE
- Recurrence of HCV after transplantation is universal.
- Twenty-five percent of patients progress to cirrhosis within 5 years, 50% within 10 years.
- The differential diagnosis of abnormal liver tests post-transplantation is broad and includes viral infection, drug toxicity, rejection and biliary obstruction.
- Anti-viral treatment is difficult for patients to tolerate post-transplantation and thus leads to a frequent need to dose reduce and terminate therapy early.
- Fibrosing cholestatic hepatitis is an infrequent occurrence and carries high morbidity/mortality, typified by hyperbilirubinemia, profound HCV viremia and specific histological features.

Section 1: Background
Definition of disease
- Recurrent HCV infection of the liver allograft occurs in all patients who are HCV-RNA positive at the time of LT. The graft is re-infected as early as the time of re-perfusion and patients may develop histologic and biochemical features of acute HCV in the first few months after transplantation, which is accompanied by a gradual rise in HCV viremia.

Disease classification
- Histologic features of chronic HCV (Figure 52.1) can be demonstrated in >70% HCV recipients after 1 year and in close to 90% 5 years after transplantation. Patients will always be viremic with recurrence being defined as histological evidence of reinfection associated with abnormal liver chemistry tests.

Incidence/prevalence
- In the USA, 45–48% of patients undergoing LT have HCV.
- If the HCV PCR is positive prior to transplantation, it is positive after transplantation.
- Fifty to 70% of patients will have histologic recurrence of HCV within 1 year of transplantation, 90% within 5 years.

Mount Sinai Expert Guides: Hepatology, First Edition. Edited by Jawad Ahmad, Scott L. Friedman, and Henryk Dancygier.
© 2014 John Wiley & Sons, Ltd. Published 2014 by John Wiley & Sons, Ltd.
Companion website: www.mountsinaiexpertguides.com

Economic impact
- The need to treat recurrent HCV with IFN-based therapy carries appreciable financial burden.
- The complications of graft failure and need for re-transplantation also bear significant economic burden.

Etiology
- Reinfection of the transplanted liver with viral hepatitis.
- The detection of HCV viremia occurs as early as the anhepatic phase of the transplantation surgery.
- Accelerated fibrosis in the transplanted liver leads to graft failure and cirrhosis and the need for re-transplantation.

Pathology/pathogenesis
- Ongoing inflammation of the transplanted liver leads to fibrosis formation. Multiple factors may contribute to this fibrosis:

Factors Associated with Accelerated Fibrosis Progression
High HCV-RNA serum levels pre- and immediately post-LT
HIV co-infection
Older donor age
Concurrent biliary problems post-transplantation
Post-transplantation diabetes mellitus
Severe inflammation/fibrosis at one year
Early histologic recurrence
Infection with CMV and HSV-6
Bolus corticosteroids to treat acute cellular rejection
Plasma cell hepatitis
Concurrent steatohepatitis

Section 2: Prevention

BOTTOM LINE
- Attempting to treat HCV pre-LT is recommended. The International Liver Transplant Society has recommended that patients with MELD scores of 15 or less undergo an attempt at HCV viral eradication prior to transplantation. Studies of early post-transplantation pre-emptive antiviral therapy have shown very poor SVR rates and for this reason the majority of transplantation centers do not pursue this.
- It may also not be practical to treat patients with antiviral therapy early after transplantation as patients may have renal dysfunction and be at great risk for infection as they recuperate from a lengthy pre-transplantation hospitalization. They may be deconditioned, have anemia and are taking a myriad of other medications in the early post-operative period, which is also the peak time for developing rejection.
- Patients with cirrhosis are complex patients to treat with IFN and ribavirin because of their increased risk for infection, liver decompensation, thrombocytopenia and anemia. Most patients require extremely close follow up as well as the use of hematopoietic growth factors, and it is difficult to achieve optimal dosing.

Screening
- Assessment of serum HCV viral loads. There may be no correlation between the degree of viremia and the amount of histologic damage.

Primary prevention
- Pre-LT anti-viral therapy can be effective in carefully selected patients.

Secondary prevention
- Pre-emptive anti-viral therapy post-LT is currently not indicated because of poor sustained viral response rates and appreciable complications.

Section 3: Diagnosis (Algorithm 52.1)

- The diagnosis is based on demonstrating HCV viremia post-LT in a patient with known hepatitis C and typical histologic findings occurring usually in the setting of abnormal liver chemistry tests.
- Patients undergoing transplantation before the early 1990s may have acquired HCV through transfusions or the transplanted graft itself.
- Genotyping gives the clinician helpful information in predicting response to treatment.
- Patients may sometimes receive hepatitis B core antibody positive livers so exclusion of hepatitis B viremia is essential in the appropriate clinical setting.

Differential diagnosis	Features
Drug-induced liver injury	Eosinophilia, suggestive histologic findings, use of known potentially hepatotoxic medications, i.e. sulfonamides
Biliary obstruction	Occurs in upwards of 10–20% of all transplantations. Cholestasis may predominate and patients may have symptoms of cholangitis
CMV and other viral infections	Patients often have constitutional symptoms, pancytopenia and fever. Typical PCR serologies and histology are seen
Acute cellular or chronic ductopenic rejection	Abnormal liver chemistry tests with neither a specific hepatocellular nor cholestatic pattern. Immunosuppressive medication levels may be sub-therapeutic. Liver biopsy is necessary to make the diagnosis
Hepatic artery thrombosis/ stenosis	High aminotransferases, diagnosed by Doppler US or arteriography

Typical presentation
- Recurrent HCV is manifested by abnormal liver chemistry tests in the presence of HCV viremia and typical histology.
- Older donor age is a strong negative prognostic factor in HCV outcome post-LT and older donors (i.e. greater than age 55) should be avoided if at all possible in the HCV recipient.
- Patients may rarely develop a rapidly progressive form of HCV recurrence known as fibrosing cholestatic hepatitis (Figure 52.2). This entity is typified by extremely high viral loads (often >10 million IU/mL) and hyperbilirubinemia. Patients with fibrosing cholestatic hepatitis or cholestasis in the setting of recurrent HCV have poorer outcomes and generally do not respond to IFN treatment.

Clinical diagnosis
- History: elevated aminotransferases in the setting of detectable serum HCV-RNA.
- Physical examination: Almost always, patients will not have any physical signs unless graft failure has already occurred, when they can present with jaundice and manifestations of portal hypertension.

Laboratory diagnosis
- Liver chemistry tests: aminotransferases are often elevated. The presence of cholestasis often portends a worse outcome and a more severe recurrence assuming that other etiologies for this have been excluded, i.e. biliary obstruction.
- Histology: liver biopsy interpretation in HCV patients post-LT is extremely challenging because of the broad range of possibilities in the differential diagnosis. Concurrence of mild histological acute cellular rejection in the setting of recurrent HCV is often not clinically relevant and is not treated. More severe degrees of acute cellular rejection should be treated with optimization of pre-existing immunosuppression with the avoidance of parenteral corticosteroids. An increase in liver tests in a patient with HCV being treated for rejection may be due to reactivation of CMV or HBV, or may be a worsening of the HCV. Typical histological changes of acute recurrent HCV include apoptotic bodies, hepatocyte unrest, activation of sinusoidal lining cells, parenchymal necrosis and portal inflammation. With chronicity, the portal inflammation increases and is accompanied by interface hepatitis, lobular inflammation and varying degrees of fibrosis.
- Imaging: although not necessary to make a diagnosis of recurrent HCV, imaging studies such as Doppler US and MRCP are useful to exclude vascular insufficiency and biliary obstruction. Several recent studies have detailed potential usefulness of fibroelastography in following the progression of hepatic fibrosis in patients with recurrent HCV.

Algorithm 52.1 Diagnosis of recurrent HCV

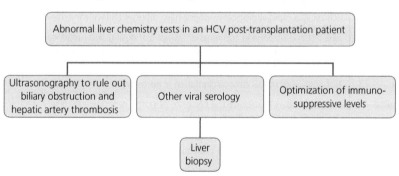

Potential pitfalls/common errors in diagnosis
- It may be difficult to histologically differentiate recurrent HCV from acute rejection.
- Tacrolimus and cyclosporine levels may rise in the setting of liver dysfunction so if these are at therapeutic or supra-therapeutic levels, rejection is not excluded.
- Plasma cell hepatitis histologically may be difficult to differentiate from recurrent HCV and/or rejection and may progress without optimizing immunosuppression.
- Recurrent HCV with concurrent biliary obstruction may histologically mimic fibrosing cholestatic hepatitis.

Section 4: Treatment
Treatment rationale
- There are no strict algorithms for the treatment of post-LT recurrent HCV.
- Most centers initiate treatment when patients have stage 1–2 fibrosis; more aggressive antiviral therapy may be pursued in the setting of early histologic recurrence, older donor age or in a patient with cholestasis.
- Predictive factors associated with SVR are similar to those in the non-transplantation patient and include early virologic response to therapy, total dose and duration of PEG-IFN and ribavirin, lower baseline fibrosis stage, genotype 2 or 3, and lower baseline HCV viral load.

When to hospitalize
- To investigate abnormal liver chemistry tests.
- Renal failure.
- Complications of portal hypertension and jaundice.

Managing the hospitalized patient
- Once patients develop cirrhosis from recurrent HCV, there is a rapid progression to hepatic decompensation and graft failure. The rate of progression thereafter to death is also accelerated with a 3-year survival of <10% following the onset of HCV-related allograft failure.

Table of treatment

Treatment	Comment
Conservative	Anti-viral treatment is precluded, i.e. renal failure. Patients achieving SVR have better long-term survival if treatment is possible. Genotypes 2 and 3 and those achieving a rapid virological response have a better chance for achieving SVR
Medical	PEG-IFN and ribavirin in combination at optimal dosing. Maintenance of therapeutic immunosuppressive levels essential. Little long-term data exists on the use of protease inhibitors in the post-transplantation setting
Surgical	Not applicable unless re-transplantation is necessary
Radiological	Imaging studies to exclude the presence of portal hypertension, biliary strictures or vascular/ischemia thrombosis
Psychological	Patients should be aware of the potential for HCV recurrence, potential graft loss, and the need for IFN/ribavirin prior to transplantation
Complementary medicine	Patients are dissuaded from using complementary medicine post-transplantation because of their unknown effects on the immune system

Management/prevention of complications
- Once patients develop cirrhosis from recurrent HCV, their management is similar to that of all cirrhotic patients, including screening for gastroesophageal varices and surveillance for HCC.

Suggested management/treatment algorithm
- Treatment of recurrent HCV has the same goal for achieving SVR. Unfortunately, SVR rates are lower in patients as compared with non-transplantation HCV patients. In part, this may

be due to the fact that many such patients have already had treatment with IFN-based therapy that has failed.

- However, the tolerability of treatment, the inability to achieve optimal dosing and the need to dose reduce or discontinue treatment is much higher in this group of patients. This may be related to the fact that glomerular filtration rates are uniformly lower in post-LT patients in large part due to the effects of CNIs.
- Dosing schedules should be similar as for non-transplantation patients using PEG-IFN and ribavirin. Anemia, however, is a significant problem post-LT with the use of IFN and ribavirin. At our institution, we use an escalating dose regimen of PEG-IFN and ribavirin both in the cirrhotic patient and in the post-LT setting. As an example, we start with half doses of PEG-IFN and ribavirin and advance to full dose over 4–8 weeks based on patient tolerability and blood counts.
- A mild histological recurrence of HCV itself does not necessitate the initiation of antiviral therapy. Many centers utilize periodic protocol biopsies to assess disease progression.

CLINICAL PEARLS
- The type of immunosuppression that patients receive does not really impact on the natural history of recurrent HCV.
- Recurrence rates are similar with the use of cyclosporine or tacrolimus as well as with other agents such as mycophenolate mofetil and oral corticosteroids.
- It remains controversial whether azathioprine and sirolimus have a salutary or negative effect on HCV recurrence.
- The use of bolus corticosteroids or monoclonal antibodies to treat acute cellular rejection is associated with a worse outcome in HCV patients. Therefore, patients should always be maintained on adequate immunosuppression to prevent the precipitation of acute cellular rejection.
- The development of concurrent biliary strictures or CMV/HSV-6 infection is also associated with a worse outcome for patients with recurrent HCV. Both of these entities need to be considered in the differential diagnosis of abnormal liver chemistry tests in HCV patients post-LT.
- Older donor age is a strong negative prognostic factor in HCV outcome post-LT and older donors (i.e. greater than age 55) should be avoided if at all possible in the HCV recipient. However, this is not logistically feasible with the current organ shortage.
- Concurrent steatohepatitis may portend a worse prognosis and a lower SVR rate.
- The development of diabetes mellitus is extremely common in post-LT HCV patients.

Section 5: Special Populations

- HIV-HCV co-infected patients appear to have higher rates of rejection and more severe HCV recurrence rates. It is difficult to manage immunosuppression in co-infected patients because of the effect of protease inhibitors on CNI metabolism.

Section 6: Prognosis

- Re-transplantation of patients with recurrent HCV carries appreciable morbidity and mortality rates; concurrent renal failure, portal hypertension and profound coagulopathy are negative

prognostic signs for survival with the most common cause of death being infection. If patients develop graft failure from recurrent HCV and have been unable to tolerate or have not responded to antiviral therapy, re-transplantation may not be an option.
- There does not appear to be any difference in outcome for HCV recipients receiving HCV antibody positive donor livers as long as there is no appreciable pre-existing fibrosis in the donor liver.
- If liver chemistry tests rise in a patient taking IFN and ribavirin, it is essential to perform liver biopsy to exclude acute/chronic rejection and plasma cell hepatitis.

Section 7: Reading List

Carrion JA, Torres F, Crespo G, et al. Liver stiffness identifies two different patterns of fibrosis progression in patients with hepatitis C virus recurrence after liver transplantation. Hepatology 2010;51:23–34

Fiel MI, Agarwal K, Stanca C, et al. Post transplant plasma cell hepatitis (de novo autoimmune hepatitis) is a variant of rejection and may lead to a negative outcome in patients transplanted for hepatitis C. Liver Transpl 2008;14:861–71

Gallegos-Orosco JF, Yosephy A, Noble B, et al. Natural history of post-liver transplantation hepatitis C: a review of factors that may influence its course. Liver Transpl 2009;15:1872–81

Gane EJ. The natural history of recurrent hepatitis C and what influences this. Liver Transpl 2008;14: S36–S44

Gordon FD, Kuo P, Vargas HE. Treatment of hepatitis C in liver transplant recipients. Liver Transpl 2009;15: 126–35

Massoumi H, Elsiesy H, Khaitova V, et al. An escalating dose regimen of pegylated interferon and ribavirin in HCV cirrhotic patients referred for liver transplant. Transplantation 2009;88:729–35

Stanca CM, Fiel MI, Kontorinis N, Agarwal AK, Emre S, Schiano TD. Increased incidence of chronic ductopenic rejection occurring in patients with recurrent post liver transplantation HCV treated with pegylated interferon alpha 2a and ribavirin. Transplantation 2007;84:180–6

Wiesner RH, Sorrell M, Villamil F. International Liver Transplantation Society Expert Panel. Report of the first International Liver Transplantation Society Expert Panel Consensus Conference on liver transplantation and hepatitis C. Liver Transpl 2003;9:S1–9

Section 8: Guidelines

- No current guidelines exist for treatment of recurrent HCV post-LT. Please see ILTS recommendations for treatment of HCV in patients with cirrhosis.

Section 9: Evidence

Not applicable for this topic.

Section 10: Images

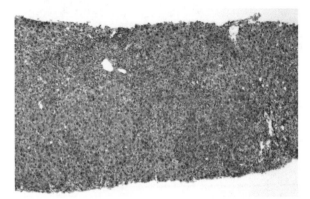

Figure 52.1 Recurrent HCV. Low-power magnification portal tracts that are expanded by dense lymphocytic infiltrates with marked interface hepatitis. There is lobular disarray with numerous foci of parenchymal necrosis and apoptotic bodies. H&E. Original magnification × 40.

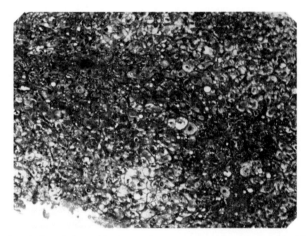

Figure 52.2 Fibrosing cholestatic hepatitis. A portal area expanded by fibrosis with delicate fibrous septa radiating into the periportal sinusoidal spaces (arrows). The severe cholestasis results in feathery degeneration of hepatocytes (arrowheads). Masson trichrome stain. Original magnification × 100.

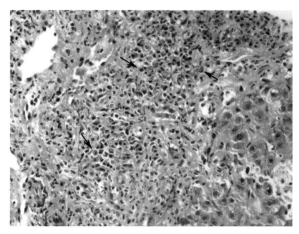

Figure 52.3 Plasma cell hepatitis in a patient receiving PEG-IFN and ribavirin. A representative portal tract with an infiltrate composed mostly of plasma cells (arrows), accompanied by interface hepatitis. The rest of the lobules also show parenchymal necrosis and often there is centrilobular hepatocyte dropout and bridging necrosis. H&E. Original magnification × 400.

Additional material for this chapter can be found online at:
www.mountsinaiexpertguides.com
This includes a case study and multiple choice questions

Recurrent Disease Post-Liver Transplantation: Autoimmune Diseases, Hepatitis B and NASH

Thomas D. Schiano

Division of Liver Diseases, Icahn School of Medicine at Mount Sinai, New York, NY, USA

OVERALL BOTTOM LINE
- Autoimmune liver conditions such as AIH, PBC and PSC all recur post-LT but graft loss is uncommon.
- Patients with HBV do extremely well post-LT because of the use of hepatitis B immunoglobulin, and now oral medications to prevent HBV recurrence.
- NASH is an increasingly common indication for LT and may recur post-transplantation. Many patients with cryptogenic cirrhosis transplanted in the past in reality may have had NASH and it has been shown to recur post-LT.
- Hepatitis B core + donor livers potentially may transmit HBV to the recipient so appropriate prophylaxis is necessary.
- LT outcomes are excellent in patients with autoimmune liver disease.
- Clinically relevant recurrence does not occur with metabolic liver diseases such as hemochromatosis and alpha-1 antitrypsin deficiency.

Section 1: Background
Definition of disease
- Most primary liver diseases that necessitate LT have the potential to recur post-transplantation.
- Recurrence of HCV is almost universal and progressive disease may lead to graft failure in upwards of 50% of patients within 10 years.
- Clinically relevant recurrence does not occur with metabolic liver diseases such as hemochromatosis and alpha-1 antitrypsin deficiency.
- Recidivism may lead to liver damage in alcoholics but rarely results in organ failure.
- PBC, PSC and AIH, as well as HBV and NASH all may recur post-LT. Transplantation outcomes overall are excellent in these groups of patients, especially those with the autoimmune liver diseases and HBV.

Incidence/prevalence
- Recurrence of PBC may ultimately occur in up to 50% of LT recipients but jaundice with a need for re-transplantation is exceedingly rare.
- PSC may recur in 20–40% of patients but true recurrence may be underestimated; up to 20% of patients with recurrent disease may develop graft failure necessitating re-transplantation.

Mount Sinai Expert Guides: Hepatology, First Edition. Edited by Jawad Ahmad, Scott L. Friedman, and Henryk Dancygier.
© 2014 John Wiley & Sons, Ltd. Published 2014 by John Wiley & Sons, Ltd.
Companion website: www.mountsinaiexpertguides.com

- AIH may recur in up to 25% of recipients during the first 5 years after transplantation and >50% of patients after 10 years.
- Prior to the advent of HBIg, HBV recurrence was universal and led to graft failure in the majority of cases. The use of HBIg and subsequently, oral medications, have almost totally prevented severe HBV recurrence. Breakthroughs of HBV while on HBIg monotherapy occur in up to 20% of cases but are easily treatable with oral combination therapy.
- The true incidence of recurrent NASH is unknown but as the number of LTs for NASH increases, it is expected that recurrent NASH will become a problem especially since obesity and the metabolic syndrome commonly occur post-LT.

Economic impact
- The true economic impact of recurrent disease after LT above is unknown but in the setting of graft failure would be associated with greater morbidity and mortality and thus, greater economic impact.
- Disease recurrence typically necessitates liver biopsy and medical treatment and in PSC, cholangiography.
- The prevention of recurrent HBV is extremely costly because of the use of HBIg prophylaxis. Most transplantation centers are now trying to convert HBIg to oral prophylaxis after the immediate post-transplantation period.

Etiology
- HBV recurs more frequently in the setting of lamivudine resistance and when patients have high viral loads at transplantation. Patients with fulminant liver failure due to HBV and those with hepatitis delta co-infection have a low risk for re-infection of the new graft.
- NASH is associated with the metabolic syndrome, which occurs commonly post-LT due to weight gain, hypercholesterolemia and diabetes mellitus that can stem from immunosuppressive medication use.
- All autoimmune liver diseases recur post-transplantation.
- Ischemic cholangiopathy resembles recurrent PSC and they may be difficult to differentiate.
- De novo AIH (plasma cell hepatitis) may occur after transplantation and appears to be a variant of rejection that can lead to graft loss.

Pathology/pathogenesis
- The diagnostic hallmark of PBC recurrence is the presence of granulomatous cholangitis or the florid-duct lesion on liver biopsy; lymphoplasmacytic inflammation may also be present.
- Biliary structuring may occur for numerous reasons in the transplanted liver. Large bile duct and anastomotic strictures may be technically related complications and amenable to stenting or surgical revision. Diffuse intrahepatic stricturing that radiologically resembles PSC can occur in liver allografts exposed to prolonged ischemia times, with the use of a donation after cardiac death donor, with ABO incompatibility or in the setting of or a history of hepatic artery thrombosis or stenosis.
- In recurrent AIH, the typical histology of prominent plasmacytic infiltration and lobular/necroinflammatory inflammation is present; significantly deranged liver chemistry tests, gamma globulin levels and autoimmune markers may not be present.
- HBV core antibody (+) allografts have the potential for transmitting HBV from donor to recipient (see Table "Transmission of HBV from a core + donor"). These donor allografts are routinely used in recipients who do not have HBV; most transplantation centers give recipients prophylaxis with lamivudine or other nucleoside analogues.

Predictive/risk factors

Transmission of HBV from a core + donor		
Recipient anti-core	**Recipient surface antibody**	**Risk of HBV transmission**
+	+	Low
−	+	Low
+	−	Intermediate
−	−	High (~ 40%)

- Some studies have suggested that PBC recurrence is much more frequent in patients receiving tacrolimus as opposed to cyclosporine as their primary immunosuppression.
- Risk factors for recurrence of PSC may include older recipient age, male gender, donor:recipient gender mismatch, the presence of an intact colon or inflammatory bowel disease post-LT, CMV infection and rejection treated with corticosteroids.

Section 2: Prevention

BOTTOM LINE
- The use of ursodiol to date has not been shown to prevent PBC recurrence.
- Treatment of overweight, diabetes and hypercholesterolemia may slow or prevent the development of recurrent NASH.
- Recurrence typically occurs in patients who are no longer receiving corticosteroids or who are being maintained on low levels of immunosuppression.
- The use of HBIg has dramatically improved the success of LT in this population to the point that HBV patients do just as well if not better than any group of recipients. Monthly use of HBIg has decreased HBV recurrence rates to less than 20% with graft loss from recurrent HBV now being exceedingly rare. The HBIg infusions typically begin intra-operatively and then often during the first post-operative week. Subsequent frequency of infusions is predicated on the achievement and maintenance of quantitative HBV surface antibody levels, ranging from 100 to 500 IU depending upon the transplantation center.

Screening
- For PBC, typically a liver biopsy is performed because of persistent mild–moderate AP elevations. There does not appear to be a correlation between the presence or titer of serum AMA and the development of recurrent disease.
- The diagnosis of recurrent PSC is based on the following criteria:
  - Confirmed diagnosis of PSC pre-transplantation.
  - Cholangiography demonstrating diffuse non-anastomotic biliary strictures >3 months post-transplantation.
  - Histology showing fibrous cholangitis and/or fibro-obliterative lesions of the large bile ducts ("onion-skinning") with or without ductopenia.
- In patients with AIH, significantly deranged liver chemistry tests, gamma globulin levels and autoimmune markers may not be present and is why some centers perform protocol liver biopsies in these patients. Recurrence typically occurs in patients who are no longer receiving corticosteroids or who are being maintained on low levels of immunosuppression.

- In patients transplanted for HBV or with a hepatitis B core + donor, hepatitis serologies and viral DNA are used to screen for recurrence of disease.

Primary prevention

- Prior to the advent of HBIg prophylaxis to prevent recurrence of HBV post-LT, survival rates for patients were extremely poor due to rapid and aggressive recurrence of disease. Recurrence was marked by profound levels of viremia, reappearance of HBSAg(+) and the development of fibrosing cholestatic hepatitis.
- The use of HBIg has dramatically improved the success of LT in this population to the point in which HBV patients do just as well if not better than any group of recipients.

Secondary prevention

- With the advent of oral nucleoside analogues such as lamivudine and their use in cirrhotic patients in an effort to stabilize chronic liver disease and slow its progression, the actual number of patients with HBV undergoing LT in the USA has steadily declined over the last decade. The combination of these medications with HBIg has further decreased the rate of HBV recurrence as compared with the use of HBIg alone.

Section 3: Diagnosis (Algorithm 53.1)

CLINICAL PEARLS
- Recurrence of PBC may ultimately occur in up to 50% of LT recipients but jaundice and the need for re-transplantation is exceedingly rare.
- Using rigorous diagnostic criteria, recurrent PSC that causes similar stricturing is estimated to occur in up to 30% of patients transplanted for PSC. The true recurrence rate of PSC may actually be higher than currently estimated when less rigorous diagnostic criteria are used.
- It can often be difficult histologically to differentiate recurrent PSC from chronic ductopenic rejection, especially as patients with PSC appear to have high incidences of rejection (like all patients with autoimmune liver disease).
- Recurrent AIH typically occurs in patients who are no longer receiving corticosteroids or who are being maintained on low levels of immunosuppression.

Differential diagnosis

Disease	Features
PBC	The histological differential diagnosis of recurrent PBC includes acute cellular and/or chronic ductopenic rejection, ischemic cholangitis and drug hepatotoxicity
PSC	Ischemic cholangiopathy may be difficult to differentiate from PSC as it is with chronic ductopenic rejection
AIH	May rarely be mistaken for acute cellular rejection; is in the differential diagnosis of chronic hepatitis occurring post-transplantation; viral hepatitides such as HBV, HCV and HEV should be excluded
HBV	Other viral hepatitides should be excluded; immunohistochemical staining for HBV antigens are specific, however
NASH	May be seen with recurrent HCV and it portends a poor prognosis and a decreased response to antiviral therapy
Plasma cell hepatitis (de novo AIH)	Appears to be a variant of rejection and can occur post-transplantation in the setting of any primary liver disease

Typical presentation

- All recurrent liver diseases post-transplantation typically manifest with abnormal liver chemistry tests that prompt additional investigations that includes serologic testing, radiologic studies and liver biopsy.
- The differential diagnosis of abnormal liver chemistry tests in this population is broad and includes acute and chronic rejection, biliary obstruction, other viral infections, drug hepatotoxicity, malignancy and vascular problems. It is important for the clinician to be mindful if the recipient received a hepatitis B core + donor liver.

Clinical diagnosis

- The timing of abnormal liver chemistry tests is extremely important, i.e. it is extremely unlikely that recurrent PBC or AIH would present in the first year post-LT.
- Knowing the type of immunosuppression and whether it has been recently lowered, if the patient was a recipient of an ABO mismatch liver or a donation after cardiac death donor, and if the patient has been compliant with all medications are all important questions to ask.

Physical examination

- Severe recurrence of autoimmune liver disease or HBV may present with jaundice.
- Recurrent PSC may present with fever, jaundice and other symptoms of cholangitis such as nausea and pruritus.
- Severe hyperbilirubinemia from any cause may be associated with pruritus and diarrhea.
- PBC and AIH may be associated with other immunologic conditions such as sprue, thyroid disease, keratoconjunctivitis sicca and rheumatoid arthritis with their attendant physical findings.

Laboratory diagnosis

List of diagnostic tests

- For recurrent PBC: liver biopsy is performed because of persistent mild to moderate AP elevations. There does not appear to be a correlation between the presence or titer of serum AMA and the development of recurrent disease.
- It can often be difficult histologically to differentiate recurrent PSC from chronic ductopenic rejection, especially as patients with PSC appear to have a high incidence of rejection (like all patients with autoimmune liver disease). Risk factors for recurrence of PSC may include older recipient age, male gender, donor:recipient gender mismatch, the presence of an intact colon or inflammatory bowel disease post-LT, CMV infection, and rejection treated with corticosteroids.
- In recurrent AIH the typical histology of prominent plasmacytic infiltration and lobular/necroinflammatory inflammation is present; significantly deranged liver chemistry tests, gamma globulin levels and autoimmune markers may not be present and is why some centers perform protocol liver biopsies in these patients.
- De novo AIH, a chronic hepatitis that histologically resembles AIH may occur in patients not transplanted for AIH.
- A small subset of patients with NASH may have accelerated fibrosis post-LT, even in the setting of normal liver chemistry tests or mild liver test abnormalities.

List of imaging techniques

- Biliary stricturing may occur for numerous reasons in the transplanted liver. Large bile duct and anastomotic strictures may be technically related complications and amenable to stenting or surgical revision. Roux-en-Y biliary anastomoses are performed in the majority of transplantations for PSC, which makes diagnostic ERCP technically challenging or not possible. PTC is the main modality for diagnosing biliary tract disease in these patients but has attendant morbidity, so MRCP is currently being used more often to first establish a diagnosis.

- In patients felt to have recurrent PBC, AIH, recurrent HBV and NASH, imaging studies such as US, MRI and CT scan are undertaken to exclude malignancy or a biliary or vascular problem.

Algorithm 53.1 Diagnosis of recurrent liver disease

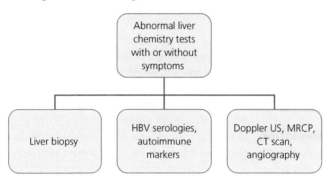

Potential pitfalls/common errors made regarding diagnosis of disease

- Recurrent PSC is not readily diagnosed by liver biopsy and is difficult to differentiate from chronic ductopenic rejection.
- Patients with HCV may have received a hepatitis B core + liver so a recurrent hepatitis may be related to HBV and not HCV.
- Awareness of plasma cell hepatitis occurring post-transplantation is paramount because if left untreated could lead to graft failure.

Section 4: Treatment (Algorithm 53.2)

Treatment rationale

- Although there have been no long-term studies of the use of ursodiol post-LT, if recurrent PBC or PSC is diagnosed, treatment with ursodiol is reasonable.
- Patients with recurrent PSC may require biliary drainage via ERCP or PTC.
- In most patients diagnosed with recurrent AIH, their biochemical and histological abnormalities may resolve rapidly after restoration of or an increase in immunosuppression. It is often necessary to maintain patients on low doses of maintenance steroids or azathioprine, as smoldering inflammation or fibrosis progression may occur with only minimal liver test abnormalities.
- De novo AIH generally responds to modification of immunosuppression; some patients may require maintenance azathioprine and corticosteroids as there may be a lack of effect with the use of CNIs.
- The combination of oral nucleoside analogues with HBIg has further decreased the rate of HBV recurrence as compared with the use of HBIg alone.
- HBV core antibody (+) allografts have the potential for transmitting HBV from donor to recipient. These donor allografts are routinely used in recipients who do not have HBV; most transplantation centers give recipients prophylaxis with lamivudine or other nucleoside analogues.

When to hospitalize

- To initiate an investigation in the setting of jaundice.
- Complications of graft failure such as cholangitis with sepsis and portal hypertension.

Managing the hospitalized patient

- Appropriate diagnostic investigations and treatment of specific complications.
- Support and maintenance of immunosuppression.
- Treatment of inflammatory bowel disease exacerbations in PSC and ulcerative colitis.

Table of treatment

Treatment	Comment
Conservative	Mild recurrences of PBC, PSC and NASH may not need to be treated and can be observed expectantly
Medical	Ursodiol for recurrent PBC and PSC, increased immunosuppression for AIH or plasma cell hepatitis, broadened antiviral coverage (and discontinuation of HBIg) for recurrent HBV and treatment of hypercholesterolemia/obesity/diabetes in NASH
Surgical	Biliary revision in patients with recurrent PSC and anastomotic strictures
Radiological	PTC or ERCP for recurrent PSC
Psychological	Counseling the patient as to the natural history of the recurrent disease and its appropriate treatments
Complementary medicine	Patients are dissuaded from using herbal and homeopathic medications post-transplantation because of their potential effects on immunosuppression

Prevention/management of complications

- Patients with PSC and ulcerative colitis are at high risk for developing colon cancer so must receive ongoing colonoscopic screening.
- Patients with AIH have already received large doses of immunosuppression throughout their lives which might place them at risk for developing post-transplantation lymphoproliferative disease.
- Patients with AIH and those with cholestatic liver conditions may have significant osteoporosis and should be aggressively screened and treated for it.
- For recurrent NASH, post-transplantation weight loss should be encouraged and patients should be alerted to this potential for ongoing weight gain early after transplantation. Medical treatment of diabetes mellitus and hypercholesterolemia should be undertaken in an aggressive manner. Statin use is not contraindicated.

CLINICAL PEARLS

- Advanced osteoporosis may be seen in patients with immunologic liver disease because of pre-transplantation predisposition and previous immunosuppression use.
- Patients with immune liver diseases all appear to be at increased risk for developing acute cellular rejection post-transplantation.
- Patients previously transplanted for cryptogenic cirrhosis may have in fact had NASH or a burnt-out AIH predisposing them to post-transplantation recurrence.
- *De novo* AIH may necessitate the use of maintenance azathioprine and corticosteroids and there may be a lack of effectiveness with the use of CNIs.

Algorithm 53.2 Management/treatment of recurrent liver disease

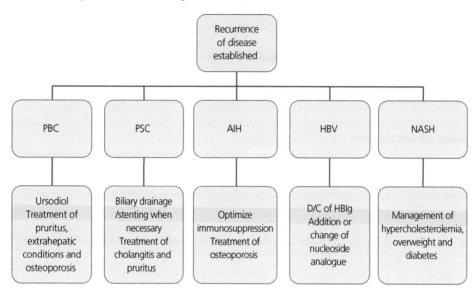

Section 5: Special Populations
Pregnancy
- Women may have successful pregnancies post-LT. This may complicate the setting of recurrent liver disease especially in patients with AIH and PSC. Immunosuppressive and anti-viral therapy may need to be modified accordingly in the setting of pregnancy.

Children
- HBV and PBC are typically not seen in the pediatric population.
- Pediatric patients transplanted for AIH and PSC may have been malnourished with growth retardation, both of which can complicate disease recurrence.
- *De novo* AIH is a well-known phenomenon in the pediatric population and may be a cause of long-term graft loss.

Elderly
- Patients may have other medical co-morbidities, i.e. coronary disease and renal dysfunction that can complicate treatment of disease recurrence.
- Osteoporosis may be even more of an issue in this patient population.

Section 6: Prognosis

BOTTOM LINE/CLINICAL PEARLS
- For PBC, the average time to recurrence is varied but appears to be between 3 and 6 years post-transplantation. Recurrence may ultimately occur in up to 50% of LT recipients but jaundice and the need for re-transplantation is exceedingly rare.
- Using rigorous diagnostic criteria, recurrent PSC is estimated to occur in up to 30% of patients. Up to 30% of patients with recurrent disease may develop graft failure

necessitating re-transplantation, either due to repeated episodes of cholangitis and biliary sepsis or to the development of portal hypertension.
- AIH may recur in up to 25% of recipients during the first 5 years after transplantation and in more than half of patients within 10 years. Patients rarely develop graft failure and the need for re-transplantation.
- Monthly use of HBIg has decreased HBV recurrence rates to less than 20% with graft loss from recurrent HBV now being exceedingly rare.
- NASH clearly can recur post-LT but to date has resulted in few instances of graft loss. A small subset of patients with NASH may have accelerated fibrosis, even in the setting of normal liver chemistry tests or mild liver test abnormalities.

Section 7: Reading List

Alabraba E, Nightingale P, Gunson B, et al. A re-evaluation of the risk factors for the recurrence of primary sclerosing cholangitis in liver allografts. Liver Transpl 2009; 15:330–40

Angus PW, Patterson SJ. Liver transplantation for hepatitis B: what is the best hepatitis B immune globulin/ antiviral regimen? Liver Transpl 2008:14:S15–S22

Cholongitas E, Papatheodoridis GV, Burroughs AK. Liver grafts from anti-hepatitis B core positive donors: a systematic review. J Hepatol 2010;52:272–9

Duclos-Vallee JC, Sebagh M. Recurrence of autoimmune disease, primary sclerosing cholangitis, primary biliary cirrhosis and autoimmune hepatitis after liver transplantation. Liver Transpl 2009;15;S25–S34

Evans HM, Kelly DA, McKiernan PJ. Hubscher S. Progessive histological damage in liver allografts following pediatric liver transplantation. Hepatology 2006;43:1109–17

Guido M, Burra P. De novo autoimmune hepatitis after liver transplantation. Semin Liver Dis 2011;31:71–81

Malik SM, deVera ME, Fontes P, Shaikh O, Sasatomi E. Ahmad J. Recurrent disease following liver transplantation for nonalcoholic steatohepatitis cirrhosis. Liver Transpl 2009;15:1843–51

O'Grady JG. Phenotypic expression of recurrent disease after liver transplantation. Am J Transplant 2010;10:1149–54

Silveira MG, Talwalkar JA, Lindor KD, Wiesner RH. Recurrent primary biliary cirrhosis after liver transplantation. Am J Transplant 2010;10:720–6

Tripathi D, Neuberger J. Autoimmune hepatitis and liver transplantation: indications, results, and management of recurrent disease. Semin Liver Dis 2009;29:286–96

Section 8: Guidelines

Not applicable for this topic.

Section 9: Evidence

Not applicable for this topic.

Section 10: Images

Not applicable for this topic.

Additional material for this chapter can be found online at:
www.mountsinaiexpertguides.com
This includes a case study and multiple choice questions

CHAPTER 54

Health Maintenance after Liver Transplantation

Lawrence U. Liu

Division of Liver Diseases, Icahn School of Medicine at Mount Sinai, New York, NY, USA

OVERALL BOTTOM LINE
- With recipients living longer after undergoing LT, it has been noted that significant causes of morbidity and mortality post-transplantation are not related to recurrent liver disease.
- The lifelong use of immunosuppressive agents places these recipients at risk for a variety of general medical conditions.
- These medical conditions include renal disease, hypertension, diabetes mellitus, dyslipidemia, obesity and osteoporosis.

Section 1: Background
Definition of disease
- With continued improvement of both graft and patient survival, long-term transplant recipients are at risk for developing general medical problems, particularly cardiovascular and metabolic diseases.
- Most of these complications are related to immunosuppressive therapy; management strategies are similar to the non-transplanted population.

Incidence/prevalence
- In long-term survivors after LT, up to a third will develop significant renal dysfunction or cardiovascular mortality.
- More than half of all LT recipients will develop some aspect of the metabolic syndrome.

Pathology/pathogenesis
- The table "Complications and associated risk factors" illustrates the common medical conditions seen after LT and their associated risk factors. In general, long-term immunosuppression medication is the primary risk factor.

Mount Sinai Expert Guides: Hepatology, First Edition. Edited by Jawad Ahmad, Scott L. Friedman, and Henryk Dancygier.

Complications and associated risk factors	
Complication	**Associated/risk factor**
Renal disease	CNIs, sirolimus, diabetes mellitus, hypertension
Hypertension	CNIs, obesity
Diabetes mellitus	Corticosteroids, CNIs, sirolimus, obesity
Dyslipidemia	Sirolimus
Malignancy	Immunosuppression
Osteoporosis	Vitamin D deficiency

Section 2: Prevention

BOTTOM LINE/CLINICAL PEARLS
- Prevention of general medical conditions after LT relies on screening appropriately (cancer screening per national guidelines, and regular dermatology assessment for skin cancer) and controlling risk factors for cardiovascular disease.

Screening
- It is appropriate to adhere to national cancer screening guidelines in LT recipients.
- It is imperative that all LT recipients have a PCP who should see them regularly and monitor for diabetes, hypertension and dyslipidemia, and other cardiovascular risk factors.
- We typically ask all patients to obtain routine laboratory tests (CBC, chemistry panel and immunosuppression level) every 3 months.
- Regular screening for bone density is recommended.

Primary prevention
- Although there are no proven primary prevention strategies for the main medical complications seen after LT, we recommend yearly cancer screening and vaccination for influenza.

Secondary prevention
- It is important to control the metabolic syndrome after LT to try and reduce the risk of cardio-vascular and renal disease.
- In patients with renal disease immunosuppression should be kept to a minimum and consideration should be given to switching to a renal sparing immunosuppression regimen.
- Osteoporosis should be treated appropriately to reduce fracture risk.

Section 3: Diagnosis

BOTTOM LINE/CLINICAL PEARLS
- LT recipients who do well after surgery are at risk for general medical conditions. They should be followed regularly by a PCP. We follow all long-term survivors annually. At office visits patients should have a complete review of symptoms, and a full medication and psychosocial history should be obtained including smoking and alcohol use.
- The examination should focus on vital signs, particularly blood pressure and weight.
- Investigations should include CBC, chemistry panel, immunosuppression level, urinalysis and other tests depending on any concerns in the history or physical examination.
- Routine imaging is not required.

Section 4: Treatment

> **CLINICAL PEARLS**
> - Long-term survivors after LT should regularly visit their PCP and be subject to laboratory tests every 3 months.
> - Regular health maintenance should include adhering to cancer screening and vaccination guidelines, dermatology assessment and bone densitometry.

Renal dysfunction

Incidence
- After LT the risk of developing CKD Stage 4 (GFR <30 mL/min) is 8% at 1 year, 18% at 5 years, 28% at 10 years.
- Mortality risk increases as GFR decreases: 5-year survival rates for patients with CKD 3, CKD 4, and ESRD were 84%, 68%, and 49%, respectively.

Risk factors
- CNI nephrotoxicity (cyclosporine).
- Mechanisms of CNI nephrotoxicity include:
  - Acute causes: afferent arteriolar vasospasm, renal hypoperfusion.
  - Chronic causes: renal hypoperfusion, obliterative arteriopathy, focal ischemia from tubular atrophy/interstitial fibrosis/glomerulosclerosis.
- All of these mechanisms can result in a decrease in the GFR.
- Diabetes mellitus.
- Hypertension.

Treatment
- Reduction of CNI dose.
- Use of immunosuppressive agents with less nephrotoxic risk (e.g. mycophenolate mofetil, sirolimus).
- Avoidance of nephrotoxic agents.

Cardiovascular risk factors

Incidence
- In LT recipients there is a threefold risk for cardiovascular events and a twofold risk for cardiovascular death.
- The mortality rate from cardiovascular disease after LT ranges from 19 to 42%.
- The presence of diabetes mellitus, hypertension or chronic renal disease each confers twice the mortality risk after transplantation.
- The risk of developing metabolic syndrome ranges from 39 to 58%.
- The table "Cardiovascular disease and associated risk factors" shows the common risk factors for cardiovascular disease after LT and their incidence.

Cardiovascular disease and associated risk factors

Risk factor	Comments	Incidence rates
Hypertension	The most common risk factor	60–70%
Diabetes mellitus	Associated with poorer post-transplantation prognosis	30–40%
Dyslipidemia	Hypertriglyceridemia and low HDL levels	50–70%
Obesity		30%

- Management of the cardiovascular risk factors is similar to that in the general population. The table "Cardiovascular disease risk factors and treatments" shows the common risk factors and treatments.

Cardiovascular disease risk factors and treatments	
Hypertension	Calcium channel blockers, beta-blockers, ACE inhibitors, angiotensin receptor blockers, loop diuretics
Diabetes mellitus	Insulin, biguanides (metformin), sulfonylureas, thiazolidinediones
Dyslipidemia	Statins, omega-3 fatty acids
Obesity	Orlistat, bariatric surgery (if benefit outweighs risk)

- Steroid reduction or steroid sparing regimens improve glycemic control, blood pressure levels, and the lipid profile, along with increasing the success of weight loss.

Metabolic syndrome after LT
- The prevalence of metabolic syndrome after LT is approximately 50% and is more than twice the rate seen in the general (i.e. non-transplantation) population.

Risk factors
- Older age.
- Pre-transplantation NAFLD.
- Pre-transplantation alcoholic cirrhosis.
- Increased BMI and pre-transplantation obesity.
- Diabetes mellitus.
- Hypertriglyceridemia.
- Decreased level of physical activity post-transplantation.
- Decreased intake of calcium, potassium, folic acid and fiber.

Risk factors for weight gain post-transplantation
- Increased oral intake.
- Recovery of health.
- Medications.
- Decreased physical activity. LT is not a reason to be sedentary; this procedure is meant to restore the person's pre-morbid level of physical activity.

Osteoporosis
Incidence
- There is a 24–55% incidence at 2 years post-LT (bone mass loss is most profound 3–6 months post-transplantation).

Risk factors
- Cholestatic liver disease (pre-transplantation).
- Corticosteroid therapy.
- CNI use.

Treatment
- The treatment for osteoporosis after LT is similar to that in the general population (calcium/vitamin D, bisphosphonates).

Quality of life
- Largest impact is on physical functioning, with less improvement in psychological health, social functioning and sexual functioning.
- Of recipients 26–57% resume working after undergoing LT.

Section 5: Special Populations
Pregnancy
- After LT, resumption of normal reproductive function among pre-menopausal women can be expected. Therefore, the appropriate use of contraception needs to be discussed and emphasized with patients of child-bearing age.
- Lower incidences of pregnancy-related hypertension and pre-eclampsia have been noted with tacrolimus-based immunosuppression when compared with cyclosporine.
- The incidence of malformations in children of mothers who have undergone LT is 3% – a rate comparable with the general population incidence.
- Although there is no clear consensus regarding the safe time interval for pregnancy after LT, most LT centers recommend waiting 1–2 years after a successful transplantation. Based on renal transplantation experience, all pregnancies in post-LT recipients should be classified as high-risk and be managed by a multidisciplinary team (including an obstetrician who specializes in high-risk cases).
- Most immunosuppressive drugs are safe during pregnancy except for mycophenolate.
- Data on transplantation outcomes can be accessed at the Pregnancy Transplant Registry (www.tju.edu/ntpr/).

Children
- See Pediatric section.

Section 6: Prognosis

> **BOTTOM LINE/CLINICAL PEARLS**
> - Cardiovascular disease carries a 19–42% mortality risk after LT.
> - Diabetes mellitus, hypertension or chronic renal disease independently increases the post-transplantation mortality risk twofold.

Follow-up tests and monitoring
- Annual physical examinations are recommended.
- Regular skin cancer surveillance (post-transplantation malignancies are reviewed in Chapter 51).
- Initiation of new medications should be assessed in terms of interaction with immunosuppressive therapy.
- Post-transplantation recipients may receive the standard vaccines (e.g. influenza) but should not receive live vaccines due to the risk of precipitation or exacerbation of the viral infection

being targeted. Patients who have undergone splenectomies need to receive vaccines against encapsulated organisms (i.e. *Haemophilus influenzae*, Pneumococcus, Meningococcus).

- Antibiotic prophylaxis recommendations for dental procedures have been recently revised to target a smaller group of patients with:
  - Artificial heart valves.
  - A history of infective endocarditis.
  - A cardiac transplant who develops a heart valve problem.
  - The following congenital heart conditions:
    > unrepaired or incompletely repaired cyanotic congenital heart disease, including those with palliative shunts and conduits.
    > a completely repaired congenital heart defect with prosthetic material or device, whether placed by surgery or by catheter intervention, during the first 6 months after the procedure.
    > any repaired congenital heart defect with residual defect at the site or adjacent to the site of a prosthetic patch or a prosthetic device.

Section 7: Reading List

Åberg F, Isoniemi H, Höckerstedt K. Long-term results of liver transplantation. Scand J Surg 2011;100: 14–21

Anastácio LR, Ferreira LG, Ribeiro Hde S, Liboredo JC, Lima AS, Correia MI. Metabolic syndrome after liver transplantation: prevalence and predictive factors. Nutrition 2011;27:931–7

Bianchi G, Marchesini G, Marzocchi R, Pinna AD, Zoli M. Metabolic syndrome in liver transplantation: relation to etiology and immunosuppression. Liver Transpl 2008;14:1648–54

Dei Malatesta MF, Rossi M, et al. Pregnancy after liver transplantation: report of 8 new cases and review of the literature. Transpl Immunol 2006;15:297–302

Jain AB, Reyes J, Marcos A, et al. Pregnancy after liver transplantation with tacrolimus immunosuppression: a single center's experience update at 13 years. Transplantation 2003;76:827–32

Johnston SD, Morris JK, Cramb R, Gunson BK, Neuberger J. Cardiovascular morbidity and mortality after orthotopic liver transplantation. Transplantation 2002;73:901–6

Kasturi KS, Chennareddygari S, Mummadi RR. Effect of bisphosphonates on bone mineral density in liver transplant patients: a meta-analysis and systematic review of randomized controlled trials. Transpl Int 2010;23:200–7

Laish I, Braun M, Mor E, Sulkes J, Harif Y, Ben Ari Z. Metabolic syndrome in liver transplant recipients: prevalence, risk factors, and association with cardiovascular events. Liver Transpl 2011;17:15–22

Laryea M, Watt KD, Molinari M, et al. Metabolic syndrome in liver transplant recipients: prevalence and association with major vascular events. Liver Transpl 2007;13:1109–14

Muñoz LE, Nañez H, Rositas F, et al. Long-term complications and survival of patients after orthotopic liver transplantation. Transplant Proc 2010;42:2381–2

Ojo AO, Held PJ, Port FK, et al. Chronic renal failure after transplantation of a nonrenal organ. N Engl J Med 2003;349:931–40

Patapis P, Irani S, Mirza DF, et al. Outcome of graft function and pregnancy following liver transplantation. Transplant Proc 1997;29:1565–6

Patel HK, Patel A, Abouljoud M, Divine G, Moonka DK. Survival after liver transplantation in patients who develop renal insufficiency. Transplant Proc 2010;42:4167-70

Tome S, Wells JT, Said A, Lucey MR. Quality of life after liver transplantation. A systematic review. J Hepatol 2008;48:567–77

Wilson W, Taubert KA, Gewitz M, et al.; American Heart Association. Prevention of Infective Endocarditis: Guidelines from the American Heart Association: A Guideline from the American Heart Association Rheumatic Fever, Endocarditis and Kawasaki Disease Committee, Council on Cardiovascular Disease in the Young, and the Council on Clinical Cardiology, Council on Cardiovascular Surgery and Anesthesia, and the Quality of Care and Outcomes Research Interdisciplinary Working Group. J Am Dent Assoc 2008;139 Suppl:3S–24S

Suggested websites

www.tju.edu/ntpr/ (Pregnancy Transplant Registry)

Section 8: Guidelines
National society guidelines

Guideline title	Guideline source	Date	Summary
The Seventh Report of the Joint National Committee on Prevention, Detection, Evaluation, and Treatment of High Blood Pressure	Joint National Committee on Prevention, Detection, Evaluation, and Treatment of High Blood Pressure http://www.nhlbi.nih.gov/guidelines/hypertension/express.pdf	2003	Guidelines for hypertension prevention and management
Guidelines for Chronic Kidney Disease Care	KDOQI http://kidney.org/professionals/kdoqi/guidelines_commentaries.cfm	2002–2012	Various guidelines on chronic kidney disease management; this includes complications from renal disease and diseases causing renal disease
Standards of medical care in diabetes	American Diabetes Association (ADA) http://care.diabetesjournals.org/content/36/Supplement_1/S11.full.pdf+html	2013	Position statement from the American Diabetes Association on diabetes management
Guidelines for management of dyslipidemia and prevention of atherosclerosis	American Association of Clinical Endocrinologists (AACE) https://www.aace.com/files/lipid-guidelines.pdf	2012	Clinical practice guidelines set by the AACE
Screening for and management of obesity in adults	US Preventive Services Task Force (USPSTF) http://www.uspreventiveservicestaskforce.org/uspstf/uspsobes.htm	2012	This topic page summarizes the USPSTF recommendation on screening for and management of obesity in adults
Screening for osteoporosis: recommendation statement	US Preventive Services Task Force (USPSTF) http://www.uspreventiveservicestaskforce.org/uspstf/uspsoste.htm	2012	An update of the 2002 USPSTF recommendation on screening for osteoporosis
Long-term management of the successful adult liver transplant	(AASLD) http://www.aasld.org/practiceguidelines/Documents/LongTermManagmentofSuccessfulLT.pdf	2012	

Section 9: Evidence

Not applicable for this topic.

Section 10: Images

Not applicable for this topic.

Additional material for this chapter can be found online at:
www.mountsinaiexpertguides.com
This includes a case study and multiple choice questions

Index

Note: Page numbers in *italics* refer to figures; page numbers in **bold** refer to tables. *vs.* denotes differential diagnosis or comparisons.

Mount Sinai Expert Guides: Hepatology, First Edition. Edited by Jawad Ahmad, Scott L. Friedman, and Henryk Dancygier.
© 2014 John Wiley & Sons, Ltd. Published 2014 by John Wiley & Sons, Ltd.
Companion website: www.mountsinaiexpertguides.com

Printed and bound by CPI Group (UK) Ltd, Croydon, CR0 4YY

27/10/2024

14580214-0003